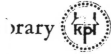

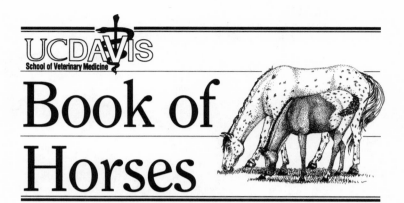

UCDAVIS
School of Veterinary Medicine

Book of Horses

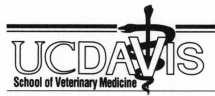

Book of Horses

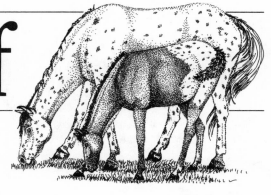

Horses

A Complete Medical Reference Guide for Horses and Foals

By Members of the Faculty and Staff,
University of California, Davis
School of Veterinary Medicine

Edited by Mordecai Siegal

Consulting Editor, Jeffrey E. Barlough, D.V.M., Ph.D.
Associate Editor, Victoria Blankenship Siegal

HarperCollinsPublishers

Figure 4 and Table 1 appearing in Chapter Six, "Equine Nutritional Requirements," were originally published as Figure 1 and Table 1 from "A Condition Score System for Horses" which appeared in *Equine Practice,* 7(8): 13–15, 1985. Reprinted with permission from Veterinary Practice Publishing Company, Nancy Bull, Managing Publisher.

HarperCollins books may be purchased for educational, business, or sales promotional use. For information, please write to: Special Markets Department, HarperCollins*Publishers*, Inc., 10 East 53rd Street, New York, NY 10022.

FIRST EDITION

Library of Congress Cataloging-in-Publication Data

UC Davis Book of Horses : a complete medical reference guide for horses and foals /by members of the faculty and staff, University of California, Davis, School of Veterinary Medicine ; edited by Mordecai Siegal, consulting editor, Jeffrey E. Barlough.—1st ed.
     p.   cm.
   Includes index.
   ISBN 0–06–270139–8
    1. Horses—Diseases. 2. Horses—Health. I. Siegal, Mordecai II. Barlough, Jeffrey E. III. University of California, Davis. School of Veterinary Medicine.
   SF951.U25   1996
   636.1'089—dc20   96-10907

96 97 98 99 00 ❖/RRD 10 9 8 7 6 5 4 3 2 1

*To the California Center for Equine Health and Performance
and all the men and women who work there.
This talented group of dedicated individuals has done much
to make life better for horses everywhere.*

Contents

Part VI: Infectious Diseases, Cancer, and Geriatrics

Contributors

Editor
Mordecai Siegal

Consulting Editor
Jeffrey E. Barlough, D.V.M., Ph.D.

Associate Editor
Victoria Blankenship Siegal

Contributing Editors
John P. Hughes, D.V.M.
Donald G. Low, D.V.M., Ph.D.

Horse Breed Illustrations
Cynthia Holmes

Photographs
Mordecai Siegal
Murray E. Fowler
Heidi Baldwin
Ruth Saada

This book represents the work of thirty-seven authors. They are:

David G. Baker, D.V.M., M.S., Ph.D., is a former resident in laboratory animal medicine at the School of Veterinary Medicine, University of California, Davis. He received his D.V.M., as well as M.S. and Ph.D. degrees in comparative pathology (specialty of parasitology), at the University of California, Davis. He is a Diplomate, American College of Laboratory Animal Medicine. He is currently an associate professor of laboratory animal medicine at Louisiana State University.

Jeffrey E. Barlough, D.V.M., Ph.D., is a postgraduate researcher in the Department of Medicine and Epidemiology, School of Veterinary Medicine, University of California, Davis. He earned his D.V.M. at the University of California, Davis, and a Ph.D. in veterinary virology at Cornell University. He is a Diplomate, American College of Veterinary Microbiologists.

Roy W. Bellhorn, D.V.M., M.S., is professor emeritus in the Department of Surgical and Radiological Sciences, School of Veterinary Medicine, University of California, Davis. He received his D.V.M. at

Michigan State University, and an M.S. in ophthalmology at New York University. He is a Diplomate, American College of Veterinary Ophthalmologists.

Ann T. Bowling, Ph.D., is an adjunct professor in the Department of Population Health and Reproduction, School of Veterinary Medicine, University of California, Davis. She received her Ph.D. in genetics at the University of California, Davis.

C.A. Tony Buffington, D.V.M., M.S., Ph.D., is an associate professor in the Department of Veterinary Clinical Sciences, College of Veterinary Medicine, Ohio State University. He earned his D.V.M. as well as M.S. and Ph.D. degrees in nutrition at the University of California, Davis. He is a Diplomate, American College of Veterinary Nutrition.

Gary P. Carlson, D.V.M., Ph.D., is a professor in the Department of Medicine and Epidemiology, School of Veterinary Medicine, University of California, Davis. He earned his D.V.M. and a Ph.D. in comparative pathology at the University of California, Davis. He is a Diplomate, American College of Veterinary Internal Medicine.

Bruno B. Chomel, D.V.M., Ph.D., is an assistant professor in the Department of Population Health and Reproduction, School of Veterinary Medicine, University of California, Davis. He received his D.V.M. at the Lyon National Veterinary School, France, and a Ph.D. in microbiology at the University of Lyon.

Lais R.R. Costa, M.V., M.S., is a resident in large animal medicine at the Veterinary Medical Teaching Hospital, School of Veterinary Medicine, University of California, Davis. She received her M.V. from São Paulo State University, Brazil, and an M.S. in virology from the University of Kentucky.

Marcelo A. Couto, D.V.M., Ph.D., is an assistant professor in the Department of Medicine, School of Medicine, University of California, Los Angeles. He received his D.V.M. at the University of Buenos Aires, Argentina, and a Ph.D. in comparative pathology at the University of California, Davis.

Noël O. Dybdal, D.V.M., Ph.D., is a veterinary pathologist in the Department of Pathobiology and Toxicology at Genentech, Inc., South San Francisco, California. She received her D.V.M. and a Ph.D. in comparative pathology at the University of California, Davis. She is a Diplomate, American College of Veterinary Pathologists.

Murray E. Fowler, D.V.M., is professor emeritus in the Department of Medicine and Epidemiology, School of Veterinary Medicine, University of California, Davis. He received his D.V.M. at Iowa State University. He is a Diplomate of the American College of Veterinary Internal Medicine, the American Board of Veterinary Toxicology, and the American College of Zoological Medicine.

Reneé M. Golenz, D.V.M., is in private practice in the Davis, California area. She received her D.V.M. at Ohio State University.

Sherril L. Green, D.V.M., Ph.D., is an assistant professor in the Department of Comparative Medicine, Stanford University. She earned her D.V.M. at Louisiana State University and a Ph.D. in neuroscience at the University of California, Davis. She is a Diplomate, American College of Veterinary Internal Medicine.

John P. Hughes, D.V.M., is professor emeritus in the Department of Population Health and Reproduction, director of the Veterinary Genetics Laboratory, and former director of the California Center for Equine Health and Performance, School of Veterinary Medicine, University of California, Davis. He received his D.V.M. at Kansas State University. He is a Diplomate, American College of Theriogenologists.

Monna F. Jordan, M.S., is a Ph.D. graduate student in physiology in the Department of Animal Science, University of California, Davis. She received her M.S. in animal science at the University of California, Davis.

Robin H. Kelly, D.V.M., is a resident in equine surgery at the Veterinary Medical Teaching Hospital, School of Veterinary Medicine, University of California, Davis. She received her D.V.M. at the University of California, Davis.

Jeffrey Lakritz, D.V.M., Ph.D., is a postgraduate researcher in the Department of Anatomy, Physiology, and Cell Biology, School of Veterinary Medicine, University of California, Davis. He earned his D.V.M. and a Ph.D. in comparative pathology at the University of California, Davis.

Irwin K.M. Liu, D.V.M., Ph.D., is a professor in the Department of Population Health and Reproduction, School of Veterinary Medicine, University of California, Davis. He received his D.V.M. at Kansas State University, and a Ph.D. in virology/immunology at the University of California, Davis.

Bruce R. Madewell, V.M.D., M.S., is a professor in the Department of Surgical and Radiological Sciences, School of Veterinary Medicine, University of California, Davis. He earned his V.M.D. at the University of Pennsylvania, and an M.S. in clinical sciences at Colorado State University. He is a Diplomate, American College of Veterinary Internal Medicine, Specialties of Internal Medicine and Oncology.

John E. Madigan, D.V.M., M.S., is a professor in the Department of Medicine and Epidemiology, School of Veterinary Medicine, University of California, Davis. He received his D.V.M. and an M.S. in animal science at the University of California, Davis. He is a Diplomate, American College of Veterinary Internal Medicine.

Mark D. Markel, D.V.M., Ph.D., is an associate professor in the Department of Surgical Sciences, and director of the Comparative Orthopaedic Research Laboratory, School of Veterinary Medicine, University of Wisconsin, Madison. He earned his D.V.M. at the University of California, Davis, and a Ph.D. in physiology at the Mayo Graduate School of Medicine, Rochester, Minnesota. He is a Diplomate, American College of Veterinary Surgeons.

John R. Pascoe, B.V.Sc., Ph.D., is associate dean for academic programs, and a professor in the Department of Surgical and Radiological Sciences, School of Veterinary Medicine, University of California, Davis. He earned his B.V.Sc. at the University of Queensland, Australia, and a Ph.D. in comparative pathology at the University of California, Davis. He is a Diplomate, American College of Veterinary Surgeons.

Charles G. Plopper, Ph.D., is a professor in the Department of Anatomy, Physiology, and Cell Biology, School of Veterinary Medicine, University of California, Davis. He received his Ph.D. in anatomy at the University of California, Davis.

Janet F. Roser, M.S., Ph.D., is an associate professor in the Department of Animal Science, University of California, Davis. She received both her M.S. in animal science and a Ph.D. in physiology at the University of California, Davis.

Mary A. Scott, D.V.M., is a postgraduate researcher in the Department of Population Health and Reproduction, School of Veterinary Medicine, University of California, Davis. She earned her D.V.M. at the University of California, Davis.

Mordecai Siegal is a journalist and author of twenty-one published books concerning animal behavior, nutritional needs, medical care, training, breed descriptions, and human/animal bonding. His articles and monthly columns on pets appear in national magazines, and he frequently appears on the broadcast media. He is also editor of the *Cornell Book of Cats* and the *UC Davis Book of Dogs*.

Barbara L. Smith, D.V.M., is a postgraduate researcher in the Department of Surgical and Radiological Sciences, School of Veterinary Medicine, University of California, Davis. She received her D.V.M. at Ohio State University.

Jack R. Snyder, D.V.M., Ph.D., is an associate professor in the Department of Surgical and Radiological Sciences, School of Veterinary Medicine, University of California, Davis. He received his D.V.M. at Washington State University, and a Ph.D. in comparative pathology at the University of California, Davis. He is a Diplomate, American College of Veterinary Surgeons.

Anthony A. Stannard, D.V.M., Ph.D., is a professor and chairman of the Department of Medicine and Epidemiology, School of Veterinary Medicine, University of California, Davis. He received his D.V.M. and a Ph.D. in comparative pathology at the University of California, Davis. He is a Diplomate, American College of Veterinary Dermatology.

Carolyn L. Stull, M.S., Ph.D., is an extension specialist in the Animal Welfare Program, School of Veterinary Medicine, University of California, Davis. She received her M.S. and Ph.D. degrees in animal science at the University of Illinois at Urbana/Champaign.

William P. Thomas, D.V.M., is a professor in the Department of Medicine and Epidemiology, School of Veterinary Medicine, University of California, Davis. He earned his D.V.M. at the University of California, Davis. He is a Diplomate, American College of Veterinary Internal Medicine, Specialty of Cardiology.

Sally L. Vivrette, D.V.M., Ph.D., is an assistant professor in the Department of Food, Animal and Equine Medicine, College of Veterinary Medicine, North Carolina State University. She received her D.V.M. and a Ph.D. in comparative pathology at the University of California, Davis. She is a Diplomate, American College of Veterinary Internal Medicine.

Johanna L. Watson, D.V.M., Ph.D., is a lecturer in the Department of Medicine and Epidemiology, School of Veterinary Medicine, University of California, Davis. She received her D.V.M. and a Ph.D. in comparative pathology at the University of California, Davis.

W. David Wilson, B.V.M.S., M.S., M.R.C.V.S., is a professor in the Department of Medicine and Epidemiology, and director of the California Center for Equine Health and Performance, School of Veterinary Medicine, University of California, Davis. He earned his B.V.M.S. at the University of Glasgow, Scotland, and an M.S. in medicine and immunology at Iowa State University.

Thomas B. Yarbrough, D.V.M., is a lecturer in the Department of Surgical and Radiological Sciences, School of Veterinary Medicine, University of California, Davis. He received his D.V.M. at Louisiana State University.

Steven Zicker, D.V.M., Ph.D., is a former lecturer and postgraduate researcher at the School of Veterinary Medicine, University of California, Davis. He received his D.V.M. and a Ph.D. in nutrition at the University of California, Davis. He is a Diplomate, American College of Veterinary Internal Medicine. He is currently in private practice in Colorado Springs, Colorado.

Joseph G. Zinkl, D.V.M., Ph.D., is a professor in the Department of Pathology, Microbiology, and Immunology, School of Veterinary Medicine, University of California, Davis. He received his D.V.M. and a Ph.D. in comparative pathology at the University of California, Davis. He is a Diplomate, American College of Veterinary Pathologists.

Acknowledgments

Those who love horses and those who are involved with them in any way at all will benefit greatly from this comprehensive medical reference guide. It may well become the most essential text on the horse person's book shelf. The contents within offer a wealth of equine medical knowledge from one of the premier veterinary schools in the world, the University of California at Davis. The book's very existence is a tribute to those members of the faculty, each an educator and scientist, who devoted a significant portion of their invaluable time, energy, and intellectual gifts to this repository of scholarship. Their presence on these pages is therefore acknowledged with gratitude and respect. They have made this book possible. It is, and will continue to be, a tribute to the invaluable work they perform as a matter of daily routine on the Davis campus.

Rarely does a veterinary school have the opportunity to make available an important portion of its resources to those who are its beneficiaries. Rarely do those who sorely need a school's academic wealth have the opportunity to avail themselves of it. The *UC Davis Book of Horses* makes these things possible. However, it required cooperation and enthusiasm at the highest levels of authority for this project to begin and develop into a tangible reality. This book exists because Frederick A. Murphy, Dean of the School of Veterinary Medicine, supported and encouraged its creation. We thank him for his nod of approval and good offices.

And we must extend a sincere expression of gratitude to Dr. Donald J. Klingborg, Assistant Dean, School of Veterinary Medicine, University of California at Davis, for his strong efforts to help this project reach fruition through its most difficult stages. His commitment and invaluable help made him an important and essential advocate.

There are no words adequate to express our appreciation for Donald G. Low, Emeritus Professor of Veterinary Medicine and former Director of the Veterinary Medical Teaching Hospital at University of California at Davis. His diligence, tenacity, and intellectual roadmap of the academic maze guided this project and transformed it from a fanciful idea to an actual book which can now be opened, read, and appreciated. During his tenure as Associate Dean for Public Programs (and afterwards, as well) he recruited the contributors for this book and for the *UC Davis Book of Dogs* as well. Throughout each phase of these projects he maintained a parental eye as work progressed and he supervised both projects on campus to their successful conclusion. We are forever grateful for his effective dedication and, perhaps most of all, for his warmth, wit, and wisdom.

The *UC Davis Book of Horses* and the *UC Davis Book of Dogs* simply would not exist if Bill Balaban had not presented the Editor's proposals to the veterinary school. He did it with intelligence, fervor, and the pleasure of knowing it was a good idea before anyone else. His enthusiasm, keen observations, and good advice have long supported many of the veterinary programs at the University of California at Davis. He is a kind, generous lover of animals whose reputation for good judgment and common sense when it comes to companion animals and their caretakers extends far beyond the campus. From start to finish, Mr. Balaban was the champion of the Davis books and in no small way was responsible for their realization. He was always there when we needed him and made all the right moves. We thank him for his help and for all the funny moments he provided. His friendship is a treasure.

Many thanks are also extended to Kelly J. Nimtz, Assistant Dean for Development, for his hard work and many efforts on behalf of this book. Good ideas for getting the word out are hard to come by and he has had more than his share.

Dr. Jeffrey E. Barlough has once again distinguished himself as Consulting Editor and as a contributing author of this book, as he did for the *UC Davis Book of Dogs* and the *Cornell Book of Cats.* He is a consummate editor, writer, educator, and scientist. Every page of this work is profoundly influenced by his editorial skill and academic judgment. Although he possesses the intellect and education of a teacher and scientist, he has the gifts of a writer. We are very grateful for his many talents and skills and for his generous devotion to this book. Dr. Barlough's invaluable contribution cannot be measured.

Our Associate Editor, Victoria Blankenship Siegal, worked harder on this project than anyone else connected with it. The endless hours she spent poring over the manuscript, giving it the benefit of her editorial judgment; her unfailing awareness of inconsistency; and her ability to find incorrect minutiae, served this book beyond expectations. Her abilities added immeasurably to the credibility of this work. The book's quality is in no small way the result of Victoria Siegal's editorial scrutiny and the skill and intelligence it represents. Her contribution was immeasurable.

We would like to express our appreciation for the fine pen-and-ink drawings of an extremely gifted artist, Cynthia Holmes. Her illustrations of the horse types and breeds are a visual feast for the browsing reader. Her love of horses and her pleasure as a rider are evident in each of her wonderful drawings. We are also grateful to Ms. Holmes for her fine renditions of the horse anatomy illustrations.

A special acknowledgment is given to devoted horsewoman and Morgan Horse owner Carole Neukamm, for her generous help in obtaining some of the photography and for her expert advice concerning the accuracy of the breed illustrations.

Many thanks to Heidi Baldwin for generously taking horse-and-rider photographs specifically for this book. Her time, effort, and good taste are greatly appreciated.

Special thanks to Ruth Saada for sharing the cherished memories of her riding vacation at Bitterroot Ranch in Wyoming. Her photographs of that wonderful time and place are scattered throughout the pages of this book and add a very pleasurable dimension to this volume.

We are also grateful to Bayard and Mel Fox for their generous cooperation with regard to Ms. Saada's photos, which were taken at their ranch. They are the owner–operators of the rugged and beautiful Bitterroot Ranch, which is nestled amid the snowcapped mountains of Dubois, Wyoming. They also direct Equitour Worldwide Riding Holidays. Their riding vacations are legendary. Thanks to David E. King for appearing in the Bitterroot photos.

The authors of Chapter 2, "Major Breeds of Horses," by Monna F. Jordan and Janet F. Roser, along with the Editor, wish to thank the following horse breed registries for providing us with important information:

Arabian Horse Registry of America, Inc., Westminster, CO; The Jockey Club, Lexington, KY; American Quarter Horse Association, Amarillo, TX; American Morgan Horse Association, Inc., Shelburne, VT; United States Trotting Association, Columbus, OH; American Saddlebred Horse Association, Inc., Lexington, KY; Swedish Warmblood Association of North America; Peruvian Paso Horse Registry of North America, Santa Rosa, CA; American Association of Owners and Breeders of Peruvian Paso Horses, Oakland, CA; American Trakehner Association, Newark, OH; American Pinto Horse Association, Fort Worth, TX; American Paint Horse Association, Fort Worth, TX; Appaloosa Horse Club, Moscow, ID; Clydesdale Breeders of the United States, Pecatonica, IL; American Shire Horse Association, Adel, IA; Percheron Horse Association of America, Fredericktown, OH; Welsh Pony and Cob Society of America, Winchester, VA.; Draft Horse & Mule Association of America, Lovington, IL; and The American Donkey and Mule Society, Denton, TX.

Many thanks are extended to the management and staff of the Riverdale Equestrian Centre in Riverdale, New York, for allowing their facilities to be photographed for this book. Thanks especially to their managers, former Olympian equestrians Rusty Holzer and Ashley Nicoll, both of whom continue to compete at the international level. We are grateful to professional Farrier Carl V. Schwarz for allowing himself to be photographed at Riverdale while hard at work in his traveling blacksmith shop. Gratitude must also be expressed to Susan Freeman and Dr. Barbara Eisner Leiman, veterinarian, for allowing themselves to be photographed with their horses.

Many thanks are also extended to Phyllis Grupe of Grupe Company Belgians; Tom Persechino of the American Quarter Horse Racing News; and to Liz Hoskinson and Mary A. Conti of the American Horse Shows Association, Inc.

We are also grateful to Linda Bentley and Eleanor Onoda for the administrative duties they performed so well. Their dedicated service contributed so much toward keeping the entire project on track.

Acknowledgment for help, assistance, advice, and service beyond the call of duty go to Mel Berger, vice-president and literary agent at the William Morris Agency; Phil Liebowitz, Esq., of the William Morris legal department; and to Kim Thornton of Fancy Publications for her advice and assistance.

A special note of gratitude must be given to the hardest-working editor at HarperReference, Trish Medved. She has moved heaven and earth to bring this book to the deserving horse owner.

Foreword

by Frederick A. Murphy, D.V.M., Ph.D.

DEAN, SCHOOL OF VETERINARY MEDICINE
UNIVERSITY OF CALIFORNIA, DAVIS

The mission of the School of Veterinary Medicine at the University of California at Davis is "to serve the people of California, the United States, and the rest of the world by providing educational, research, clinical service and public service programs of the very highest quality that advance the health and care of animals and public health." The faculty and staff of this School have kept this mission before them every day as they have gone about educating generations of outstanding veterinary students, carrying out innovative research projects to solve important animal disease problems, and providing world-class clinical care for an ever-increasing patient population. This book, the *UC Davis Book of Horses*, represents yet another way by which my colleagues are carrying out our unique mission. I think it is clear that in the future they will continue their devotion to this mission in increasingly effective ways as the profession of veterinary medicine continues to advance.

This book represents a special tribute to the horse as one of our most important domestic animal species, a species that serves as companion and as compatriot in so many sporting and recreational activities. This book also represents a special tribute to caring owners who strive to be educated and responsive regarding the health of their favorite horses. Owners today, more than ever before, seek knowledge about their horses' health and performance, and the preventive measures needed to improve their horses' overall well-being and quality of life.

This School has one of the largest equine health programs in the country. Through the Veterinary Medical Teaching Hospital and especially through our interdisciplinary California Center for Equine Health and Performance, many of our faculty are working to advance our knowledge of equine diseases, nutrition, reproduction, and other health- and performance-related subjects. Our goal is to assure that horses have the high quality of life and the high level of performance that is inherent in the genetic base of the species and its breeds. Over the years, the School's faculty have identified the causes of many equine diseases, created novel equine medical treatments, developed innovative equine surgical techniques, and promoted advanced equine diagnostic tests.

The development of new knowledge is essential to the continued well-being of our horses and improvement of their health. Developing new knowledge may best be described using the metaphor of "the three-legged stool"—all three legs are needed if the stool is to function. The faculty of the School, the private veterinary practitioner, and the horse-owning public form these three legs. All are essential, all depend upon each other, and all share the common goal of providing the best health care possible for our equine companions. You, the readers of this book, people who know and love horses, contribute every day to our understanding of equine health. The excellent relationship between faculty members at the University of California at Davis, and your veterinarian build upon your insights and innovation in the development of new knowledge. This collaborative relationship helps everyone, not the least your horses. This book is an attempt by the faculty to give back to those dedicated people some of the knowledge and tools which have been developed as a result of these collaborations.

Throughout the past decade an explosion of knowledge has substantially improved the understanding and application of medical principles that has greatly improved the general health of horses. This has been particularly evident in the rise of equine clinical specialties (i.e., specialized surgery, reproduction and newborn care, dermatology, infectious diseases, ophthalmology, genetics and inherited diseases, and so forth). This is just the beginning. People who care about horses can expect much more in the future, for medical science is undergoing a grand revolution that will pay off in better and better prevention, care, and treatment approaches in the future.

To deal with this new expansion in the scope of equine medicine and surgery, the faculty of the School have had to develop a new perspective, a new view of the sciences that underpin clinical veterinary medicine. Whereas in earlier years the classic disciplines of veterinary medicine such as anatomy, physiology, and pathology described a unidimensional perspective, today all of the disciplines of biomedicine—such as molecular biology, cell biology, developmental biology, and so forth—have been added to the classical base. All of these disciplines and their technologies are brought to bear as we educate our students and solve the problems that society has assigned to us. This multidimensional approach has served the School well, but more importantly, it has greatly improved the capability of veterinarians to help animals of all species in all the different stages of life.

The School has proudly developed this reference book, the *UC Davis Book of Horses,* with the goal of providing basic, everyday information to horse owners who want a more complete understanding of their animal's health, well-being, and performance. Many faculty members have participated in the writing of this book; their hard work, in my view, is evident in the quality of the chapters. This book would never have come to be without the hard work of Dr. Donald G. Low, who organized and coordinated the project. I wish to thank Dr. Low and all of his colleagues for a job well done. We hope that this book will provide horse owners with helpful information and will promote improved animal health, well-being, and performance. The *UC Davis Book of Horses* is one more way in which the School of Veterinary Medicine is striving to be of service to society.

A Word from Dr. John P. Hughes

by **John P. Hughes, D.V.M., Diplomate A.C.T.**

PROFESSOR EMERITUS, SCHOOL OF VETERINARY MEDICINE
UNIVERSITY OF CALIFORNIA, DAVIS

There exists a need for a book about horses and their diseases that is up-to-date, comprehensive, and understandable to us all. The new *UC Davis Book of Horses* fills this need.

The horse has played an important but changing role in the life of humans for some 10,000 years before the birth of Christ. The first use of horses was, undoubtedly, for food. They then played an important role in warfare, transportation, farming, ranching, and a variety of performance events. Today most horses are used for pleasure and recreational purposes. Often quoted was the old Arabian proverb, "The outside of the horse is good for the inside of man." This is probably even more true today.

This text will take the reader on a journey that covers the horse from its origin, behavioral patterns, husbandry, nutritional requirements, reproduction, anatomy, disorders of the various body systems, infectious diseases, geriatrics, horse care, vaccination programs, parasites, and medical emergencies to its modern-day existence in our society. We need to understand the "pitfalls" that may occur along this journey if we are to benefit the horse. The *UC Davis Book of Horses* has combined into one volume the most recent information that will give owners a more complete understanding of what is normal and abnormal concerning their horse's health.

Many faculty members, graduate students, residents—present and past—have contributed to writing this book. We are grateful to them all. Dr. Donald G. Low, as in the *UC Davis Book of Dogs,* played a key role in organizing and coordinating the writing of the *UC Davis Book of Horses.*

Preface

by W. David Wilson, B.V.M.S., M.S., M.R.C.V.S.

PROFESSOR OF VETERINARY MEDICINE AND DIRECTOR,
CALIFORNIA CENTER FOR EQUINE HEALTH AND PERFORMANCE
SCHOOL OF VETERINARY MEDICINE
UNIVERSITY OF CALIFORNIA, DAVIS

Horses in the wild demonstrate a profound ability to survive and are well adapted to searching out shelter, water, and forage on which to graze. Within a few hours of birth foals already have a very effective flight response and they quickly develop the strong herding instinct necessary for survival of the group. Through domestication we have removed horses from the natural range environment of the wild and by enclosing them in pastures or stalls have eliminated much of their ability to exercise the choices necessary for survival. In addition, the conditions we impose on horses—through manipulation of their management, feeding, housing, and use—frequently promote diseases or injuries to which they are not subject in the wild. It is clear that in the act of domesticating horses we have necessarily assumed a heavy responsibility for their health and welfare. This is a responsibility we must take seriously and, to carry it out effectively, we need to develop, through experience, a true appreciation for the needs of the horse. We also need to seek out the best possible advice and information regarding management and preventive health care. As in other aspects of life, education to optimal care for horses is a lifelong process and demands both a desire to learn and the ready availability of sources of accurate and current information. Many impressive books on horsemanship have been published, and a great deal of useful new information regarding equine health is available to horse owners through an expanding array of high-quality horse magazines and journals. However, it is currently difficult to find in one place information covering a broad range of horse health issues. We believe that the *UC Davis Book of Horses* will go a long way to fulfilling this need.

The UC Davis Book of Horses was written by thirty-seven authors, most of whom are present or past faculty members, graduate students, or residents at the University of California at Davis School of Veterinary Medicine. These dedicated educators are veterinary clinicians, teachers, specialists, and researchers involved in educating future equine veterinary practitioners and they are committed to finding solutions to health and performance problems facing our equine companions. Many of the authors are also experienced horsemen and horsewomen who know firsthand the impact of disease and injury on a horse owner's enjoyment of his or her horse and of the anguish experienced when a painful condition such as colic or laminitis afflicts the horse. While I believe it would be difficult to find a more comprehensive source of up-to-date information regarding horse health care than is found in this book, the objective is not to train you, the horse owner, to become your own veterinarian. Rather, the goal of this book is to improve your ability to identify problems or potential problems at an early stage and recognize when it is necessary to call your veterinarian, realizing that he or she is a crucial member of your horse's health-care team. As well as providing a readable source of health information to enhance your knowledge base, this book is also meant to serve as a handy comprehensive source of information you can turn to in times of need. In addition, it is hoped that this book will help you to better understand the rationale behind recommendations and advice provided by your veterinarian. From the experience I have gained through almost twenty years working as an equine veterinarian, there is no doubt in my mind that well-informed clients are the ones with whom it is most enjoyable to work. These horse enthusiasts are inquisitive, receptive to new ideas and, because they seek to understand disease processes, they are likely to diligently follow through on recommendations for treatment and prevention.

Despite my introductory remarks regarding horses in the wild, it is clear that horses would not have survived in the numbers and diverse types we encounter today had it not been for the fact that they have adapted to a role of serving humans in various forms of work. Thus, unlike the situation pertaining to many domestic pets, the serviceability of a horse for its intended use (its *soundness*) is a crucial aspect of equine health. The importance of performance, be it in the show-jumping area, in the dressage ring, on the endurance trail, on the racetrack, in the rodeo arena, or on the breeding farm, is emphasized throughout this book by highlighting strategies to prevent and treat diseases or injuries that have their primary impact on performance. Recent advances in veterinary care,

preventive medicine, nutrition, and management have helped to prolong the useful life of horses and so enhance the enjoyment horse owners derive from their equine companions.

In preparing for the writing of this book, a major effort was made to assemble the most knowledgeable and enthusiastic group of veterinarians and animal scientists possible to author sections in their primary areas of specialist expertise. Each of the chapters is underpinned by the enormous amount of insight, clinical experience, and research information necessary to address ever-burning questions of how to better diagnose, treat, manage, and prevent specific diseases of horses. Much of this research has been, and continues to be, conducted at the California Center for Equine Health and Performance (CCEHP) and other centers for horse research throughout the world. In some respects, the trail leading to the creation of this book is superimposed on the trail leading to the establishment and evolution of the CCEHP. The first step along the way was the visionary decision in 1973 of Dr. William R. Pritchard, then Dean of the School of Veterinary Medicine, to establish the Equine Disease Research Laboratory (EDRL) in recognition of the need for research into equine health, reproduction, performance, and disease. The name of the unit was later changed to the Equine Research Laboratory (ERL), and in 1995 the current name, California Center for Equine Health and Performance, was adopted to help more accurately reflect the current scope of the research, educational, public outreach service, and development programs of the Center. The CCEHP is not only the administrative and academic umbrella under which horse research is performed in the School of Veterinary Medicine, it is also a physical facility occupying a 60-acre site on the southern edge of the Davis campus. The Center's facilities now include a 4-stallion barn, three additional barns with a total of 51 stalls and adjoining runs, two foaling stalls, numerous covered individual pens and portable stall structures, outdoor paddocks, 50 acres of irrigated pasture, laboratories, treatment rooms, an administrative office building, and a security facility which houses three students who serve as the Center's security and night treatment crew. During the height of research activity, particularly during the foaling season, up to 300 horses are maintained at the facility. Most of the Center's horses are acquired through donations with a small number having been sired by CCEHP stallions and raised at the facility. In addition, the Center has since 1982 served as the United States Department of Agriculture's federally designated West Coast Quarantine and Treatment Station for Contagious Equine Metritis (CEM). In this capacity, the Center quarantines recently imported mares and stallions and tests them to prevent introduction of this potentially devastating disease into the horse population of the United States.

Much of the enormous progress that has been made in the twenty-three years since the founding of the Center is attributable to the visionary leadership of Dr. John P. Hughes, an internationally recognized equine reproduction specialist who served as Director from 1980 until his retirement in 1995. Since no federal moneys are allocated to the CCEHP to support research, facilities' development and upkeep, maintenance of the horse herd, and staff salaries, funds must be generated from outside sources. To meet the goals of expanding a viable and innovative research program, Dr. Hughes turned to the private sector of the horse industry for support. From the early years the Oak Tree Racing Association and, since 1988, the State of California Satellite Wagering Fund have been the major sources of funds to support research at the CCEHP. The Horsemen's Benevolent and Protective Association has also been helpful in supporting CCEHP projects. In recent years this Thoroughbred racing industry support has been increasingly supplemented by gifts and grants from individuals representing many breeds and disciplines within the equine industry, as well as both private and corporate foundations. A vital source of funds from individual donors comes through the Silver Stirrup Society, the current membership of which exceeds 80 individual association or corporate donors.

Recognizing the crucial importance of input from members of the horse industry in determining research priorities, an Industry Advisory Board was established in 1987 to advise the Center on future directions and goals for equine research, to disseminate equine-related information and research finds to horse enthusiasts in California and throughout the country, and to generate interest in and support for the Center through both public and private resources. The Industry Advisory Board currently consists of fourteen members representing broad segments of the equine industry. Funds generated through grants, gifts, and donations and from the stallion breeding program are applied directly to research. A call for research proposals is issued to faculty researchers once each year. Proposals are reviewed by the Director and a Scientific Advisory Committee composed of nine faculty members from the School of Veterinary Medicine, three members of the Industry Advisory Board, and two faculty members from the California State University system. This rigorous peer review process ensures that only the best and most relevant projects are funded so that the return on precious research dollars is maximized. Since 1984 the Center has funded over 300 research projects with total budgets running to several million dollars. Today, more than 50 researchers are active in studies involving virtually all disciplines including orthopedics, surgery, reproduction, neonatology, radiology and other imaging modalities, medicine, gastroenterology, physiology, sports medicine, anatomy, anesthesiology, genetics, immunology, pathology, microbiology, clinical pathology, pharmacology, toxicology, drug testing, and nutrition. Examples of current research pursuits include studies to better diagnose and treat horses with colic and improve survival following intestinal surgery; studies to better define factors predisposing to breakdown injuries in performance horses; development of new approaches to diagnose and treat infertility in mares and stallions; and investigation of new approaches to diagnose and prevent, perhaps with novel vaccines, important infectious diseases such as equine viral arteritis (EVA), equine protozoal myeloencephalitis (EPM), influenza, and equine ehrlichiosis.

It is my intention to further develop the research and educational mission of the Center by building on the solid foundation established by Dr. Hughes and the School's faculty and administrators. To achieve this goal it will be important to continue to engender support from the equine industry by demonstrating a commitment to solving important problems impacting equine health, performance, and welfare and communicating our findings to horse enthusiasts in a timely and understandable manner. Our breakthroughs in equine research are well known in veterinary academic circles through presentation of new research findings at meetings throughout the world and extensive publication by investigators of results in major scientific journals and applied veterinary journals. Several CCEHP publications and presentation of seminars to groups of horse enthusiasts serve as the primary vehicles through which we educate members of the equine industry regarding new research developments. Our publications include: (1) *The Horse Report*, a long-standing quarterly newsletter with a current circulation of over 25,000; (2) "CCEHP Updates," articles that appear monthly in *The Thoroughbred of California*, and on a routine basis in numerous other national and international industry publications; and (3) *CCEHP News Briefs*, which highlight late-breaking equine research findings. By dissemination of information through these channels, results of research conducted at the Center not only benefit the horse industry of California but also are made available to the national and international equine and veterinary medical communities.

To help contribute to the funding base of the California Center for Equine Health and Performance, the School of Veterinary Medicine has designated the Center as the recipient of royalties from the sale of this book. This will greatly facilitate the Center's mission of improving horse health, performance, and welfare through innovative research and education. Should you be interested in exploring other avenues through which you can contribute to furthering this mission, you are encouraged to contact the Develop-ment Office, School of Veterinary Medicine, University of California, Davis, CA 95616. We also welcome your comments on the *UC Davis Book of Horses*. Acquisition and dissemination of new information is an ongoing process. We recognize that your comments and suggestions will prove invaluable in our efforts to make the next edition even better!

Introduction

by Mordecai Siegal, Editor

Few pleasures in life compare to a horse's warm face nuzzling your cheek and gently pushing your shoulder, insisting on a hug, a word or two of affection, and maybe, just maybe, half an apple. Those who love horses, which is just about everyone who gets near them, know they are lucky to have a relationship with one or more and feel complemented by the experience as well as being enriched as human beings. Through the millennia to the current moment vast numbers of horsemen and horsewomen continue to enjoy and adore their horses and value them as much as people, maybe more so. To such *equephiles* horses are more than transportation, entertainment, recreation, or carters and haulers. To the lovers of all things *equus,* a horse is a majestic, larger-than-life presence that resides in the human environment with a distinct personality, with likes and dislikes, good habits and bad habits and noble aspects and not-so-noble aspects.

There was a time, not too long ago, when the horse was the most useful, the most necessary of all domestic animals. Nothing moved without a horse to carry it, pull it, or draw it to its desti-

nation. Wars were won, new lands explored, and countries developed by men and women on horseback or horse-drawn vehicles, all were transported from one place to another by the ubiquitous horse. It is a fact, however, that horses are no longer an important means for moving people and their possessions from one place to another. Yet the horse continues as a presence of considerable importance and status everywhere. As times have changed, so has the focus placed on today's horses. Although they are not seen on the streets and roads as they once were, they are still with us in great abundance. The equine presence in contemporary times is not merely an indulgent flight of nostalgia or a wistful desire to connect with simpler times. Horses are very much an important part of today's culture in both recreational and occupational activities. There is a good reason why industry uses the term "horsepower" for measuring mechanized energy output. Some small farms still use the horse's strength and vigor to pull plows, hay balers, combines, and many other farming implements. Mounted police and army units exist throughout the world for a variety of purposes and are considered essential. Few cattle ranches exist without horses to do what they always did. Modern-day cowboys continue to work on horseback as they move and control cattle. It seems that there will always be an important job for horses.

The greatest focus on horses today is in the areas of recreational riding and horse-related sports. Horses are no longer the exclusive domain of the military, the wealthy, or of working ranches and farms. Riding academies and commercially operated stables are available everywhere that will board privately owned horses for a fee or provide horses for hire to anyone wanting a pleasant ride on local trails. Of the millions of horses in the United States, many are privately owned and maintained at home, be it humble or grand. The importance of the equine presence becomes obvious when considering the 3 to 5 million horses that are thriving throughout this country and in many parts of the world.

The most important sporting events involving horses are the wide variety of horse shows that exhibit great examples of breeding, training, horsemanship, and many forms of competition. Horse shows range from local events to those of international prestige, not the least of which is the Summer Olympic Games. Jumping, dressage, conformation, and the art of horsemanship are the most important aspects of competition in the show ring. Other respected horse sports are polo and various hunting events. Of course, horse racing is possibly the oldest continuing sport in existence and promotes the creation of large numbers of horses and everything necessary for their maintenance. It is now, as it always has been, a contest of speed and endurance among horses with both small and large sums of money wagered on the outcome. Harness racing is an equally engaging sport with the horses hitched to lightweight, two-wheel vehicles called *sulkies*. This, too, is a contest of speed and stamina with betting on the outcome as an incentive for its large audience.

A horse can be enjoyed for riding, hunting, competition, or just for his friendship. He is a living being that inspires deep feelings of love, respect, and a sense of responsibility for all his needs, in those who share their lives with one. Taking care of a horse requires a commitment to being a presence in the animal's life and seeing to it that he's fed properly, kept clean, maintained in appropriate surroundings, protected from his own misbehavior and that of others, and given preventive and curative medical attention as it is needed. Like the rest of us, horses are vulnerable to illness and injury. Because a horse is easily panicked, he is likely to injure himself if he tries to escape what he perceives to be an immediate danger. As a result he may cut his skin, pull a muscle, or even break a bone. The experience will cause bodily pain and damage to the horse unless medical treatment is provided.

The equine body is a warm-blooded mammalian organism and as such is subject to invasion by viruses, bacteria, and funguses that range from irritating to painful to life-threatening. Although the body's immune system defeats hundreds, perhaps thousands, of such invaders on an hourly basis, it occasionally loses a battle and falls prey to disease which can only be defeated, if at all, by a highly trained professional. That is when we must reach out to the animal doctor, the veterinarian. The science of veterinary medicine alleviates the suffering of animals to a very great degree and promotes longer, healthier lives.

Suffering is greatly reduced and life is extended because of the sophisticated training of veterinarians, highly skilled professionals who are essential to horses and those looking after them. The veterinarian is as much a part of our lives as the family doctor. Like general practitioners, veterinarians too must have a working knowledge of all aspects of the body and be prepared to treat as wide a range of disorders as heart disease, broken bones, cancer, and skin allergies. Unlike general practitioners, they must also be prepared to diagnose and treat the medical problems of many different species, only one of which is the horse. Veterinary medicine is among the most remarkable professions in the world and those who teach it or those who go into private practice have the respect and undying gratitude of animal lovers everywhere.

How young men and women become veterinarians is not a mystery. First and foremost, they must possess intellectual gifts. They must express a thirst for highly technical and complex knowledge, demonstrate their willingness to perform hard, often grimy work, and choose to sacrifice many of the pleasures available to other young people during the time of their education and training. Through an unyielding schooling process consuming all of their time and a great deal of money, they systematically learn the medical sciences and healing arts that are taught at veterinary colleges. After four years of undergraduate school and four years of veterinary school, they become doctors of veterinary medicine. It is a considerable accomplishment. Many veterinarians then become board-certified specialists by completing a minimum of three years' additional training, by entering and concluding a residency program in their field of study, and by passing state examinations in their specialty. That is an even greater accomplishment.

The School of Veterinary Medicine of the University of California at Davis and its impressive faculty have educated and trained many of the world's finest veterinarians. Horses and their human caretakers have benefited enormously from these highly trained doctors. Thanks to this great institution and others like it, medical riches are available to all animal lovers, especially those who live with horses. Nevertheless, devoted horse owners also require a source of veterinary information at their fingertips that enables them to act quickly, properly, and in the best interests of their equine family members when they become sick or injured. The *UC Davis Book of Horses* offers a highly sophisticated source of medical information that is difficult to find outside the campus of veterinary colleges. This is a medical reference book written for horse owners, breeders, exhibitors, judges, trainers, grooms, stable operators, and just about everyone in the world of horses, including veterinarians themselves. This unique sourcebook was written by those who teach veterinary medicine to veterinary students.

The *UC Davis Book of Horses* makes available medical information pertaining to horses in a form that is concise, understandable, but not shallow or oversimplified. It represents a major

body of sophisticated information for those with a need or desire to understand the medical disorders of horses and how they are dealt with by veterinarians. *This reference book cannot enable any horse person to diagnose an illness or treat an ailing horse*. It cannot, nor should it, attempt to replace professional veterinary care. Its purpose is to impart to those who conscientiously care for horses, especially those involved with horses on a professional basis, medical information about the diseases and disorders that threaten the equine body and its various systems. Within the pages of this book is an important portion of collected knowledge from one of America's major learning institutions of veterinary medicine.

The purpose of the book is to clarify to the horse person what his or her veterinarian is trying to explain within the constraints of time and emotion. When a veterinarian tries to explain a complicated disorder or disease to a horse owner who may be distraught or distracted, it is difficult for that person to come away from the experience with a full understanding of the veterinarian's discussion. The *UC Davis Book of Horses* hopes to fill the gap and provide the horse owner and the veterinarian with the communication needed to explain and clarify the patient's illness. It is hoped that this book will function as an aid to both veterinarian and horse person, serving both as a consulting reference tool.

When a horse owner fully understands what the veterinarian is trying to explain, the horse's chances for improvement are greatly enhanced. It is in the spirit of creating a partnership between owners and veterinarians that this book is added to the existing body of horse literature. All those responsible for this book, especially the contributing authors, who are on the faculty at the School of Veterinary Medicine at the University of California at Davis, believe that horses in good health are an important source of pleasure and happiness to those fortunate to have a horse in their lives. Your horse's good health is the principal theme running through this volume.

The *UC Davis Book of Horses* is divided into eight parts, each offering a unique aspect of medical information. Consistent with the central issue of this book, the health of your horse, PART I: "GETTING A HORSE" and PART II: "LIVING WITH YOUR HORSE" offer the prospective owner the proper introduction to starting out right by learning how to choose a good horse along with a brief description of the major breeds. "EQUINE HUSBANDRY," "EQUINE BEHAVIOR," AND "MISBEHAVIOR" are chapters for both the new and experienced horse owner and help to avoid the mistakes that often lead to medical problems. PARTS III and IV offer chapters on nutrition and reproduction, which have a great influence on equine health; these topics will be of special importance for those entrusted with the care of a horse. PART V offers fourteen medical chapters describing the equine body, how its respective internal and external systems work and the various disorders that are associated with them. PART VI: "INFECTIOUS DISEASES, CANCER, AND GERIATRICS" will become a valuable part of the horse owner's

arsenal of knowledge. PART VII: "HOME CARE" presents six highly useful chapters for the owner of sick or convalescing horse. PART VIII consists of four appendices, each in their own way describing important aspects of horse ownership: "ZOONOTIC DISEASES" (the illnesses you can get from your horse); "VACCINATIONS AND INFECTIOUS DISEASE CONTROL" (schedules and types); "DIAGNOSTIC TESTS" (what they are and what they do); "TRANSPORTING HORSES" (how to do it without injury). The extensive Glossary of medical terms in the back of the book is the key that opens the door to the entire work. It can serve independently as a concise dictionary of equine medical terms or as a supplement to the information described within each chapter. A glossary of this length and breadth will be invaluable in the pursuit of veterinary medical knowledge.

In the course of producing this medical reference, it was my great pleasure to visit the University of California at Davis. As I entered each of the various buildings on campus I was profoundly impressed and quietly overwhelmed by the teaching and medical facilities, and especially the California Center for Equine Health and Performance which is so prominent a part of the School of Veterinary Medicine on the Davis campus. The enormous barns, fields, treatment rooms, operating rooms (they are immense with highly sophisticated equipment), and the horses themselves are an impressive sight. Most stirring of all was the obvious dedication and devotion of the faculty and students to the well-being of the horses in their care and the extraordinary quality of their work. I remember thinking at the time that all this is an enrichment of the lives of horses everywhere. The quality of this great school and those who give it life and significance is, I believe, imparted to all who use this book, page after page after page.

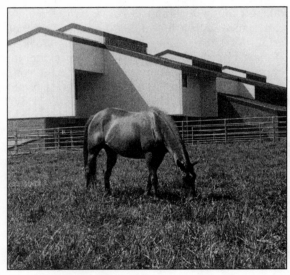

Photo by Mordecai Siegal.

PART I

Getting a Horse

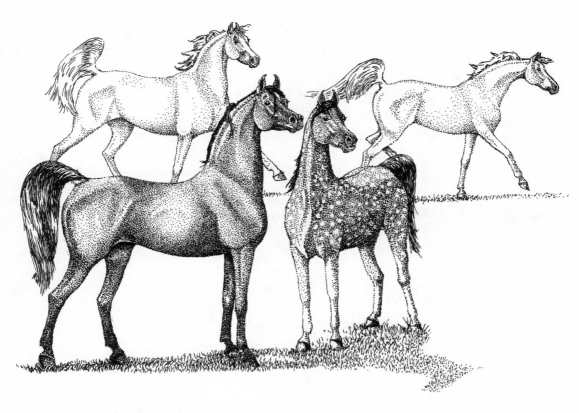

A horse! A horse! My kingdom for a horse!

—WILLIAM SHAKESPEARE
RICHARD III, V, iv

CHAPTER 1

Origins, Sources, and Selection

by Janet F. Roser

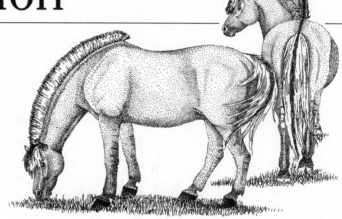

Origins

EVOLUTION

According to Darwin's theory, changes that occur in animals during evolution may be caused by natural selection and/or by mutation. In a given environment animals with an inherited ability to survive in that environment are favored, and so will flourish and transmit this ability to their offspring. Those without this ability (or having it to a lesser extent) are correspondingly less fit to compete, so their chances for survival and production of offspring are diminished. This is the process of **natural selection.** The horse and its kin are unique among mammals, for in no other mammalian group is Darwin's theory of evolution so well substantiated and documented by paleontological finds from the fossil record (*see* TABLE 1).

The horse's ancestral chain can be traced back in unbroken links for approximately 58 million years to the Eocene epoch and the famous ***Eohippus*** (Greek, "dawn horse"), now more correctly known as ***Hyracotherium***. This was a rabbitlike animal about 12 inches high that had four toes on each fore foot and three

toes on each hind foot. A slender, graceful animal with an arched back, short neck, narrow limbs, and a long tail, it was adapted for living in a swampy terrain. The teeth were soft and low-crowned, more suitable for browsing leaves than for grazing grass.

Although fossil remains of *Eohippus* have been found scattered throughout North America, Great Britain, and Europe, it appears that only in North America did this animal survive and develop for another 20 million years into its next evolutionary form, ***Mesohippus***. *Mesohippus* ("middle horse") was an animal the size of a Collie Dog but with longer legs and a straighter back. It had three toes on each foot, with the middle toe being distinctly larger. The fourth toe on the front foot had been reduced to a splint. All toes touched the ground and shared in carrying the animal's weight. Although *Mesohippus* was still a browser, its intelligence and agility had increased.

By approximately 28 million years ago, in the Miocene epoch, *Mesohippus* had evolved into the next form, ***Merychippus*** ("rudimentary horse"). *Merychippus* also had three toes on each foot, but

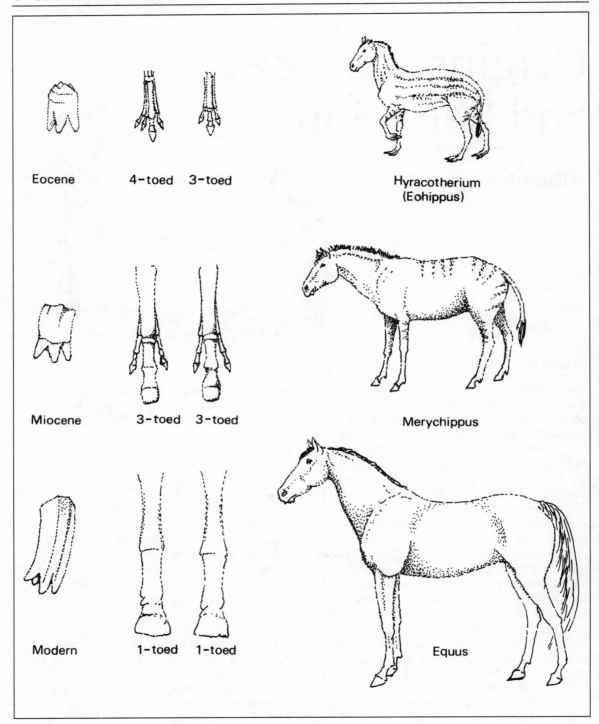

Eocene   4-toed   3-toed   Hyracotherium (Eohippus)

Miocene   3-toed   3-toed   Merychippus

Modern   1-toed   1-toed   Equus

Figure 1. Evolution of the Horse.

the middle toe was much heavier and the only one of the three that touched the ground. *Merychippus* was about the size of a Shetland Pony, and its high-crowned teeth were more suitable for grazing prairie grass. The first one-toed horse was

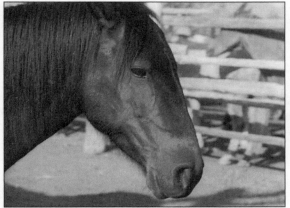

Photo by Ruth Saada.

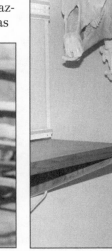

Photo by Mordecai Siegal.

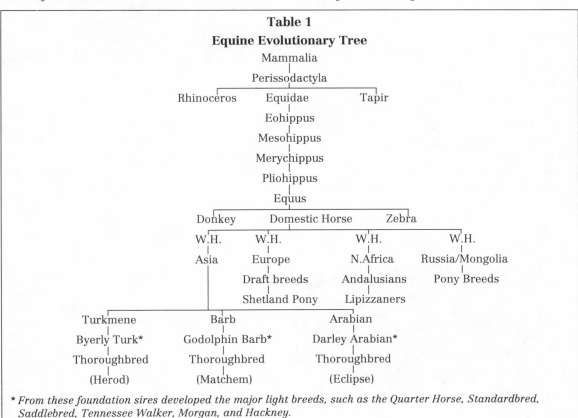

Table 1
Equine Evolutionary Tree

Mammalia

Perissodactyla

Rhinoceros — Equidae — Tapir

Eohippus

Mesohippus

Merychippus

Pliohippus

Equus

Donkey — Domestic Horse — Zebra

W.H. Asia — W.H. Europe — W.H. N.Africa — W.H. Russia/Mongolia

Draft breeds — Andalusians — Pony Breeds

Shetland Pony — Lipizzaners

Turkmene — Barb — Arabian

Byerly Turk* — Godolphin Barb* — Darley Arabian*

Thoroughbred — Thoroughbred — Thoroughbred

(Herod) — (Matchem) — (Eclipse)

* From these foundation sires developed the major light breeds, such as the Quarter Horse, Standardbred, Saddlebred, Tennessee Walker, Morgan, and Hackney.

Pliohippus ("more horse"), which lived 12 million years ago. This animal was the immediate predecessor of modern horses. Like *Merychippus* it was about the size of a pony and had high-crowned teeth suitable for grazing. But it also exhibited greater speed and stamina compared to other competing animals. (The word "horse" is derived from the Anglo-Saxon *hors*, meaning "swiftness").

Thus over many millions of years the horse developed from a rabbit-hopping swampland browser to a long-legged, single-toed, swift and agile prairie grazer. About 1 million years ago the modern horse *Equus* arose in North America. Historians believe that *Equus* all but died out about 10,000 years ago, perhaps because of climatic change, competition, disease, or a failure to adapt. Luckily, a few horses survived by migrating into Asia across the Bering land bridge, which at that time connected Alaska with Siberia. The horse remained absent from North America until it returned 500 years ago, bearing the Spanish conquistadors.

DOMESTICATION

By about 25,000 years ago, during the Paleolithic era ("Old Stone Age"), early humans were hunting horses and using them as a source of food. It appears that the horse was probably the last of the present-day farm animals to be domesticated. According to early records, first came the ox, then the sheep, goat, ass, camel, and finally the horse.

Horses were domesticated by nomadic tribes in Central Asia or Persia around 3000 B.C. A

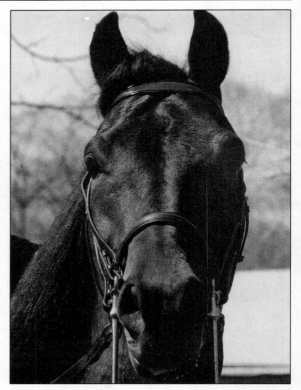

Photo by Heidi Baldwin.

Persian tribe, the Sumerians, were the first people to invent the wheel. To their wheeled carts they hitched the onager, or wild ass, and conquered Babylon in about 2000 B.C. Although the Egyptians had used the ass from earliest times, the horse did not enter Egypt until about 1680 B.C., when horses and war chariots thundered into the valley of the Nile under the command of the Asiatic Hyksôs, nomadic conquerors of uncertain affiliation. The Egyptians rapidly became outstanding charioteers and horse-breeders, and spread the use of horses to other countries.

By 1000 B.C. the Greeks were using horses in battle. It was the Greeks who probably coined the term "No foot, no horse," meaning no matter how good the horse was, without good feet, he could not perform; and it was the Greeks who developed the snaffle bit. Horse racing had long existed in Greece, but it wasn't until the 25th Olympic Games (750 B.C.) that chariot races were included along with gymnastic events.

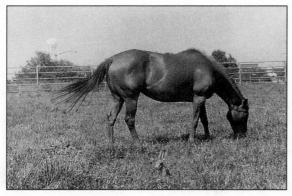

Photo by Mordecai Siegal.

From Greece the horse was exported to Rome and other parts of Europe. The Romans, who were known as excellent equestrians, were the first to invent the curb bit. When Julius Caesar invaded Britain in 55 B.C., it is believed that his infusion of Roman horses onto the island laid the foundation for the blood horses of today.

According to legend, around A.D. 600 the prophet Mohammed identified five mares that were to serve as the foundation dams for all pure-bred Arabian horses as we know them today. The legend relates how Mohammed ordered a herd of horses to be confined and left without water for seven days. When the gates of the enclosure were opened the dehydrated animals ran for the watering hole. But then the prophet sounded the call of battle; five mares turned and raced back to him without taking so much as a drop of water. This story may have some truth in it, since Mohammed was stringently careful when selecting horses for breeding and demanded that the blood lines be absolutely pure.

FORMATION OF THE ANCIENT HORSE TYPES

Even before the horse was domesticated it was self-diversifying, i.e., it was forming natural sub-populations whose physical characteristics were determined not by humans but by the local terrain and environmental conditions. As a result, many of today's breeds developed from a few ancient types that were already in existence about 10,000 years ago. Records indicate that there were probably four primitive "building blocks" of the modern horse population. These wild groups of horses can be characterized as follows:

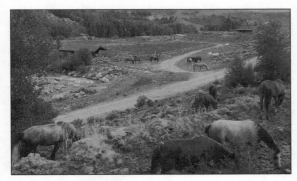

Photo by Ruth Saada.

The Wild Horses of Asia

These horses are also referred to collectively as the hot-blooded Oriental horses of the Asiatic deserts. They probably stood 13 or 14 hands (a *hand* is a 4-inch unit of length used to measure a horse's height), and were thin-skinned and very refined, with a delicate bone structure. No doubt they had a rather dished face, a small muzzle, great speed, and were anatomically and physiologically adapted for endurance. Historical records indicate that these horses developed into the swift and slender breeds of the modern era. Domestication began in the Near East, where the first riding horses developed into three major lines:

- *The Turkmene*, a tall racing type
- *The Barb*, a coarse but speedy animal
- *The Arabian*, a swift horse with a high-set tail

From these lines were developed the three foundation sires of the Thoroughbred in late seventeenth-century England: the Byerly Turk, the Godolphin Barb, and the Darley Arabian.

The Wild Horses of Europe

The cold-blooded European horses, sometimes referred to as the European forest type, lived in the forests of Germany and Scandinavia until historic times. Pure strains of this type developed into the "great war horse" of the Middle Ages. Living in the cold, dense forest regions, these horses survived by developing into large, strong, hardy, shaggy-coated beasts. Instead of fleeing they hid in the dense woods or fought their predators. Records indicate that these horses developed into the various draft-horse breeds, as well as the Shetland Pony.

The Wild Horses of North Africa

These were light, long-legged horses with ramlike heads, that lived in the bleak mountains of North Africa. Records indicate that they developed into the parade horses of the Baroque period and were used as the basis for breeding Andalusians. Because of their stamina and sure-footed abilities, they were said to be the forerunners of the Lipizzaners and the American Mustang.

The Wild Horses of Russia and Mongolia

The now-extinct *Tarpan*, of dun or buckskin coloring, is said to have been the forerunner of the European Pony types. Found in southern Russia and Central Asia, these small animals were constantly devouring or trampling crops and becoming a problem for local farmers. By 1870 the Russian farmers had destroyed all the wild Tarpans; the last captive specimen died in 1919. Thus, any remaining "Tarpans" are said to be of mixed breed. Records indicate that the wild horse of Mongolia, referred to as *Przewalski's horse*, is the last true remaining wild horse of today. Discovered by a Russian explorer in 1879 in the northwest corner of Mongolia, these small, stocky, coarse, dun-colored horses with an erect mane and no forelock can be found in captivity at zoological parks around the world, including the San Diego Zoo in southern California. Although the Przewalski's horse carries a set of 66 chromosomes in each cell and the domestic horse (***Equus caballus***) carries 64, the two animals can cross-breed and produce fertile hybrid offspring, demonstrating that the Przewalski is a very close relative of the domestic species.

Uses

The horse has diligently served humankind throughout the ages. Horses have served as a source of food and have proven themselves invaluable for military purposes, for agricultural and commercial pursuits, and for sport and recreation.

Source of Food

The cracked and dismembered bones of more than 40,000 horses, 25,000 years old, found outside a rock shelter at La Solutré, in the valley of the Rhône in southwestern France, provide mute testimony of early humans' dependence on the horse. During the New Stone Age, it is thought that the horse was used as a source of milk, providing up to 4½ gallons per day. Today horse meat is a common dinner item in countries such as France, Belgium, and Switzerland. In the United States the horse is considered more of a companion, performance, or work animal, rather than a food-and-fiber source.

Military Purposes

For 4,000 years the horse was used primarily for purposes of war. One of the earliest events involving horses and warfare occurred around 1500 B.C.., when the Egyptians pursued the Israelites to the Red Sea in horse-drawn chariots. Between 900 and 600 B.C. the Assyrians became the first military power to deploy both mounted archers and war chariots in battle. From 334 to 325 B.C. Alexander the Great (riding his great steed, Bucephalus) and the Greek cavalry successfully conquered the Persians, who had been a pervading threat for 150 years. Soon many groups became proficient on horseback and proceeded to mount the horse in war. These included the Romans, the Vikings, and the Normans. To protect themselves soldiers began to wear heavy armor. The Age of Chivalry (A.D. 1000–1600) gave birth to the image of "knights in shining armor." To carry both rider and armor (350 to 425 pounds), horses had to be of great size and strength. Thus the great war horse of the Middle Ages, the heavy draft-type horse from European stock, made its appearance.

It was the military operations of the Spanish conquistadors that brought the horse back to North America, roughly 10,000 years after it had mysteriously disappeared from the continent. Between 1500 and 1600 Cortez and others landed in America, bringing with them many military horses that later escaped domestication to become the wild Mustangs, or "feral horses" of North America. These animals were subsequently captured by the Native Americans and trained for hunting and war. Only one tribe of Native Americans actually bred their horses in a systematic way: the Nez Percé, who established the Appaloosa breed in the Palouse valley in what is now Idaho. It was the Civil War (1861–1865), and the Indian Wars that followed, that gave the U.S. Cavalry (soldiers on horseback) a prominent place in history. The horse also played a substantive role in both World War I and World War II, conflicts in which several million horses lost their lives.

Agricultural and Commercial Pursuits

During the last 4,000 years, while the horse was employed in military service, it was also serving humankind by transporting food and goods from one campsite or village to the next. Horses were used to draw loads in harness and to pull traveling chariots. In the eighteenth and nineteenth centuries horses pulled light coaches and elegant vehicles for business and pleasure trips. The horse was the last of the domestic animals to be used for work on the farm; there is no evidence to indicate that it was used in Europe to draw the plow earlier than the tenth century. The slower teams of oxen worked the land from medieval times up until the end of the eighteenth century. The growth of road systems served to introduce the draft horse onto the farm—a quicker and more agile animal that could sow, cultivate, and harvest the crop effectively and efficiently. Between 1900 and 1910 there were over 5,000 breeders of Percherons alone in the United States, and the number of registered horses reached a massive 31,900. (*See* CHAPTER 2, "MAJOR BREEDS OF HORSES.") Then came the tractor and automobile, with the result that the number of work horses dwindled from 21 million in 1910 to 3 million in 1960. Sporting and recreational pursuits have since revived and effectively rejuvenated the horse population. Today there are over 10 million horses in the United States—over 1 million just in California—generating a 15.3-billion-dollar industry.

Sport and Recreation

The horse was introduced to the world of competitive sports as early as 750 B.C. during the Olympic

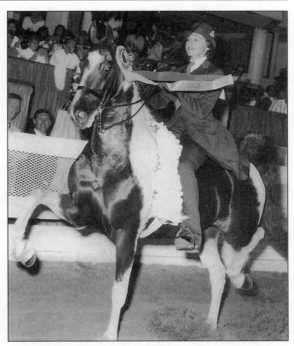

Photo by Sargent (courtesy of American Saddlebred Horse Association).

Games in Greece. The major events included both chariot and horse racing. Polo is probably one of the oldest team sports in the world. It originated in Persia long before the birth of Christ and became popular in India and China as well. Returning crusaders introduced the sport into France as early as 1200, but it did not become really established in Europe until 1872 when English soldiers brought it back to the British Empire and established the Monmouthshire Polo Club. In the American West of the 1800s, rodeo events and ***gymkhanas*** (equestrian athletic meets) became very popular.

The biggest sport involving the most money has been Thoroughbred racing. In the 1600s the Stuart kings of England James I and Charles I fostered the development of racing as a sport. Under Charles, the town of Newmarket, England, became the center of the horse-racing scene. In 1752 the English Jockey Club was founded with the objective of laying down strict rules to regulate racing and breeding.

Fox hunting, a recreational sport, had its ori-

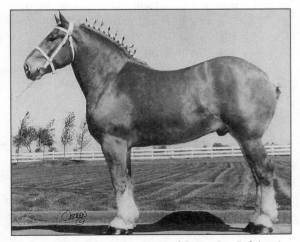

Photo by Rick O'Steen (courtesy of Grupe Co., Belgians).

gins probably toward the end of the second millennium B.C., when the Egyptian pharaohs used dogs and horse-drawn chariots to hunt gazelles, hares, and hyenas. Their dogs were slender, long-legged greyhounds which seemed as nobly bred as their small, finely-limbed horses. The Romans also had high standards for hunting and considered their dogs of the finest breeding. When the Empire collapsed and the Romans withdrew from England, English noblemen took over the sport of hunting, established strict rules and laws, and introduced the fox as the prey of choice because of its extremely cunning nature and athletic abilities.

Today the combination of available money, leisure time, and emphasis on the outdoors has fostered an interest in light horses for recreation and sport such as dressage, jumping, endurance riding, team penning, and horse packing in the wilderness.

Sources

WHERE DO I GO TO BUY A HORSE?

Breeding and Training Farms
Perhaps the best starting-point in the search for the right horse is a farm that specializes in breeding, training, and selling finished horses. Here you can see a number of horses typical of the breed you are interested in, including perhaps the dam and sire of the horse in which you are interested. On the same farm may be found some of the sire's and/or dam's records of accomplishments in the show arena or some history of their offspring over the years. Most breeders are trying to promote their breed and want to be sure that their clients are satisfied with the horses they purchase. A satisfied client spreads the word and often comes back for additional purchases. This kind of farm is not found in large numbers, but by writing your local horse clubs or associations you may be able to obtain a record of the farms in your area, as well as an updated list of horses currently offered for sale.

Further information on breeding registries, local horse clubs, and local horse councils can be found in the *Horse Industry Directory*, published by the American Horse Council, 1700 K Street,

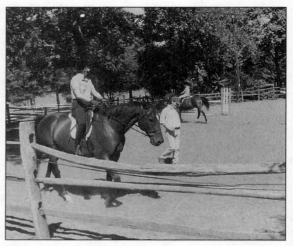

Photo by Mordecai Siegal.

N.W., Suite 300, Washington, DC, 20006–3805. Phone: (202) 296–4031.

Dealers, Trainers, Farriers, and Veterinarians
Horse dealers and trainers, local farriers (horse shoers), and veterinarians are another good starting-point in your search. Contrary to popular belief, dealers can be honest. Successful dealers realize that only satisfied customers will give them return business and word-of-mouth advertising. Local horse dealers keep a variety of horses on hand, and if they do not have the horse you are looking for they may be able to tell you where one is available. Many professional trainers are actively selling horses they are training. Trainers will make an effort to find the appropriate horse for you, especially if they feel that you might want them to train you and your new horse. Although farriers and veterinarians are not in the business of selling horses, they do have opportunities to see many horses and to interact with a lot of horse people, and so may be of some help to you.

Advertisements
There are probably more than 150 horse magazines and newsletters currently on the market. Many of them are free and can be obtained at the local tack or feed store. Classified ads can be of some help in locating a horse. Veterinary clinics, feed and tack stores, and boarding and

training stables often provide bulletin boards listing horses to buy or sell. Once you have identified a potential purchase, be sure to take the time to visit the horse and seller in person. Bring a knowledgeable friend or trainer with you when you go, and ride or lunge the horse if at all possible.

Auction or Production Sales

A public auction is usually not a very satisfactory venue for purchasing a horse, because you must make a quick decision without having sufficient time to examine a horse thoroughly. Although quality horses are sold at auction every day, the law governing these sales is *caveat emptor* ("buyer beware!"). Younger animals—weanlings and yearlings—are usually less of a risk because they have not suffered the wear and tear of older, more experienced horses. Breeding or training farms that have auctions once or twice a year usually sell more quality horses than do the local, weekly, or monthly auctions "down the road." Some auctions do not require a veterinary check before the sale. If at all possible, bring a veterinarian with you so that you can obtain a better on-site assessment of the animal you are buying.

Human Resources

A knowledgeable friend may be a good source of information, but if the recommended horse fails to meet your expectations it may affect your friendship. On the more positive side, friends are generally more available than other people in your life. State horse specialists, Department of Agriculture marketing specialists, county extension agents, Extension 4-H leaders, or 4-H members are also good resource people.

Selection

CRITERIA FOR SELECTING THE RIGHT HORSE

Purchase Price

How much can you afford? Set your purchase-price ceiling before you start your search. In some cases the seller will want to be paid the entire amount at purchase; others may work out a payment plan. Don't forget that a cheap horse

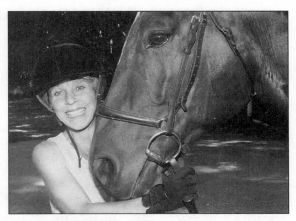

Photo by Mordecai Siegal.

will cost just as much to maintain as an expensive horse.

Age and Experience of the Rider

Is the horse for a 7-year-old or an adult? How much riding experience has the person had? Physical limitations as well as past riding experience are equally important in selecting the right horse. The rider's size and physical condition may have a profound influence on his or her ability to make a horse perform. By contrast, the young rider who has had three to four years of riding lessons may be more prepared to take on a high-spirited horse than is the adult with no experience at all. To put an inexperienced 7-year-old on a 16-hand Thoroughbred just off the track is asking for trouble; a gentle, well-trained Welsh pony would be more suitable.

Use

Perhaps the single most important criterion in the selection process is the purpose for which the horse is to be used. Is the horse going to be used for Western pleasure, cutting, three-day eventing, saddle-seat equitation, polo, dressage, or just plain trail riding? To what level of accomplishment do you want to take the horse? The intended use determines the importance of other considerations, including temperament and manners, movement or way of going, conformation and soundness, blemishes, health, size, quality, pedigree, color and markings, age, sex, and breed or type.

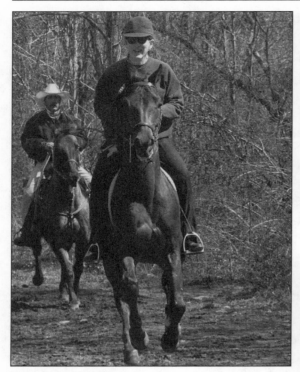

Photo by Heidi Baldwin.

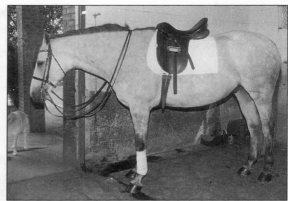

Photo by Mordecai Siegal.

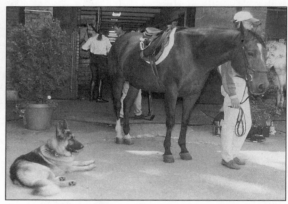

Photo by Mordecai Siegal.

Of these considerations, which one do you start with? The breed or type of horse is an extremely important criterion. Certain breeds are more suitable for certain sports or recreational activities. For example, a Warmblood (such as a Hanoverian or Trekehener) or Thoroughbred would be more suitable for three-day eventing than a gaited horse such as the American Saddlebred or Tennessee Walker. Within a breed, certain types of horses may have better conformation for jumping or dressage.

Breed and Type

The breed or breed-type of the horse to be selected will usually be based on the interests of the prospective buyer. If the buyer is interested in racing the horse, then he or she might want to choose a Thoroughbred, Arabian, or Quarter Horse. Within each breed, conformation, pedigree, and/or training might dictate the type of horse to choose. By contrast, if the buyer is interested in showing the horse in harness, then he

or she might want a gaited horse such as a Tennessee Walker, Hackney, or Saddlebred. There is no ideal breed for a particular sport; some are better suited for one sport than another. However, there is considerable variation in type and ability within all breeds. Breed-type is usually based on such characteristics as head shape, neck carriage, body structure, color and markings, or gaits. The more desirable these characteristics are, the more valuable the horse. (*See* CHAPTER 2, "MAJOR BREEDS OF HORSES.")

Temperament and Manners

Temperament can be defined as the inherent physical and mental nature of a horse. Is the horse willing to please, or is it uncooperative, mean, or stubborn? Is the horse aggressive or passive? The temperament generally is expressed by the eyes and ears and implemented by the feet or teeth. A horse with a good temperament will have its ears forward and be readily receptive to handling and training. A mean horse will pin its ears back, strike, bite, or kick in an unpredictable fashion while being handled. A horse with bad habits or vices can be dangerous, especially for the beginner. (*See* CHAPTER 4, "EQUINE BEHAVIOR," and CHAPTER 5, "MISBEHAVIOR.")

Conformation and Unsoundness

The term **"conformation"** refers to the overall physical appearance of a horse, the result of the arrangement of its muscles, bones, and other body tissues. Unsoundness is any deviation in structure or function that interferes with a horse's intended use or performance. Conformation drives the functional aspects of the horse and can dictate superior performance in certain sports or recreational activities. Good conformation is a blending together of all the body parts to form a superb athlete, while poor conformation predisposes a horse to unsoundness.

Good conformation does not always mean a "beautiful" horse. Beauty is in the eye of the beholder, and since breeds were formed by human selection each breed organization has identified its "ideal" horse, based on a set of conformational traits selected over time by a group of individuals. The following brief description of desirable conformation applies to all horses regardless of breed.

Head and neck The head and neck play a major role in determining the horse's balance, stability, freedom of stride, and agility. The head should be in proportion to the body and be refined, with a pleasing profile, prominent eyes, and small ears. When viewed from the front the head should have a triangular appearance, tapering down to a fine muzzle with large flaring nostrils and lips that meet evenly. The head should join the neck in such a manner as to provide ample movement and flexion without impairment of the air passages. The neck should be fairly long and smooth, lean and muscular, and slightly arched. It

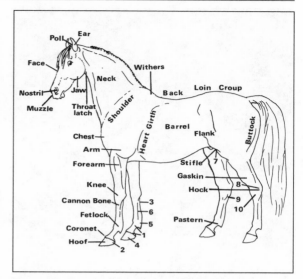

Figure 2: Parts of the horse. Common leg unsoundnesses: *Forelegs:* 1) Ringbone; 2) Sidebones; 3) Bowed tendons; 4) Navicular disease; 5) Osselets; 6) Splints; *Hindlimbs:* 7) Stifled; 8) Thoroughpin; 9) Bone spavin; 10) Bog spavin

should neatly join the shoulder with a definite line of demarcation.

Withers and shoulders Well-defined withers increase the area of attachment for the neck and shoulder muscles and are associated with good depth and angle of the shoulder, freedom of movement, and a longer stride. Coarse or low withers reflect a lack of liberty and range of shoulder movement. The shoulder should be long and sloping at about a 45- or 50-degree angle to the ground. A long, sloping shoulder increases stride and absorbs concussion, whereas a short, upright shoulder shortens the stride and increases concussion in the foot.

Chest Viewed from the front, the chest should not be too wide or too narrow. A horse with a wide chest may have a waddling gait and paddle (swing the foot outward) in front. A horse with a narrow chest may interfere in front and strike its forelegs. The chest should have good depth to allow plenty of room for the heart and lungs.

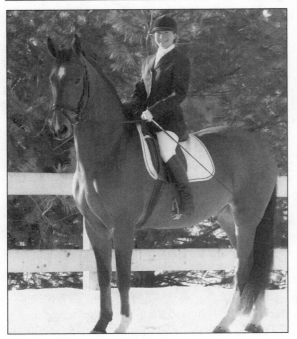

Photo by Heidi Baldwin.

Arm The arm extends from the point of the shoulder to the point of the elbow. The arm should be moderately long, well-muscled, and fairly upright to allow for maximum extension of the forearm. It should be in a parallel plane with the spinal column. If the elbow is set too near the body, the toes will turn out and the horse will be splay-footed. If the elbow is turned outward, the horse will stand pigeon-toed.

Forelegs The forelegs of a horse carry 60–65 percent of the horse's body weight, plus the rider's weight, and therefore are very susceptible to injury if they are not well formed. The forearm should be long, with smooth muscles tying in just above the knee. The knee itself should be wide and flat and void of lumps and bumps. The cannon bone below the knee should be shorter than the forearm and should have well-defined tendons and ligaments. When viewed from the front, the cannon should be straight and centered from the knee. The fetlock joint, located between the cannon and pasterns, should be wide, thick, well directed, and free of

lumps and bumps. The pastern should be moderately long and slope at a 45- to 55-degree angle to the ground. Both the shoulder and pasterns should have similar slopes. Long, weak pasterns predispose a horse to injure the tendons behind the cannon bone and the small bones behind the fetlock joint. By contrast, a short, upright pastern leads to excessive concussion in the foot, predisposing the horse to bone and soft-tissue damage.

The forelegs should be set square and straight for normal functioning of the limbs. Viewed from the front, an imaginary plumb line dropped from the point of the shoulder to the ground should bisect the forearm, knee, cannon, fetlock, pastern, and foot. From the side, a plumb line dropped from the middle of the forearm to the ground should bisect the knee and cannon equally and touch the ground about 1 inch behind the heel. Crooked limbs will alter the way of going or gait of a horse, predisposing it to unsoundness and poor athletic performance. Some of the more common unsoundnesses due to crooked legs are:

- Ringbone (new bony growth between and/or around the pastern and coffin joints)
- Sidebones (bone formation in the lateral cartilage attached to the wings of the coffin bone)
- Bowed tendons (stress or tear of the deep and/or superficial flexor tendons behind the cannon bone. *See* "TENDINITIS" in CHAPTER 22,

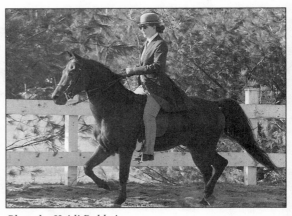

Photo by Heidi Baldwin.

"THE MUSCULOSKELETAL SYSTEM AND VARIOUS DISORDERS," on page 209.)

- Navicular disease (inflammation of the navicular bone, located between the small pastern and the coffin bone)
- Osselets (puffiness around the fetlock joint. *See* "SESAMOIDITIS" in CHAPTER 22, "THE MUSCULOSKELETAL SYSTEM AND VARIOUS DISORDERS," on page 223.)
- Splints (inflammation and calcification of the interosseous ligament that attaches the splint bone to the coffin bone. *See* FIGURE 2, and CHAPTER 22, "THE MUSCULOSKELETAL SYSTEM AND VARIOUS DISORDERS")

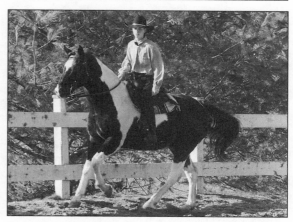

Photo by Heidi Baldwin.

Body The back and loin of the horse should be short, straight, strong, and muscular to support the weight of the rider. The ribs should be long and well sprung to provide vital capacity of the heart, lungs, and digestive system. The ribs should be felt but not seen.

Hindquarters The hindquarters should be well muscled and powerful to provide the force necessary to propel the horse forward. The length and width of the *croup* (area between the hips and the point of the buttocks) should be given consideration, because long muscles are related to speed and endurance, while width of muscling is associated with strength and power. The slope of the croup varies with the different breeds. A long, flat croup and high-set tail allows for long, low, effortless striding from behind and is desirable in the Arabian breed, from which come the superior endurance horses. A slightly sloping croup and lower-set tail allow the hindlimbs to step underneath the horse for quick starts and turns. This type of conformation is desirable in the Quarter Horse and Thoroughbred breeds. The hips should be well-defined and their width a bit narrower than the distance between the stifles. Excessively prominent hips indicate poor conditioning and lack of strength and endurance.

Hindlimbs The role of the hindlimbs is to propel the horse forward. Most of the work of the hindlimbs is carried out by the joints, particu-

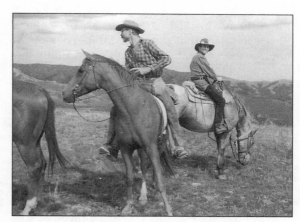

Photo by Ruth Saada.

larly the hock joints (joint between stifle and fetlock). Strong, well-muscled thighs and gaskins (portion of hindlimbs between the stifle and hock), along with a proper leg set as viewed from the back and side, are critical in preventing serious arthritic conditions in the joints. As viewed from behind, a plumb line dropped from the point of the buttocks to the ground should bisect all parts of the hindlimb equally. As viewed from the side, the line should touch the hocks, run parallel with the cannon (long bone between fetlock and hock), and drop to the ground 3 or 4 inches behind the heel. The hocks should be wide and flat. The pasterns (area between the fetlock and coronet) should be shorter and slightly less sloping than the front pasterns. Some of the more common unsoundnesses found in the hindlimbs include:

- Upward fixation of the patella (kneecap)
- Thoroughpin (stress on the deep digital flexor tendon, with puffiness in the web of the hock. *See* "ACQUIRED FLEXURAL DEFORMITIES" in CHAPTER 22, "THE MUSCULOSKELETAL SYSTEM AND VARIOUS DISORDERS," on page 201.)
- Bone spavin (bony enlargement that develops on the inside and front of the hock)
- Bog spavin (distension and swelling of the joint capsule of the hock. *See* FIGURE 2, and CHAPTER 22, "THE MUSCULOSKELETAL SYSTEM AND VARIOUS DISORDERS").

Blemishes A blemish is defined as an acquired physical defect that does not interfere with the horse's way of going but may be unsightly and decrease the animal's value. Examples of old injuries that can turn into blemishes are:

- Splints (hard bump along the splint bone)
- Capped elbow (soft to firm swelling over the point of the elbow, usually involves subcutaneous bursa. *See* "OLECRANON BURSITIS" in CHAPTER 22, "THE MUSCULOSKELETAL SYSTEM AND VARIOUS DISORDERS," on page 230.
- Capped hocks (soft to firm swelling over the point of the hock, usually involves subcutaneous bursa)
- Windpuffs (small puffy area slightly above and to the rear of the fetlock joint. *See* CHAPTER 22, "THE MUSCULOSKELETAL SYSTEM AND VARIOUS DISORDERS.")

Health The overall appearance of the horse should be considered. A healthy horse is alert, ready to eat and work, displays a shiny coat, and is in good body condition. An unhealthy horse is dull, lethargic, has a pot belly and a rough hair coat. A pre-purchase veterinary examination is an extremely important consideration for the prospective horse buyer. The buyer's veterinarian thoroughly examines the horse for both health and soundness and determines the suitability of the horse for the rider and its

potential use. Additionally, the buyer can request the horse's previous vaccination and deworming schedules as well as other health records.

Level of performance and accomplishments Training is time and training is money. The more accomplished the horse, the higher the price tag. An experienced rider may want to buy a high-level performance horse that not only meets the rider's abilities but continues to learn from the rider's training. By contrast, an inexperienced rider may not capitalize on the talents of an accomplished horse, in which case the extra money paid was poorly spent and the horse may end up at the same level of accomplishment as the rider. However, an inexperienced rider should *not* buy an inexperienced horse with the idea that they will learn together. Such a relationship usually fails in frustration. Ideally, the buyer should identify a horse that fits his or her ability, talent, and ambition.

Size The size of the horse should fit the size of the rider, and be adequate for the desired purpose and appropriate for the task. Bigger horses usually cost more because they can accommodate a wider variety of rider sizes and appear to have more presence in the show arena.

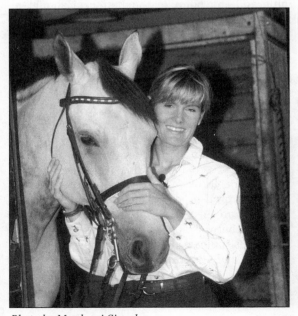

Photo by Mordecai Siegal.

Quality and pedigree Quality and pedigree seem to go hand in hand. Quality refers to the refinement in a horse, as evidenced by the texture of the hair, hide, bones, and joints. The more attractive, more refined, "classier" horse will probably come with a higher price tag. The pedigree is an historical record of a horse's ancestry. A horse is usually bred for its look and ability to perform. Bloodlines can dictate a horse's quality and suitability to perform a particular task. The higher the level of performance and accomplishments recorded, the higher the sale price on a newborn foal with those bloodlines.

Age The age of a horse can in part influence its value. A young horse will usually cost less because of its lack of training and the risk involved in potential unsoundnesses or injuries when put to work. Horses in their prime—5 to 8 years of age—will probably command the highest prices because they usually have some training, have shown some years of service, and are relatively mature both mentally and physically. An older horse (15 years and above) may only have a few more years left to perform but may be a perfect choice for a novice rider, so the price range may vary.

Color and markings Color and markings are usually the first thing one notices about a horse, but are really the least important factors to consider when making a purchase, unless the horse is to be shown in halter in one of the color breeds.

Sex Stallions are usually more difficult to handle than geldings or mares. Mares can be brilliant but may be moody, owing to hormonal changes. Overall, geldings are more consistent in their day-to-day behavior.

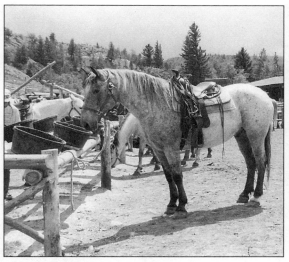

Photo by Ruth Saada.

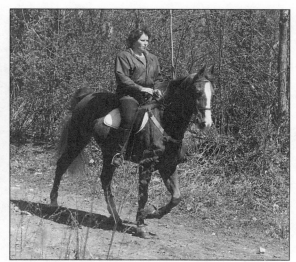

Photo by Heidi Baldwin.

CHAPTER 2

Major Breeds of Horses

**by Monna F. Jordan and
Janet F. Roser**

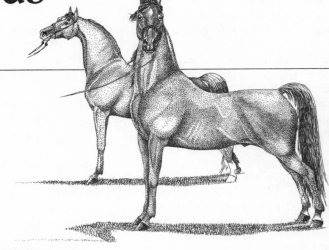

The purpose of this chapter is to provide a broad overview of the major breeds of horses found throughout the world. Because there are over 150 breed registries in existence, it would be a difficult task to present the characteristics and history of every breed in one single chapter. The authors have chosen instead to present a selection of the major breeds existing today, to give the reader some insight into the incredible range of horse and pony types that have evolved since the days of *Eohippus*. We would like to thank all the breed registries acknowledged at the end of the chapter for providing us with the excellent information presented here.

What is a breed? The usual definition of a **"breed"** is a group of animals with certain distinguishable characteristics involving conformation, size, action, function, and, in some cases, color. The characteristics are a result of either *natural selection* (i.e., they are shaped naturally by the geographical terrain and environment) or *artificial selection* (shaped by human desire). Breed organizations register horses as a fixed type with common ancestry in the breed's

studbook. In most cases a horse must be born of parents belonging to that breed and exhibit typical breed characteristics.

Equine breeds are divided into ponies, light

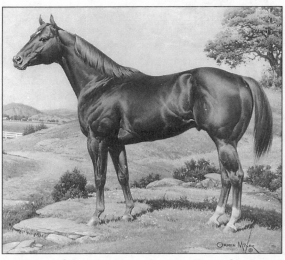

Drawing of the American Quarter Horse by Orren Mixer.
Courtesy of American Quarter Horse Racing News.

Table 1
Coat Colors and Patterns of the Horse

Basic Colors

Note:"points" are mane and tail, lower legs, ear tips, muzzle

bay	reddish brown body color with black points
black	uniform black
brown	between bay and black; shaded black over a brown base
chestnut	various shades of reddish brown with self colored or lighter points
liver	used for the darkest chestnut shades; the color of raw liver
sorrel	varies with breed or region of country; may be darker or lighter chestnut
piebald	British term for black and white coat
skewbald	British term for white and any color but black
white	pink skin, white hair coat, brown eyes

Dilution

Cream dilutes

palomino	gold or tan with white or near-white mane and tail
buckskin	more or less tan body color with dark points
cream, cremello	pink skin, blue eyes, near-white hair coat

Dun dilutes

"dun pattern"	darker points, stripe along spine, and more or less striping across withers and on upper legs
red dun	pinkish or orange shades with darker red dun pattern
buckskin (yellow)	dun similar to buckskin with addition of dun pattern
grulla (blue dun)	uniform slate gray body with black dun pattern

Patterns

gray	progressive silvering; white hairs mixed into any body color and increasing with age to eventual white or flecked state
roan	white hairs mixed into any of the base colors but not increasing with age

Appaloosa (see own section for "Appaloosa characteristics" in addition to coat pattern)

blanket	any body color with white over loin and hips
snowflake	small white flecks over the entire darker coat
roan Appaloosa	resembles ordinary roan but has Appaloosa characteristics
leopard	mostly white with small regularly scattered colored spots; spots are larger than those of flecked gray, and has Appaloosa characteristics

Paint/pinto

tobiano	"dorsal" pattern with white usually crossing backline between ears and tail; usually white on all four legs; usually not much white on face; may give effect of white horse with dark patches
overo	"ventral" pattern, white does not usually cross backline; face usually has more white than that of tobiano, legs may be minimally or much marked; may give effect of dark horse with white patches

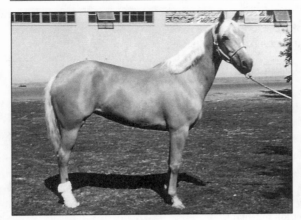

Palomino.
Photo by Murray E. Fowler.

horses, and draft horses (heavy horses), with further subdivisions by geographical origin and human direction. Horses are further described as being "hotbloods," "warmbloods," or "coldbloods." These terms have nothing to do with the animals' regulation of their body temperature; rather, they are descriptive of horses' origin and temperament. The Arabian and the Thoroughbred breeds typify the hot-blooded horses. These light-boned, quick-footed animals evolved in the desert climates or as the result of human selection and are known for their volatile temperaments. Heavy draft horses such as Shires and Clydesdales typify the cold-blooded horses. They originated in the forests of northern Europe and are characterized by large, strong bodies and calm natures. Horses in which strains of hot-blooded and cold-blooded ancestors are mixed are referred to as warmbloods.

Visualizing coat color from words is difficult but the descriptions in Table 1 may be helpful (assume dark skin and eyes unless noted).

The Breeds

Arabian

TEMPERAMENT: Highly strung

QUALITIES: Speed, endurance, intelligence, courage, gentleness

FUNCTION: Riding horse, light draft

ACTION: Free easy stride with stylish, natural, balanced action

HISTORY: The origin and early history of the Arabian horse are obscure and shrouded in legend. Most scholars regard the Arabian as the oldest breed of horse and the fountainhead of all the other light horse breeds. Some believe the breed originated in Turkey or Syria, or perhaps southern Arabia. There is some archaeological evidence that Arabian horses may have existed before the year 3000 B.C. in the deserts of Saudi Arabia. Certainly there are a number of legends surrounding the development of the Arabian. According to one tradition, King Solomon selected five horses from among the 40,000 chariot horses and 12,000 riding horses he owned. Five strains developed through the female lines from these ancestors: the Koheilan, the Maneghi and a substrain called the Hadraj, the Saqlawi, the Jilfan, and the Hedban. Popular folklore also holds that the Arabian descends from the five mares of Mohammed that were the first to reach Mecca, of the 85 sent by the Prophet to bring news of victory.

The *asil* is the horse of the true Bedouin Arab. The desert Bedouin people treasured their Arabians as their own flesh and blood. They lived in close contact with their horses, sharing their food and tents. The Bedouin tribes believed the Arabian horse was a gift from God; legend

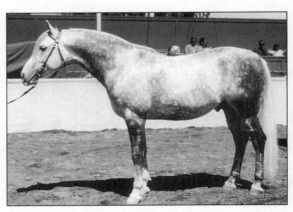

Arabian.
Photo by Murray E. Fowler.

relates how God fashioned the desert wind into a creature that "shall fly without wings." Bedouins distinguish their horses as being *asil*, of known breeding stock, or as non-*asil*, *tref* (as in "not Kosher"), meaning the horse was probably captured in a raid or at least its heritage is unknown. The Arabian breed includes animals whose precise origins are uncertain, or whose pedigrees reflect the influence of the Berber, the Persian, the Syrian, the Egyptian Arab, or other related breeds.

Imported to England, the Arabian became the progenitor of the English Thoroughbred, and through the Thoroughbred the progenitor of the Hackney, Standardbred, and American Saddle Horse breeds. In Russia, Arabian blood contributed to make the Orloff Trotter; in France, the Percheron; and in America, the Morgan.

The largest Arabian registry is the Arabian Horse Registry of America, Inc. It was founded in 1908 and has registered over 400,000 Arabians. The second largest registry is the International Arabian Horse Association (IAHA), which registers purebred Arabians, half-Arabians, and Anglo-Arabians. The IAHA was founded in 1950 and has approximately 300,000 registered horses. It will accept any horse that has at least 25 percent recorded Arabian blood.

CONFORMATION: The Arabian stands between 14.1 and 15.1 **hands** (4-inch units of length used to measure horses) and weighs between 800 and 1,000 pounds. Its coat may be gray, bay, chestnut, black, or more rarely, roan. The head should have a slightly **dished** (concave) profile, a broad, protruding forehead (called the "**jibbah**"), small alert ears, large expressive eyes, flared nostrils, and a small fine muzzle. The neck should be long and arched, set high and run well back in to the **withers** (area between shoulders, neck, and back). The withers should be prominent and set well back over a long, sloping shoulder. The back should be straight and short (some Arabians have fewer thoracic and/or lumbar vertebrae and some do not) and the loins short (five lumbar vertebrae instead of six) and broad.

Two of the most distinguishing characteristics of the Arabian horse are its flat **croup** (pelvis) and naturally high tail carriage. These conformational traits provide a long low stride, moving the Arabian across desert lands with ease. The legs should be muscular in the forearm and **gaskin** (second thigh). The **cannons** (metatarsals) should be short, flat, clean, and of good size, showing strong, heavy tendons. The **fetlock joints** (ankles) should be bold and clean, extending into long, sloping elastic and **strong pasterns** (phalanx bones). The hooves should be relatively large, round, wide, and low at the heels. Legs should be set parallel when viewed from the front, straight from the side, and point squarely ahead.

Thoroughbred

TEMPERAMENT: Highly strung, energetic

QUALITIES: Speed and stamina

FUNCTION: Racing, jumping, dressage

ACTION: Free easy stride with stylish, natural, balanced action

HISTORY: The origins of the Thoroughbred extend back to the turn of the seventeenth century with the importation into England of three stallions from the Mediterranean Middle East. These three stallions, the Darley Arabian (a bay from the Maneghi tribe of Allepo named after its

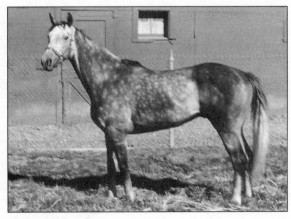

Thoroughbred.
Photo by Murray E. Fowler.

owner, Thomas Darley), the Godolphin Barb (a brown Jilfan, again of asil origin, named after its owner, Lord Godolphin), and the Byerly Turk (a bay horse named after its owner, Capt. Robert Byerly), became the foundation sires of the Thoroughbred breed. The stallions were subsequently bred to stronger but less precocious English broodmares. These mares, known as the "royal mares," were the result of a closely supervised, selective breeding program involving consistent input from oriental blood. The end result was an animal that could carry weight with sustained speed over extended distances, a quality that brought a new dimension to the growing, aristocratically supported sport of horse racing.

In 1791 James Weatherby published the first volume of *The General Stud Book*, the first breed registry for any species of livestock, listing the pedigrees of 387 mares, each of which could be traced back to Eclipse (1764), a direct descendent of the Darley Arabian; Matchem (1748), a grandson of the Godolphin Barb; and Herod (1758), whose great-great-grandsire was the Byerly Turk. The *General Stud Book* influenced the form of pedigree record keeping worldwide, and is still published in England by Weatherby and Sons, Secretaries to the English Jockey Club.

As racing spread to the North American continent, a need for an American-bred Thoroughbred registry became clear. Colonel Sanders D. Bruce, a Kentuckian who had spent almost a lifetime researching the pedigrees of American Thoroughbreds, published the first volume of *The American Stud Book* in 1873. Guardianship of the *American Stud Book* is today a responsibility of the American Jockey Club.

Over the years the sport of horse racing has evolved from a pursuit of the wealthy to a multi-million-dollar industry where for some owners with limited incomes, dreams do come true. The Thoroughbred is sought after not only for its speed on the racetrack, but for its courage, stamina, agility, and intelligence in other sports, such as show jumping, hunting, dressage, three-day eventing, and polo. In 1962 the approximate world population of Thoroughbreds was 233,000 horses. By 1991 the American Jockey Club alone had 1,241,442 Thoroughbred horses registered.

CONFORMATION: The average Thoroughbred stands 15 to 17 hands and weighs between 1,000 and 1,200 pounds. Its coat may be gray, bay, chestnut, brown, black, and occasionally roan. The head should have a straight profile, well-defined ears, wide-set intelligent eyes, flared nostrils, and a fine muzzle. The neck should be long and straight, with long flat muscles that tie smoothly into the shoulder. The withers should be high and well defined, leading to an evenly curved back. The shoulder should be deep, well muscled, and sloped along the same parallel as that on which the head is carried, at about 45 degrees from the vertical. From the point of the shoulder, the forearm should be well muscled and taper into a clean flat knee which in turn tapers into the full width of the cannon. The cannon area should be relatively short and comparatively flat, with the tendons distinctly set out and clean. The pastern should be set at an angle of a little less than 45 degrees to the vertical and should be neither too long, too weak, nor too short. The legs should be straight and parallel when observed from the front and side, respectively. The stride should be long, smooth, and easy. The powerful muscling of the hip, thigh, and buttocks and the slight slope of the croup help propel the horse forward, allowing for that initial burst of speed from the starting gate.

Quarter Horse

TEMPERAMENT: Pleasing disposition and gentleness, remarkable instinct for working with cattle

QUALITIES: Agile, fast, quick to start and "turns on a dime"

FUNCTION: Riding horse, cow pony, quarter-mile sprinter

ACTION: Free easy stride, natural, balanced action

HISTORY: The history of the Quarter Horse began in America in the early 1600s when the English colonists, particularly those in Maryland, Virginia, and the Carolinas, crossed their own

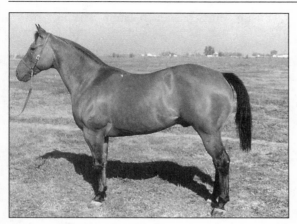

Quarter Horse.
Photo by Murray E. Fowler.

stallions on mares gained from the Chickasaw. Early documentation of the English importations, which first arrived in 1609 in the form of one stallion and nine mares, listed them as Hobby and Galloway horses. The Hobby horses of Ireland that developed during the thirteenth, fourteenth, and fifteenth centuries were relatively small and compact, and noted for their lightning speed in battle and on the racecourse. The Galloways were Spanish Barbs that escaped from the ill-fated Spanish Armada when it was driven ashore in England in 1588. These horses gained popularity in the district of Galloway, on the shores of Solway Firth in the south of Scotland. The Galloways were 14 hands high or more, bay or brown, with a small head and short neck, and deep, clean black legs. Their special qualities were speed, stoutness, and surefootedness. Together, these horses formed the bulk of the early English importations into the colonies.

For lack of other entertainment, English colonists took their leisure by match-racing horses on Sunday afternoons. Races were often run through the main street of a settlement or town, since this was often the only straight stretch of clear ground available. Thus, the distance was often one quarter mile or less.

By the mid–eighteenth century progeny of the Godolphin Barb, one of the three foundation sires of the Thoroughbred, were being shipped to the colonies and crossed with native hybrids.

One of these imports was Janus, a grandson of the Godolphin Barb. A powerful, strong, compact horse of short stature (14 hands), Janus galvanized the Quarter Horse breed into a distinct form. The most important stallion to influence the Quarter Horse after Janus was a son of the imported stallion Diomede called Sir Archy. Born in 1805, Sir Archy was a bay that stood 16 hands; on the track he beat all the outstanding racers of his day.

The American Quarter Horse was bred not only for speed but for its utility as a working farm animal. Quarter Horses went west with the wagon trains, with cowboys and trail hands using them for both transportation and recreation. In Texas more than any other state, the Quarter Horse became the working cow horse as the cattle industry flourished. As Mexicans moved north into California they began crossing Quarter Horses with Mustangs, combining speed with intelligence, stamina, and hardiness—the last significant genetic alteration of the Quarter Horse. A famous stallion from this crossing was Steel Dust. Known for his superb conformation and swiftness, Steel Dust became a legendary sprinter throughout the West; for a long time after, Quarter Horses were known simply as "Steel Dusts."

For many years ranchers bred Quarter Horses without giving much attention to pedigree or lineage. On 15 March 1940, a historian named Robert M. Denhardt gathered a group of ranchers in Fort Worth, Texas, to organize a breed registry for the Quarter Horse. This was the beginning of the American Quarter Horse Association (AQHA), which is presently headquartered in Amarillo, Texas. Today the AQHA is the largest breed registry in the world, with over 3 million registered horses.

CONFORMATION: The Quarter Horse is a sturdy, powerfully built horse of medium size, standing 14.1 to 16 hands at the withers and weighing 900 to 1,200 pounds. Coat colors include sorrel, bay, brown, black, liver, chestnut, dun, red dun, buckskin, grullo, palomino, gray, blue roan, and red roan. Quarter Horses with Paint, Pinto, Appaloosa, or American Albino markings are not eligible for registration. The head of the Quarter Horse is short, the profile straight, the

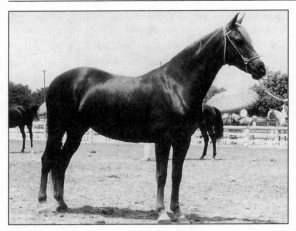

Morgan.
Photo by Murray E. Fowler.

jowls large, and the ears small but alert. The neck is muscular, well formed, and slightly arched. The chest, shoulders, forearms, thighs, gaskins, and hindquarters are well muscled. The croup is long and sloping, with the tail set on quite low. The cannons are short, clean, and well defined.

Morgan

TEMPERAMENT: Energetic and willing, yet docile

QUALITIES: Incredible endurance and versatility

FUNCTION: Riding, harness, light draft

ACTION: Natural, easy stride, may also exhibit more action when shown

HISTORY: The Morgan is possessed of a past rich in history and legend, some of it true and some exaggerated, owing to a scarcity of accurate records. What is known for certain is that a colt was born to a mixed-breed mare and a Thoroughbred stallion named True Briton (also called Beautiful Bay) in Massachusetts in 1790. This colt, originally called Figure, was bartered to one Thomas Justin Morgan. The colt's name was subsequently changed to Justin Morgan, as it was customary at that time to name a horse after its owner.

Justin Morgan soon became a local hero. It was said that he could outrun, outpull, outtrot, and in every way just outdo any other horse. This remarkable animal was only 14 hands tall, but what he lacked in size he more than made up in spirit, endurance, and strength. Over the 32 years of his life Justin Morgan became famous, particularly for his prowess at contests of strength, especially pulling. Because of this fame he was much sought after as a sire. Many, many foals were fathered by this incredible little horse—yet another truly American breed was born.

The Morgan quickly became an extremely popular horse, owing to its strength, intelligence, and versatility. By the 1850s the Morgan was the most popular breed in the United States, and included among its numbers many Civil War cavalry mounts. The American Morgan Horse Register was formed in 1894 with the assistance of Morgan enthusiast Colonel Joseph Battell, who donated a farm in Vermont to the United States Department of Agriculture in 1907 for the sole purpose of improving and preserving the Morgan breed. The Morgan Horse Club was founded in 1909, becoming the American Morgan Horse Association in 1971. The Morgan has influenced other American breeds by contributing foundation blood to the Standardbred, Saddlebred, and American Quarter Horse.

CONFORMATION: Although Justin Morgan was himself a small horse, the modern Morgan may be 14.1 to 15.2 hands tall (with occasional examples over or under) and weigh 800 to 1,200 pounds. The most common colors are bay, black, brown, and chestnut. White may be present on the face and also the legs—but not above the knee or hock. The head is of average size with a straight profile, prominent jaw, small, pointed ears, and expressive, wide-set eyes. The muscular and slightly arched neck blends well with the muscular, sloping shoulders and well defined, although not overly prominent, withers. The breed's probable Arabian ancestry is evident in the wide, short, strong back. The croup should be long, rounded and muscular, indicative of the ability to pull heavy loads. The chest is deep and powerful and the legs are solid with dense bone, well defined tendons, and tough feet. The Morgan should give the appearance of a strong, powerful horse with overall substance and refinement.

Standardbred

TEMPERAMENT: Willing and competitive

QUALITIES: Great speed and endurance

FUNCTION: Trotting and pacing races

ACTION: Long, extended, natural strides whether trotting or pacing

HISTORY: The continued growth of the United States during the mid–1800s elicited a need for long-distance transportation, engendering the expansion of the railroads. The horse remained the preferred means of transport for shorter distances, although people were beginning to become impatient to travel faster and more efficiently. The Standardbred, or American Trotter, became the right horse for that job.

The Standardbred developed from a Thoroughbred stallion named Messenger, imported to North America from England in 1788. Messenger's great-grandson, Hambletonian 10, is considered the true foundation sire of the breed. From 1851 to 1875, Hambletonian 10 sired 1,335 foals, thereby exercising a substantial influence on the conformation and style of the breed. Today 99 percent of all Standardbreds trace back to Hambletonian 10 and Messenger.

Although the Standardbred was utilized extensively for transportation, owners discovered that the horse possessed great speed, and harness racing soon became a popular exhibition of this talent. Today harness racing is still very popular in the United States and elsewhere. Standardbred racing includes two different styles of racing, based solely on the gait by which the horse is raced. Some horses are raced at the trot, a two-beat diagonal gait wherein the opposite hind and fore feet move at the same time. Other horses are pacers. The pace is a two-beat lateral gait wherein the hind and fore feet on the same side move in unison. Horses

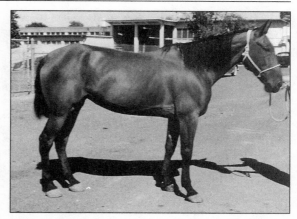

Standardbred.
Photo by Murray E. Fowler.

that pace are faster than trotters because of the variation between the two gaits; for this reason pacers and trotters do not race against each other. Each horse is either a natural trotter or a natural pacer.

The name "Standardbred" evolved from the qualifications or standards that horses had to meet to be considered a member of the breed. These qualifications were based solely on time trials. In 1806 horses had to be able to complete one mile in under three minutes. By 1879 the required time had dropped considerably. Trotters must have completed the mile in under two minutes and thirty seconds, while pacers were limited to two minutes and twenty-five seconds. Until 1892 racing sulkies consisted of heavy carts with wheels five feet in diameter. That year an advanced, lighter sulky with 30-inch wheels was introduced, and following this, racing times continued to drop. Breaking the two-minute mile became an attainable goal; a pacer named Star Pointer broke the barrier in 1897 with a time of one minute, fifty-nine and one-quarter seconds. In 1903 a mare, Lou Dillon, became the first trotter to accomplish this, taking one minute, fifty-eight and one-half seconds. Today many horses can accomplish a mile in under one minute and fifty seconds.

The United States Trotting Association (USTA) in Columbus, Ohio, is the governing body of the Standardbred industry. The USTA keeps official racing and breeding records and also verifies pedigrees. Only foals born to two already-registered parents are eligible for registration.

CONFORMATION: The Standardbred is a horse of medium size, standing 14.2 to 16 hands at the withers and weighing 900 to 1,200 pounds. Bay is the most common color; however, black, brown, chestnut, gray, and roan are also seen. The head is refined and cleancut with a broad forehead, alert eyes, and active ears. The neck should be long and straight, flowing smoothly into sloping, muscular shoulders. The chest and girth are deep and the ribs well sprung, allowing for incredible respiratory capacity and stamina. Muscling in the front and rear quarters should be smooth and long. Muscling, together with long, clean-boned legs, assures a long-reaching, fluid stride—a necessity in a quality Standardbred.

American Saddlebred

TEMPERAMENT: Intelligent, energetic, and docile

QUALITIES: Strong, with good endurance

FUNCTION: Riding and harness

ACTION: Grand stride with knee and hock action, yet comfortable to ride

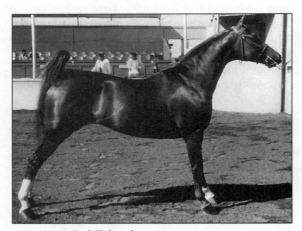

American Saddlebred.
Photo by Murray E. Fowler.

HISTORY: The settlers of the southern United States developed the Saddlebred as their vision of the ideal all-purpose horse, one that was capable of pulling a plow during the week and taking the family to church on Sunday. The original ancestors of the Saddlebred were easy-gaited riding horses known as Hobby and Galloway horses, which were imported from Britain in the 1600s. The characteristic stride of an easy-gaited horse follows a lateral broken cadence in which the legs on the same side of the body move together. This stride yields a most comfortable ride when compared to the jolting experienced at the trot.

The breed truly developed in the early nineteenth century by crossing the Thoroughbred, Morgan, and Narrangansett Pacer, the latter an easy-gaited horse found mostly in Rhode Island and Virginia. The foundation sire for the Saddlebred was a Thoroughbred, Denmark F.S., foaled in 1839. His breeding to a mare known only as the "Stevenson Mare" produced Gaines Denmark, to whom most Saddlebreds can be traced. Much of the early selection and breeding occurred in Kentucky; therefore, the breed has also been referred to as the Kentucky Saddler.

The American Saddlebred gained in popularity during the 1800s. Among its many and varied uses was as a Civil War mount. Robert E. Lee's Traveller, Ulysses S. Grant's Cincinnati, and Stonewall Jackson's Little Sorrel were all Saddlebreds of particular note. In 1891 a group of breeders met in Louisville, Kentucky, to form the National Saddle Horse Breeders' Association. In 1899 the name was changed to the American Saddle Horse Breeders' Association.

Today the Saddlebred is used primarily as a pleasure horse. Many Saddlebreds are exhibited at shows as either three-gaited (walk, trot, canter) or five-gaited (walk, trot, canter, slow gait, the rack) horses. This versatile breed is shown at both Western and English styles, fine harness, dressage, and jumping, and is even used in endurance riding, thereby taking advantage of its strength and stamina.

CONFORMATION: The Saddlebred is a medium to tall breed, measuring 15 to 16 hands and weighing 1,000 to 1,200 pounds. As registration is based solely on pedigree and not on color, coat colors are many and varied and include chestnut, bay, brown, black, palomino, gray, roan, and spotted. The head is well shaped with small, close-set, alert ears, a broad forehead, bright, wide-set eyes, and a straight profile. A clean throatlatch (where the head joins the neck) and long arching neck are also desirable. The withers are well defined, the back short, and the croup level with short, strong coupling. A sloping, well-muscled shoulder, lengthy, clean legs and long, sloping pasterns that give spring to the stride are also characteristic.

Peruvian Paso

TEMPERAMENT: Calm, but lively and eager to please

QUALITIES: Strong and willing, excellent stamina, elegant

FUNCTION: Riding horse

ACTION: Natural four-beat lateral gait; smooth, rolling action in the forelegs

HISTORY: The Peruvian Paso can be recognized by its beautiful, characteristic gait. The bloodstock that was combined to develop the breed in Peru was introduced by the Spanish and included the Andalusian, Spanish Jennet, Barb, and Friesian. The Andalusian contributed conformation, action, beauty, and pride. The Spanish Jennet provided an even temperament and smooth gait, while energy, stamina and strength were the traits passed on from the Barb and Friesian. Peruvians called their beloved horse the "Caballo Peruando de Paso." These horses helped the conquistadors defeat the Incas, and were considered so valuable that many were shod in silver. Instead of having to walk, foals were carried in hammocklike devices during long marches.

No outside breeding has been allowed for centuries. One hundred percent of the offspring have the characteristic gait, which is inherited rather than learned. These horses have an excellent temperament and demeanor, which can be attributed to a particular breeding practice: Horses with undesirable dispositions are excluded from the breeding stock in order to keep the breed calm and pleasant.

The Paso is one of the smoothest and most pleasurable riding horses in the world, owing to its distinct four-beat gait. The stylish action of the breed is known as the *termino*. This graceful, fluid movement is an outward rolling of the forelegs that originates from the shoulder (much like a swimmer's arms) with high knee lift, fetlock flex, and foreleg extension. Two gaits that emphasize the beauty of the *termino* are the *paso llano*, a slow, equally-spaced four-beat gait, and the *sobreandando*, a faster, more lateral gait.

Another characteristic of the breed is much more intangible than the flashy action of its gait. These animals exhibit *brio*—a quality of spirit, an almost arrogant pride, that is rooted in their war-horse ancestry and gives them an aura of greatness. The Peruvian Paso is one of the most distinctive breeds of horse and is gaining great popularity today.

CONFORMATION: The Peruvian Paso is a small to medium-size horse reaching 14.1 to 15.2 hands, with an occasional individual over or

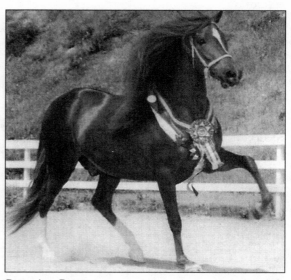

Peruvian Paso.
Courtesy of Peruvian Paso Horse Registry of North America.

under, and weighing 900 to 1,100 pounds. Nearly all solid colors are seen including bay, black, brown, chestnut, gray, and variations of dun, palomino, and roan. The skin should be dark; white markings are acceptable on the legs below the knees, and on the face between the eyes and above the lower lip. The head should be proportional to the body with a straight or slightly concave profile. The muzzle is small, and the ears are medium in length with fine tips that curve slightly inward. The neck is of medium length with a graceful arch, yet may be slightly heavier than most saddle-type breeds. The neck should blend nicely with nonprominent withers and the short, strong back. The breed's strength is shown in the wide and muscular chest, the strong, round hip and croup, and the depth of girth and spring of rib. The legs are straight and clean with long, muscular forearms that set well into a long, sloping shoulder, allowing for the graceful motion of the *termino*.

Hanoverian

TEMPERAMENT: Calm, very willing to work, quiet

QUALITIES: Very good jumpers, courageous, deliberate

FUNCTION: Riding (dressage, eventing, jumping); also light draft

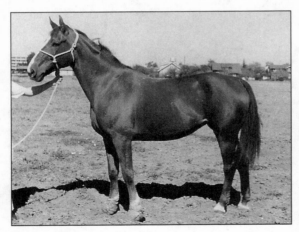

Hanoverian.
Photo by Murray E. Fowler.

ACTION: Long, extensive strides with suspension, may move heavily

HISTORY: The Hanoverian originated in the fertile lowlands of northern Germany, where dukes and farmers alike bred these warmbloods for cavalry mounts and agricultural work. In 1653 the Memsen stud was started to breed the Hanoverian creams. These white or cream-colored horses were used in England to pull royal coaches. In 1735, when the Elector of Hanover became King George I of England, he sent Thoroughbreds back to Germany to improve the Hanoverian stock. Landgestut, the German state-operated stud, was opened to make quality stallions available for breeding to local farmers' mares at a low fee in an attempt to produce better horses. From these breedings two types of Hanoverians developed: the "robust" horses used to pull large carriages and military vehicles and for other draft labor, and the "riding" horses, cavalry mounts that were refined even more by the incorporation of Thoroughbred blood.

European breeders formed the first Hanoverian breed society in 1867, following up in 1888 with the development of a stud book that noted which horses had been bred and graded the quality of their offspring. In 1922 the breed society evolved into the current *Verband Hannoverscher Warmblutzüchter*. A foal born to approved and registered parents is automatically registered. If the dam is a European warmblood or a Thoroughbred, the foal is inspected and evaluated. If it passes muster, it is registered and placed in the stud book.

The breed has developed into a notable sport horse somewhat out of necessity, as mechanization on the farm has replaced working animals. Hanoverians won medals at the first equestrian events in the modern Olympics and still dominate in international competition today. The International Equestrian Yearbook World Ratings of 1988 rated the Hanoverian as the top breed in the world, based on performance in dressage, eventing, and stadium jumping. There are approximately 3,000 Hanoverians in North America, many of which have been imported from Europe over the last 20 years. The American Hanoverian Society was formed in 1974.

CONFORMATION: Although the Hanoverian can be rather large—15.2 to 17 hands tall and weighing 1,100 to 1,900 pounds—it is still an extremely elegant mover and grand jumper. The most common colors are black, bay, chestnut, brown, and gray, with white on the face and legs a frequent occurrence. The head should be well proportioned to the rest of the body, with well-defined jaws and a straight or slightly convex profile. A long, well set-on neck ties in smoothly to the pronounced withers, and the straight back is somewhat long. The croup should be long, wide, and rounded, indicative of the great propulsory power of the hindquarters. The shoulder is long and sloping. The legs should be strong and well muscled, and of more substance than those of a Thoroughbred, with broad, flat, clean joints and large feet.

Trakehner

TEMPERAMENT: Quiet, yet dynamic

QUALITIES: Competitive, with great stamina and endurance

FUNCTION: Riding (dressage, eventing, jumping), some light draft

ACTION: Flowing, balanced gait with elongation and extension evident

HISTORY: The Trakehner is one of the oldest of the German warmbloods, originating 400 years ago in what was eastern Prussia. It was developed from the Schweiken, a native heavy breed used in the Middle Ages. King Friedrich Wilhelm I founded the royal stud office, Trakehnen, in 1731 to refine the Schweiken. Later King Friedrich II incorporated Thoroughbred and Arabian blood to add balance and beauty to the breed and to make it nobler. Area farmers brought their mares to Trakehnen to breed to the stallions there; eventually the breeding was restricted to selected mares for the improvement of the breed as a whole. The first stud book was arranged in 1878. This selective breeding program produced animals that were elegant, versatile, and highly sought after.

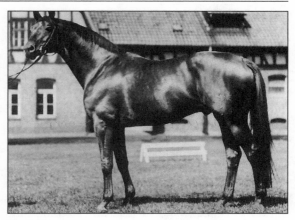

Trakehner.
Photo by Dr. Fritz Schilke. Courtesy of American Trakehner Association.

Trakehners were originally grouped by color (black, brown, chestnut) and use (carriage, riding) because royalty preferred black carriage horses over the other varieties of the breed. The Trakehner was also used extensively in the cavalry and was the premier German military mount during the nineteenth century.

Social unrest plaguing Germany and the rest of Europe did not ignore the Trakehner. Somehow these horses managed to survive the trying times forced upon them by two world wars—although World War II almost eradicated this aged and noble breed. In the chaotic aftermath of the war, only 1,000 Trakehners escaped to the safety of West Germany. The remainder were not so fortunate, and what was once the most populous breed in Prussia was now scattered and declining. Luckily, those who remembered the past and cared for the breed kept it alive. Today the Trakehner is regaining popularity in Europe and other parts of the world as a talented and competitive sport horse.

The Trakehner was introduced into the United States in 1957 by a German, Gerda Friedrichs, who has helped to establish the breed on this side of the Atlantic. The American Trakehner Association was founded in 1974, followed closely by the North American Trakehner Association in 1977—proving that this German import has discovered a place in America.

CONFORMATION: Although somewhat more refined than other warmbloods, the Trakehner is still a large horse, usually 16 to 17 hands tall and weighing 1,000 to 1,200 pounds. They are most often bay, brown, black, chestnut, or gray, with some white markings. The well-proportioned head is refined, with a broad forehead and slightly dished face in some animals. The neck, setting easily into prominent withers, should be well formed and slim, the back straight, and the croup slightly sloping, yet strong. Trakehners exhibit a deep chest and heart girth with a full-sprung rib, evidence of the great respiratory capacity necessary for stamina and endurance. The shoulders are well muscled, long and sloping, giving much extension to the stride, and the legs are of compact bone with broad, flat joints and adequate muscle.

Swedish Warmblood

TEMPERAMENT: Quiet, yet spirited, intelligent

QUALITIES: Competitive, good endurance

FUNCTION: Riding (dressage, eventing, jumping)

ACTION: Springy gaits with rhythm, exceptionally long-strided trot

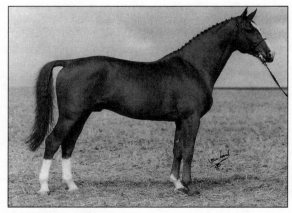

Swedish Warmblood.
Photo by Rik van Lent. Courtesy of Swedish Warmblood Association of North America and The National Stud Flyinge [of Sweden].

HISTORY: As its name implies, the Swedish Warmblood was developed in Sweden. In the seventeenth century King Charles X ordered the establishment of a royal stud at Flyinge where the Swedish Warmblood was derived from crosses with such breeds as the Hanoverian, Trakehner, Thoroughbred, Andalusian, Friesian, and Arabian. Stallions still stand at Flyinge today, where there is an active breeding program.

By the late 1800s a very distinct breed had been developed for both riding and driving. The government began to regulate breeding in 1874 when the first stud book was opened. The breed was the exclusive mount for the Swedish military and was praised for its endurance and athleticism. The military-trained horses became world-renowned and won all the dressage medals at the 1912 Olympics. The government wanted to perfect the Swedish Warmblood even more and so opened the stud book again in 1918 to allow improvement by incorporating Thoroughbred, Trakehner, Hanoverian, and Arabian blood. The Swedish Warmblood Association was established in 1928 as the breed increased in popularity. Swedish Warmbloods remained the horse of choice for the cavalry until its decline in the 1940s. Since then the ever-flexible Warmblood has gone on to enjoy widespread acceptance as an international sport horse. The Swedish Warmblood is recognized as an exceptional dressage mount owing to its intelligence and unique springy gaits, especially the trot, which exhibits remarkable extension.

CONFORMATION: As with other sport horses, the Swedish Warmblood is a large athletic animal, standing 16 to 17 hands and weighing 1,000 to 1,200 pounds. Colors are usually bay, brown, chestnut, or gray, with some white markings. The head is proportional to the body, with lively eyes and an expressive head. The neck is long and slender, yet muscular. Prominent withers lead into a strong back of medium length and a long croup. The shoulder should be strong and sloping and the chest deep and well muscled. The legs are shorter than a Thoroughbred's, yet strong and muscled, with broad, clean joints. The Swedish Warmblood is not considered to be as substantial or robust as other warmbloods, possibly owing to the influence of the slighter Trakehner. It is also described as having more spirit than the quieter German breeds.

Pinto

TEMPERAMENT: Pleasant personality, depends upon the type of horse

QUALITIES: Many, based upon the individual horse

FUNCTION: Many varied uses

ACTION: Depends upon the type of horse

HISTORY: Horses with interesting and variable color patterns have always been very popular with owners searching for an aesthetically pleasing and unique mount. Parti-colored horses were the "orphans" of the horse world for a long period, as no breed associations would allow these animals to be registered. For this reason, lovers of these horses formed the Pinto Horse Association in 1956. The Pinto Horse Association accepts all breeds into its registry as long as the animals exhibit the appropriate coloration. The Pinto is primarily a color breed and will register anything from draft horses to ponies and everything in between.

Particolored horses have existed for nearly as long as horses have been on the earth. Paintings in Egyptian tombs from the fourth century B.C. depict these intriguing spotted animals. The history of this horse in North America is nearly as colorful as the animal itself. It is documented that one or two of the horses brought to Mexico in 1519 by Cortez and his conquistadors was a Pinto. (The name "Pinto" comes from the Spanish *pintado*, meaning "painted".) These horses were subsequently bred in Mexico; some escaped or were stolen by native peoples. Over the years Pintos continued to escape and formed herds of Mustangs with other feral horses. Native Americans highly favored these horses; many believed that

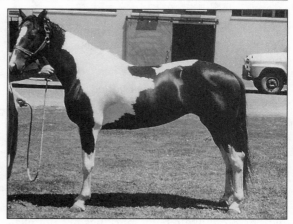

Pinto.
Photo by Murray E. Fowler.

the Pinto had magical powers, such as the ability to protect its rider in battle. The American cowboy also enjoyed these colorful animals, and much Western art depicts the cowboy astride a Pinto.

CONFORMATION AND COLOR PATTERNS: The conformation of the Pinto is entirely breed-dependent, so characteristics of that breed are what the horse should exhibit.

The color patterns of the Pinto are much easier to describe than its conformation. General terms are *piebald* and *skewbald*. A piebald horse is black and white, while a skewbald is white and any color other than black. There are two genetically different color patterns that have been described: tobiano and overo. *Tobiano* is the dominantly inherited color pattern, and is expressed as a white base coat with colored patches on the body. The legs are usually white, and white normally crosses the back. The colored areas are regular, usually oval or round. The head is colored, as are the flanks. An *overo* normally has a colored base coat with white patches and colored legs. The white markings are more irregular than the colored patches of the tobiano; white does not cross the back and the head is mostly white. If the horse shows coloration indicative of both the tobiano and overo, it may be referred to as **tovero**. (*See* CHAPTER 13, "GENETICS.")

Paint

TEMPERAMENT: Docile, yet energetic, similar to the Quarter Horse

QUALITIES: Robust and versatile

FUNCTION: Riding and driving

ACTION: Free, easy stride with natural action

HISTORY: With the increasing popularity of attractive, versatile parti-colored horses, specialization was bound to occur. Stock-type horses with extreme white body markings are not eligible for registry with the American Quarter Horse Association even if they are from registered Quarter Horse parents. Nevertheless such "loud"

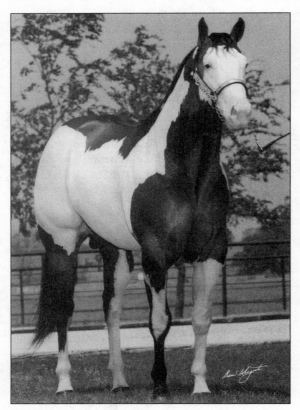

Paint.
Photo courtesy of the American Paint Horse Association.

coloration was popular with those fortunate enough to have one of these beautiful animals, and so in 1962 the American Paint Horse Association was born.

The various coat coloration patterns of the Paint, *tobiano* and *overo*, are genetic traits inherited from the parents (*see* "Pinto," above, and CHAPTER 13, "GENETICS"). The original Paints were Quarter Horses that expressed these two traits, which they had inherited from colorful Mustangs that roamed the American West. During the development of the Quarter Horse, foundation animals were crossed with the Mustangs and the coloration patterns were passed on. Quarter Horse standards do not allow particolors. Horses with these colorful coat patterns are registered with the American Paint Horse Association.

While any horse with a coloration pattern of white and any other color can be registered as a Pinto, only foals born to two registered Paint parents, or one registered Paint parent and one registered Quarter Horse or Thoroughbred parent, are eligible for registry with the American Paint Horse Association. The Paint is based upon breeding, conformation, and color.

CONFORMATION AND COLOR PATTERNS: The Paint has been bred to be a stock-type horse and has been influenced greatly by the Quarter Horse. For this reason Paints possess many of the same conformational qualities as the Quarter Horse, especially the definitive muscling of the chest, shoulders, forearms, gaskins, and hindquarters.

The color patterns of the Paint are the same as those of the Pinto. The two genetically different color patterns are tobiano and overo. Tobiano, dominantly inherited, is a white base coat with colored patches on the body. The legs are usually white, and white normally crosses the back. The colored areas are regular, usually oval or round, and the head and flanks are colored. The overo normally has a colored base coat with white patches and colored legs. The white markings are irregular, white does not cross the back, and the head is mostly white.

Appaloosa

TEMPERAMENT: Docile and quiet, but with a lively and pleasant demeanor

QUALITIES: Versatile, good endurance, intelligent, athletic

FUNCTION: Riding, racing, sport horse

ACTION: Free, easy stride with natural balanced action

HISTORY: The horse has coexisted with humans for centuries, yet somehow the spotted horse has acquired a special place in our hearts. French cave drawings dating back 20,000 years depict our ancient ancestors and their colorful horses. Very old Asian art features these spotted animals as well. A modern breed that exhibits these special spots is the Appaloosa. Spotted horses were introduced to North America by the Spanish conquistadors. Herds of wild Mustangs that roamed Mexico and the American Southwest began to show spotting, supposedly from breeding with escaped Spanish imports. Native Americans captured these spotted horses and traded among the various tribes.

The Nez Percé of eastern Washington, Oregon, and Idaho were revered horsemen who treasured their spotted mounts and purposefully bred them as great warhorses with definitive coloring. White settlers to this area, which was known as the northern Palouse from the Palouse River that flowed through the region, named the Native American horse "a Palouse horse." This name was subsequently corrupted to "appalousey," and finally "Appaloosa."

The late 1800s was a trying time for both the tribe and their horses with the occurrence of the Nez Percé War. Under the command of their venerable and peaceful leader, Chief Joseph, the Nez Percé avoided battles and eluded the United States cavalry for months. The tribe fled through 1,300 miles of rugged mountain terrain with the help of their trusted horses. The Nez Percé finally surrendered in Montana after the cavalry had eradicated many members of the tribe and many of their Appaloosas. The remaining horses were dispersed.

A group of horsemen dedicated to rescuing and preserving the breed and its rich heritage founded the Appaloosa Horse Club in 1938. The popularity of this versatile breed continues to rise as more people discover that the Appaloosa can be used for riding, ranch work, racing, and jumping, among other purposes. Today the Appaloosa Horse Club is the third largest horse registry in the world with 500,000 registered horses and annual increases of 10,000 animals.

CONFORMATION AND COLOR: The Appaloosa is most widely used as a stock-type horse; therefore, its conformation is similar to that of the Quarter Horse, which has been extensively utilized in cross-breeding. Other Appaloosas exhibit a look closer to that of the Thoroughbred and are used as sport horses. Overall, the conformation should be correct and sound. The head should be proportional, well set-on, and exhibit much character. The profile is straight, the eyes large, and the ears nicely pointed. The long, muscular neck should tie in smoothly with nonprominent, muscular withers and a strong, sloping shoulder. The back should be short and straight, leading to a slightly sloping croup which is heavily muscled for propulsion. The chest and girth are deep, and muscling through the gaskin and forearm should be evident. Solid legs with good bone structure and flat, clean joints are also a must.

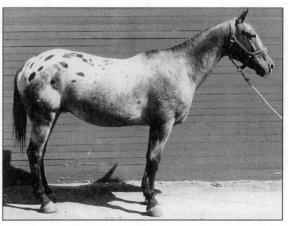

Appaloosa.
Photo by Murray E. Fowler.

Appaloosa coat colors and patterns are as many and varied as the horses that wear them. Any coat color with contrasting spots is acceptable. Some of the color patterns include: blanketed, leopard, roan, roan with blanket, and solid. Spots, however, do not always make an Appaloosa, for other criteria are necessary. To be eligible for registry the horse must exhibit a recognizable coat pattern and the following characteristics:

MOTTLED SKIN: A mixture of dark pigmented skin and light non-pigmented skin. Usually seen on the muzzle, around the eyes, and on the anus, vulva, sheath, scrotum, or udder.

WHITE SCLERA: White area of the eye surrounding the cornea. Should be readily visible and not associated with white facial markings.

STRIPED HOOVES: Vertical light and dark stripes on the hooves. Not associated with white leg markings. Should see striped hooves with solid colored legs.

Clydesdale

TEMPERAMENT: Calm, sociable, willing to work

QUALITIES: Strong and hardy

FUNCTION: Heavy draft, farm work, parades

ACTION: Natural high-lifting of all feet cleanly off the ground

HISTORY: The Clydesdale originated in the eighteenth century in the Lanarkshire district of Scotland surrounding the river Clyde. Influential foundation-sire bloodstock was imported from Flanders very early in the history of the breed. The Clydesdale was used for heavy draft work in virtually every area of Scotland, from the farm to the coalfield, to the bustling streets of Glasgow and other cities.

The first official public recognition of the breed came in 1826 when horses debuted at the Glasgow Exhibition. A selective breeding program, implemented in 1837, made great progress to standardize the characteristics of the Clydesdale and establish breed standards. The young breed had become so popular by this time that it had eclipsed the Shire (*see* below) as the most common carriage horse in Scotland.

The Clydesdale Horse Society was founded in 1877 and has done much to promote the breed throughout the world. The American Clydesdale Association was formed in 1879. The Clydesdale is such an impressive and favored horse that it has become quite familiar as a commercial trademark in the United States and abroad.

CONFORMATION: Like most heavy draft breeds, the Clydesdale is a very large horse; however, breeders have succeeded in producing an overall look of power, strength, and weight in an animal that remains well balanced and not overly bulky. Clydesdales are usually 16.2 to 18 hands tall and weigh 1,600 to 1,800 pounds (although stallions and geldings may be taller and weigh up to 2,200 pounds). The color most often associated with the Clydesdale is the characteristic bay, but there are also browns, blacks, chestnuts, and roans. Four white socks to the knees and hocks are common, as is a white blaze or bald face. The face is broad, especially between the eyes, and the head has a flat-to-convex profile with large nostrils. A long, well-arched neck that ties in smoothly to high with-

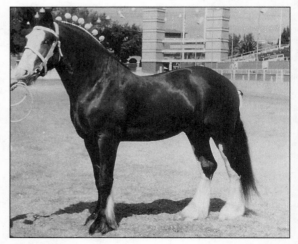

Clydesdale.
Photo by Murray E. Fowler.

ers and a muscular, sloping shoulder is desirable. The back should be short and lead to a well-muscled, wide, sloping croup that exhibits the remarkable power of the hind quarters. A wide chest, deep heart girth, and well-sprung rib also indicate a stalwart animal. Robust legs with broad, clean hocks and knees are a necessity. The hocks are frequently set closely together, which allows for greater pulling capacity. The legs also possess the characteristic feathers (silky hair on the back of the legs) and spats (hair on the front of the legs). Feet are a very important asset and should be broad with wide, springy heel bulbs and short toes.

Shire

TEMPERAMENT: Docile and good natured, willing to work

QUALITIES: Very strong, good endurance

FUNCTION: Heavy draft and farm work

ACTION: Moves with force and presence, notable use of knees and hocks

HISTORY: The Shire is another breed whose origin and history are shrouded in mystery. It is believed that the Shire is descended from the great English war horse of the Middle Ages that carried soldiers to battle in suits of armor weighing nearly 400 pounds. Around the year 1200, magnificent black stallions were imported from the lowlands of Holland to be bred to the English horses. Special attention was paid to the breeding and raising of these mighty creatures during the reign of King Henry VIII from 1509 to 1547. Acts were passed prohibiting the breeding of horses less than 15 hands tall, and exportation was banned. Thus the large, native-bred Shire flourished during this period in history.

The Shire probably arose in the marshy areas of Lincolnshire and Cambridgeshire in eastern England. The early horses were stouter of bone and thicker of hair than the later Shires of Yorkshire and Lancashire. The latter animals were noted for their finer texture and superior endurance compared to other Shires. Shires of

every type were utilized for many purposes. They were used in times of war and in times of peace. Shires plowed the fields and hauled cargo on the streets and docks of many British cities, where a horse of formidable strength but remarkably docile temperament was a special treasure. Only horses of considerable soundness and quality were able to be used extensively; owners selected for those traits that kept their horses healthy and able to work for many years. The American Shire Horse Association, founded in 1885, was elemental in establishing the breed in the United States. Selectivity in breeding and adherence to standards helped to improve the Shire and make it the grand breed it is today.

CONFORMATION: The standards of this formidable breed require that horses stand no less than 16.2 hands tall. There is no upper limit, though the breed average is 17.1 hands. Shires can weigh 1,700 to over 2,200 pounds. Many colors are common, among them black, brown, bay, chestnut, and gray. Excessive roaning is not desired. White occurs frequently on the legs and face. The head is small compared to the rest of the body, with pronounced jaws, a broad forehead, large expressive eyes, and a somewhat convex profile. The neck should be long, muscular and somewhat arched, and the withers wide

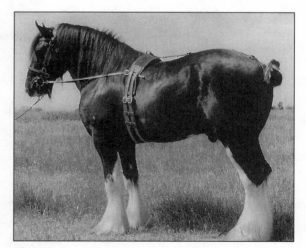

Shire.
Photo by Sharon McLin. Courtesy of the American Shire Horse Association.

yet not prominent. A short muscular back and sloping croup give the Shire great strength for pulling, as do the wide chest, deep girth, and well-muscled, sloping shoulder. The legs are muscular with fairly long cannons and moderately sloping pasterns. Joints are flat and broad, and the hocks are set close for increased pulling force. The feet are of the utmost importance, being very sound and large with springy heel bulbs. Stylish feathering from the knees and hocks to the ground is the finishing touch on a horse known both for its style and strength.

Percheron

TEMPERAMENT: Willing and energetic, yet very docile and quiet

QUALITIES: Strong with great endurance, long-lived

FUNCTION: Heavy draft and farm work, can also be ridden

ACTION: Balanced, natural easy gait, and light on its feet for its size

HISTORY: The province of La Perche in northern France, near Normandy, is the native home of

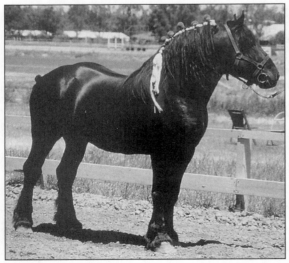

Percheron.
Photo by Murray E. Fowler.

the Percheron. There these grand horses were derived from an ancient indigenous breed, possibly of Flemish ancestry. The breed was refined very early by the infusion of Arabian blood, from horses acquired after the French defeat of the Saracens at Poitiers in 732. A thousand years later the Arabian was utilized again, its influence evident in the stylish head and velvety coat of the Percheron. The foundation sire for all modern Percherons was foaled a La Perche in 1823. The stallion was named Jean Le Blanc, and all of today's bloodlines trace directly to him.

The first Percherons were imported into the United States in 1839 by Edward Harris of New Jersey. The breed immediately began to gain in popularity. Two famous stallions, Normandy and Louis Napoleon, were imported into Ohio in 1851. The year 1876 saw the formation of the Norman-Percheron Association and the opening of the stud book. This was the first purebred livestock association formed in the United States and still exists today, although the name has been modified several times. The word "Norman" was dropped in 1877, and the association became the Percheron Society of America in 1905. In 1934 the name was changed to the Percheron Horse Association of America, which is the name still in use today.

Breeders in the United States imported thousands of Percherons in the second half of the nineteenth century. By 1930 there were three times as many Percherons in this country as the four other most popular draft breeds combined. Unfortunately the mechanization of the agricultural world after World War II greatly decreased the need for draft animals, and Percheron numbers declined. A handful of traditional farmers, including many Amish, continued to utilize this great breed and helped to preserve it. Today the breed has regained popularity and is being used for more diverse tasks, including riding, since it has been discovered that some Percherons are excellent jumpers.

CONFORMATION: Although the Percheron is not the largest of the draft breeds, the world's largest known horse was a Percheron—Dr. Le Gear, who towered 22 hands high and tipped the scales at an astonishing 3,024 pounds. Normally Percherons are 15 to 19 hands tall and weigh between 1,700 and 2,600 pounds. The Percheron is known as the breed of blacks and grays because 90 percent of all Percherons are one of these two colors. The other 10 percent are bay, brown, chestnut, or even roan, which is possible but very rare. The head is very attractive and refined for a draft breed, indicative of its Arabian ancestry. The forehead is broad, the eyes large and expressive, and the profile straight with a strong jawline. A well-muscled, slightly arched neck should tie in smoothly with slightly prominent withers and a muscular, sloping shoulder. The back is strong and slightly hollow, leading to a long, level, muscular croup and large, round hip. Short, robust legs, heavily boned with broad clean joints and short pasterns, are representative of the breed. Some feathering may be present. The chest is deep and wide. The incredible muscling of the gaskin and forearm exemplifies the power and strength of the Percheron.

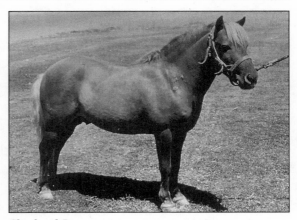

Shetland Pony.
Photo by Murray E. Fowler.

Shetland Pony

TEMPERAMENT: Sensible and docile

QUALITIES: Sturdy, sure-footed and strong

FUNCTION: Riding for children and harness work

ACTION: Springy action, thinner neck, narrower body and more sloping shoulder

HISTORY: The smallest American pony is the Shetland. It developed on the often cold and damp Shetland Islands in northern Scotland hundreds of years ago. As a result it is extremely hardy. The Islanders used the ponies for transportation and hauling. Some were used in coal mines in the mid-nineteenth century. By 1888, a stud book was established in the United States. The conformation of American ponies at that time still reflected their Scottish origins. Until World War I, Shetland stallions stood at a maximum of 42 inches (or 10.2 hands; Shetlands were measured in Scotland in inches, not hands). The ponies had long, strong necks, short backs, deep girths, sloping shoul-

ders, and strong legs. Since that time, the ponies have been bred for narrower bodies with a nearly level top line. Approximately 90 percent of the Shetlands in America today are of this American type. King Larigo, a show pony in the 1920s, and Curtiss Frisco Pete, his direct descendent in the 1950s and 1960s, are the most noted examples of the new American Shetlands.

CONFORMATION: American Shetlands should be strong and versatile ponies that blend the original Scottish Shetland Pony with the refinement and quality that has resulted from American care and selective breeding. The height limits are: yearlings 10.1 to 10.3 hands; two-year-olds 10.2 to just over 11.0 hands (44½ inches); and three-year-olds 10.3 to 11.2 hands (46 inches). All coat colors and eye colors are accepted. Shetland Ponies should have flat-boned, muscular legs, strong, springy pasterns, and of course good, strong feet. The back should be short and level, with a flat croup. The barrel should be well rounded, the shoulders sloping, the withers high. A Shetland should have a small muzzle with flaring nostrils, a fine jaw line leading to a refined throatlatch, prominent eyes, short, sharp, erect ears, and a full mane and tail.

Welsh Pony

TEMPERAMENT: Lively and intelligent

QUALITIES: Hardy, sure-footed, elegant mover

FUNCTION: Riding and light draft

ACTION: Free, fast action in front, well-flexed hocks and powerful behind

HISTORY: Equines are quite adaptive in their ability to survive in extremely severe climates, and the Welsh Pony is no exception. The pony's original home is the hills and valleys of Wales, where the breed survived tempestuous weather and sparse vegetation and shelter. Such adversity created a hardy breed of great endurance, strong character, and intelligence. The Romans discovered the Welsh Pony when they invaded the British Isles in 55–54 B.C., and Julius Caesar soon took an interest in them. He crossed Welsh mares with Arabian stallions, producing an obvious refinement of the head, neck, and overall carriage.

Not every great ruler, however, appreciated the Welsh Pony. King Henry VIII issued an edict stating that all horses under 15 hands be destroyed. Fortunately the Welsh lived in such an inhospitable clime that people did not want to go there—so the breed flourished despite the King of England's attempt to eradicate it.

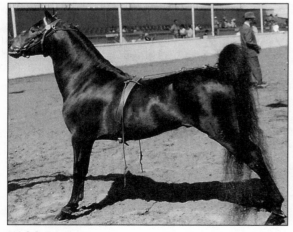

Welsh Pony.
Photo by Murray E. Fowler.

The versatility of the pony is shown clearly in the many roles it has played throughout history, experiencing every extreme as the pampered carriage ponies of the rich to the cherished plow ponies of the poor. The plucky Welsh survived the terrible conditions of the coal mines, where they pulled carts underground, and endured the hard life of a cart pony on the unforgiving cobblestone streets of the cities.

The Welsh Pony was first imported into the United States by George E. Brown in the 1800s. Interest in the breed rose during the early 1900s. The Welsh Pony and Cob Society of America was founded in 1907. The pony population dropped during the Depression but experienced a resurgence in the 1950s. The breed is very popular today as a children's mount and harness pony.

To categorize this versatile equine, breed divisions based upon size variation have been established. Type "A" ponies are no larger than 12.2 hands (12 hands in Britain), while "B" ponies are no larger than 14.2 hands. The "C" type are considered Welsh Ponies of Cob type and are no taller than 13.2 hands, while type "D" animals are known as Welsh Cobs. They must be at least 13.2 hands tall and are considered to be different owing to their body type. The Cob has shorter legs and a sturdier build than a horse, yet it still possesses the refined head and definitive character of the pony. Type "C" ponies are simply smaller versions of the type "D" Cobs.

CONFORMATION: The size of the Welsh Pony varies greatly depending upon the type of animal being considered. Overall they can be no larger than 14.2 hands, and many are much smaller than that. Any color is acceptable except piebald and skewbald. The head is quite characteristic and should be small, well set-on with a broad forehead, slightly dished profile, small, pricked ears, and large, expressive eyes. The neck is lengthy and quite arched. The head and neck are indicative of the past Arabian influence on the breed. Withers are somewhat pronounced, and shoulders are long and sloping, allowing for the ponies' strides to be nicely extended. The back should be muscular and well coupled, and the tail set high and carried gaily. A broad chest and deep girth show that the pony can work as well as be pleasing to the eye. Legs are sturdy with flat, broad, and very clean bones and joints. The feet are small with flintlike hooves. The Cob and Cob-type pony may have some feathering.

Miniature Horse

TEMPERAMENT: Quiet, yet spirited, intelligent

QUALITIES: Quite strong for its very small size

FUNCTION: Light harness, pet

ACTION: Graceful, natural balance and light stride

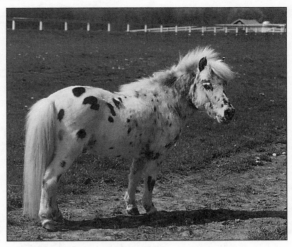

Miniature Horse (Falabella).
Photo by Sally Anne Thompson.

HISTORY: Miniature horses have been bred for centuries as novel pets and companion animals. The miniature horse is not a pony because it does not possess ponylike characteristics, but is more horselike in its body proportions and character. A good example of the modern miniature horse is the Falabella. The Falabella family of the Recreo de Roca Ranch in Buenos Aires, Argentina, developed the Falabella in an attempt to create the perfect equine specimen in miniature. They first crossed very small Shetland Ponies with small Thoroughbreds, and then selectively inbred the smallest of the offspring. Many Falabellas are beautiful examples of tiny horses. Some breeding selections for miniature horses, however, made primarily for size without regard to conformation and/or dwarfism have resulted in the surfacing of conformational defects as well as loss of vigor and good health. The novelty of such an animal has made the miniature horse a popular pet in North America. The American Miniature Horse Association was formed in 1978. The smallest horse on record is Sugar Dumpling, who belonged to Smith McCoy of Roderfield, West Virginia. This most minute of mounts was 20 inches tall and weighed only 30 pounds.

CONFORMATION: The Falabella can be no more than 34 inches tall at the withers. Any and all colors in any combination are acceptable; a spotted coat is particularly desirable and sought after. The head should be proportionally small with a straight or slightly dished profile and small, alert ears; however, the head also may be relatively large and lack refinement. The neck should be well formed and well set-on to fairly flat withers, although ewe neck (more concave on the upper line and convex on the lower line) is not uncommon. A short, straight back, angled croup, deep girth (waist), and sloping shoulder are all characteristic of the breed. The legs are slender and clean throughout the joints; however, inbreeding has caused flaws to emerge, such as weak legs caused by a lack of well-formed bone. The countenance and style of the refined little Falabella are accented by its flowing mane and tail and its spritely personality.

Mule

TEMPERAMENT: Excellent personality, highly intelligent

QUALITIES: Great endurance, strong, sure-footed

FUNCTION: Pack animal, light or heavy draft, riding, harness

ACTION: Easy stride with natural action, will have stride similar to dam

HISTORY: The first mules accompanied the explorer Christopher Columbus to what is now Haiti in 1493. Mules were also present in Mexico, owing to the breeding of horses and donkeys brought to the New World by the Spanish conquistadors. George Washington was an avid horseman and also had a great interest in mules. The first quality donkey jack (male) used for the production of mules in the newly formed United States was a gift to Washington from the Marquis de Lafayette in 1787. This jack, named Knight of Malta, and another jack received from the King of Spain, aptly named Royal Gift, became the foundation sires for most mules in the United States. Washington, and later Henry Clay, helped to establish the practice of breeding quality mules in this country.

A mule is defined as a hybrid produced by breeding a **jack** (male donkey) with a **mare** (female horse). The resulting offspring (**horse** or **john mule** if male, **mare** or **molly mule** if female) is sterile because it has 63 chromosomes. The unbalanced chromosome number, 32 from the horse and 31 from the donkey, usually does not allow the sex cells to function properly, leaving the mule unable to reproduce.

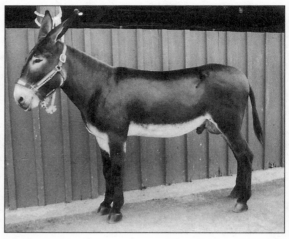

Donkey.
Photo by Juanita Snyder. Courtesy of The American Donkey and Mule Society.

Remarkably, there have been a few rare occurrences over the years in which a mare mule did produce a foal. A **hinny** is a hybrid resulting from a mating between a **jennet** (female donkey) and a **stallion**. The offspring of this cross have the same characteristics as a mule; however, these are not as common as the mule nor are they usually known to reproduce.

During the active expansion of the United States in the 1800s, mules gained in popularity owing to the diverse number of tasks at which the animals excelled. Hardy animals were needed for the difficult work being done at the time. Mules were used on farms and plantations to pull heavy machinery (plows, planters, mowers, and threshing machines). They were also useful in the mines because of their ability to work very well under adverse conditions. The United States Army used mules extensively for nearly two hundred years, from 1775 to 1957, to transport supplies and perform many other difficult tasks.

The mules of today are used for a vast range of jobs, some traditional and others very new. They serve as pack animals for hunters and campers in the mountains. Park officials in the Grand Canyon still use mules for challenging excursions into the back country. Some mules pull wagons for trail rides and parades, while

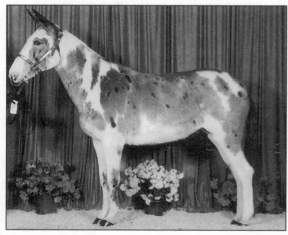

Mule.
Photo by Marc Robins. Courtesy of the American Donkey and Mule Society.

others have shed the rough pack-animal persona and are being ridden both Western and English and shown at dressage and jumping. The extremely versatile mule is often chosen over a horse because of its greater physical endurance and intuitive nature. Mules stand heat better than do horses, are less likely to overeat, usually work to an older age, have tougher feet, and are more sure-footed and careful.

CONFORMATION: There are only two traits that really define the look of a mule. First (and most obvious), mules have long ears passed down from the donkey parent. Second, mules have an almost streamlined look, owing to a lack of bunchy muscling and muscle definition. The conformation type of the mule is based considerably on the dam. Size and body type vary greatly among the animals and they are categorized accordingly. The draft mule is produced when crossing a mammoth jack with a heavy draft mare. Mating a saddle-horse mare with a jack similar in size results in a saddle-type mule. Work or pack mules result from the breeding of a mammoth or large standard jack and a part-draft mare. The miniature mule was developed by mating a pony or miniature horse mare with a standard or miniature jack.

As with size, mules frequently inherit the color of the dam. Nearly any color may be seen including chestnut, bay, gray, white, roan, dun, spotted, and even the leopard Appaloosa-type color pattern.

PART II

Living with Your Horse

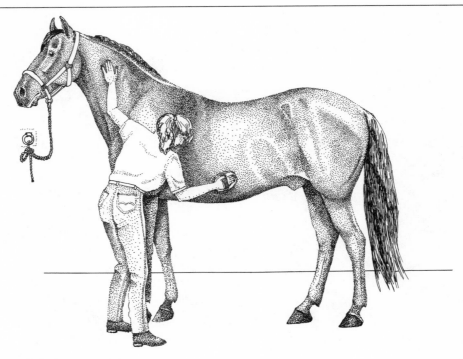

A little neglect may breed mischief...
for want of a nail the shoe was lost;
for want of a shoe the horse was lost;
and for want of a horse the rider was lost...

—BENJAMIN FRANKLIN
POOR RICHARD'S ALMANAC

CHAPTER 3

Equine Husbandry

by Reneé M. Golenz and
Janet F. Roser

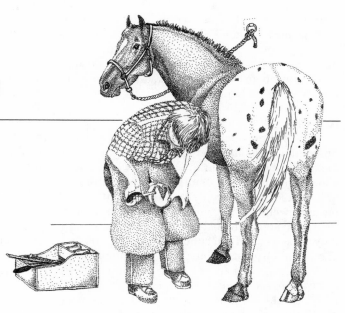

S ome horse farms seem to have all the "bad luck" when it comes to injured or sick horses, while other farms, even those with a large number of horses, may go for months without any serious health problems. What makes the difference? A high-quality equine husbandry program. The following chapter provides an overview of various aspects of equine husbandry, such as feeding, grooming, and housing, as well as dental, ear, and foot care.

Routine Care

Routine daily care may seem like hard, time-consuming work (and it is!), but it is essential for maintaining a healthy and happy horse. A dedicated horse owner must apply the basic principles of good sanitation, nutrition, exercise, and grooming. Keeping good records of a horse's health, foot care, work schedule, and insurance will also contribute to the efficiency of caring for a horse.

SANITATION AND WASTE MANAGEMENT
Cleaning stalls and paddocks on a daily basis will help control insects, parasites, and odor. Remove the fresh manure and store it in a pile in a suitable area away from horses, humans, other animals, lakes, or streams. Either have the manure hauled off the premises periodically, or spread it thinly over areas not grazed by horses.

DISEASE AND PARASITE CONTROL PROGRAM
All horses should be vaccinated and dewormed on a regular basis. (For more detailed information on these procedures, *see* CHAPTER 33, "INTERNAL PARASITES," and APPENDIX B, "VACCINA-

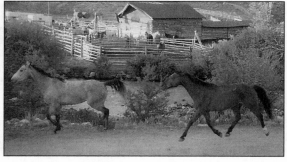

Photo by Ruth Saada.

tions and Infectious Disease Control..") Horses arriving at a new place for breeding, showing, or training should be housed initially in an isolation barn or paddock that is at least 500 yards away from other animals. Isolated horses should be monitored for signs of ill health for at least 14–21 days before they are mixed with the other members of the herd.

Nutrition

Proper feeding management will ensure that a horse maintains its good health and receives the maximum benefit from the ration. A feed ration should be modified to suit the individual horse, and should match the daily requirements based on age, weight, and type of activity. In general the ration should be balanced between **roughage** (hay, pasture) and **concentrates** (grain). The feed should be of good quality. The ration should be fed on a regular basis at least 2–3 times a day. Always provide free access to fresh, clean water and a salt block. (For more detailed discussions, *see* Chapter 6, "Equine Nutritional Requirements," and Chapter 7, "Feeding Horses.")

Exercise

Daily exercise is essential for a horse's physical and mental well-being. A minimum of 30 minutes of exercise a day is recommended. Complete stall confinement is not appropriate unless a horse has a medical problem that warrants stall rest. Types of exercise programs will vary with age and intended use. Free exercise in a pasture situation is very beneficial if the handler is unable to exercise the horse.

Insurance

Several kinds of equine insurance programs are available. Insurance companies offer equine mortality insurance, medical and surgical insurance, disuse insurance, and live foal insurance. The economic value of the horse and the type of insurance policy desired will determine the annual premium. Most policies require a pre-insurance health examination by a veterinarian. Under a typical policy, the owner agrees to seek veterinary care and notify the insurance company in the event of injury or illness.

Records

An individual horse record should contain space for identification of the horse, daily feed ration, medical history, vaccination and deworming schedule, hoof and dental care schedule, and breeding, racing, or show record, if applicable.

Grooming Horses

Regular grooming cleanses the hair and massages the skin and underlying musculature. Grooming increases the blood circulation to the skin, promotes a healthy hair coat, and enhances the appearance. Grooming also gives the horse owner a regular opportunity to examine the horse for wounds, skin disorders, swellings or masses, and parasite eggs that might be present. Ideally a horse should be groomed daily, and should always be groomed before and after exercise.

The usual grooming procedure involves currying and brushing the horse's coat, brushing and/or combing the mane and tail, cleaning debris from around the eyes, wiping out the nostrils, and cleaning the feet.

A rubber or plastic curry comb is used first in a circular or back-and-forth motion over the horse's body. (The curry comb is *not* used on the head or legs of the horse.) This loosens caked dirt and brings loose hairs to the surface. In addition, the curry comb massages the hide and muscles.

A stiff brush is used after the curry comb. Short, vigorous strokes in the direction of the

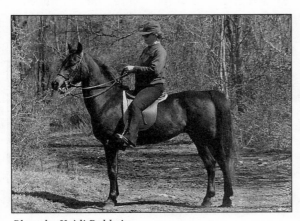

Photo by Heidi Baldwin.

hair growth are made over the horse's body and legs. A soft brush follows the stiff brush and is used to smooth down the coat and remove the scurf brought to the surface by the stiff brush. The soft brush is used in the direction of hair growth over the horse's body, legs, and face. The mane and tail may be brushed with a comb, regular hair brush, or stiff brush. The feet are always cleaned with a hoof pick (*see* below).

Horses can be bathed with a mild shampoo or with available horse shampoo products. A hose is normally used over the horse's body and legs and a wash cloth or sponge is used on the head. After the final rinse, the excess water can be removed from the horse's body with a sweat scraper.

Body-clipping is often performed on show horses and horses with long hair coats that are worked regularly. Body-clipping allows the horse owner to cool down a horse properly after a hard workout, and makes it easier to keep the hair coat clean during the winter and spring months when most horses grow a long coat. During cold or rainy weather, a clipped horse should wear a warm blanket or sheet. Clipping the hair from the inner ears, muzzle, and bridle path is optional and usually done for horse shows.

Care of the Teeth

Dental care is an important component of an equine husbandry program. When the teeth are neglected, a horse may experience difficulty in eating, excessive salivation, **halitosis** (bad breath), weight loss, biting problems, and gastrointestinal disorders. Seeing a dentist regularly may be as important for your horse as it is for you! Routine dental examinations at 6- to 12-month intervals are recommended.

NUMBERS AND TYPES OF TEETH
A horse's teeth are well adapted to cope with a normal equine diet. The **incisor** teeth are specially developed for prehension and cutting food, whereas the **premolars** and **molars** ("cheek teeth") serve to grind the food. The total number of **deciduous** (temporary) teeth include 12 incisors and 12 premolars. (*See* TABLE 1.) The average adult male horse (5 years old) has 40 to 44 teeth, while the average adult female horse

has 36 to 40 teeth. The major difference between the two sexes is that males usually have 4 canine teeth whereas most females do not have any canines. (*See* FIGURES 1 and 2.)

The horse has high-crowned teeth that continue to grow and push out as they wear. The

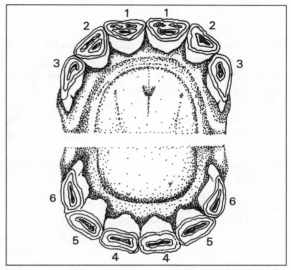

Figure 1. Horse's incisor teeth: 1) upper central; 2) upper intermediate; 3) upper corner; 4) lower central; 5) lower intermediate; 6) lower corner

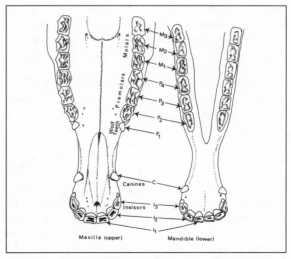

Figure 2. Upper and lower arcades of a mature male horse's mouth.

average adult horse has a total of 12 incisors, 12–16 premolars, and 12 molars. The inconsistency in the number of premolars is due to the variable presence of the vestigial first premolar (**"wolf tooth"**). This tooth is much more likely to be present in the upper jaw than in the lower, but can be found in either.

Aging a Horse by Its Teeth

A horse's age can be estimated by examining the number and types of teeth present. After a horse is 10–12 years of age, however, it becomes progressively more difficult to determine an exact age. It must also be realized that a horse's diet can affect the wear on its teeth. Hard, pelleted feeds can cause the teeth to wear more rapidly than soft, succulent feeds. Unusual wear of the teeth can also be altered by malocclusion and cribbing (*see* below).

The 6 upper incisors and 6 lower incisors each include 2 central, 2 intermediate, and 2 corner incisors. Between birth and 6 days of age the central incisors are present, then at 6 weeks the intermediate incisors erupt, and by 6 months the corner incisors are present. The deciduous premolars erupt during the first 6 months. The deciduous incisors are shell-shaped with a distinct neck at the gum line, whereas the permanent teeth are rectangular and larger. The permanent incisors erupt at 2.5, 3.5, and 4.5 years (proceeding from the central to corner incisors). The molars become visible at 1, 2, and 3.5 years of age. The canine teeth appear between 4 and 5 years. At 5 years of age a horse should have all its adult teeth.

The biting surface of the incisor teeth has a single depression or cup. As the adult teeth wear with age, the cups on the lower **arcade** (row of teeth) disappear (between 6 and 8 years), beginning with the central incisors and moving out to the corner incisors. Between 9 and 11 years the cups disappear on the upper arcade in a similar fashion.

Other estimations of age can be made by observing the angle of **occlusion** (bite), the shape of the surface of the tooth, and observing **Galvayne's groove.** With advancing age the angle of the incisors, when viewed from the side, changes from the nearly perpendicu-

lar to a sharp forward slant. The cross-sectional shape of the incisors also changes progressively from rectangular to round to triangular (Figure 3). Galvayne's groove is the dark line that forms on the outside of the corner incisors, starting at the top of the gum line and advancing downward (Figure 4). At 10 years of age the groove is at the gum line; by 15 years it is down to the middle of the tooth; by 20 years it reaches the bottom of the tooth. By 25 years of age the initial half of the groove from the gum line has disappeared, and by 30 years of age the entire groove is gone.

Table 1
Average Times When Teeth Erupt

Deciduous	
Tooth	Eruption
1st incisor (or centrals)	Birth or first week
2nd incisor (or intermediates)	4 to 6 weeks
3rd incisor (or corners)	6 to 9 months
Canine (or bridle)	
1st premolar	Birth or first 2 weeks for all premolars
2nd premolar	
3rd premolar	
Permanent	
1st incisor (or centrals)	2 years
2nd incisor (or intermediates)	3 years
3rd incisor (or corners)	4 years
Canine (or bridle)	4 to 5 years
1st premolar (or wolf tooth)	5 to 6 months
2nd premolar	2 years
3rd premolar	3 years
4th premolar	4 years
1st molar	9 to 12 months
2nd molar	2 years
3rd molar	3 to 4 years

Dental Abnormalities

MALOCCLUSIONS

An overshot jaw (**parrot mouth**) and an undershot jaw (**sow mouth**) are the two most commonly encountered *malocclusions* in horses. (A malocclusion is an improper bite.) They are thought to be inherited traits and are seen consistently in certain bloodlines. On first glance parrot mouth would appear to be caused by an overgrowth of the **maxilla** (upper jaw); instead, it is actually caused by a shortening of the **mandible** (lower jaw). The overbite of the incisors is more noticeable than the corresponding abnormality in the cheek teeth. The upper second premolar and the lower third molars have little if any opposing (**occlusal**) wear and therefore grow unopposed, creating large sharp hooks. This may lead to soft-tissue trauma within the oral cavity, and to other problems associated with **mastication** (chewing). The reverse conditions occur with undershot jaw. (*See* "DENTAL DISORDERS OF THE ORAL CAVITY," in Chapter 26, "THE DIGESTIVE SYSTEM AND VARIOUS DISORDERS.")

ABNORMALITIES OF ERUPTION

The retention of deciduous teeth (**caps**) after eruption of the permanent teeth is a common condition. Retained caps of premolar teeth may cause pain in a young horse and should be removed. Deciduous incisor teeth that have not been lost after the eruption of the corresponding permanent incisors should also be removed to prevent interference and trauma to the lips.

Horses sometimes develop more teeth than is considered normal. Extra incisors are more common than extra premolars or molars. Extra teeth should be left in place unless they are causing problems for the horse. Occasionally, an incisor or cheek tooth erupts and grows in an abnormal direction, usually because of trauma to the developing tooth bud.

WOLF TEETH

Wolf teeth are the first premolars and can cause localized irritation owing to pressure from the bit. Wolf teeth erupt from the gum line when the horse is 5 or 6 months of age. Due to their shallow roots, however, they usually are shed by about 2½ years of age, when the permanent premolars emerge. Wolf teeth can cause pain even if they have not erupted through the **gingiva** (gums). Should the wolf teeth not fall out on their own, the veterinarian should surgically remove them before the horse is put into training.

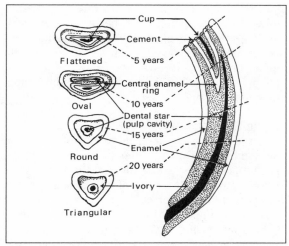

Figure 3. Anatomy of the incisor tooth of the horse. The permanent middle incisor tooth at different ages and stages of wear. Changes in shape from oval to angular are shown in the cross-sectional views as wear progresses toward the root.

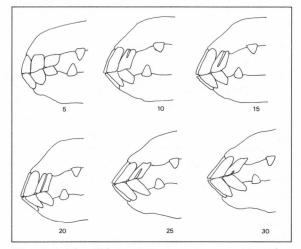

Figure 4. The Galvayne groove comes at 10 and is gone at 30. It is about the only means of estimating the age of an older horse.

TOOTH-ROOT ABSCESS

The cause of tooth-root abscesses remains controversial. The upper first molar is the most common tooth to become abscessed, followed by the upper second molar, upper fourth premolar, and lower first molar. It is rare to find an abscess involving the incisors. Tooth-root abscesses may produce substantial discomfort, causing a horse to stop eating and become depressed. More specific clinical signs will be dependent on which tooth is involved. Such signs can include upper or lower jaw swelling, a draining tract, foul breath, nasal discharge, and secondary sinus infection.

SHARP ENAMEL POINTS

One of the most common dental problems is the development of sharp enamel points, owing to the normal positioning and growth of the teeth in the horse's mouth. The rows of cheek teeth in the lower arcade are normally closer together than those in the upper arcade. When the horse grinds its food by moving the jaws from side to side, the inner surfaces of the teeth in the lower arcade and outer surfaces of the teeth in the upper arcade frequently develop sharp enamel points. These sharpened teeth can potentially produce abrasions on the tongue and cheeks. Pain in these areas may cause a horse to go off feed, drop food while eating, lose weight, and predispose the horse to colic. The condition can be corrected by having a veterinarian grind down the sharp points with a special instrument called a *dental float*.

Older horses often require more frequent dental attention owing to the progressive loss of teeth, uneven wearing of the cheek teeth creating "**wave mouth**" (mismatched bite), excessive tartar build-up, tooth decay, and **periodontal disease** (disease of the gums). Older horses that are missing several teeth may need to be fed a diet of soft foods such as alfalfa and molasses meal, water-soaked alfalfa cubes, or other grain-mix mashes or gruels. (*See* CHAPTER 26, "THE DIGESTIVE SYSTEM AND VARIOUS DISORDERS," and CHAPTER 35, "THE AGED HORSE.")

SCHEDULING EQUINE DENTAL CARE

Between birth and 3 months of age, foals should be checked for malocclusions such as parrot mouth. Unless there is a problem, real dental care doesn't start until a horse is 1 or 2 years old. At this time wolf teeth and retained caps can be removed and the teeth can be floated for the first time. Until the age of 5 years, horses should be checked for erupting teeth and retained caps. Floating the teeth should be performed as required. Most horses should have their teeth floated once a year. If a malocclusion or wave mouth (uneven wearing of the teeth) is found or teeth are lost, dental care may need to be performed every 6 months. Dental attention at regular intervals, along with specific examinations when problems arise, will ensure that a horse maintains a healthy mouth for life.

Care of the Feet

To take proper care of the feet, it is important to be familiar with the external structures of the normal equine foot (*see* FIGURE 5), since each structure may need to be cared for individually. Inadequate foot care can result in many orthopedic problems and lamenesses. Ideally, the bottom of the feet should be cleaned on a daily basis, and *always* before and after exercise. The feet are usually cleaned with a hoof pick, which is used to scrape away debris from the soles, sulcus

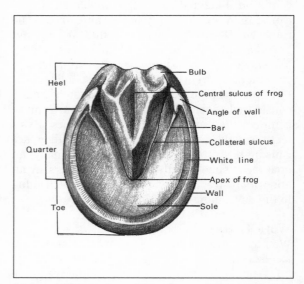

Figure 5. The external structures of the normal forefoot of the horse.

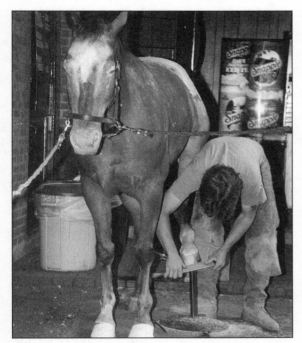

Photo by Mordecai Siegal.

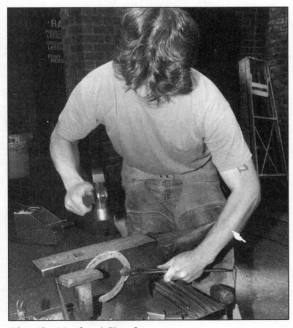

Photo by Mordecai Siegal.

of the frog, and bars of the heel. At the same time the feet can be examined for abnormalities such as a sole bruise or abscess, cracks involving the hoof wall, foreign bodies, or infection.

Foot care begins at birth. Early signs of infection, foot abnormalities, or congenital flexural or angular limb deformities can be detected during the post-foaling veterinary examination. Mild angular and flexural deformities of the legs often benefit from corrective trimming during the first week of life, continued at 1- to 2-week intervals until correction is achieved. More severe abnormalities may require further evaluation and more involved corrective measures, such as the application of glue-on-shoes, splinting, casting, or surgery. The limbs and feet of foals should be examined daily and the feet trimmed at intervals of no more than 6 weeks, in order to optimize the development of normal feet and limbs. (*See* CHAPTER 22, "THE MUSCULOSKELETAL SYSTEM AND VARIOUS DISORDERS.")

Trimming and shoeing should be performed every 4 to 6 weeks on horses that are shod. Shoeing is usually performed at 2- to 4-week intervals on race horses and horses with orthopedic problems involving the foot. The object of proper trimming is to make the shape of the foot, the angle of the foot axis, and the level aspect of the foot as normal as possible (*see* FIGURE 6).

Overgrowth of the hoof increases a horse's susceptibility to foot infections. An unbalanced foot created by improper or infrequent trimming may cause secondary trauma to the joints and soft-tissue structures of the limbs. Improper foot care can predispose a horse to such lameness conditions as ringbone, sidebone, pedal osteitis, laminitis, fractured coffin bone, and navicular disease. (*See* CHAPTER 22, "THE MUSCULOSKELETAL SYSTEM AND VARIOUS DISORDERS.")

Horseshoes provide protection, support, and balance to the foot. They also may improve the gait of the horse and correct underlying orthopedic abnormalities. The type of shoe applied to the foot will depend on the use of the horse, breed regulations of shoeing, and the presence of any gait disturbances.

Horseshoes are made of iron, steel, aluminum, rubber, or plastic. Iron and steel shoes are used

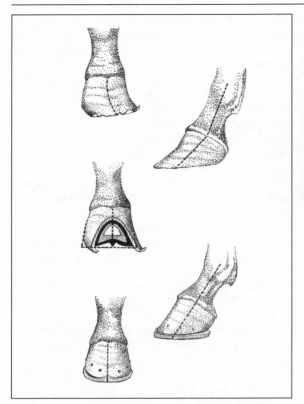

Figure 6. Principles for shaping the hoof *(from top to bottom)*: Rough untrimmed foot; broken angle of foot axis; diagram of trimming; correct foot axis; trimmed and shod.

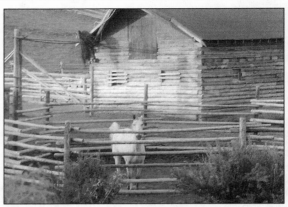

Photo by Ruth Saada.

in many types of performance horses, while aluminum shoes are used primarily for racing. Rubber or plastic shoes can be employed for therapeutic purposes. Weighted shoes alter the gait at high speed and are most often used for gaited horses and trotters. Toe weights cause the horse to reach farther, while heel weights cause the horse to lift the foot higher in its action. Weighted shoes reduce speed, decrease agility, and increase fatigue to the limb. Therefore, the lightest shoe possible for the task to be performed should be used.

Shoe pads are used to decrease concussion to the bottom of the foot and irritation of a tender sole. Pads can be made of leather, plastic, or rubber, and are classified as full pads or rim pads, and as flat pads or wedge pads. A full pad covers the entire sole, whereas a rim pad is shaped like a horseshoe. Wedge pads are commonly used to raise the heels in order to balance the hoof.

A variety of corrective shoes are available for orthopedic problems. Shoes used to facilitate easy break over at the toe include roller toe, square toe, and rocker toe shoes. There are many types of bar shoes available, including full bar, diamond bar, egg bar, V bar, heart bar, and half bar shoes. In general, bar shoes increase ground-surface contact, distribute the weight over a greater surface area, protect certain areas of the foot, provide selective pressure, and add stability to the foot. Shoes that improve traction include heel calks and toe grabs. Trailer shoes decrease foot rotation by extending one or both heels. Quarter clips and toe clips are used to reinforce the toe or quarter regions in the event of hoof cracks or to secure the shoe to a weak-walled hoof.

Care of the Ears

The ears of the horse are an often-neglected area of routine care. A regular examination of the ears for signs of trauma, inner-ear infection, external parasites, and tumors should be performed. Veterinary care may be required for further diagnosis and treatment of conditions affecting the ear if a horse exhibits the following signs: head-shaking, a head-tilt to one side, loss of balance, incoordination, unusual growths or masses

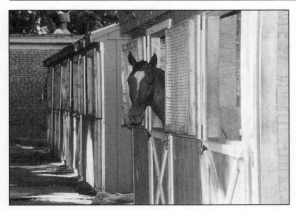

Photo by Mordecai Siegal.

involving the ear, or skin infection or irritation. A damp-dry sponge or towel may be used to clean the outer and inner surfaces of the ear. Avoid putting anything inside the ear (e.g., medication) without first consulting a veterinarian.

Housing and Facilities

Horses seem to thrive best in mild weather, with well-drained pastures, plenty of shade, and a good supply of fresh water. Such considerations are important when selecting the best site for a horse facility. Cost, durability, usefulness, flexibility, location, and suitability for the intended purpose are important points to consider when establishing a horse operation. The primary consideration for any horse facility should be safety for both the horse and rider. Many horses are injured as a result of neglect or poor farm maintenance, such as the presence of protruding nails, sharp edges, unscreened glass, exposed electric wires, sagging fences, broken gates, or barbed-wire fencing.

PASTURES

The ideal pasture contains high-quality forage, providing an excellent source of protein, vitamins, and minerals while lowering the cost of feed and labor. Horses on pasture are sure to receive exercise and often have improved dispositions.

A pasture should provide shade. If trees are not present, open sheds can be provided. A fresh-water source should always be available. Pastures should be carefully surveyed for any deep holes, foreign objects, and poisonous plants. Avoid overcrowding the pastures; ideally 1 or 2 acres of land per horse is recommended.

FENCES

Fences should be designed and built with safety in mind. The smaller the enclosure, the more likely a horse will come in contact with the fence. The ideal fence should have strength, height (5 to 6 feet), and tightness (which can be provided by correctly setting the posts). The most popular and most traditional type of fencing for horses is board fencing. Other types include post and rail, pipe, chain-link, post and cable, pre-cast concrete, rubber nylon, electric, and woven wire-mesh fence. The most dangerous fencing is made of barbed wire; its use should be avoided. Detailed pamphlets on building fences can usually be obtained from local agricultural colleges and fence suppliers.

BARNS

The type of barn depends on the climate and the specialized needs of the farm. Considerations for designing a horse barn include attractiveness, ventilation, fire resistance, safety, durability, and cost. The types of barns available range from a simple open-front shed to a show stable with office, box stalls, indoor arena, tackroom, feed room, wash rack area, and lounge.

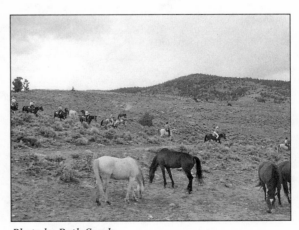

Photo by Ruth Saada.

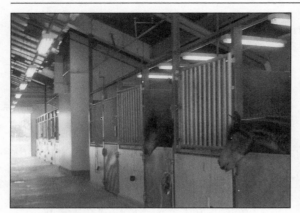

Photo by Mordecai Siegal.

A variety of materials are available for the construction of stalls, wood being the most popular. Oak and other hard woods will withstand chewing from bored horses longer than will soft woods. (*See* Chapter 5, "Misbehavior.") The wood may be treated with an "anti-chew" product. No sharp edges or nails should be exposed. The minimum size of a box stall for a gelding or mare is 12 feet × 12 feet. Foaling stalls are usually 12 feet × 16 feet, 14 feet × 14 feet, or 16 feet × 20 feet. Stallion stalls should be a minimum of 14 feet × 14 feet. Feeders and waterers should be placed out of the way in corners of the stall. Ideally each stall should have proper safety lights and a built-in drainage system.

Hard-packed clay is the most popular material for stall floors. Wooden planks, roughened concrete, and asphalt are also available. Rubber floor mats will add extra comfort but can be expensive and labor-intensive to keep clean. Stalls should be heavily bedded with either wood shavings or straw.

CHAPTER 4

Equine Behavior

by Carolyn L. Stull

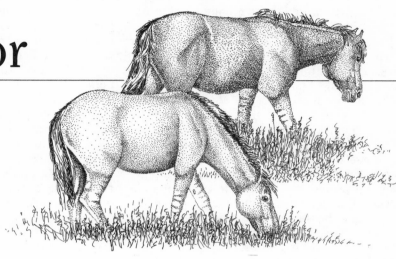

Normal equine behavior is a fascinating phenomenon and is influenced by many different factors. Evolution, genetics, domestication, training, age, sex, and environment all exert a profound effect on the behavior of an individual horse. The welfare of the domesticated horse depends on satisfying both the physiological and psychological needs of the animal. The physiological needs of the horse (e.g., nutrition, health care, exercise) have been extensively researched. The psychological needs and preferences are less well understood, and may be more difficult to satisfy.

The value of the performing equine athlete depends on the horse's behavioral responses to both training and management. For an individual horse to become a successful performer, physical capability must be linked to behavioral responses. Much time, effort, and money are spent in training a horse for both physical fitness and appropriate behavioral responses. Sometimes, misbehavior can result in dismissal of a horse that is perfectly capable of performing a specific activity. (*See* CHAPTER 5, "MISBEHAVIOR.") Knowledge and incorporation of a horse's natural behavior, instincts, needs, and responses

can assist in the training, management, and enjoyment of all types of performance horses.

Evolution and Domestication of the Horse

Evolution has had a substantial impact on the domesticated horse's ability to react to novel situations and environments. All horses behave in a manner designed to maximize survival and propagation of the species. This behavior is expressed through horses' social organization, communication, and sexual relationships. Some equine behavior patterns are genetically "programmed" and have evolved so that horses can better cope with challenging environmental conditions.

As a browsing or grazing animal, the horse is adapted physically to its environment. Horses must be capable of identifying plants for ingestion, harvesting the identified plant material, and digesting it into an absorbable form. The shape of the horse's nose evolved to help identify different species of plants through sight, smell, and touch, while the long, flexible neck developed in order to reach the foliage of trees. The gastrointestinal tract expanded and acquired an ample supply of microorganisms for digesting the cell walls of plants and grasses. The horse's teeth are not sharp and pointed for flesh tearing, but instead are large, flat structures designed for nibbling and grinding.

Horses did not evolve claws, horns, or sharp teeth for fighting and defending themselves against attacks by predatory **carnivores** (meat eaters). Instead they developed keen senses of hearing and sight, along with marvelous legs and hooves that enabled them to flee for long distances over the roughest terrain. In most threatening situations, the evolving horse's tendency was to escape rather than fight. Thus, running away became a powerful self-protective reaction to any situation perceived as startling, frightening, or dangerous. If the horse could not run, it usually turned to face the threat or else kicked out with one or both hind limbs.

This same "flight or fight" behavior is apparent in domestic horses today, even though they have few natural enemies. The flight or fight pattern is also displayed in management and training situations. The horse that is difficult to catch in the field (and therefore flees its handler) may perceive an unpleasant situation in being caught. Likewise a horse tied by its halter and unable to flee may kick out at any unexpected noise or startling commotion.

SOCIAL ORGANIZATION

Horses and ponies are naturally social animals, a quality that has enhanced their survival both as individuals and as species. Social groups evolved mainly to reduce the risk of attack by predators. The chances of being alerted to a stalking predator are obviously improved if the senses of a large number of individuals within a herd are attuned to the surrounding environment. Much of the research on the social organization of the horse has been conducted on **feral** (wild) horses rather than on domesticated horses. However, some of the behaviors of feral horses are readily apparent in their domesticated counterparts, particularly in groups of horses grazing on pasture. Feral horses are organized into **harems**, with one mature stallion living with several mares and their offspring. The size of a harem can vary from a few to over ten mares. If the harem is large, two stallions may remain in permanent association with the herd. The strongest bond is between a mare and her foal, and together they comprise the focal center of the herd. Mares usually foal on average once every two years, usually in late spring when sources of forage are plentiful for both the lactating dam and her offspring. Immature males, known as "**bachelor stallions,**" usually leave the herd when they are two or three years of age. Some of these bachelor stallions prefer to lead a solitary existence, while others band together to form bachelor herds.

DOMINANCE

Both domesticated and feral horses exhibit *dominance hierarchies*, which can be readily observed when feeding a group of horses. Typically the more dominant individuals will display aggressive behavior in obtaining food or water, while submissive horses will seek alternate feeding areas, or wait until the dominant horses have finished eating and then consume any remaining feed. Feeding horses individually can help eliminate aggressive behavior, thus lessening the chances of the horses' injuring one another. Providing an extra portion of hay for a group will assure that both dominant and subordinate horses receive an appropriate amount of feed and have enough time to consume it. Another strategy involves feeding from a single trough, using head partitions to separate the horses. Scientists have shown that partitions

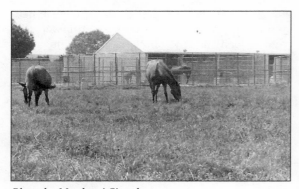

Photo by Mordecai Siegal.

can facilitate proper feeding of subordinate horses in the presence of dominant pen mates, thus providing a more equitable distribution of feed.

The introduction of a new horse to an established herd usually represents a challenge to the group's hierarchical structure. The new horse may be the object of behaviors ranging from mild threats to seriously aggressive kicking, squealing, rearing, and biting. In less contentious situations, threats by the dominant horse are effectively conveyed by a laying back of the ears, which is then followed by a retreat of the new (submissive) member of the herd. Regardless of the likely outcome, the introduction of any new horse to an established group should always be closely monitored.

NEED FOR COMPANIONSHIP

Horses have evolved for millions of years in a predominantly social, herd environment. Thus it is not surprising that strong attachments can spring up between horses housed in stables or on pasture. The bond between a mare and her newborn foal has already been noted as the strongest among horses. In general, horses prefer the company of other horses to isolation. If other horses are not available, the company of a member of a different species (such as a goat or cow) may suffice. Horses often form strong bonds to their companions, which may cause apprehension when they are separated from them. Separation anxiety may be manifested by whinnying, nervousness, and in some cases uncontrollable behavior. Such displays are obviously disruptive when training, riding, or showing. The safety of both horse and handler should always be taken into consideration before separating a horse from its companions.

Communication

VOCAL

Horses signal herd mates (and possibly human beings) using three different communication systems based on sight, smell, and hearing. Vocal communication is the system most easily recognized by handlers. It is used by feral horses to communicate with one another over large distances. The whinny, nicker, squeal, and snort represent common vocalizations of the horse. The **whinny** is the vocalization a mare produces when separated from her foal, while the soft **nicker** is given by the mare when the foal has been located and returns to her. **Snorting** is usually elicited under frightening or threatening conditions as an alarm call to others, while **squealing** is associated with an aggressive or painful situation, such as being the recipient of a powerful kick. Stallions also utilize many of these same vocalizations during the courtship and breeding of mares.

VISUAL

Visual signals communicated by horses may be more difficult for handlers to detect. They include the placement and position of the ears, head, body, and tail. An easily recognized visual cue is the flattening or "**pinning**" of the ears back against the head, signaling aggression or agitation. This behavior often is expressed by dominant horses. Ears placed forward indicates attentiveness or friendliness, or may be a response to a visual stimulus. **Snapping**, which involves a repetitive opening and closing of the mouth, exposing the teeth and tongue, is often observed in suckling and weaning foals. This behavior, which normally is associated with suckling of the mare, is sometimes directed instead at mature horses other than the dam. Submissive body posture is displayed when the tail of the horse is tucked close to the body, the head is held low, and the ears droop in a sideways position. A

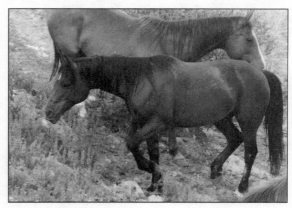

Photo by Ruth Saada.

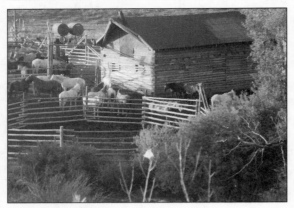

Photo by Ruth Saada.

playful horse, by contrast, will hold its head and neck upright, elevate the tail, and prick its ears forward.

OLFACTORY

Olfactory signals (signals involving the sense of smell) are used in the marking of territory with urine and feces, possibly for the purpose of identifying horses passing through an area. A

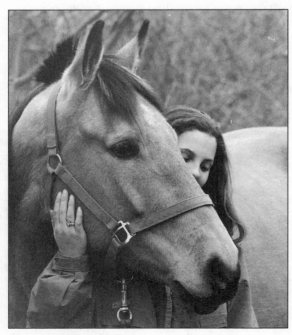

Photo by Heidi Baldwin.

unique behavior involving the horse's sense of smell that is often observed by horse owners is the **Flehmen reaction** or *lip curl*, wherein the horse extends its head and neck and curls back the upper lip while drawing air into the nasal cavity. Flehmen is usually expressed by a stallion attempting to detect **estrus** ("heat") in a mare, but may also be exhibited by the mare following **parturition** (giving birth), or after a horse sniffs feces, urine, and sometimes even feed.

Daily Behavior

TIME BUDGET

The amount of time horses spend on their various daily activities is a direct result of the evolution of the species, horses' needs, and the opportunities afforded by the surrounding environment. Extensive studies of feeding behaviors have revealed that feral horses spend 25 to 80 percent of their waking hours grazing, depending on the availability of grass and its nutritive value. The remainder of their time each day is spent resting (20 to 25 percent) and performing **ambulatory** (involving locomotion) activities, mainly at the walk (10 percent).

EATING

The stomach of the horse is relatively small in size, probably reflecting ancestral habits of eating small quantities of forage throughout the day rather than single large meals. The expansive *large intestine* with its **cecum** (a blind pouch located at the junction of the small and large intestines) is essentially a mixing vat for the digestion of fiber by intestinal microorganisms, resulting in the release of absorbable nutrients. Modern stable management usually provides horses with two or three meals per day of comparatively low-volume, nutrient-dense feed. Although this may supply all the necessary nutrients for performing horses, such a feeding regime can promote digestive upsets and certain behavioral vices. (*See* CHAPTER 5, "MISBEHAVIOR," and CHAPTER 7, "FEEDING HORSES.")

The amount and type of feed a horse ingests also may reflect the animal's psychological state. Excitement, agitation, fear, apprehension, or nervousness may depress the appetite, i.e., the horse will "go off" feed. Health problems including dental irritation may also contribute to a decreased appetite.

URINATION AND DEFECATION

Normally, horses urinate every four to six hours. Some horses prefer to urinate in a stall or another familiar place and will not urinate in a trailer or other unfamiliar area. Thus the nature of the environment should be taken into consideration when any performing horse exhibits a reluctance to urinate.

The normal interval between bowel movements in the horse is two to three hours. Nervousness, illness, colic, exercise, and other factors may lengthen or shorten the defecation interval or alter fecal consistency or the amount of manure produced. **Coprophagy** (the eating of feces) can be observed in young foals or adult horses. In foals coprophagy may aid in establishing the normal microbial population of the digestive tract and thus is considered a normal behavior. In mature horses coprophagy represents an abnormal behavior and may reflect a lack of roughage or nutrients in the diet. Coprophagy in mature horses is more likely to occur in horses that are confined than in those that are exercised. In both foals and mature horses, coprophagy also provides a mechanism for the transmission of parasites. (*See* CHAPTER 33, "INTERNAL PARASITES.")

SLEEP

The two states of consciousness are alertness and sleep, with several gradations in each state. Horses sleep about seven hours each day, most of the time in a standing position. There are two forms of sleep: **slow-wave sleep** and **paradoxical sleep.** Slow-wave sleep can occur while the horse is standing. Paradoxical sleep, also known as **rapid-eye-movement sleep,** is a deeper sleep requiring the horse to be recumbent. Horses may whinny, snore, or twitch their eyes or limbs during paradoxical sleep. Whether horses dream or experience nightmares, however, is unknown. Horses sleep mostly at night, although they frequently take short naps during the day. This pattern of nocturnal sleep, like many other behav-

ioral characteristics, is probably a result of the horse's evolutionary history, i.e., most predators being active during the daylight hours, horses could safely retreat for sleep during the night.

Typically a horse spends approximately 5 hours a day in slow-wave sleep, 2 hours in paradoxical sleep, and another 5 hours in a drowsy stage. In the drowsy stage the horse is in a conscious or "awake" state but appears very relaxed and inactive. The remaining 12 hours each day are spent in a wakeful, active state, usually searching for food, playing, or if necessary, avoiding predators.

PLAY

Both younger and older horses engage in play activity. Foals interact first with their mothers and then with other foals. Playing involves running, bucking, and the friendly exchange of nips and squeals. Feed tubs, sticks, and balls are favorite objects for horses to pick up, carry, or toss. For a horse confined to a stall, a ball or a one-gallon plastic jug suspended from the ceiling at about the height of the **withers** (ridge between the shoulder blades) can be a useful play object for warding off boredom.

GROOMING

Horses enjoy rolling on soft ground, especially after exercise and during the seasons when they are shedding their coats. Two horses may also engage in mutual grooming, with each horse

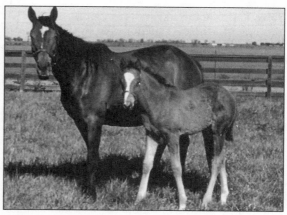

Photo by Murray E. Fowler.

gently nibbling the partner's withers, neck, and **croup** (hindquarters) areas. The duration of time spent in mutual grooming may last for several seconds or for over ten minutes. Several horses may also stand close together, using their tails to switch off flies and other irritating insects from members of the group.

SEXUAL BEHAVIOR

Stallions are fertile all year round, although **libido** (sexual drive) may be slightly reduced in the fall and winter months. Mares begin to cycle through estrus as day length increases, usually in early spring. During estrus a mare will urinate frequently, raise her tail, and open and close the lips of the **vulva** (the external genitalia of the female, representing the entrance to the vagina). She may position her hindquarters facing a male horse and assume a breeding stance with the hind limbs slightly apart and the tail raised. She may also accept mutual grooming from another horse. When she is no longer in estrus, she may react aggressively to any advances by other horses. Such erratic behavior can be readily observed in relationships among pasture mates, and may be of some importance during training or riding. (*See* CHAPTER 9, "REPRODUCTIVE PHYSIOLOGY," and CHAPTER 10, "BREEDING MANAGEMENT.")

Perception

A horse, like most mammals, utilizes its senses of hearing, smell, sight, touch, and taste to perceive and react to its environment. It is said that the lips of a horse function like the fingers of a person. The lips are the manipulating and investigating instrument of the horse. A horse's lips, tongue, and muzzle are extremely sensitive and delicate instruments. Many a horse, while exploring the stall door with its muzzle, has even learned to slide open the door latch!

Horses utilize their sense of smell for assessing the suitability of feed, recognizing herd mates, identifying their young, and possibly for recognizing their caretaker. Most horses enjoy such sweet-tasting treats as sugar or molasses and abhor sour or bitter substances like vinegar. Many oral health-care products are flavored with a sweet substance such as peppermint or licorice to increase their acceptability to the discriminating horse.

EYES

Most mammals rely on vision to perceive their environment, more so than on any other sense, and horses are no exception. The location of the eyes in the skull is important in determining an animal's range of vision. Because most predators would attack by running at ground level rather than by leaping from a tree, it was crucial that the field of vision of the evolving horse should be focused on the surrounding ground. Sharp forward vision was also needed, not only for seeking forage and water but for guiding placement of the hooves while fleeing from a predator.

The large eyes of the horse provide it with a wide range of peripheral vision. Each eye boasts a field of 215 degrees of **monocular fixation** (focusing of one eye on an object), the two fields overlapping in front of the horse to produce 60 to 70 degrees of **binocular fixation** (ability to focus both eyes on a single object). The area of binocular fixation enables the horse to view the ground ahead more sharply and with the added advantage of depth perception or **stereopsis**. Small "blind spots" directly in front of and behind the horse can be accommodated for by a slight turn of the head or body, providing an image in monocular vision. Any stationary object in the rear blind spot may seem to "jump" when its image moves in and out of the

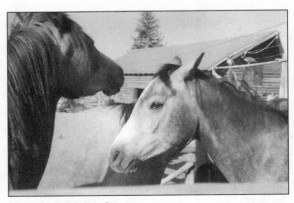

Photo by Ruth Saada.

peripheral field of vision, as the horse turns its head in an attempt to focus. This can result in a typical fleeing or "spooking" behavioral response. (*See* CHAPTER 19, "THE EYE AND VARIOUS DISORDERS.") Unlike a human being, a horse must move its head up and down to focus its eyes on an object. When a horse holds its head upright and high, it is usually focusing on an object in the distance and cannot clearly see the ground directly beneath its nose. The vision of a trotting or galloping horse is not as acute as that of a stationary horse. A horse's range of vision along with its degree of visual acuity should always be taken into consideration when training, especially in such events as jumping.

The **nocturnal vision** (night vision) of a horse is superior to that of human beings but not as acute as that of a bat or cat. The extent to which horses see color is not fully known. Some studies have concluded that horses can indeed discriminate colors, with yellow being most easily identified, followed by green, blue, red, and purple.

EARS

Horse owners often rely on the ears of the horse as an indicator of the animal's attentiveness and emotional state, and to provide clues to behavioral responses. A horse's reaction is often based on hearing along with sight. Horses can discriminate between different words, different human voices, and different herd-mate vocalizations. Horses can also detect a higher frequency of sound vibrations than can people. However, as a horse grows older this higher end of the sound range is gradually lost. Horses may be capable of hearing softer tones as well. The larger range of perceivable sound is partially due to horses' ability to receive sound vibrations through their large, funnel-shaped ears. The ears are capable of rotating independently in response to sound without having to move the head or body. This is especially important to a grazing animal for perceiving threats and detecting predators. The horse positions its body to prick both ears forward in the direction of a particularly alarming noise. Trainers and handlers often follow the direction where the ears are pointing to locate the source of a sound that may be frightening a horse.

Learning and Training

INTELLIGENCE

The intelligence of any animal species is difficult to assess. Brain size in relation to body weight is often used as a measure for comparing intelligence levels between species. The ratio of brain size to body weight of the horse is smaller than that of the cat, dog, or rat but larger than that of the pig. Researchers believe that basing intelligence solely on such ratios has many pitfalls, however, because different abilities exist for different activities in each species. For example, horses do not compare favorably to rats or monkeys in problem-solving tests, such as a maze challenge. Learning by association, however, can be successfully incorporated into a horse's training program, especially if it involves locomotion. Horses have excellent memories once a defined task has been learned, but they can also recall unpleasant experiences equally well!

Much of a horse's worth depends on its level of training. Training, in turn, depends on the ability of the horse to learn. The extent to which the ability to learn is passed from parent to offspring tends to be low in horses, when compared to the heritability of purely physical traits such as racing speed or conformation.

IMPRINTING

The first learning that occurs after birth is known as **imprinting**, wherein the foal learns to recognize and follow its mother. Bonding begins with the licking of the foal by the mare soon after birth. Social bonding and mutual recognition then intensify to a peak within two hours. Human contact with a foal within the first one or two hours of its birth may be beneficial for later handling of the foal. Interestingly, orphan foals have been known to imprint onto other species, such as goats or human beings.

AVERSION CONDITIONING

Horses learn to adapt to their environment and to training protocols. **Aversion conditioning** refers to the learned avoidance of unpleasant situations, such as an encounter with an electric fence (or a veterinarian!). Aversion conditioning is based on the premises that the horse can identify the source of the averse stimulus, that it is able to flee the stimulus, and that the stimulus is consistent. Taste aversion, for example, is important for distinguishing poisonous plants from edible grasses. Some poisonous plants do not produce unpleasant tastes or reactions, however, and horses may learn to seek them out. For example, certain plants of the genus *Senecio* (e.g., **tansy ragwort**) can produce permanent liver damage in horses, yet some horses will actively search for these plants, particularly when pasture is sparse.

HABITUATION

Habituation is a learning process wherein the response to a repeated stimulus gradually declines, resulting eventually in the total absence of the response. Horses pastured next to a railway line, for example, become habituated to the passing of trains. After the first train the horses may be extremely alert, gallop around, even snort and prance. But after the passing of the hundredth train, the horses may not even raise their heads from grazing. The process of teaching a horse to accept a saddle or cart incorporates this habituation principle. Trailering is another example of habituation, the horse becoming calmer and more relaxed with each subsequent trip.

ASSOCIATION LEARNING

Classical and operant conditioning are two types of association learning utilized in training. **Classical conditioning** is the association between a stimulus and a response. An example of classical conditioning in stabled horses is the sight of the person who feeds them followed by the nickering and pawing of the horses. **Operant conditioning** is "trial and error" learning and usually involves a reward. The reward may be food, praise, or termination of the request. There are numerous examples in training, such as teaching a horse to pick up its feet and then feeding it a lump of sugar. Continuous rewarding of the horse is necessary for the horse to learn the task; once learned, however, the reward becomes more variable.

Varying the reward schedule has been shown to provide the highest rate of response and the slowest extinction of the response, probably because the horse cannot predict when it will be rewarded.

Negative reinforcement involves the use of an unpleasant stimulus, such as a whip or bit, if a task is not performed. Use of a whip on a horse that refuses a jump, excessive use of a bit on a horse that doesn't promptly stop, and use of a chain across the nose while leading an unruly horse, are examples of negative reinforcement.

SHAPING

The process of **shaping** occurs as a task or movement is refined or improved. Rewarding all improvements towards the goal will help to refine the task. Most training of high-level performance maneuvers utilizes this shaping concept. Teaching a horse to stop initially may require the use of the voice and considerable pressure on the bit. As the horse is shaped, however, the rider may need simply to squeeze the reins or utter a softly spoken command.

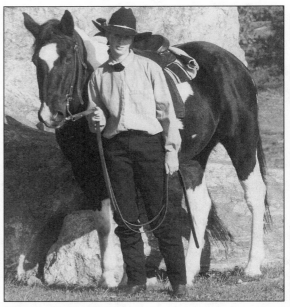

Photo by Heidi Baldwin.

MIMICRY

Horses also learn from each other through mimicry. Often the behavior learned through mimicry is undesirable; the stable vices of wood-chewing and cribbing, for example, are thought to be learned from neighboring horses (*see* CHAPTER 5, "MISBEHAVIOR"). If one horse learns to open a stall door or to chew wood, other horses may soon acquire the same habit. Mimicry is also displayed in pasture situations, as when horses splash and play at the water trough or in rain puddles. It is often a good idea to use mimicry when teaching young horses to load and haul in a trailer, by utilizing an experienced, well-mannered horse for the young ones to observe and learn from.

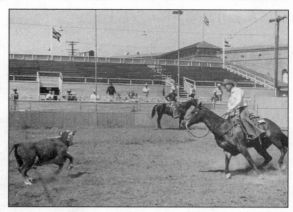

Photo by Murray E. Fowler.

CHAPTER 5
Misbehavior

by Carolyn L. Stull

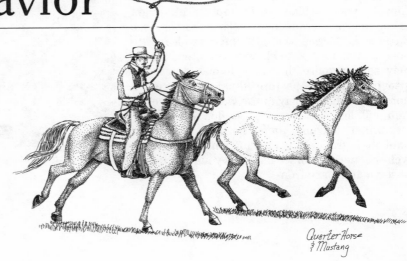

Quarter Horse & Mustang

Misbehavior in horses can assume many different forms, such as disobedience to a command, aggression, a repetitive or stereotypic behavior, or a behavior that the owner just finds annoying. Some normal behaviors can become misbehaviors when they are performed with increasing frequency or intensity. In some cases misbehavior can become so severe as to cause injury to both handler and horse, and wreak havoc in the stable. Too many vices can also drastically decrease the potential value of a horse.

Most horses exhibit some form of misbehavior at some time in their lives. Generally, vices tend to emerge during a horse's younger years, while it is undergoing intensive training and is housed in confinement. Although they are often easy to identify, misbehaviors are not always easy to correct. Solutions or treatments for misbehavior often produce inherently inconsistent results, because no two horses have the same background, genetics, or training. Such solutions may involve punishment, prevention, changes in management or environment, or correction of underlying physiological deficiencies.

The various types of misbehaviors can be classified into either of two major groups: *temperament problems* and *stable vices*. **Temperament problems** include aggression and withdrawal (depression), while **stable vices** include repetitive behaviors and general management problems.

Temperament Problems

AGGRESSION
Aggression often is exhibited when horses are initially grouped together, as the dominant–submissive relationships ("pecking order") among them become established. Aggressive behavior may also be associated with fear and with protection of the young. Warning behaviors, such as a switching or clamping of the tail or pinning of the ears back against the head, often precede more violent displays of kicking and biting. Aggression was a behavior of key importance in the survival of the horse throughout its evolutionary history, and as such remains a dominant factor among **feral** (wild) horses of today.

Rewarding suitable behavior is sometimes an effective treatment for aggression. If **negative**

reinforcement (the use of an unpleasant stimulus, such as a whip or bit, if a task is not performed) is employed, the punishment must be delivered within seconds after the misbehavior occurs in order to be effective. Otherwise, the horse will perceive whatever innocent behavior it may have been engaged in at the time of punishment as inappropriate. Mares with suckling foals have a tendency to be aggressive in order to protect their young, but such behavior usually diminishes as the foal grows older. Stallions in general are more aggressive than either mares or **geldings** (castrated males) owing to the presence of the male hormone **testosterone**.

WITHDRAWAL OR DEPRESSION
Withdrawal or depression is usually associated with illness, pain, or psychological disturbances. Depressed horses exhibit a marked reduction in general activity, become unresponsive to stimuli such as food, and have a reduced awareness of their environment. Lack of social interaction and loss of maintenance behaviors such as eating and grooming often are associated with depression. The depressed horse may isolate itself from the group, assuming a quiet, relaxed posture with its head hung low. Older horses may experience depression resulting from the loss of a long-time companion. (*See* CHAPTER 4, "EQUINE BEHAVIOR.") Significant changes in the environment and drastic reductions in stimulating activities also can cause depression.

Treatment of depression caused by illness or injury will be dictated by the nature of the underlying problem. Psychologically induced depression also must be treated on the basis of the cause, if it can be identified, with appropriate changes incorporated into the horse's daily management through nutrition, companionship, or training regimes.

Stable Vices

Stable vices are stereotypic behaviors that are repeated without any apparent or obvious purpose or function. Such behaviors involve a need-related drive that develops in an environment with inadequate opportunities for satisfying the need. Once established, a stereotypic behavior may become a need in itself.

Stereotypic behaviors tend to occur more often in horses that are confined for long periods of time. They may result from a complex interplay of factors including genetics, stress, social deprivation, frustration, fear, composition of the diet, and the rigors of confinement. Horses kept on pasture usually do not develop stereotypic behaviors.

Many horses appear to develop stable vices as a way to keep themselves busy. Many of the vices involve either investigative exercises using the mouth, lips, or tongue, or **ambulatory** (involving locomotion) types of repetitive movements. Modern stable management tends to isolate horses in individual stalls and to provide a limited feed that is energy-dense and low in fiber. Horses in confinement spend many unoccupied hours alone, without any form of external stimulation. Horses may learn stable vices through mimicry, usually from a neighboring horse, and such habits tend to be self-rewarding (*see* CHAPTER 4, "EQUINE BEHAVIOR.") Once established, vices are extremely difficult to cure permanently.

CRIBBING AND WIND-SUCKING
Cribbing and *wind-sucking* are perhaps the two most familiar vices occurring in the stable. The horse **cribs** by placing its upper teeth on the edge of a feeder or fence, arching its neck, inhaling, and often producing a grunt or belching sound. This habit can result in digestive

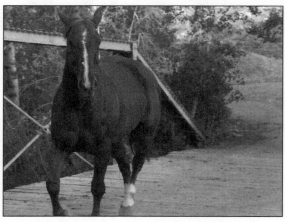

Photo by Ruth Saada.

problems, including colic and loss of body condition. The telltale sign of a cribber is a noticeable wearing of the upper *incisors* (the teeth most forward in the mouth). Often, the wooden edges of the stall or board fence will have a scalloped appearance from repeated cribbing. **Wind-sucking** is somewhat like cribbing; rather than placing its teeth into wood, however, the horse simply flexes its neck while forcibly swallowing air. A distinct belching sound may then be produced as air is expelled. Wind-suckers often exhibit marked muscular development along the underside of the neck as a result of their habit. Horses that wind-suck or crib usually are fit show or race horses that are confined in individual stalls for a large portion of the day.

No one solution for these vices has emerged. Less time spent with "nothing to do," the companionship of another horse (or possibly a goat or chicken), access to pasture, and reducing the number of potential cribbing surfaces, may help minimize their expression. Early detection and treatment are important. Young horses in the initial stages of fitness training are likely candidates to develop such habits (it is rare for older horses to develop them). Once either vice has become established, a horse may exhibit the habit for the rest of its life. Established cribbers

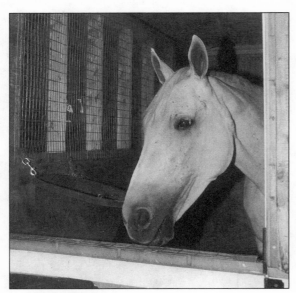

Photo by Ruth Saada.

subsequently kept on pasture have been observed to crib on fence lines, even though plenty of forage was available for consumption.

In severely affected horses, cribbing or wind-sucking may cause a reduction in food intake, loss of physical condition, and emaciation. Milder cases of cribbing may be controlled by applying a bitter-tasting substance to cribbing surfaces. A wind-sucking or cribbing strap can be worn snugly behind the **poll** (back of the head) to prevent the horse from using its muscles to suck air. The strap makes it uncomfortable for the horse to arch and flex its neck muscles, but allows it to breath, eat, and drink normally. A surgical procedure to prevent cribbing has been used in extreme cases, but the success rate of this procedure has been variable.

WEAVING AND STALL-WALKING

Weaving is a repetitive rocking motion made by rhythmically swinging the head and neck from side to side while transferring the weight back and forth from one foreleg to the other. It is easily learned from stable mates and usually is performed each time in the same location in the stall. Weaving is a habit of light-horse breeds and has not been observed in the draft or pony breeds. The closely related habit of **stall-walking** is characterized by constant circling, the horse's feet describing a roughly circular path through the bedding material on the floor of the stall.

The origins of weaving and stall-walking have been attributed to frustration and boredom. Horses are rarely seen weaving or walking continuously in circles while turned out on pasture. Such vices are hazardous to the horse because they produce uneven wearing of the shoes, put stress on leg joints and muscles, and ruin the floor of a stall. Weight loss, fatigue, and even physical exhaustion are characteristics of weaving or stall-walking horses.

Weaving can be controlled by placing a horse in **cross-ties** (fixed lines attached to each side of the halter) for short periods of time to limit lateral movement of the head. The best solutions for this vice, however, include the following:

• Decreasing the amount of time a horse spends confined to a stall

- Availing the horse of pasture
- Providing companionship (another horse, a chicken, or a goat)

Stall-walking can be discouraged by placing rubber tires on the floor of the stall or by hanging a plastic bottle or other object from the ceiling.

HEAD-SHAKING AND HEAD-NODDING

Head-shaking is a normal behavior that developed as a defense mechanism against irritating and often biting insects. It can become a misbehavior, however, when it is displayed during placement of the halter or bridle or becomes a repetitive nuisance during training. **Head-nodding** is a repetitive bobbing motion of head, usually performed alone in a stall while in a drowsy state of consciousness. Underlying ear disorders and nasal irritations have both been shown to provoke head-shaking and head-nodding.

PAWING

Pawing leads to holes in dirt or clay stall floors and to uneven wear of the horse's hooves or shoes. Horses paw:

- When they are restrained or confined
- In anticipation of feeding or other activity
- During trailering

The behavior should not be inadvertently rewarded by feeding a pawing horse, or by removing a horse from its stall while it is pawing. In extreme cases pawing can be prevented by **hobbling** the horse (tying its legs together).

KICKING

Kicking is one of the most dangerous vices, particularly when it occurs in a confined situation. The "flight or fight" instinct is strong in horses, and in kicking, horses are exhibiting the "fight" aspect of this response (*see* CHAPTER 4, "EQUINE BEHAVIOR"). Horses kick for a variety of reasons, including aggression, frustration, playfulness, or just to attract attention. Some horses will kick the wall of the stall prior to being fed or in anticipation of being handled, or for the loud, attention-getting noise it produces. Often the horse is inadvertently rewarded for such behavior as handlers investigate the cause of the commotion. An aggressive horse may kick out at its handler if it feels threatened, or may show its dislike of a neighboring horse by kicking. Repetitive kicking is harmful to the joints of the hind legs, and can cause **lacerations** (tears in the skin and underlying muscle) if the kicking destroys wall partitions or other objects.

Mild cases of kicking can be controlled by sharp verbal reprimands, while severe cases may require **kicking chains**. These are commercially available and are placed on the hind leg above the fetlock. As the horse kicks out, the chain immediately strikes back and stings the horse. The effectiveness of this measure is due to the instant disciplinary reaction that the horse self-inflicts.

BITING

Biting can be either an aggressive or a playful act. Teasing, brushing a ticklish spot, eliciting pain, or threatening a horse can elicit a biting response. Young foals often bite their pasture mates during play, while mares may nip to reprimand their offspring. Stallions will aggressively bite when defending their territories and harems. Biting directed against a horse's handlers, however, is a misbehavior that can be quite dangerous.

Correction of a biting misbehavior depends on the nature of the underlying problem. Regardless of the cause, reform should be initiated as soon

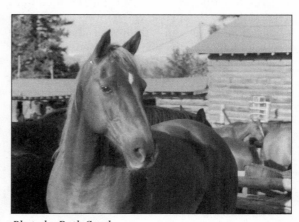

Photo by Ruth Saada.

as possible after the first occurrence. Care should be taken to avoid striking the horse in the head because this may cause the horse to become head-shy. A shouted reprimand can be an effective deterrent for many mildly aggressive horses. Muzzles are available to prevent biting in more severe cases.

TAIL-CHEWING AND MANE-CHEWING

Tail-chewing and mane-chewing are two vices exhibited primarily by yearlings and two-year-olds. Although some cases may be caused by a nutritional deficiency, it is more likely that the youngsters simply are curious or bored, or that the behavior represents an extension of mutual grooming. Typically, large portions of the victim's tail are missing, while the mane will have holes chewed throughout it. Placing a disagreeable substance (such as hot chili pepper powder) on the victim's tail and mane may deter the habit. However, isolation of the chewing horse remains the only completely reliable solution.

THROWING FEED ABOUT AND EATING TOO FAST

Horses may throw feed about their stalls, a messy and costly habit that can result in consumption of an unbalanced diet. Feeding hay from an elevated rack, or a change to feeding on the ground or in a trough with bars across it, can minimize feed wastage. Some horses get into the habit of eating too fast, bolting their feed with only minimal or no preparatory chewing. Digestive upsets and decreased digestibility of the feed may result. Some horses bolt their feed only in the presence of other horses, so separation at feeding time will diminish the habit. Grain can be fed in a feeder with an inside lip to prevent the horse from pushing the feed out. Placing several stones or salt blocks in the bottom of the feeder can also assist in keeping the grain inside the tub. Mixing chopped hay or other roughage with the grain will promote normal chewing and can also slow a fast eater, since more chewing is required as the fiber content of the feed increases.

WOOD-CHEWING

Wood-chewing is a misbehavior in which the horse grasps the edges of wood surfaces in its mouth and actually ingests the wood. Horses prefer softer types of wood such as pine rather than hardwoods (oak, for example). Lack of roughage in the diet has been implicated as a cause of wood-chewing. Pelleted diets are more likely to predispose the horse to wood-chewing than are diets containing ample roughage. Boredom may also play a role. Wood-chewing is extremely destructive to the surfaces of stalls, feeders, mangers, and board fences. Corrective measures include:

- Increasing the roughage component of the diet
- Covering wood surfaces with metal
- Painting wood surfaces with unappetizingly flavored substances
- Using electrified wire on wood surfaces to deliver a mild shock

Treatment of Misbehavior

The approach taken in treating a particular misbehavior or vice depends on the cause, intensity, frequency of expression, and time of development of the behavior. Causes of misbehaviors may be rooted in disease, environment, social needs, previous training, dietary requirements, or other factors. Lack of roughage in the diet and boredom from an unstimulating, confining environment are commonly cited causes of stereotypic behaviors and other stable vices.

Treatment of a misbehavior involves removal or alleviation of the inciting cause. This often can be accomplished by:

- Providing the horse with a companion, such as a pony, goat, or chicken
- Increasing the duration and/or frequency of exercise
- Formulating the feed ration to include abundant roughage
- Using cribbing straps, muzzles, or other restraining devices (in extreme cases only)

Behavior modification using **positive reinforcement** (giving a reward, such as food, for suitable behavior) may be successful with some aggressive horses. **Aversion conditioning** or negative reinforcement (such as an electric shock, a foul-tasting substance, or pain infliction [e.g., kicking chains]) may be required in more severe cases. (*See* CHAPTER 4, "EQUINE BEHAVIOR.")

The best approach to managing vices and misbehaviors is to prevent their development at the outset. Stable vices can be prevented by providing a stimulating stable environment and designing management and training schedules around a horse's natural instincts and needs. A horse has the behavioral and physiological needs of a constantly grazing, socially interactive herd animal, not an animal that is fed rigidly twice a day and kept isolated from its companions in a darkened box stall. Proper stable management can usually balance a horse's needs with the requirements of handlers and the necessary training schedules.

Individual variation undoubtedly plays a significant role in the onset, treatment, and prevention of misbehaviors in horses. Of course, the acceptability of a behavior in an individual horse will ultimately be decided not by the horse itself but by its owner or handler.

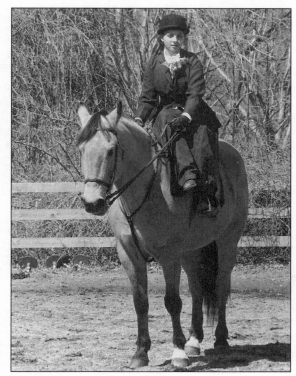

Photo by Heidi Baldwin.

PART III

Nutrition

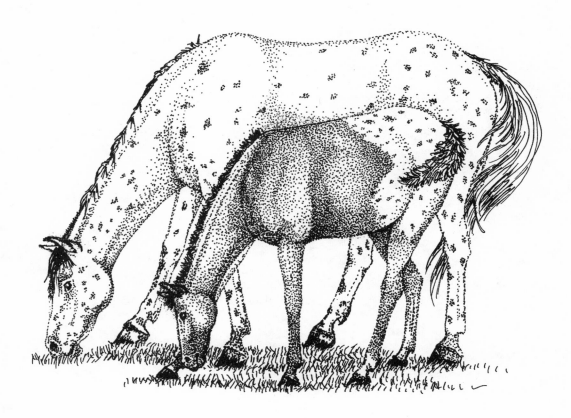

The horse loves his oats more
than his saddle.

—RUSSIAN PROVERB

CHAPTER 6

Equine Nutritional Requirements

by C.A. Tony Buffington

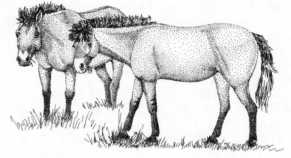

Feeding horses combines both science and art. Some understanding of the sciences of nutrition, physiology, and agronomy allows one to appreciate the influence of the equine digestive system on horses' nutritional requirements and utilization of various feeds. The art of feeding is the skill to recognize high-quality feeds, to purchase them at an economical price, and to store them in a way that retains their quality. Combining these elements into a feeding program that maintains healthy stock is the mark of successful equine husbandry.

Horses' specific nutritional needs may be best understood in light of some general principles of nutrition that can be applied to many different species of animals. The first principle is that a nutrient "requirement" represents a range of dietary nutrient concentrations that result in adequate function. Thus the need for any individual nutrient is better represented graphically by a plateau ("optimal range") rather than a peak, as shown in Figure 1. Once one adds enough of the nutrient to a diet, no further response will be detected as more of the nutrient is added until toxic levels are achieved. The width of the plateau varies with the nutrient itself, with other components of the diet that interact with the nutrient, and with the age and physiological status of the animal.

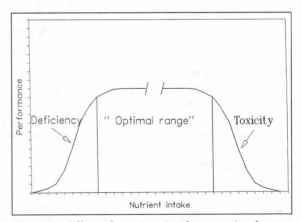

Figure 1. Effect of nutrient intake on animal performance. The gap in the plateau phase indicates that the range of intake between deficiency and toxicity varies with the nutrient in question, the overall diet, and the physiological state of the animal.

Table 4 demonstrates the important distinction between the nutrient concentration of a feed and the amount of nutrient actually eaten. The concentration or **density** of a nutrient in a feed is reported as a percent (parts per hundred) or parts per million (**ppm**, which is equivalent to milligrams per kilogram), while the nutrient needs of horses are expressed in amounts (grams, milligrams, or units) per horse per day. Thus the recommendation to feed a yearling a diet containing 14 percent crude protein assumes that the animal will ingest 12–13 pounds of the feed in order to obtain the 800 grams of protein it needs every day. If an owner mistakenly assumes that a diet containing 14 percent crude protein is sufficient *regardless of the quantity actually eaten*, then he or she may not be providing sufficient protein to meet an animal's needs.

Another important principle of nutrition is that nutrient requirements change during an animal's life. The influence of age and physiological status on a horse's need for one nutrient, energy, is presented in Figure 2. Because many nutrient needs vary with energy requirements, this pattern is worth remembering because the risk of nutrition-related problems is greatest during periods when nutrient requirements are high. From Figure 2 one would predict that the greatest care in diet formulation should be taken early in periods of growth and **lactation** (production of milk by the mare), and in animals subjected to intense work. In addition to these, careful attention to diet must be provided for mares in the final trimester of pregnancy owing to the rapid growth of the fetus during this time.

The partition and utilization of dietary energy to maintain horses are shown in Figure 3. From the figure it is evident that not all food energy is available to animals, since some of it is lost in the feces and urine. Moreover, the needs of maintenance must first be met before energy can be used for productive purposes such as growth, reproduction, or work.

Although these general principles provide a useful framework, they apply to groups of animals better than they do to individuals. Feeding individual horses requires the discerning "eye of

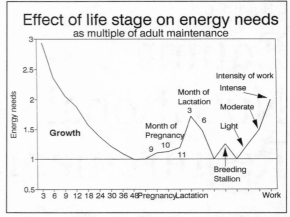

Figure 2. Effect of physiological state on energy needs, expressed as a multiple of average adult maintenance.

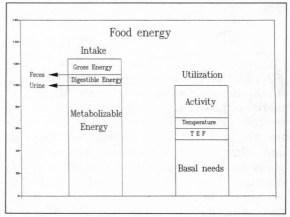

Figure 3. The "balance" between energy intake and energy utilization at maintenance in animals. A horse's needs for energy for basal functions, to assimilate food (TEF), to maintain body temperature, and to support some activity must be met before productive activities such as growth, reproduction, and work can be performed.

the master" in order to maintain optimum body condition during changing physiological and environmental circumstances. A system of body-condition scoring devised for horses is presented in Table 1, with the body areas emphasized being shown in Figure 4.

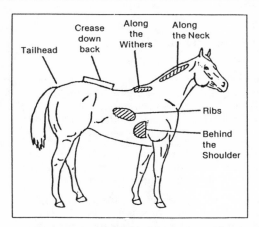

Figure 4. Diagram of the body areas emphasized in body-condition scoring (TABLE 1).
Source: Reprinted, by permission of the publisher, from: D.R. Henneke, "A condition score system for horses," Equine Practice 7(8) (1985): 13–15.

Nutrient Needs of Horses

WATER

After oxygen, water is the nutrient most essential for life. Horses can live for weeks without food but only for days without water. Daily water needs are greatest in young foals, lactating mares, working horses, and animals residing in hot climates. Increasing protein and/or mineral intake will increase water requirements, in order to provide the fluid needed to excrete excess quantities of these compounds in the urine.

Horses obtain water from their food and its **metabolism** (breakdown and utilization by the body) as well as by drinking. Horses grazing succulent pastures may consume sufficient water in their food to meet their requirements, while those consuming dry forages may take in only 2–4 quarts of water per pound of dry feed.

To ensure adequate water intake, horses should have access to clean, fresh water at all times. Water consumption will decline if the water is unpalatable, too hot, or too cold. This in turn will decrease food intake. To ensure availability and palatability, water buckets, bowls, or troughs should be cleaned and replenished frequently, particularly during the winter months

when water freezes. Electric water heaters must be properly grounded to avoid any shock hazard.

One measure of suitability of water for horses is the *total dissolved solids*, or total mineral content of the water, which can be measured in most testing laboratories. Good water should have fewer than 2500 ppm of total dissolved solids. Horses should not be permitted to consume water containing more than 7000 ppm of total dissolved solids in order to avoid diarrhea and decreased performance. Horses hot and tired after work should not be offered water until hay and a rest period of 30–60 minutes have been provided. If a horse drinks too much water too soon after exercise, colic or founder (**laminitis**) may result. (*See* CHAPTER 22, "THE MUSCULOSKELETAL SYSTEM AND VARIOUS DISORDERS;" CHAPTER 26, "THE DIGESTIVE SYSTEM AND VARIOUS DISORDERS;" and CHAPTER 40, "PROCEDURES FOR MEDICAL EMERGENCIES.")

ENERGY

Horses use energy for their basic body functions, to digest and utilize food, to maintain body temperature, and for growth, reproduction, and activity (FIGURE 2). Large individual variation exists among horses in the amount of energy needed to maintain normal body condition; "hard" keepers may need to consume twice as much feed to maintain themselves as "easy" keepers.

Energy is contained in the carbohydrate, protein, and fat portions of the diet. **Carbohydrates—** the starches inside plant cells and the fiber that

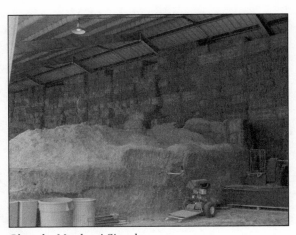

Photo by Mordecai Siegal.

Table 1
A Body-Condition Scoring System for Horses

Score	Description
1	POOR: Emaciated. Prominent spinous processes, ribs, **tailhead and hooks** (the bony prominences on each side below the tail) and **pins** (the bony prominences of the tuber coxae, i.e. pont of the hip). Noticeable bone structure on withers, shoulders and neck. No fatty tissues can be palpated.
2	VERY THIN: Emaciated. Slight fat covering over base of spinous processes. Transverse processes of lumbar vertebrae feel rounded. Prominent spinous processes, ribs, tailhead and hooks and pins. Withers, shoulders and neck structures faintly discernable.
3	THIN: Fat built up about halfway on spinous processes, transverse processes cannot be felt. Slight fat cover over ribs. Spinous processes and ribs easily discernable. Tailhead prominent, but individual vertebrae cannot be visually identified. Hook bones appear rounded, but easily discernable. Pin bones not distinguishable. Withers, shoulders and neck accentuated.
4	MODERATELY THIN: Negative crease along back. Faint outline of ribs discernable. Tailhead prominence depends on conformation, fat, can be felt around it. Hook bones not discernable. Withers, shoulders and neck not obviously thin.
5	MODERATE: Back is level. Ribs cannot be visually distinguished but can be easily felt. Fat around tailhead beginning to feel spongy. Withers appear rounded over spinous processes. Shoulders and neck blend smoothly into body.
6	MODERATE TO FLESHY: May have slight crease down back. Fat over ribs feels spongy. Fat around tailhead feels soft. Fat beginning to be deposited along the sides of the withers, behind the shoulders and along the sides of the neck.
7	FLESHY: May have crease down back. Individual ribs can be felt, but noticeable filling between ribs with fat. Fat around tailhead is soft. Fat deposits along withers, behind shoulders and along the neck.
8	FAT: Crease down back. Difficult to palpate ribs. Fat around tailhead very soft. Area along withers filled with fat. Area behind shoulder filled in flush. Noticeable thickening of neck. Fat deposited along inner buttocks.
9	EXTREMELY FAT: Obvious crease down back. Patchy fat appearing over ribs. Bulging fat around tailhead, along withers, behind shoulders and along neck. Fat along inner buttocks may rub together. Flank filled in flush.

Reprinted with permission from: Henneke, D.R.: A condition score system for horses. *Equine Practice* 7(8):13–15, 1985.

makes up their cell walls—are the chief source of energy in horse feeds. Protein also provides energy, in addition to the essential amino acids and nitrogen that horses need for maintenance. Fat is the most concentrated form of energy, containing 2.25 times the energy content per gram of either carbohydrate or protein. Fat also provides essential fatty acids needed for a variety of body functions.

The energy derived from food can be quantified in units known as *calories*. A **calorie** (abbreviated **cal**) is defined as the amount of energy needed to raise the temperature of 1 gram of water 1 degree **Celsius (centigrade)**. Because this amount of energy is very small, nutritionists prefer to use the term **kilocalorie** (abbreviated **kcal**; also referred to as a **Calorie**, with a capital "C"), which represents 1000 calories. A **megacalo-**

rie (abbreviated **mcal**) is defined as 1000 kcal and is a useful term for quantifying the energy in rations.

The energy content of feeds usually is reported as the *total digestible nutrients* (**TDN**) or *digestible energy* (**DE**). The TDN content of a feed represents the sum of the digestible carbohydrate (called *nitrogen-free extract*), protein, fat (× 2.25 because of its higher energy content), and fiber. TDN is determined by subtracting the content of these nutrients in the feces from that in the feed. Values for TDN are reported in pounds of TDN per hundred pounds of feed, or percent. The DE content of feeds is determined in a similar fashion, except that only the total energy content of feed and feces is considered. Determinations of the TDN content of feeds have been made by animal nutritionists for many years, and values are available for a large number of feeds. More recently DE has come into increasing use to describe the energy content of feeds. The DE content of some feeds has been measured, while for others it has been approximated by multiplying TDN (in pounds) by 2.2 to obtain DE in megacalories.

Fiber, the portion of dietary carbohydrate that cannot be broken down by the horse's digestive enzymes, provides both energy and physical stimulation to the intestine. The energy in **fermentable** (able to be digested by intestinal microorganisms) fiber only becomes available after breakdown to fatty acids by the microbial population of the equine large intestine. In addition to providing energy, these fatty acids aid in sustaining the health of the cells lining the large intestine. Nonfermentable fiber, the inert portion of fiber not degraded by the horse or its intestinal bacteria, also aids in maintaining normal function by providing physical stimulation, which promotes the movement of food through the digestive tract.

PROTEIN

The **amino acids** (nitrogen-containing molecules forming the structural backbone of proteins) that make up dietary protein are used by horses to maintain normal body structure and function. Amino acids can be divided into two categories: **essential amino acids** (those that cannot be synthesized in sufficient quantities by the body and must be provided in the diet) and **dispensable** or **nonessential amino acids** (those that can be synthesized by the body so long as a source of nitrogen is present in the diet).

Proteins themselves can be classified as either *structural* or *functional*. Muscles, **cartilage** (specialized connective tissue especially important in bone growth and the formation of joints), **ligaments** (strengthening bands of fibrous tissue that support and stabilize joints), **tendons** (fibrous tissue attaching muscle to bone), and bone all contain structural proteins. Functional proteins include enzymes, **blood carrier proteins** (proteins that transport substances in the blood), and **antibodies** (specialized proteins produced by cells of the immune system in response to the presence of foreign material). Body proteins are constantly being broken down and resynthesized; replacement amino acids from dietary protein are needed because this process is not completely efficient. Dietary protein is also needed for the manufacture of new proteins during pregnancy, lactation, and growth.

Protein deficiency, owing either to insufficient intake or to ingestion of **poor-quality protein** (any protein that is deficient in one or more essential amino acids), may result in decreased weight gain, a rough hair coat, small offspring at birth, reproductive dysfunction, and depressed immune function. Excessive amounts of protein in the diet are not beneficial, however, because amino acids that are not actively required for making body protein are broken down and not stored; the result is an increase in urine volume in order to excrete the excess nitrogen. Although work does increase protein requirements, the increased food intake required to meet the increased energy demand of the working horse usually will supply any additional protein needs.

Contrary to popular belief, stallions do *not* require more protein during the breeding season, because the protein loss in **spermatozoa** (sperm; the mature reproductive cells of the male) is small. Neither is there evidence to support the notion that the addition of **methionine** (a sulfur-containing amino acid), gelatin, or a kelp-based product to the feed will improve hoof growth, nor that excessive protein levels contribute to metabolic bone disease or "protein bumps."

MAJOR MINERALS

The major minerals include calcium, phosphorus, sodium, chloride, potassium, magnesium, and sulfur, quantities of which are usually stated as a percentage of the diet. Of these, nutritionists are concerned primarily with the calcium and phosphorus content in the rations of growing horses, because of these minerals' profound effects on growth and development.

Calcium and phosphorus are the chief mineral constituents of bones and teeth. Calcium is also important for blood clotting and for the transmission of nerve impulses. Phosphorus is essential for the activation or inhibition of many enzyme systems, the generation and transfer of energy, and for many other metabolic processes. An upset in the dietary ratio of calcium to phosphorus (**Ca:P ratio**) can result in severe physical abnormalities, including deformed and excessively fragile bones (*see* CHAPTER 8, "DISEASES OF DIETARY ORIGIN"). The recommended ratio of calcium to phosphorus in the diet ranges from 1:1 to 2:1. Horses cannot tolerate absolute calcium or phosphorus deficiencies or low Ca:P ratios. Growing horses reportedly can tolerate a higher Ca:P ratio, up to 6:1, if the total mineral content of the diet is adequate, but Ca:P ratios greater than 3:1 are not recommended. It is important to remember that grains are not high in phosphorus, and as much as 70 percent of the phosphorus present may be unavailable for absorption. Grains have a lower Ca:P ratio than either alfalfa or mixed hay, but alfalfa and oats in a diet do not "balance each other out." Fertilization methods and species of forage grown both can affect the phosphorus content of a hay or pasture. Chemical analysis is the only way to determine the phosphorus content of forage.

Commercial concentrates usually have a calcium–phosphorus content that is compatible with legume, grass, or mixed hay. For owners with a small number of horses, using an appropriate commercial concentrate feed from a reputable manufacturer along with mixed grass-legume hay is a convenient way to ensure an adequate diet for their animals.

Sodium and chloride needs can be met by provision of iodized, trace mineral-containing salt blocks, which should always be available to horses. Potassium, magnesium, and sulfur usually are present in adequate quantities in most equine diets and supplementation is not considered necessary.

TRACE MINERALS

Trace minerals are minerals required in the diet in very minute amounts. For horses these usually include copper, iodine, iron, manganese, selenium, and zinc. Exact requirements of these minerals for horses have not been determined, and are difficult to define owing to the many interactions that exist among the minerals in the body. For example, when zinc, sulfur, or molybdenum intakes are high, the dietary requirement for copper is increased. This interaction is of growing importance because of the increased use of alfalfa hay in the rations of growing horses in some areas of the country. Fertilizing alfalfa fields with lime to increase top yields increases the molybdenum content of the forage and so may decrease the amount of available copper, inducing a copper deficiency in horses ingesting the forage.

The iron content of roughage-grain diets is usually adequate under most conditions, making iron supplementation an undesirable practice. Iron toxicities have resulted from the frequent intravenous injection of iron preparations. Formation of red blood cells requires three trace minerals (iron, copper, cobalt) and three vitamins (B_6, B_{12}, folic acid). **Anemia** (low red-blood-cell count) can result from a deficiency of any of these (and also some other) nutrients. If anemia is suspected, the cause should be investigated by a veterinarian before a specific treatment is initiated.

Current daily nutrient recommendations for growing horses for copper, manganese, and zinc are 10 ppm of copper and 40 ppm each of manganese and zinc. Recent concern over an apparent increase in bone disease in young horses has prompted a reconsideration of the role of trace-mineral deficiencies in skeletal disorders. A survey conducted by Ohio State University suggests that a higher concentration of these nutrients may be of benefit for the health and integrity of growing bone and cartilage. Preliminary results indicate that bone defects begin at a very early age, as has already been shown to occur in pigs. Weanling diets containing 25 ppm of copper, 50 ppm of manganese, and 80 ppm of zinc have been beneficial on farms where bone and cartilage problems such as **epiphysitis** (disorder of the growing ends of long bones) and **osteochondrosis** (degeneration of bone underlying the cartilage of joint surfaces) are of concern.

All rations should contain iodine and selenium at appropriate concentrations; current recommendations are 0.1 ppm of iodine and 0.3 ppm of selenium. The wide variation in soil iodine and selenium content in the United States requires that horse owners follow local recommendations for the addition of these two nutrients to diets. Relatively small excesses of either of these minerals may be toxic. **Goiter** (enlarged thyroid gland) may develop in horses suffering either iodine excess or deficiency, while horses with selenium toxicity may appear stiff-gaited or **ataxic** (incoordinated), exhibit hair loss about the mane and tail, and develop hoof cracks. As a historical sidelight, selenium toxicity in their horses may have cost George Armstrong Custer and his men the Battle of the Little Big Horn. Custer's horses had been maintained in a region of high soil selenium content and were lame, whereas those of the Sioux chief, Sitting Bull, originated elsewhere and were sound.

The use of hair analysis for determining the mineral status of horses has recently been proposed. Unfortunately this has little validity owing to the great variation in mineral content attributable to hair color, rate of hair growth, season of the year, and environmental contamination of horses' hair.

VITAMINS

Vitamins are required in very small quantities in the diet because horses cannot synthesize sufficient amounts to fulfill their daily needs. Vitamins are second only to protein among the nutrients most often abused and overfed. Good-quality forage, coupled with the normal synthesis of B vitamins by intestinal microbes, usually supplies a sufficient vitamin intake for most horses. Animals maintained on pasture apparently need no vitamin supplementation at all. Horses involved in strenuous activity, however, may require additional B vitamins, especially if feed quality is poor. Brewer's yeast at 0.5–1 percent (0.5 oz. per horse per day) of the grain mix can be added to horse rations as a source of vitamins and trace minerals.

Vitamins are classified as either **fat-soluble** (vitamins A, D, E, K) or **water-soluble** (B vitamins, C). Fat-soluble vitamins are stored in the body and their absorption is facilitated by the presence of moderate levels of fat in the diet. Water-soluble vitamins, except for vitamin B_{12}, are not stored to any extent.

Current recommendations for fat-soluble vitamins for adult maintenance are 2000 international units (IU) of vitamin A, 350 IU of vitamin D (as D_3), and 50 IU of vitamin E, per kilogram (2.2 pounds) of the diet. These vitamins should be supplemented in regions where the hay quality varies. However, recent research at the University of Pennsylvania has shown that the use of some vitamin supplements, even at recommended levels, can produce vitamin A toxicity in a short period of time. This finding is of particular significance because some horse owners provide several supplements "just to be sure," thinking that a little is good and so more must be better. Horses consuming more than 60,000 IU of vitamin A or 10,000 IU of vitamin D per day may develop toxicities over time. Horses are capable of storing enough vitamin A and vitamin D in the liver to get them through the winter months until adequate pasture is available; supplementation may only expand their normal stores of these vitamins to toxic levels. (*See* CHAPTER 8, "DISEASES OF DIETARY ORIGIN.")

Sources of Nutrients

PASTURE AND HAY

The most common sources of nutrients for horses are pasture and hay, which are classified by nutritionists as roughages or forages. Roughages may be further subdivided into legumes and grasses. **Legumes** are plants that can directly absorb or "fix" nitrogen from the air, that have a taproot, and whose leaves are supported by a stalk attached to the main stem. Examples of legumes include alfalfa, clovers, bird's-foot trefoil, lespedeza, and the vetches. Grasses have a fibrous root system and their leaves originate directly from the main stem. Examples of grasses include timothy, orchard grass, bromegrass, bluegrass, and fescue. Legumes are higher in protein and calcium and in general are richer sources of nutrients than are grasses. None of the forages contains much phosphorus. Nutrient content varies widely with stage of maturity as well as with soil fertility, availability of water, and curing and processing.

It is important to be able to recognize good-quality hay. In general, hay should be harvested as immature as possible without sacrificing too much yield in order to maximize protein content and digestibility. It should be leafy and weed-free. The criteria presented in Table 2 may be used to guide purchase of the best-quality hay available. As an adjunct to visual evaluation, chemical testing of forages for nutrient content is relatively inexpensive and available. Veterinarians and extension agents can provide advice on sample collection, laboratory availability, and interpretation of results.

CONCENTRATES

Concentrates are rich sources of individual nutrients and are used to enhance the quality of the diet. Concentrated feeds are subdivided into energy, protein, and mineral and vitamin supplements. Criteria for evaluation of concentrate feeds are presented in Table 2.

Energy Concentrates Grains are the most common energy concentrate fed to horses. The protein content of grains is moderate to low. Grains are poor sources of calcium but moderate sources of phosphorus. For many, oats are the "grain of choice." Oats are highly palatable but vary in digestibility and quality owing to hull content and method of processing. They are

---

Table 2
Criteria for Visual Appraisal of Horse Feeds

Evaluating hay quality

1. *Type of plant*: The higher the percentage of legume present, usually the higher the nutrient content.

2. *Stage of maturity when cut*: Early-cut hay assures the maximum content of proteins, minerals, and vitamins, and the highest digestibility.

3. *Percentage of leaves present*: Leaves contain the highest nutrient content, so a high leaf-to-stem ratio indicates high quality.

4. *Green color*: Although not essential, a bright green color generally indicates a minimum of bleaching and leaching losses of carotene and other nutrients, and also high palatability.

5. *Aroma and fragrance*: High-quality hay has a pleasing fragrant aroma to most people. Moldy feeds have undesirable smells.

6. *Steminess*: Large, woody stems reduce acceptability and quality. High-quality hay is finely stemmed and pliable. The stems should not cause pain when the hay is squeezed in the hand.

7. *Foreign material*: Hay should be free of weeds, stubble, sticks, dirt, twine, and other foreign material.

Characteristics of good grains and other concentrates

1. Seeds are not cracked or split.

2. Seeds are low in moisture. Processed grains (e.g., rolled barley) are likely to "sweat" and mold if the moisture content is too high before entering storage.

3. Seeds have a good color, characteristic of the species.

4. Free of mold, rodent and insect damage, foreign material, and rancid odors.

lower in energy and higher in protein than corn. Oats are relatively "safe" to feed and there is nothing chemically in oats (or any grain) that makes horses "high." Corn is highly palatable and more energy-dense than oats. Caution is necessary when switching from oats to corn: Replace oats in the ration with the same *weight* of corn, not the same volume. Corn is not a "hot" feed, as some owners may claim, provided it is fed according to its caloric value, which is based on weight. Horses derive more heat from digesting hay than grain. The DE content of wheat is almost the same as that of corn. Wheat kernels are hard and small, however, and should be crushed or ground to medium degree and mixed with a bulky feed (the ration should not exceed 20–25 percent wheat) to prevent digestive disturbances.

Protein Concentrates In addition to legume forages, a variety of protein supplements are available. Most such supplements contain low to moderate amounts of calcium but are good sources of phosphorus. The quality of a protein supplement is related to the digestibility of the amino acids in the supplement. Most sources are readily digested by horses, but excessive heating of protein supplements during processing will greatly decrease the availability of the amino acids for absorption from the digestive tract. Although studies of amino acid requirements for horses are few, lysine has been shown to be one of the primary limiting amino

Table 3
Approximate Calcium and Phosphorus Contents of Selected Mineral Supplements

Supplement	% Calcium	% Phosphorus
Calcium carbonate	40	0
Oyster shells	36	0
Limestone	35	0
Tricalcium phosphate	31	17
Bone meal	24	13
Dicalcium phosphate	23	19
Monosodium phosphate	0	24

acids. Soybean meal contains the highest level of lysine of all the vegetable proteins. Soybeans should not be fed raw, however, because they contain a digestive-enzyme inhibitor that lowers the digestibility of protein. Milk products and fish meal also are good sources of lysine but are generally more expensive. Linseed meal is low in digestibility and lysine. Cottonseed meal also is low in lysine but may contain **gossypol**, a toxic fatty acid. Horses can utilize some **urea** (a nitrogen-containing compound) as non-protein nitrogen for making amino acids, but the efficiency of this process is much less than simply feeding pre-formed protein.

Mineral and Vitamin Supplements Mineral supplements include trace-mineralized salt and a variety of sources of calcium and phosphorus (TABLE 3). Although these may be offered in boxes to horses, it must be remembered that horses (or any other species) cannot choose a balanced diet from among a *smorgasbord* of individual nutrients. This is why mineral and vitamin supplementation of a sweet feed is a more effective way to ensure consumption of an adequate diet in those circumstances wherein supplementation is necessary.

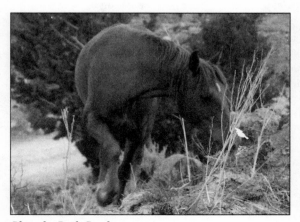

Photo by Ruth Saada.

DETERMINING NUTRIENT REQUIREMENTS OF INDIVIDUAL HORSES

The nutrient needs of horses are presented in a National Research Council publication entitled *The Nutrient Requirements of Horses*. This publication also contains a computer disk that may be used to estimate the nutrient needs of horses at maintenance and during growth, reproduction, and performance. An example of the output of this program is presented in Table 4.

Table 4
Sample Computerized Printout of National Research Council Recommendations for an Adult Horse (1,000 lb) at Maintenance

National Research Council
Nutrient Requirements of Domestic Animals
Equine Nutrient Requirements (1989)
Body Weight (lb): 1000

Horse Description
Class: Maintenance Horse

Requirement Basis

Nutrient	Total	Percent
Dry Matter Intake	16.5 lb/day	1.65 & of BW
Digestible Energy	15.0 Mcal/day	0.91 Mcal/lb
Crude Protein	600 grams/day	8.00 %
Lysine	21.0 grams/day	0.28 %
Calcium	18.1 grams/day	0.24 %
Phosphorus	12.7 grams/day	0.17 %
Magnesium	6.8 grams/day	0.09 %
Potassium	23 grams/day	0.30 %
Sodium	7.5 grams/day	0.10 %
Sulfur	11.3 grams/day	0.15 %
Iron	300 mgs/day	18.1 mg/lb
Zinc	300 mgs/day	18.1 mg/lb
Copper	75.0 mgs/day	4.5 mg/lb
Manganese	300 mgs/day	18.1 mg/lb
Iodine	0.8 mgs/day	0.05 mg/lb
Cobalt	0.8 mgs/day	0.05 mg/lb
Selenium	0.8 mgs/day	0.05 mg/lb
Vitamin A	13608 IU/day	822.6 IU/lb
Vitamin D	2251 IU/day	136.1 IU/lb
Vitamin E	375 IU/day	22.7 IU/lb

CHAPTER 7

Feeding Horses

by C.A. Tony Buffington

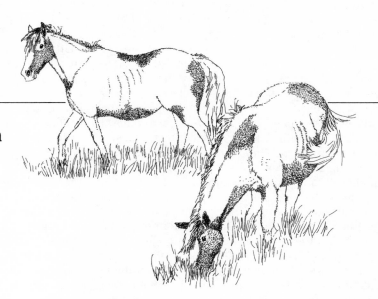

Most horses should be allowed to eat all the good-quality roughage they want. Consumption of large quantities of a poor-quality hay, however, will encourage the development of a "hay belly," which is particularly unacceptable in halter and performance horses. Horses that are strenuously exercised (racing, polo, eventing, endurance rides) or that are in their rapid-growth phase (1–6 months of age) cannot consume enough hay to meet their energy requirements, so the remaining energy must be supplied by a concentrated feed, which should also contain supplementary protein, vitamins, and minerals. (*See* Chapter 6, "Equine Nutritional Requirements.") When small numbers of horses are maintained, a concentrate containing the percentage of protein required by the youngest animal should be adequate. Adult horses may be fed a hay of lower quality and protein content, along with small amounts of concentrate as necessary to meet any increased needs.

Feeding During the Reproductive Cycle

PREGNANCY AND LACTATION

The nutritional needs of pregnant mares remain at maintenance for the first 7 months of **gestation** (pregnancy). Most mares can sustain themselves on pasture and/or an excellent- or good-quality hay. During the final 3 months of the pregnancy, however, supplementation of the diet (particularly with minerals) should be considered. At this time the foal begins to increase rapidly in size and weight. In the tenth month of gestation calcium, phosphorus, copper, manganese, and zinc are transferred from the mother to the foal. If nutrient demand outstrips dietary intake during this period, the mare may draw upon her own body stores of nutrients to meet the needs of the developing foal. Mares consuming deficient diets during the final trimester of pregnancy run the risk of producing foals having low tissue stores of nutrients at birth. These stores may be quickly depleted during the foal's early rapid-growth phase if another nutrient source is not available. Mare's milk is very low in trace minerals, and very few foals are offered significant quantities of **creep feed** (feed provided in a separate area where the foal can eat without interference from the mare) to help meet their nutrient demands for growth. The perceived increase in bone problems among rapidly growing foals and weanlings may be caused by an inadequate supply of trace-mineral stores. Trace minerals are needed for the development of a solid foundation upon which bone mineralization can occur; without them, the quality of bone may be compromised. Research has suggested that defects in bone and **cartilage** (specialized connective tissue, especially important in bone growth and the formation of joints) can begin at a very early age, even before birth. Offering the mare a fortified trace-mineral salt free-choice or feeding 1–2 pounds of a protein–vitamin–mineral supplement daily should help provide "nutrient insurance" for the developing foal.

During the first 4 months of life, mare's milk is the major nutrient source for the foal. **Lactation** (production of milk by the mare) places great nutritional demands on the mare. Water consumption can soar 50–100 percent above the level required for maintenance, and energy intake will nearly double to meet milk-production demands. Calcium and phosphorus requirements also rise to account for losses in the milk. Each kilogram of milk contains approximately 1 gram of calcium and 0.5 gram of phosphorus. Depending on the amount of milk produced, an additional 11–18 grams of calcium and 6–9 grams of phosphorus *above maintenance* may be required.

The best gauge for determining the quantity of feed needed by a lactating mare is to assess her body condition (*see* TABLE 1 and FIGURE 4 in CHAPTER 6, "EQUINE NUTRITIONAL REQUIREMENTS"). Because of the common practice of providing feed at a fixed rate to all horses on a premise, mares that are good milk-producers are sometimes underfed and can lose a considerable amount of weight during lactation. Mares that are poor producers occasionally are fed more

feed in the hope that their production will increase. Milk production is genetically determined, however, and such a practice will only lead to obesity.

As lactation progresses beyond 13–24 weeks **postpartum** (after birth of the foal), milk production decreases from 3 percent to approximately 2 percent of the mare's body weight, which concomitantly decreases her nutrient needs. The amount of food offered to the mare should be decreased during this period to maintain optimum body condition.

FOALS

The nutritional needs of foals younger than 3 months of age have not been well characterized. Healthy nursing foals that are growing at an acceptable rate are presumed to be receiving proper nutrition. However, both the quantity and quality of the milk decrease as lactation progresses, while the foal's body size and nutrient requirements increase. Assuming that approximately 35 pounds of milk are consumed at the peak of lactation, mare's milk may only provide half the energy, protein, and mineral needs of the foal. Additional nutrients needed to meet the requirements for growth come from the nutrient stores acquired during the last trimester of gestation, as well as from consumption of grain (creep feeds) and hay.

Foals that are thin or that appear to be developing bone problems should receive supplemental feed. This can be easily accomplished by tying the mare and foal in separate corners of their stall and providing separate feed to each. Alternatively a **creep feeder** (a feeder to which the foal but not the mare has access) may be provided.

Supplemental feed also helps prepare the foal for the dietary change that will occur at weaning. Before 4 months of age, up to a pound of milk-based pellet should be included as part of the supplement. Research suggests that the foal's digestive system is better able to digest milk-based than grain-based feeds early in life. If the region has a history of bone problems such as epiphysitis, osteochondrosis, or contracted tendons in its foals, the copper, manganese, and zinc concentrations in the foal's feed may be increased, based on local recommendations. Water, an appropriate calcium phosphate supplement if necessary, and iodized salt also should be available free-choice. Horse owners should not permit creep-fed foals to become obese during this time as this tends to aggravate limb problems. This is particularly true if the foal has relatively straight (upright) pasterns. Maintaining growing horses at a body condition closer to 4 than to 5 (*see* TABLE 1 in CHAPTER 6, "EQUINE NUTRITIONAL REQUIREMENTS," page 76) and providing plenty of exercise is cheap and effective insurance against many of the bone disorders that can afflict foals.

WEANLINGS

Foals usually are weaned at 4–6 months of age. By this time most growing horses are able to consume 6–8 pounds of grain and 4–5 pounds of hay daily. As mentioned in the previous chapter, surveys conducted by Ohio State University have suggested that a greater concentration of copper, manganese, and zinc, rather than an increase in total food, energy, or protein intake, may help promote the health and integrity of growing cartilage and bone. Feeding weanling diets containing the nutrient concentrations shown in Table 1 have been found helpful on farms where bone and cartilage disorders have been a problem.

YEARLINGS AND TWO-YEAR-OLDS

Because the young horse continues to grow through its second and third years (as illustrated in FIGURE 1), it is important to continue supplying adequate nutrition to support this growth. Excellent-quality hay should always be fed to eliminate reliance on large amounts of supplemental feed to make up for dietary deficiencies. When a large proportion of the diet consists of grain products, the rate of passage of food through the intestinal tract is increased, with a concomitant decrease in nutrient digestibility and absorption. At this age most horses will be consuming a diet that is 50% hay and 50% grain by weight. Horses should be permitted to exercise freely every day to encourage proper muscular and skeletal development. As with the earlier growth phases, a body condition of less than 5 should be maintained if possible.

Feeding Horses for Performance

Increasing interest in equine exercise physiology has renewed research efforts in the area of nutrition and the equine athlete. Surveys of feeding practices at both Thoroughbred and Standardbred tracks indicate that 35–42 megacalories (mcal) of digestible energy per day were fed to horses in training. Feed intake ranged from 28 to 33 pounds of grain and hay

Table 1
Approximate Feeding Schedule for Orphan Foals

Age	Milk replacer	Milk-based pellets	Grain mix	Hay
Birth to 2 weeks	3–4 oz/lb body wt. per day, divided into 2 feedings	0	0	0
2–4 weeks	"	½ lb per day	0	¼ flake
4–6 weeks	"	1 lb per day	0	½ flake
6–8 weeks (2 mo.)	STOP	2 lbs per day	½ lb per day	1–1½ flake
8–16 weeks	0	Decrease	Increas	
16 weeks (4 mo.)	0	STOP	2 lbs per day	
24 weeks (6 mo.)	0	0	6–7 lbs per day	

Clean fresh water and trace-mineralized salt should be available at all times.

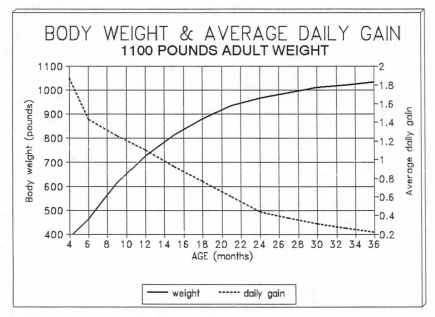

Figure 1. Body weight and average daily gain of growing horses.

per day, roughly 2.5–3.5% of body weight. The proportion of grain in the diet was close to 45% of total intake.

The increased feed intake necessary to meet energy needs should contain sufficient quantities of all other nutrients needed by performance horses. Although protein, mineral, and vitamin needs are increased by performance, the increases are not greater than the rise in energy needs. Feeding supplements of these nutrients is expensive, rarely necessary, and of benefit primarily to the manufacturers of the supplements. The money often would be better spent on better-quality feed, training, and genetics.

A trace-mineralized salt block should be available at all times to replenish minerals lost in the sweat. **Hematinics** (compounds that improve the quality of the blood: "blood builders") containing high levels of iron are rarely necessary; iron deficiency in horses is uncommon owing to the high levels of iron already present in conventional feedstuffs. Such products are no substitute for appropriate husbandry and veterinary care.

Feeding the Older Horse

Many horses, like other animals and people in our society, are living longer as a consequence of improved nutrition and health care. No definition of "old" is applicable to all horses, because variation abounds among individual animals. As the saying goes, "It's not so much the age as the mileage." The physical signs of aging—decreased activity and/or loss of hearing and eyesight—are more reliable indicators of advanced age in any particular horse than is its chronological age. The presence of these signs reflects a diminution of the reserve capacities that allow young animals to adapt readily to changes in their environment.

If older horses are healthy and their teeth are properly cared for, dietary changes are usually not necessary. Closer attention should be paid to food intake, however. The increased risk of health problems in older animals makes once- or twice-daily hand-feeding advisable. An unexplained decrease in food intake could be an early sign of disease that should be investigated. Spontaneous activity often decreases in older animals, so their feed intake should be adjusted accordingly in order to avoid obesity. Activity should be encouraged in older horses, however, for the beneficial effects on well-being that exercise provides.

Feeding Orphan Foals

It is occasionally necessary for the horse owner to raise a foal in the absence of its mother. Orphan foals must be strong, vigorous, and healthy to resist disease early in life. They should receive at least 2 pints of high-quality **colostrum** (the mare's first milk, which contains important *antibodies* necessary to protect the foal from infection) *within the first twelve hours of life*. The mare's best-quality colostrum is produced in the first 8 hours after foaling. If colostrum feeding is delayed beyond 24 hours, a transfusion of **plasma** (the fluid portion of the blood, containing antibodies among other things) to the foal may be necessary.

Orphan foals may be fed by a nursemare or trained to drink from a bucket. Most nursemares are excellent mothers, and feeding is less labor-intensive once the foal and mare have been **grafted** (bonded). Nursemares are used for foals that are older than 2 weeks of age and that will not readily accept milk replacers. A nursemare will protect the foal, provide plenty of milk, and can be turned out with other mares and their foals to introduce the orphan to the "rules of equine etiquette." The major disadvantages of nursemares are their cost and limited availability.

Feeding foals from buckets is simple and inexpensive, requiring only a small amount of time to mix formula and clean buckets. A separate area for exercise should also be provided if other horses are present. Turning out orphan foals with the herd often results in injury to the foals as they attempt to find a mother.

There are several milk replacers available that have been used to raise young foals successfully. The cold calf formulas have been popular owing to their availability, low cost, and acceptability by foals. Lamb milk replacers and goat's milk also have been used, and products designed specifically for foals have recently become available. Veal-calf replacers should not be fed, owing to their low iron content (*anemia*—low red blood cell count—has been observed in foals fed these products) and to the antibiotics present in some formulas.

A kitchen whisk is very valuable for mixing powdered milk replacers. Dissolve the powder in a small quantity of hot water and mix to the consistency of thin pancake batter (to reduce the lumps and shorten preparation time), mixing only what is needed for each feeding. Once a replacer is chosen one should stick with it unless problems arise, because switching formulas often causes the foal to develop diarrhea. Foals generally consume about 20 percent of their body weight in milk each day; this will be approximately 3–4 ounces per pound of body weight. One gallon is approximately 128 ounces which is adequate for about 40 pounds of body weight.

The foal can be trained to drink from a bucket by encouraging it to nurse on a finger as its head is directed toward the milk. Offer milk in a bucket after the foal has been alone for approximately 4 hours (hungry foals become very cooperative and learn quickly). A plastic pail containing about 2 gallons of lukewarm milk may be offered during the first attempt. Persistence is the key. Hang the bucket on the wall at the level of the foal's chest and work with the foal frequently until it attempts to drink on its own. Tipping the bucket toward the foal will help it to make contact with the milk. Once the foal has consumed some milk leave it alone, but observe it occasionally to be sure it is drinking. As the foal begins to drink on its own, milk can be fed at room temperature twice a day. Begin with 1 gallon per feeding and increase "to appetite" (as the foal's appetite improves or increases). Any milk not consumed should be discarded and the bucket scrubbed clean after each feeding.

The foal's feces may be soft initially as the intestinal tract adapts to the diet. As long as the foal appears to be healthy and is gaining weight there should be no difficulty with diarrhea. If the foal becomes depressed, decreases its milk intake, develops a fever, or appears bloated or exhibits abdominal pain, a veterinarian should be summoned immediately.

Fresh water and free-choice iodized, trace-mineralized salt should be available at all times. Small quantities (¼ **flake**, a unit of baled hay weighing between 5 and 10 pounds) of a good legume or mixed grass-legume hay may be provided beginning at 2 weeks of age, along with a milk-based pellet (Table 1). Milk-based pellets can be started at ½ pound per day and increased by ½-pound increments up to 2 pounds per day. Pellets can be put into the milk for the first day or two to stimulate consumption. By 2 months of age milk consumption can be decreased or stopped altogether, but milk-based pellets should remain a staple of the diet for the first 3–4 months of life. Hay may be increased by ½ to 1 flake during this period.

Once the foal reaches 2 pounds of milk-based pellet feed per day, ½-pound increments of a 16–18% crude protein creep feed may be fed as described previously. Feeding of milk-based pellets can be discontinued when the foal is 12–16 weeks old. There is no benefit to feeding milk-based feeds to older foals. At about 12 weeks begin decreasing the milk-based pellet by ½ pound per week, replacing it with grain. Hay intake should be increased to 1 or 1½ flakes per day.

By 12 weeks of age foals may be eating 3–4 pounds of feed per day. By 6 months, 6–7 pounds of grain and 1–1½ flakes of hay per day may be consumed. If foals are fed in groups they should be observed daily. Sick or submissive foals may not eat within the group, but may gorge themselves on grain when able to eat. Foals should not be permitted to become fat or "slick"; this is frequently a problem in young horses destined for halter futurities.

Foals, including orphans, should have *plenty of exercise* to encourage growth and skeletal development. Orphan foals should be put with other foals of similar age as soon as possible to encourage bonding with other horses. Some owners may wean another foal early (3 months of age) as a companion to an orphan foal, while others allow the orphan to come into contact with dam-reared foals through the fence of a neighboring paddock, and then pair the orphan with the other foals at weaning time.

CHAPTER 8

Diseases of Dietary Origin

by C.A. Tony Buffington

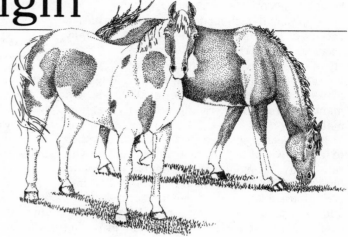

A variety of nutrition-related diseases occur in horses. These disorders may be caused by an inappropriate diet or improper feeding practices, or may be the result of a genetic predisposition. Various combinations of these factors may be involved in any individual case. Unfortunately, many diseases of dietary origin in the horse are not well understood.

This chapter presents descriptions of some of the more common diseases of dietary origin afflicting horses. Included in the descriptions are the presenting clinical signs and strategies for prevention. Once dietary disorders occur they may be difficult or even impossible to treat, and some may be fatal. Fortunately, all are preventable by feeding an appropriate diet in a proper manner.

Diseases of Dietary Origin in Foals

Diet-related diseases caused by deficiencies, toxicities, or nutrient imbalances usually occur during periods of greatest nutritional stress, e.g., rapid growth in foals. The common diseases of growing foals include nutritional secondary hyperparathyroidism, developmental orthopedic disease, and contracted tendons.

NUTRITIONAL SECONDARY HYPERPARATHYROIDISM

Nutritional secondary hyperparathyroidism is caused by an imbalance in the quantities of calcium and phosphorus in the diet. Diets rich in organic phosphorus and low in calcium can trigger the release of *parathyroid hormone* (**PTH**) from the parathyroid glands. The action of PTH is to stimulate the removal of calcium from the bones in an attempt to maintain normal blood levels of this mineral. The calcium lost from the bone is replaced not by calcium but by connective tissue, resulting in an enlargement of the bones of the head. Because of this abnormality the disease is often called *big head*. Another common name is *miller's disease*, because the disorder historically was often observed in horses owned by wheat millers, who fed their animals large quantities of bran. The disease is easily preventable by ensuring that growing animals consume appropriate amounts of calcium and phosphorus. Because horses, like other animals, cannot choose a balanced diet if individual nutrients are provided separately, it is important that these nutrients be balanced in the feed and that consumption be monitored to assure an appropriate intake. (*See* Chapter 7, "Feeding Horses.")

Developmental Orthopedic Disease

Developmental orthopedic disease describes a variety of bone abnormalities that occasionally occur in young, rapidly growing horses. A variety of causes have been reported—environmental, genetic, and nutritional. It is likely that there is no one single cause in all cases, i.e., many factors may interact to produce an abnormality.

It has been suggested that excessive amounts of feed provided to foals to achieve rapid growth rates may promote developmental orthopedic disease. It also has been suggested that deficiencies of trace minerals, including copper, zinc, and manganese, may play a role. Whatever the cause, sufficient evidence exists that providing moderate quantities of a nutritionally balanced diet is the best insurance against diet-induced developmental orthopedic disease. Significantly, there is no evidence to suggest that foals must be fed large quantities of feed and maintain rapid rates of growth in order to achieve their maximal final size as adults. Young horses that maintain a lean body condition through appropriate amounts of feed and exercise appear to have the best chance of avoiding diet-induced orthopedic diseases. (*See* Chapter 22, "The Musculoskeletal System and Various Disorders.")

Contracted Tendons

Contracted tendons in foals have been associated with rapid growth rates and **high planes of nutrition** (large quantities of high-energy, low-fiber feed, e.g., oats or barley). Contracted tendons can develop quite rapidly; a concavity can develop in the hoof wall and the heel begin to rise within 24 hours. The name "contracted tendons" refers to an apparent contraction of the flexor tendons of the foot. In actuality it is more likely that development of the flexor apparatus does not develop at the same rate as the rest of the limb, resulting in a pointed-toe appearance.

As with developmental orthopedic disease, contracted tendons are best prevented by providing moderate amounts of feed and exercise. When mares and foals are confined to stalls for long periods of time, it is particularly important to monitor their food intake closely to avoid overfeeding. (*See* Chapter 22, "The Musculoskeletal System and Various Disorders.")

Diseases of Dietary Origin in Horses of Any Age

Ingestion of Poisonous Plants

A wide variety of plants may be poisonous to horses. Toxic plants grow in most areas of the country. It is important for horse owners to develop the ability to recognize poisonous plants in their own area, because some horses will not avoid consuming them. Information concerning recognition and management of toxic plant growth can be obtained from local veterinarians and agricultural extension agents. (*See* Chapter 41, "Poisonous Plants.")

Some of the more common poisonous plants in the western United States include the common groundsel (*Senecio vulgaris*), which can cause permanent liver damage, and yellow star thistle (*Centaurea soltitialis*), which affects the brain. Oleander (*Nerium oleander*), a common ornamental in the west, is highly toxic to horses, causing convulsions, diarrhea, colic, irregular heartbeat, and death.

The yew (*Taxus* spp.), a common ornamental plant in many areas of the country, is sufficiently toxic that consumption of only 3 or 4 ounces of the plant may cause death by stopping the heart. Another common ornamental plant toxic to horses is the horsetail (*Equisetum* spp.), which can produce a deficiency of vitamin B_1. Signs of horsetail intoxication include weakness, decreased appetite, and loss of coordination. The seeds of a number of legumes, such as some beans and peas, also can be toxic for horses. The clinical signs depend on the toxin in the particular seed and may involve many organ systems. A variety of sorghum plants, such as Sudan grass (*Sorghum vulgare*), can cause incoordination and staggering as well as bladder inflammation.

Ingestion of tall fescue (*Festuca arundinacea*) by pregnant mares can result in a variety of reproductive disorders, including abortion, difficulties during birth, thickened or retained fetal membranes, depressed milk production, and an increased risk of foal death. The problem with fescue is actually not the plant itself but a fungus that grows on the plant. Identification and removal of infected plants are necessary to prevent the disease. Pastures should be replanted with fungus-free fescue seed. Another disease-causing fungus associated with plants is ergot (*Claviceps* spp.), which infects the seeds of a variety of cereal grains (rye, oats, wheat) and can cause abortion, **gangrene** (death and decay of tissue, usually caused by loss of blood supply and subsequent invasion by bacteria), and neurologic disorders. Another fungus, *Aspergillus flavus*, produces a toxin (**aflatoxin**) in grains and peanuts, causing decreased growth and severe liver disease.

In general, the signs of plant intoxication depend on the particular plant and the amount of toxin ingested. Preventing exposure to poisonous plants is the best defense against their toxic effects. If consumption of a toxic plant is suspected, a veterinarian should be consulted immediately.

Blister Beetle Poisoning
A common insect poisoning of horses is caused by consumption of hay infested with blister beetles (*Epicauta* spp.). Blister beetle poisoning usually occurs during the late summer in the western and southwestern states, where the swarming insects infest alfalfa hay pastures. A toxin in the beetle, called **cantharidin**, is absorbed and excreted in the horse's urine, causing severe irritation and inflammation of the digestive and urinary tracts. After consuming infested hay, horses may develop abdominal pain (**colic**) and may play continuously in their water. Other signs include increased temperature and heart and respiratory rates, together with depression, sweating, and diarrhea. Prevention is by avoidance of hay cut in areas known to be infested with blister beetles, and by purchasing hay at pre-bloom stage (blister beetles apparently are attracted by alfalfa flowers).

Monensin Toxicity
A feed additive called **monensin**, commmonly used to increase feed efficiency in cattle and poultry, is toxic for horses. Clinical signs of toxicity include decreased feed intake and mild colic. When larger amounts of monensin are consumed, the horse becomes weak, staggers, sweats profusely, and eventually is unable to rise. With large overdoses death may occur within 12–24 hours. Monensin toxicity is best avoided by ensuring that horses are not fed grains that are formulated for cattle or poultry or that have been processed with equipment at feed mills where such mixes have been recently used.

Diet-related Allergies
Diet-related allergies also occasionally occur in horses. Horses may become sensitized to *allergens* (substances inducing allergy) in soybeans, grains, bran, or molds present in feed. Signs of diet-related allergies are not specific and may include *urticaria* (acute, usually localized skin swellings caused by an increased permeability of capillaries, producing a net outflow of fluid into the tissue spaces: "hives"), rashes, diarrhea, and *dyspnea* (difficulty breathing). As in other species, allergies in horses are treated by avoidance of the causative allergen(s).

OBESITY, COLIC, AND LAMINITIS ("FOUNDER")
Nutritional problems more commonly associated with feeding practices rather than the diet itself include obesity, colic, and *laminitis* ("founder").

Obesity Although many horses are overweight, the health significance of this condition in the equine species is unknown. In other animals (and in people) a variety of medical problems have been linked to obesity; fortunately, most obesity-related diseases are not commonly seen in horses. Overweight horses do seem to be less exercise- and heat-tolerant and more prone to founder than horses of normal weight, however. Obesity will also increase the risks of surgery should it be necessary for any reason.

Although horses may gain weight for a variety of reasons, the most common seems to be lack of attention by the owner to the animal's body condition, combined with a lack of exercise and access to large quantities of palatable feed. Inexperienced horse owners often mistakenly believe that their animals should receive a fixed amount of food daily, regardless of the animals' environment or level of exercise. Horses are more appropriately fed by adjusting their intake to maintain body condition at approximately 4 to 6 on the body-condition scoring system, depending on one's personal preference (*see* CHAPTER 6, "EQUINE NUTRITIONAL REQUIREMENTS," and CHAPTER 7, "FEEDING HORSES").

Inactive adult horses often are fed a variety of concentrated feeds and treats in addition to their usual roughage ration. Such animals often need little more than access to fresh water, a good-quality grass hay, and an appropriately formulated trace-mineralized salt. Additional feed should be provided *at the expense of* a portion of this diet, rather than *in addition to* it. Moreover, if highly palatable grains or concentrates are provided with relatively unpalatable forage, horses may consume them instead of the forage. In many species of animals obesity is a notoriously difficult problem to treat, often because it requires changing deeply entrenched habits and beliefs on the part of the owner regarding diet and feeding practices. Obesity is a problem that is more easily prevented by feeding "to the eye of the master" rather than the fullness of the hayrack and grain bucket, and by avoiding a relationship with a horse based largely on provision of large quantities of food treats and rewards above and beyond the animal's normal diet.

Colic Another common disease of horses that can be caused by diet is **colic**, i.e., abdominal pain. A horse with colic appears restless and uncomfortable, and may look at or paw its abdomen. In more severe cases animals lie down and stand up repeatedly or roll and thrash on the ground. Heart and respiratory rates may increase and the horse may sweat. *A veterinarian should be called as soon as these clinical signs are recognized.* Colic can be caused by many different conditions, including twists of the intestine, parasitic worms, disease of any abdominal organ, and diet. (*See* CHAPTER 26, "THE DIGESTIVE SYSTEM AND VARIOUS DISORDERS.")

Diet-related types of colic include gas colic, impaction colic, sand colic, and spasmodic colic. **Gas colic** is caused by overconsumption of lush grass feed, resulting in excessive gas production in the intestine. **Impaction colic**, due to blockage of the intestine, can result from sudden changes in feed, excessive consumption of grain or lush pasture, or by ingestion of foreign material. Ingested grain or grass may produce by-products that suppress the normal movements of the intestinal wall, while foreign material, such as wood chewed from fences, can become lodged in the intestine and block the passage of gut contents. **Sand colic** occurs when horses are fed on the ground in areas where the soil is sandy, or when they develop the vice of eating soil. **Spasmodic colic** is characterized by increased numbers of bowel movements and episodes of pain following sudden changes in environmental temperature, diet, or activity level. These diet-related causes of colic, like those of other diet-related disorders, are more successfully prevented than treated.

Laminitis ("Founder") Excessive consumption of grains can also cause founder (laminitis). Depending on severity, horses with founder may be reluctant to move and appear to "walk on eggs" when forced to move. The foot often is warm to the touch and the horse may appear anxious and tremble. The underlying cause is swelling (inflammation) of the tissue between the foot bone and the wall of the hoof. When this soft tissue swells, it is compressed between the hard underlying bone and the overlying hoof. If the swelling is severe, blood flow to the hoof may cease and the tissue may die. When this happens the foot bone becomes disconnected from the hoof and may rotate downward, while the tip of the hoof curls upward. (*See* CHAPTER 22, "THE MUSCULOSKELETAL SYSTEM AND VARIOUS DISORDERS.")

Many cases of founder are unrelated to nutrition; such cases may be the result of running on hard ground, abortion, high fever, infections, or exposure to certain drugs. Nutritional causes of founder include rapid consumption of excessive amounts of grain, cold water after exercise, or lush grass or legume pastures. *If one of these circumstances has occurred, a veterinarian should be called at once (before signs develop) to care for the animal.*

Like obesity, founder can be difficult to treat and is better prevented. Locking up grains, cooling horses out before permitting them access to water, feeding hay to decrease appetite before horses are turned out onto lush pastures, and restricting access to such pastures, should prevent most diet-related cases of founder.

Conclusion

Horses have been designed by nature to be relatively continuous consumers of plants over relatively large areas of land. Many American horses currently are kept in environments of unusually high feed quality and nutrient density, with unusually restricted opportunities for exercise—similar to the situation faced by many American people! These are precisely the circumstances that will increase the likelihood of diet-related diseases. Effective prevention requires an understanding of the causes of these diseases and vigilance to see that opportunities for their development are not presented.

PART IV

Reproduction

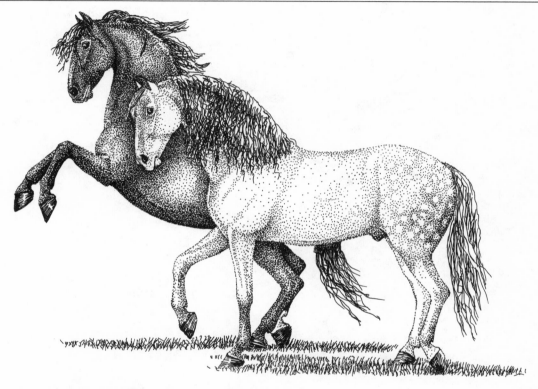

Round-hoof'd, short-jointed, fetlocks shag and long,
Broad breast, full eye, small head and nostril wide,
High crest, short ears, straight legs and passing strong,
Thin mane, thick tail, broad buttock, tender hide:
Look, what a horse should have he did not lack,
Save a proud rider on so proud a back.

—WILLIAM SHAKESPEARE
VENUS AND ADONIS, PREFACE

CHAPTER 9

Reproductive Physiology

by John P. Hughes

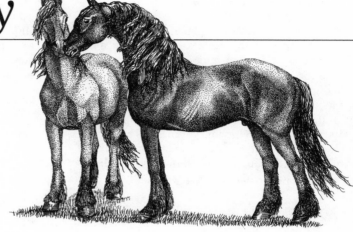

The Normal Mare

The reproductive system of the mare consists of the *vulva*, *clitoris*, *vagina*, *cervix*, *uterus*, the paired **oviducts** (also known as the **uterine** or **fallopian tubes**), the paired *ovaries*, and the **mammary glands** (one mammary gland for each of two teats, and each of four quarters). (*See* CHAPTER 16, "ANATOMY.") The **cervix** acts as a barrier to the entry of contaminants into the uterus, as do the constrictor muscles of the vulva and vagina. The **uterus** consists of a *body* and two **uterine horns** arranged in a "Y" or "T" form, and is suspended from the upper abdominal wall by the **broad ligaments**. The ovaries are attached along the forward border of the broad ligaments, near the tips of the uterine horns, and so are quite mobile.

Some mares will mate with a stallion during any season of the year, but on the whole mares must be classified as **seasonal breeders**. Puberty normally occurs by 18 months of age but has been reported as early as 10–12 months. Light has a major influence on the mare's **estrous cycle,** the recurrent, rhythmic cycle of sexual receptivity that is characteristic of most female mammals. The mare responds to increasing periods of light in the spring by slowly establishing cyclic ovarian activity, and to decreasing periods of light in the winter by slowly terminating ovarian activity. During **estrus** ("heat") the mare **ovulates** (releases an egg from the ovary), secretes a watery, lubricating fluid into the lower genital tract, and becomes sexually receptive to the male. The egg passes down into the oviduct, where fertilization with **sperm** (male reproductive cells) from the stallion takes place. The fertilized egg or **zygote** moves down the uterine tube and thence into the uterus by day 6 post-ovulation. It then migrates throughout the uterus until about day 16, when it becomes fixed at the base of either the left or right uterine horn.

In California the physiological breeding season extends from April through October. The length of the estrous cycle averages 21–22 days, with estrus itself lasting for 5–7 days and ovulation occurring 24–48 hours before the end of estrus.

A major problem in equine reproduction is that breed associations have imposed a breeding season on mares that does not necessarily coincide with the physiological breeding season. The "universal birthdate" of January 1 results in the start of a breeding season in February which is not the physiological season for mares. Only 20–25% of mares develop signs of heat and ovulate in January and February; by contrast, fully 90+% of estrous periods occurring during the summer months result in ovulation. The farther north or south of the equator one is, the more pronounced is the absence of ovarian activity during the winter months.

Irregularities in the estrous cycle of the mare, while strongly tied to season, are also affected by nutrition and climatic factors. Variations in patterns of cyclic behavior can include an erratic cycle length, erratic estrous behavior, failure of ovulation, and failure to develop ovarian **follicles** (egg precursor forms in the ovaries).

The Ovarian Cycle

Mares can be classified into three general groups on the basis of estrous behavioral patterns and season. Neither breed, nor size, nor genetic makeup determine which category a mare falls into. Considerable overlap exists in both behavior and ovarian activity among these three groups.

Polyestrous mares
A few mares cycle regularly throughout the year, i.e., they are **polyestrous**. While there may be some variability in the duration of the estrous cycle and its component elements, particularly in winter, the variation is within normal limits. On occasion the cervix may fail to relax or secretions may remain scant or sticky, particularly at the end of the winter period.

Seasonally polyestrous mares
Mares in this group have a definite cyclic period and a rather definite noncyclic or **anestrous** period. There is a transitional phase coming out of winter anestrus that may be prolonged, and during which the degree of intensity of sexual receptivity varies until **standing heat** (the full behavioral signs of estrus) with ovulation is observed. A regular cyclic ovulatory pattern is

then established following this ovulation. The noncyclic or **anovulatory** period varies greatly in length (40–120 days, rarely as long as 8 months) and in the month of occurrence, so far as individual mares are concerned. The response of mares when teased during anestrus may vary considerably. Anestrous mares with little if any ovarian follicular activity often respond passively to the stallion, neither rejecting nor participating in his advances. Upon **vaginoscopic** examination (visual examination of the female reproductive tract, with the aid of a viewing instrument), the cervix appears pale, free of mucus, and in some instances is partly to fully dilated. Other mares have considerable ovarian activity during winter anestrus, with ovarian follicles growing to moderate size and then regressing, to be replaced by others. These mares actively resist the advances of the stallion. The cervix is pale, dry, tight, and sticky.

Once they begin to come out of the winter anestrus, some mares may start cycling abruptly. More commonly, however, there is a prolonged period during which the degree of sexual receptivity varies until an intense standing heat is evident. Mares will stand to be covered by a stallion for periods of 15–60 days or more during this phase. The ovaries during these periods of prolonged heat may have little if any detectable follicular development, or they may have small follicles, a few larger ones, and finally one or two follicles that progress to ovulation.

Seasonally polyestrous mares with erratic reproductive patterns
This group includes mares exhibiting irregularities in all characteristics of the estrous cycle in winter and early spring. Irregularities may include heat without ovulation, ovulation without heat, variations in length of the estrous cycle and heat, intensity of heat, and variable responses to the stallion when teased.

It is important to remember that mares in anestrus, mares in prolonged estrus, mares in the transitional phase of erratic reproductive behavior from winter anestrus to regular cyclic ovarian activity, and mares with a prolonged *corpus luteum* (*see* below)—though not a pathologic state—are all in a nonfertile condition.

Given time, such mares will eventually resume regular patterns of estrous cycling.

ESTRUS

The reproductive cycle of the mare is more easily understood if it is divided into a **follicular phase** (or **estrus**) and a **luteal phase** (or **diestrus**). The follicular phase is characterized by the growth of follicles in the ovary, their secretion of the hormone **estrogen**, and by signs of sexual receptivity in the mare. The length of time a mare is in heat decreases from February through June, with a shortening of the interval from the onset of estrus to ovulation.

Determination of estrous behavior in the mare by use of a teaser stallion is one of the most important functions of broodmare management. Teasing should be carried out daily or every other day using a stallion with good **libido** (sexual drive). There are a number of different teasing methods. Mares can be teased in a stock, at a teasing bar, or even in some instances out in the pasture. Whatever the method, each mare must be teased as an individual, unless she breaks down with the usual signs of estrus at sight or sound of the stallion. A common practice is to put a stallion in a pen or stall in one corner of the paddock, so that mares can come up to him and exhibit signs of estrus of their own volition. (*See* CHAPTER 10, "BREEDING MANAGEMENT.")

The usual response of the mare in heat is one of interest in, and acceptance of, the stallion. Although there may be an initial rejection of the teaser, most mares accept his advances without agitation. In a typical estrous mare the tail is elevated without switching, the legs are spread apart, the pelvis is flexed, and kicking at the stallion is not observed. The lips of the vulva contract and relax, accompanied by urination and eversion of the **clitoris** (the female equivalent of the penis). The mare stands to be mounted by the stallion. Behavioral changes of less intensity are often observed just before and after true heat.

During the luteal phase (diestrus), the ovarian follicles grow and regress. Those destined for ovulation begin to increase in size and become prominent before the mare comes into heat.

Usually only one follicle continues to grow to ovulatory size (35–60 mm, average of 45 mm), but on occasion two or more follicles may grow at a similar rate so that a double ovulation occurs. Occasionally, a follicle will rupture when a second smaller (20–30 mm) follicle is on one of the ovaries. The second follicle will then grow rapidly and be released 24–48 or more hours later.

In a group of mares studied at the University of California, Davis, multiple ovulations were found to occur approximately 25 percent of the time. Some mares have a much greater tendency for multiple ovulation than do other mares. The interval between multiple ovulations averages 1 day, but it is not uncommon for it to be 2 or 3 days. Multiple ovulations are not significantly different between the same and opposite ovaries, and there is no reason to believe that multiple ovulations appearing on the same ovary are not just as likely to result in twins as are multiple ovulations occurring on opposite ovaries. Most mares ovulate within 48 hours prior to the end of estrus, usually between the hours of 4:00 P.M. and 8:00 A.M.

Failure of ovulation during the physiological breeding season is rare. Ovulatory failure during estrus is most often observed at the onset of winter anestrus. Ovulation without estrus during the follicular phase occasionally occurs, most often in mares with a young foal.

Estrogens secreted by the follicle are responsible for sexual receptivity (**heat**). They are also responsible for changes in the female reproductive tract that permit passage and transport of the sperm, and they have a role in initiating the release of **luteinizing hormone (LH)** from the brain's **pituitary gland,** which leads to ovulation. These events all must take place according to a defined time sequence if mating is to occur and sperm from the stallion are to be available when the mature egg reaches the oviduct. Failure of any one or combination of these events, or of timing, can result in **infertility** (diminished ability to produce offspring). The rate of failure is greatly affected by seasonal changes.

Characteristic visual changes in the female reproductive tract are noted during estrus. While considerable variation exists among mares, individual mares are fairly consistent. Usually, just prior to or at the onset of estrus, the cervix undergoes a progressive softening and relaxation, increases in color from pale to shades of pink or red, becomes **edematous** (swollen), and its secretions become more abundant and fluid in consistency.

(In a few mares the cervix fails to relax during heat. Such a condition may contribute to infertility.)

While the greatest degree of cervical change usually occurs near ovulation, such changes are sometimes present either earlier or later; thus, these physical changes alone are not an accurate indication of the time of ovulation. Within 5 days after ovulation the cervix reverts to its diestrus condition. The best estimate of when to breed a mare is derived from a combination of factors:

- The behavior of the mare when teased by the stallion
- The condition of the cervix when **palpated** (felt with the hands) and viewed with a **speculum** (viewing instrument)
- Follicle development on the ovary as determined by palpation and **ultrasonography** (noninvasive diagnostic technique for visualizing internal body structures by means of sound [echo] reflections; also called **ultrasound**).

DIESTRUS

Each ovarian follicle, after discharging its egg, matures rapidly into a hormone-producing **corpus luteum** (plural = **corpora lutea**) before eventually degenerating. The diestrous phase of the estrous cycle is initiated by ovulation and the formation of the corpus luteum, which secretes the hormone **progesterone**. Diestrus in the horse averages 15 days in length and is characterized by active resistance of the mare to a teaser stallion. The mare often will lay her ears back, wring her tail, squeal, bite and kick at the stallion. Some mares may be only slightly agitated, however, and then only when aggressively teased.

The corpus luteum has a functional life span of about 14 days. Progesterone secreted by the corpus luteum takes the mare out of heat and is responsible for sealing the uterus off from the outside world and preparing its tissues for the support of pregnancy, should it occur. During diestrus the cervix is tightly constricted, white in color, with no swelling and only a scanty amount of viscous mucus present. Mares will ovulate during the diestrous phase of the estrous cycle, but these ovulations are not accompanied by signs of estrus, while the cervix remains pale, dry, tight, and sticky.

On occasion, after ovulation the cavity of the collapsed follicle continues to fill with blood and forms what is termed a **hematoma**. Hematomas may reach a size of 10–12 cm and can persist beyond the next ovulation without affecting cycle length. One must be careful not to confuse a hematoma occurring after ovulation—and which occasionally persists for several months—with an ovarian tumor. For diagnostic purposes it is important to recognize that a mare with a hematoma of the ovary will continue to cycle normally, while a mare with an ovarian tumor of any duration seldom if ever cycles normally.

Hormonal control of the estrous cycle involves a complex series of biochemical reactions leading ultimately to ovulation. Briefly, **gonadotropin-releasing hormone (GnRH)** produced by the **hypothalamus** area of the brain acts on the pituitary gland to release LH and **follicle-stimulating hormone (FSH)**. These two hormones, along with **inhibin** and **prostaglandin**, control the development of ovarian follicles, ovulation, and the formation of corpora lutea. The follicle produces estrogen, which peaks just before ovulation and is accompanied by inhibin. Inhibin suppresses FSH and is probably responsible for inhibiting the growth and ovulation of follicles other than the dominant one present during estrus. LH not only assists in bringing follicles to maturity and ovulation but also plays a role in the formation of the corpus luteum. Regression of the corpus luteum in the nonpregnant mare is brought about by **prostaglandin PGF2$_a$** released from the uterus.

It is not uncommon for the corpus luteum to fail to regress at the expected time, resulting in persistence of the luteal phase. Spontaneous prolongation of the corpus luteum can last for as long as 2–3 months before regression finally occurs and ovarian cyclicity is re-initiated. A prolonged corpus luteum is an important clinical problem, since the mare will fail to cycle normally or exhibit signs of heat as long as the corpus luteum remains active. Injection of prostaglandin $PGF2_a$ or one of its synthetic analogs is the treatment of choice to cause regression of a persistent corpus luteum.

The Normal Stallion

The reproductive system of the stallion consists of the *penis*; the paired **testes** or **testicles** (in which the sperm are produced); the **scrotum** (dependent pouch of skin containing the testicles); the **vas deferens** (one in each testicle; the duct that serves as a transport conduit for the sperm from the testis to the urethra [*see* below]); the **epididymis** (one in each testicle; the duct that connects the vas deferens to the testis); the paired **seminal vesicles** (pouches attached to the urinary bladder); the paired **bulbourethral glands** (located near the ischial arch); and the **prostate gland,** which surrounds the urethra where it joins the bladder.

The testes are the site of production of **testosterone,** the major sex hormone of the male. The **prepuce** or *sheath* is a protective fold of skin that encloses the penis in its nonerect state. The **urethra,** a long hollow tube, runs through the penis from its origin at the neck of the bladder and serves to transport urine to the exterior. It also acts as the final conduit for the **semen**, the thick, milky white fluid containing sperm that is deposited in the female's vagina during an **ejaculation.** The sperm or *spermatozoa* are produced in the **seminiferous tubules** within the testes but are incapable of fertilizing an egg until they mature and become motile in the epididymis, where they are stored until ejaculation.

The mare and stallion each contribute 50 percent of the genetic makeup of their offspring. The stallion however is usually mated to many mares and therefore his overall contribution to the genetic pool is more than that con-

tributed by a single mare. Puberty in the stallion usually is attained by 18–20 months of age, with sexual maturity occurring at about 3.5 to 4 years of age.

Season affects the reproductive activity of the stallion but not to the same degree observed in the mare. The stallion will mate with mares at any time of the year; however semen volume, sperm concentration, and total number of sperm are lowest in January and February. These parameters gradually increase in the spring and peak in June, with sperm output increasing almost 50 percent during this period.

Stallions should possess good libido to mate with a mare. Erection of the penis, mounting, **intromission** (insertion of the penis), copulatory movements followed by ejaculation, relaxation of the penis, and dismounting from the mare should all occur in an orderly manner. A lack of desire to mount the mare, failure to obtain an erection, failure to ejaculate, dismounting and remounting numerous times before ejaculation, or ejaculation while dismounting from the mare are undesirable traits in a breeding stallion and can be difficult to overcome.

Spermatogenesis is the process whereby sperm cells within the testes of the stallion undergo cell divisions and cellular changes that result in the production of mature spermatozoa. The process occurs in a cyclical pattern with a total duration of about 57 days. Because another 4–8 days are required for the sperm to travel through the epididymis, a total of about 61–65 days are needed for spermatozoa to develop to the point of ejaculation.

Testosterone is produced by specialized cells within the testes called **Leydig cells** and is under the control of LH from the pituitary gland. GnRH from the hypothalamus influences the pituitary to produce LH and FSH, which stimulate the testes to produce sperm and testosterone as well as estrogen. FSH is also thought to act on other cells in the testes (**Sertoli cells**) to produce hormones (**inhibin** and **activin**) whose roles in the male reproductive cycle are currently unknown. The concentration of estrogen in the stallion's testes is very high and is quite unique among the domestic animals.

CHAPTER 10

Breeding Management

by Marcelo A. Couto

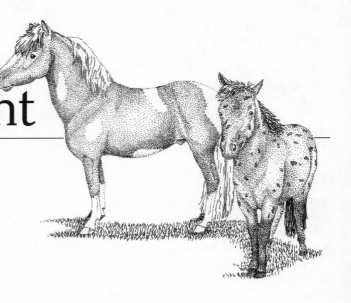

A successful breeding program rests on three fundamental pillars:

- Health care and preventive medicine
- Accurate detection of *estrus* (heat)
- Proper management of the services

This chapter will cover the latter two aspects of a breeding operation. In a reproductively sound horse population, accurate detection of estrus is perhaps the single most important factor leading to the overall success of the breeding season. Failure to detect estrus precludes the mating of mares at the height of their fertility (i.e., around **ovulation** [egg release from the ovary] time), resulting in an unacceptably low pregnancy rate, multiple matings per mare, increased stallion and personnel utilization, and increased risk of exposure to genital infections and accidents. The farm manager must ensure that safety and hygiene are observed during the services in order to prevent accidents and the spread of infectious conditions.

Detection of Estrus: Teasing

Teasing is best accomplished by exposing individual broodmares to an active teaser stallion on a daily basis. Although it can be a dull and time-consuming task, teasing should be supervised by a skilled and interested person—usually the breeding manager—who is familiar with the mares and who is capable of detecting even the subtlest of behavioral changes.

Special consideration should be given to the selection of the teaser stallion. Although the extent to which a stallion's aggressiveness affects estrous behavior in the mare remains controversial, it is generally accepted that the ideal teaser is gentle but vocal, exhibits the right amount of aggressiveness and enthusiasm, is easily controllable by the handler, and does not give up too quickly. While it would be ideal to maintain a horse specially dedicated to teasing, most small operations cannot afford such a luxury and have no choice but to use their regular stallion. However practical, this latter situation presents some serious drawbacks, such as undue exposure of a farm's primary (or only) stallion to injury and the risk of inducing abnormal sexual behavior. As an alternative, pony stallions or mares treated with the male hormone testosterone have been used as teasers, with varying degrees of success.

THE MARE'S BEHAVIORAL CHANGES THROUGHOUT THE ESTROUS CYCLE

Estrus Although most mares display characteristic signs of estrus in the presence of a teaser stallion, the intensity of the signs can vary considerably depending on a number of factors. Among these factors the natural disposition of the mare and her previous breeding experience, the ability of the teaser stallion, and the teasing method employed can all play significant roles. By and large the most consistent signs of estrus include rhythmic contractions of the lips of the **vulva** (female external genitalia) ("**winking**"), squatting, tail-raising, urinating, and failure to kick at the stallion. (*See* CHAPTER 9, "REPRODUCTIVE PHYSIOLOGY.") Although considerable variation exists among different mares, individual animals are quite consistent in their estrous manifestations from cycle to cycle. One should keep in mind that the presence of the mare's foal, as well as the separation of the mare from her offspring during teasing, can completely mask the usual signs of heat, especially at the first estrus after birth of the foal ("foal heat"). In such cases the mare may appear agitated and even react violently to the stallion's advances, yet at the same time squirt urine and "wink." Such mares often accept the stallion once a **twitch** (an instrument consisting of two handles and a loop utilized as a means of restraint) has been applied to the upper lip of the mare's mouth.

Diestrus Diestrus is the quiescent period between one heat period and the next and is characterized by an overt rejection of the teaser stallion. Mares appear clearly angry and act accordingly by switching the tail, squealing, moving, jumping, and kicking or striking at the stallion.

TEASING TECHNIQUES

The choice of technique depends primarily on the number of mares to be teased, whether they are dry or **lactating** (producing milk), the availability of teasing facilities, personnel, and personal preference. Whatever the method selected, it must be safe (for both horses and people), effective, and labor-saving. Broadly speaking, teasing can be done either on individual mares or on groups of mares.

Individual teasing can be carried out by exposing the mare to the stallion in an *ad hoc* facility such as a chute or a rail, or in the mare's stall. In this setting each mare is individually exposed to the teaser stallion across a rail or the bottom half of a stall door. In a variation of this technique known as **pen-teasing** the stallion is brought to the mare's pen. (The use of this latter technique should be discouraged for mares kept in metal pens because of the risk of leg injury from kicking or striking).

Group teasing allows the detection of estrus in a large number of mares at one time. Mares in a paddock or pasture are teased by a stallion being handled on the other side of the fence. Alternatively the teaser can be placed in a small enclosure adjacent to or within the paddock. A major disadvantage of group teasing is that dominant and aggressive mares, whether in heat or not, will tend to monopolize the stallion's attention and keep shy estrous mares from approaching the teaser. Most nonlactating mares, though, will exhibit normal estrous behavior, even in the presence of other mares, and thus are amenable to group teasing. Mares that fail to display the usual signs of estrus when other mares are present should be teased individually.

Lactating mares, especially those in foal heat with a newborn at their side, often fail to exhibit signs of estrus to the stallion. These mares must be teased individually and may even require the application of a twitch to the mare's upper lip. Lactating mares should not be teased in groups unless the safety of their offspring can be ensured.

Individual teasing is safer and far more effective than group teasing but is quite time consuming. For this reason many farms use both group and individual teasing methods. For this system to succeed, the person in charge of teasing must be familiar with the individual mares' manifestations of estrus and with their normal reactions to the stallion.

Management of the Services

BREEDING SOUNDNESS EXAMINATION
Thorough reproductive examinations of mares and the stallion(s) should be carried out in the fall of each year so that any problems can be diagnosed and corrected well ahead of the foaling and breeding seasons. Special emphasis should be placed on the stallion's general health, soundness of the musculoskeletal system (particularly the hind limbs), **libido** (sexual desire), reproductive system (penis and testicles), and quality of the **spermatozoa** (sperm; mature reproductive cells of the male). Two **ejaculates** (expulsion of semen, the milky fluid containing the sperm) collected one hour apart, followed by a third collection 7 days later, will usually be adequate to evaluate sperm numbers, their concentration and **progressive motility** (ability to swim forward), and also to predict with reasonable accuracy the daily sperm output. (*See* CHAPTER 12, "REPRODUCTIVE DISORDERS.") This information is useful for determining the number of mares that can be bred and the frequency with which the stallion can be mated or his semen collected. Although excellent semen quality favors fertilization, it should be recognized that other factors such as lack of libido can interfere with successful breeding.

Barren mares must be carefully examined to ascertain why they have failed to become pregnant. Pregnant mares should not be bothered before foaling unless there is a problem. The only procedure that might be necessary to perform just before the mare gives birth is a temporary **episiotomy** (surgical enlargement of the vulvar opening) if the mare's vulva has been previously **sutured** (stitched) in a **Caslick's operation** (surgical procedure to decrease the aspiration of air and contaminants into the female reproductive tract). The pre-breeding reproductive exam for foaling mares should be delayed until the foal heat, at which time the veterinarian must examine the mare's reproductive tract visually and manually for lacerations, tears, bruises, or other abnormalities.

BREEDING FACILITIES
Whether or not a farm uses natural service or artificial insemination, there are certain general rules that can be applied to any sound breeding operation. The three main considerations are safety, hygiene, and efficiency. Mares should be mated quickly and efficiently, all the while ensuring the safety of both horses and their handlers. The breeding shed should be spacious enough to allow for the unobstructed flow of animals and personnel, and for the rapid maneuvering of the stallion away from a nonreceptive mare. Light fixtures and ceiling beams must be placed high enough so they will not interfere with a stallion mounting a mare. Cabinets, racks, and other wall-mounted structures should be kept away from the breeding area proper. If there is a "phantom" or "dummy" mare (*see* below) permanently positioned in the shed, it must not get in the way of stallions covering live mares. The flooring material should be nonslippery, should be kept dust free by misting with disinfectants, and should allow for adequate drainage of water. Surface materials conforming to these requirements include crushed rocks, pebbles, rubber mats, and Fibar. To offer additional protection, the walls of the breeding shed can be padded with heavy sheets of urethane foam.

Some mares are significantly taller than the stallion, which transforms the act of mating into a test of the stallion's balancing skills. This height disparity can be minimized by creating a small depression in the flooring material for the mare's hind limbs. If the floor does not allow for such excavation, coconut mats can be used to raise the height of the stallion.

PREPARATION OF THE MARE
The mare should be led to the breeding shed using a shank and must be teased again immediately before mating. In some cases there will be a padded chute in one corner of the breeding shed where the mare can be washed and pre-

pared for mating. This area should be nonslippery and adequately drained. Prior to washing, the mare's tail is firmly wrapped from its base to the end of the tail bone using nonsterile disposable gauze. The wrap minimizes contamination and prevents laceration of the penis during mating. After the tail has been wrapped, the mare's vulva and all those areas likely to come into contact with the stallion's penis should be gently but thoroughly washed with warm water and a mild soap such as Ivory, and dried with paper towels. Water can be conveniently dispensed from a hand-held hose equipped with a spray nozzle, thus eliminating the need for buckets (a potential source of contamination between mares, unless plastic bags are utilized to line the buckets). Washing is best accomplished by scrubbing the vulva and the region around the anus with the back of the hand, working from the vulvar lips outward. If the mare has had a Caslick's operation or if she has a breeding stitch, one must carefully wash around each suture where feces tend to accumulate and harden. Following this wash it is important to scrub the area below the vulva and between the thighs and to moisten the top and sides of the hips. Finally, the depression around the **clitoris** (the small mound of erectile tissue that represents the female analog of the penis) should be everted and cleansed, and a moist piece of cotton inserted into the lips and stroked upward to clean the vaginal entrance. This is a good time also to evaluate the vulvar lips for conformation, sealing action and tilt, and to decide whether an already sutured mare needs to be opened to allow natural service, needs a breeding stitch before mating, or will require a Caslick's operation after breeding.

PREPARATION OF THE STALLION

The stallion is led from his stall to the breeding shed using a leather shank with a chain over the bridge of the nose or through the mouth. Alternatively, a snaffle bit or a lip chain can be used. Frequently, by the time the stallion has reached the breeding shed and seen the mare he will already have an erect penis. If a visible accumulation of a grayish, oily material (**smegma**) is present on the surface of the penis, it should

be gently washed off with clean, warm water and cotton, and dried with disposable paper towels. If the stallion is mated at least once a day, washing before breeding may not be necessary, i.e., rinsing and drying after each mating should be sufficient.

RESTRAINT AND SAFETY FEATURES

After the mare has been prepared she is led to the mating area and a twitch is applied to the upper lip. Some form of restraint is usually applied to either the front or hind legs (e.g., leg strap, breeding hobbles). Additional safety devices sometimes used on the mare at mating include rubber boots applied to the hind feet to prevent injury to the stallion if kicked by the mare, and a leather apron placed over the neck and poll areas. The latter will protect the mare's skin from a stallion's bite and may improve the stallion's balance by providing him with an extra grip. Another important safety device is the **breeding roll,** a padded, tapered cylinder that is placed between the base of the penis and the belly wall and acts to limit the depth of penetration of the penis into the vagina. This device is especially important to prevent vaginal tears when breeding small mares, maiden fillies, or any mare with a short vagina relative to the size of the stallion's penis. An effective breeding roll can be improvised with a clean roll of cotton similarly positioned. A leather muzzle can be used on those stallions that savage their breeding partners by biting. Because stallions frequently react to a squealing or uncooperative mare by striking or kicking, it is a good idea to remove the stallion's shoes during the breeding season.

THE MATING ACT (NATURAL COVER)

Whether the stallion is going to live-cover a mare or his semen is to be collected with an artificial vagina, he should be allowed to approach from behind on the left side at a slight angle, in order to avoid direct kicks from a frightened or nonreceptive mare. The experienced stallion will first tease the mare by rubbing his nose over her rump, flanks, and vulvar area, occasionally reaching as far forward as the neck and head. Because many mares object to the latter, it is advisable to restrict the stallion's advances to the rear and sides of the mare.

Once the stallion is fully erected he should be encouraged to mount. At this time each member of the breeding crew must attend to his or her own specific responsibilities. The *mare handler* must keep the twitch on the mare, maintain the mare's balance, and observe her responses to the stallion in order to anticipate any sudden movements. The mare handler is also responsible for warning the rest of the crew if the mare is about to jump, fall, or otherwise compromise the completion of the act. The *stallion handler* is essentially in charge of the breeding and should keep the stallion under control at all times. It is up to the handler, not the stallion, to decide when the mount should take place, since many stallions will mount prematurely with an incomplete erection.

Once the stallion is on top of the mare, the stallion handler will stand at the level of the mare's left flank and may hold the stallion's front fetlock to help prevent premature dismount. As the stallion mounts, a third crew member (the *tail handler*), standing to the right of the mare and wearing disposable gloves, should quickly move the mare's tail out of the way and, if needed, help the stallion introduce his penis by gently guiding it into the vulva. The tail handler is then free to help maintain the mare's balance and to control the stallion's right foreleg.

The stallion should be allowed to proceed with the copulatory movements that lead to ejaculation. Ejaculation is usually marked by **flagging** (rhythmic up-and-down movements of the stallion's tail) and by the stallion's resting his head lightly on one side of the mare's neck. The stallion should be allowed to stay on the mare for a reasonable length of time after ejaculation, i.e., he should not be pulled off the mare as soon as he ejaculates. Most stallions will stay on the mare for 5 to 10 seconds and then quietly dismount. At this time the mare handler turns the mare to the left so that her hind legs now point away from the dismounting stallion. Simultaneously a crew member steps in holding a disposable plastic cup and collects a dismount semen sample from the penis, then rinses the penis with clean warm water and dries it with paper towels. Since flagging is not *always* indicative of ejaculation, the microscopic detection of **motile** (moving) sperm in the dismount semen sample serves as confirmation of the completed act. Stallion and mare are then led back to their respective quarters.

Artificial Insemination (AI)

The preparation of the "jump mare" and stallion is identical to that described above for live cover. An alternative to a live jump mare is the use of a "phantom" or "dummy" mare, which is a structure that simulates the mare's back and rump. The phantom is firmly bolted to the floor of the breeding shed or anchored into the ground, and is usually tilted slightly from back to front. Periodically washing the phantom and keeping it covered when not in use will minimize contamination and spread of disease. While most stallions adapt easily to a phantom, some require extensive training before they will use a dummy mare; others will not adapt at all and will require a live mare. Some will accept mounting a phantom so long as a live mare is standing alongside. Many variations exist in the successful training of an individual stallion to a phantom, and different techniques should be tried until the one most successful for any particular case is found.

An essential component in AI is the **artificial vagina (AV).** There are many different models of AV on the market and each stallion may exhibit a preference for one or another. We have found that one particular type, the Missouri model, is almost universally accepted by stallions. This lightweight AV consists of a leather carrying-case containing a rubber jacket which is filled with water warmed to about 115°F (46°C). The volume of water in the jacket determines the tightness of the AV on the stallion's penis and is adjusted according to both the size of the penis and the stallion's personal preference as determined from experience. The opening of the AV must be lightly lubricated with a nonspermicidal jelly such as K-Y. A bottle or disposable plastic bag (Whirl-Pak) is firmly attached to the other end of the AV to collect the ejaculate. Semen must be protected from sunlight and from extremes of heat and cold, as these can adversely affect sperm quality.

Once the jump mare or the phantom has been prepared and the temperature of the AV has been adjusted, the stallion is brought in and washed (if necessary). As the stallion mounts, its handler moves forward on the left side of the mare and allows the AV handler to step in on the same side. The AV handler gently guides the stallion's penis into the AV, using a disposable glove. The AV handler must sense the reaction of the stud to the AV and allow him to thrust into the AV. The stallion then ejaculates and dismounts.

The semen is kept in a water bath at 86°F (30°C). Immediately upon collection the gelatinous fraction normally present in the ejaculate is removed by aspiration with a disposable 60-cc syringe, and a small volume is quickly evaluated microscopically for sperm motility and con-

centration. Semen is diluted 1 to 1 or 3 to 1 with a seminal *extender* containing antibiotics. The total volume is then divided into the number of mares selected for insemination, making sure 500 million progressively motile sperm are in each dose inseminated.

By the time the semen is ready, each mare to be inseminated must have had her tail wrapped and her genital area scrubbed. After an assistant parts the vulvar lips, the inseminator, wearing a light lubricated disposable sleeve, introduces a sterile pipette through the vagina and cervix into the uterus and deposits the insemination dose from a syringe. To increase the chances of the mare's ovulating within 48 hours, an intravenous dose of **human chorionic gonadotropin (hCG)** (hormone produced by the placenta that can stimulate ovulation) may be administered at the time of breeding.

CHAPTER 11

Pregnancy, Parturition, and the Young Foal

by Sally L. Vivrette

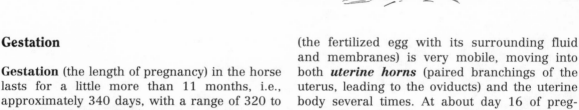

Gestation

Gestation (the length of pregnancy) in the horse lasts for a little more than 11 months, i.e., approximately 340 days, with a range of 320 to 360 days. The length of gestation does not vary significantly among the different breeds of horses. The nutritional status of the mare—except for marked undernutrition—does not significantly influence gestation length. The length of gestation is typically longer for mares bred in the winter and spring, compared to mares bred in the summer and fall. Foals born after less than 320 days are considered premature and may require various degrees of veterinary assistance. A very small percentage of equine pregnancies may be prolonged, exceeding 370 days. Prolonged gestation may be seen in mares grazing endophyte-infected fescue pastures.

After breeding, fertilization of the **ovum** (egg) occurs in the mare's **oviduct** (**uterine** or **Fallopian tube**), with the fertilized ovum reaching the uterus 5 to 6 days after **ovulation** (release of the egg from the *ovary*). During the first week after arrival in the uterus, the **embryonic vesicle** (the fertilized egg with its surrounding fluid and membranes) is very mobile, moving into both **uterine horns** (paired branchings of the uterus, leading to the oviducts) and the uterine body several times. At about day 16 of pregnancy the embryo becomes fixed to the uterine wall, usually at the base of one of the uterine horns.

During the first 2 weeks of pregnancy, a dramatic increase in the tone of the mare's uterus may be detectable when the uterus is **palpated** (felt with the hands) through the rectum. A bulge in the uterus, representing the embryonic vesicle, may be detected 18 to 19 days after ovulation. The embryonic vesicle, often called a **conceptus** at this stage of pregnancy, grows and gradually fills the uterus much like an expanding balloon. After day 40 of pregnancy, the **umbilical cord** (blood-vessel connection between the mother and offspring) is formed and the conceptus is then referred to as a **fetus**. The head and body of the fetus can be palpated at about day 85 of gestation. Fetal age and development have been recorded by measuring body weight, crown–rump length, and development of external features such as eyes, external genitalia, and hair. Such measurements are usually obtained only after a foal has been aborted or the mare has died, however. Accurate assessment of fetal age and fetal growth while the foal is in the womb is difficult, even with **diagnostic ultrasound** (noninvasive diagnostic technique for visualizing internal structures of the body by means of sound [echo] reflections).

Hormonal Changes During Early Pregnancy

After ovulation, the **corpus luteum** (the endocrine structure which develops within the follicle after ovulation; *see* CHAPTER 9, "REPRODUCTIVE PHYSIOLOGY") within the ovary produces the hormone **progesterone**, which promotes an environment in the uterus supportive of the developing embryo. Between day 35 and 40 of gestation, specialized cells from the embryonic vesicle attach to the uterus, invading deep into the uterine tissues and developing into **endometrial cups**. The endometrial cups produce the hormone **equine chorionic gonadotropin (eCG)** (formerly known as **pregnant mare serum gonadotropin [PMSG]**). Equine chorionic gonadotropin causes an increase in the production of progesterone by the ovary. The endometrial cups produce eCG until about day 130 of gestation, even if the pregnancy is terminated before that time.

Controversy exists concerning the practice of supplementing mares in early pregnancy with progesterone. *There is essentially no scientific evidence that early abortion in mares is associated with a subnormal concentration of progesterone.* Nevertheless, many mares are routinely supplemented with progesterone during early pregnancy, either orally or by injection. This is most often done for mares that habitually lose their pregnancies during the first 40 days of gestation. Some veterinarians or stud farm managers maintain that progesterone supplementation will help such mares maintain their pregnancies.

During gestation the fetal **gonads** (reproductive organs) increase markedly in size and participate in the production of hormones for the maintenance of the pregnancy. The fetal gonads work in cooperation with the **placenta** (the tissue in the uterus physically connecting the mother and offspring) to produce high concentrations of **estrogens** (general term for female sex hormones)—specifically **estrone sulfate**—which are important for promoting fetal and uterine growth.

Diagnosis of Pregnancy

Beginning at about day 10 after ovulation, pregnancy can be diagnosed by identification of the embryonic vesicle during an ultrasound examination of the mare's uterus. This examination is usually delayed until day 15 or 16, however, owing to the mobility of the early embryonic vesicle. The embryo can be visualized within the embryonic vesicle at day 22 postovulation, and the embryonic heartbeat can be detected beginning at day 24. Ultrasound examination allows for the diagnosis of pregnancy at all stages of gestation. During late pregnancy the fetus can be evaluated by an ultrasound examination through the underside of the mare's abdomen.

Pregnancy can also be diagnosed by palpation of a bulge in the uterus between days 20 and 60 of gestation. After day 60 the fetus may occasionally be palpable within the uterus, becoming consistently palpable after 120 days of gestation.

Hormonal tests for the diagnosis of pregnancy include measurement of estrone sulfate concentrations in the blood of the mare. This test can be performed with good accuracy after day 45 of pregnancy. Estrone sulfate measurement is very useful for pregnancy diagnosis in mares that cannot be examined by ultrasound or uterine palpation. Estrone sulfate concentrations decrease soon after a fetus dies or is aborted. Equine chorionic gonadotropin also can serve as an indicator of pregnancy in the mare; as indicated earlier, however, eCG production by the endometrial cups can continue even if a pregnancy is terminated.

Measurement of serum progesterone concentrations is *not* a good indicator of pregnancy in mares. Some nonpregnant mares may have elevated progesterone levels caused by a prolonged corpus luteum, while some pregnant mares may have low progesterone levels and yet carry a foal to term.

It is sometimes assumed that because a mare shows heat during the first 3 weeks after breeding she is not in foal. For the most part this is true; up to 10 percent of mares, however, will show heat and be pregnant.

Twins

Twins represent a special problem in the horse. They are most often aborted or born dead, owing to the inability of the uterus to supply nutrition to both fetuses. Occasionally one or both twins may be born alive, but often do not grow to expected size as adults. Twins occur in 1–2 percent of equine pregnancies and are theoretically caused by the ovulation of more than one follicle. They may result from a single ovulation that splits early in embryonic development but this is very rare in the mare. About 60 percent of pregnancies with twins will undergo natural reduction to a single fetus by day 20 of pregnancy. If diagnosed early in pregnancy, especially while the embryonic vesicle is still in the mobile phase, one of the twins can be manually compressed, allowing the mare to continue on with a single pregnancy.

Abortion

About 10–20 percent of pregnant mares undergo pregnancy loss early in gestation. The causes of such losses are often undetermined, but may include physical or genetic abnormalities of the embryo, maternal stress, and increased maternal age. The presence of twins is a common cause of late-gestation abortion. Bacterial, fungal and viral infections are sometimes diagnosed in cases of late-gestation abortion. Less common causes of abortion include nutritional imbalances, and placental or umbilical-cord problems. Fetal or placental tissues recovered after abortion should be submitted to a veterinarian or veterinary diagnostic laboratory to determine, if possible, the underlying cause of the abortion.

Management of the Pregnant Mare

During the first 8 months of gestation, broodmares can be fed the same ration as their non-pregnant herdmates. In the final 3 months an increasing amount of grain should be added to high-quality legume (e.g., alfalfa) and non-legume (e.g., oat) hay. A vitamin-mineral supplement designed to complement the type of hay being fed may be provided. Broodmares should *not* be allowed to become overweight during pregnancy.

Pregnant mares should be up-to-date on their vaccinations. It is common practice to vaccinate for equine viral rhinopneumonitis (which can cause abortion) during the fifth, seventh, and ninth months of gestation. Four to 6 weeks before foaling, the mare should receive a toxoid/encephalomyelitis/equine influenza booster vaccine. (*See* APPENDIX B, "VACCINATIONS AND INFECTIOUS DISEASE CONTROL.")

A regular schedule of deworming can be followed. Most commercially available dewormers are safe for use in pregnant mares; nevertheless the product labels should be scrutinized carefully for warnings. Dewormers containing organophosphates—associated with abortion when administered to mares late in gestation—should be avoided.

Pregnant mares should receive daily exercise, either by turnout in large pastures or light riding, lunging, or hand-walking. A regular hoof-care program should be followed as well.

Predicting Parturition

It is not possible to predict with accuracy the delivery date of a foal based on gestation length alone. Instead, gestation length should be considered along with the physical signs of impending **parturition** (giving birth): softening of the muscles over the croup, relaxation of the vulva, and udder development.

About one month prior to foaling, the mare's udder begins to increase in size ("**bagging up**"). In the final week of gestation, the teats begin to enlarge and *may* develop a small bead of wax ("**waxing up**") at the openings. (Contrary to popular belief, not all mares wax up before foaling). Prior to foaling a small amount of milk can be expressed from the teats and evaluated for color and viscosity. About one week before foaling, the milk changes in appearance from watery and serum-colored to thick and honey-like. This reflects the udder's production of the antibody-rich **colostrum** (first milk), which helps to protect the newborn from infectious diseases. (*See* CHAPTER 29, "THE IMMUNE SYSTEM AND VARIOUS DISORDERS.") In maiden mares the physical signs of impending delivery may be more subtle.

The milk prior to foaling can be evaluated for other changes that may indicate when the mare will deliver. For example, commercial kits are available that can detect changes in calcium concentration in the blood. The accuracy of such kits can vary, however, so test results should be interpreted in conjunction with the observed physical signs. Kit tests may be most useful for deciding when to begin observing the mare more closely for foaling.

In some cases owners may become frustrated after sitting up many nights waiting for a mare to foal. In such situations the attending veterinarian may be asked to give the mare an injection to induce foaling. Mares must be selected carefully for induction of parturition. It is generally inadvisable to induce foaling in mares, however, as this may result in the delivery of a foal that appears premature and may require extra days of special care.

Delivery of the Foal

Six weeks before the anticipated foaling date, the mare should be taken to the premises where she is to foal. Once an increase in udder development has been detected, the mare should be housed at night in a box stall so that she may be closely monitored. The foaling stall should be bedded in straw, measure at least 14 feet by 14 feet in size, and have solid walls and gates. A veterinarian should be asked to open the upper portion of the mare's vulva if she has had a **Caslick's operation** (*see* CHAPTER 12, "REPRODUCTIVE DISORDERS"). If the mare has a history of delivering a foal that was ill or died of **neonatal isoerythrolysis** *(hemolytic disease of the newborn)*, a blood sample can be drawn and submitted to the laboratory to determine if it is safe for the newborn to ingest the mare's colostrum (*see* below, and also CHAPTER 29, "THE IMMUNE SYSTEM AND VARIOUS DISORDERS").

Delivery of the foal usually occurs at night and is typically divided into three stages of labor:

Stage one
The mare may appear uneasy, look at her flank, sweat, and pace around. Mares in stage one may progress immediately into stage two or may postpone delivery of the foal for hours or days.

Stage two
The beginning of stage two is marked by the "breaking of the water," which represents rupture of the **chorioallantois** membrane of the placenta. The breaking of the water may occur with the mare standing or lying down. It is not normal for the velvety-red chorioallantois to appear at the vulvar lips without rupturing. *If this occurs the membrane should be quickly opened.*

The majority of mares deliver their foals while lying down, and utilize both uterine contractions and abdominal muscle contractions to push the foal out. The mare may rise to her feet and circle a few times, presumably in an effort to position the fetus properly. Most mares deliver their foals without assistance; thus, observers should remain quietly outside the stall. If, however, it appears that the mare is going to deliver the foal while standing, gentle assistance should be provided to deliver the foal and prevent it from falling to the ground.

Normal labor always proceeds in a progressive fashion after the breaking of the water with the appearance of the shiny-white **amnion** (the placental membrane immediately surrounding the foal) through which one and then both of the foal's forelimbs can be seen, followed by the foal's muzzle and head. Once the foal's shoulders become visible the rest of the body is delivered quickly. Second stage labor usually lasts less than 20 minutes in most mares, but in some it may last up to 60 minutes. If more than 60 minutes have elapsed before the foal is delivered, or if labor is not proceeding in a progressive fashion, a veterinarian should be called. In such cases the mare may be experiencing **dystocia** (abnormal delivery). Dystocia may be caused by an abnormal positioning of the foal, such as a **breech** presentation (rear end first), or by problems with the mare (e.g., uterine inertia).

After the foal has been delivered, the amnion should be gently removed from the foal's head. The mare may remain **recumbent** (lying down) for up to an hour after delivery, during which time the umbilical cord remains unbroken. In most cases the umbilical cord is broken as the mare rises to her feet or through the efforts of the foal as it struggles to stand. After the umbilical cord has been broken it should be dipped in an antiseptic solution such as chlorhexidine, povidone-iodine, or weak iodine, to prevent serious infection in the foal (*see* below).

Stage three

In the third stage of labor the placenta is expelled, usually within an hour after foaling. During this time the mare may lie down and appear a little uncomfortable. If the placenta has not been expelled within 6 hours a veterinarian should be called. Unlike cows, horses can become severely ill if the placenta is retained.

The Normal Newborn Foal

Immediately after delivery the newborn foal will usually lie very quietly behind the mare, with its hind limbs still in the mare's vagina. After a few minutes it will begin to struggle away from the mare. At birth the foal's ears are limp, but as it gains the strength necessary to stand the ears will become more erect.

The foal usually will stand within an hour after birth (range: 15 minutes to 2½ hours). Soon after this the foal will begin searching for the mare's udder. It will investigate dark places in the immediate vicinity, including the area between the mare's front legs and, to the frustration of people observing, dark corners of the stall. Eventually the foal finds the udder and begins to suckle. It is often tempting to assist the foal in finding the udder; this is usually not necessary and may actually delay the foal's first meal. Foals will usually begin to nurse the mare within 2 hours after birth (range: 35 minutes to 7 hours). If the foal's attempts to stand and nurse exceed the upper limits of these ranges, veterinary attention should be obtained.

When the mare stands after delivery, or during the struggling movements of the foal after birth, the umbilical cord is usually broken about 1 inch from the foal's body. The umbilical stump should be dipped in chlorhexidine (diluted 1:4 with water), povidone-iodine (diluted to a weak tea color), or weak iodine solution soon after it is broken and monitored closely for moistness during the first week of life. If any moistness or swelling is observed, the veterinarian should be notified.

The foal usually passes the **meconium** (the contents of the first bowel movement) during the first 24 hours of life. The foal may strain slightly during passage of the meconium; excessive straining or signs of colic may indicate a meconium impaction, which requires veterinary attention. It is common practice to administer an enema to the foal soon after birth. Either a commercial enema or a mild soapy-water enema may be used.

It is often advisable for a veterinarian to examine the newborn foal within the first 24 hours of birth. During this initial visit the foal is inspected for birth defects or trauma associated with delivery. Practices vary concerning injections administered to the foal at this time. If the mare was not vaccinated during the last month of gestation, it is advisable to give the foal a tetanus antitoxin injection. (Horses are exquisitely sensitive to tetanus toxin). It is generally *not* necessary to administer antibiotics to a newborn foal in the absence of specific signs of infection. After the foal is 12 hours old, a blood sample may be drawn and evaluated for adequacy of maternal antibody transfer in the colostrum (*see* below).

Newborn foals follow a basic behavioral routine that includes frequent napping, nursing, and exploration of the mare and stall. Deviation from these normal sorts of activities, such as excessive sleeping or failure to nurse the mare, is cause for concern.

During the first 3 days of its life, the foal should be confined to a box stall with the mare. Then, weather permitting, the pair can be turned out into a small, private, well-fenced paddock or small pasture. It is very useful to work gently with the foal during its first days of life and to acclimatize it to normal handling by human beings, such as picking up the legs and rubbing the bottom of the hooves.

Newborn foals do not require nutritional supplements and do quite well on a diet of mare's milk. The foal may begin to chew hay along with the mare as early as 3 days of age. **Creep feed** (supplemental concentrates provided exclusively to the foal) may be made available. Care should be exercised not to overfeed the foal, as this may cause bone and joint problems later in life. (*See* CHAPTER 8, "DISEASES OF DIETARY ORIGIN.")

The foal usually receives its first immunizations at 3 to 4 months of age, followed by a booster 4 weeks later. This should include the administration of tetanus toxoid, encephalomyelitis, and equine influenza vaccines. Vaccination against other disease agents prevalent in the area may be recommended by the veterinarian. (*See* APPENDIX B, "VACCINATIONS AND INFECTIOUS DISEASE CONTROL.") Foals may be dewormed beginning at 1 month of age, and then at 1- to 2-month intervals thereafter.

Diseases of Foals

PREMATURITY

A foal is considered to be premature if it is born before 320 days of gestation. The foal is referred to as **dysmature** if it is born after 320 days of gestation but appears immature. A premature or dysmature foal is at risk for developing infectious, respiratory, and metabolic problems that may require costly, intensive veterinary care.

FAILURE OF MATERNAL ANTIBODY TRANSFER

While in the uterus the foal is protected from disease by the mare's immune system and the barrier provided by the placenta. The placenta does not allow antibodies to pass from the mare to the foal, however, so the foal is born without protection from bacterial and viral disease agents. *It is thus of paramount importance that the foal receive colostrum, the antibody-rich first milk produced by the mare.* It is common practice to draw a blood sample from the foal at 12–18 hours of age to determine if the foal has received an adequate amount of antibodies from the mare. If antibody levels in the sample are low, a plasma transfusion may be necessary to boost antibody levels. If the foal is still less than 24 hours old, additional colostrum can be administered orally. (After this time the foal is no longer able to absorb the antibodies present in colostrum).

INFECTION

Prior to or shortly after birth, the foal may become infected with disease-causing bacteria that may spread to many parts of the body, a problem referred to as **septicemia**. Foals with septicemia usually are lethargic and infrequently nurse the mare. The rectal temperature may be *below normal, normal,* or *elevated.* In severe cases the foal may develop swollen joints, diarrhea, respiratory distress, or neurologic problems such as convulsions or coma.

Depending on the severity of the condition, a variety of diagnostic tests (complete blood count, blood culture, serum antibody concentration, serum chemistry profile) may be performed. Intensive therapy, often including intravenous antibiotics and fluids, is then begun. Foals with septicemia usually require several days of treatment and are at risk for developing complications that can include infected joints, diarrhea, stomach ulcers, and abscess formation in the umbilical stump. The prognosis is generally fair to poor, depending on the individual circumstances of each case.

Foals may become infected in the uterus with equine herpesvirus type 1 (**equine rhinopneumonitis virus**), particularly if the mare was not vaccinated against this agent during gestation. Affected foals may be aborted or born weak with pneumonia. In foals born alive the disease can progress to severe respiratory distress. The prog-

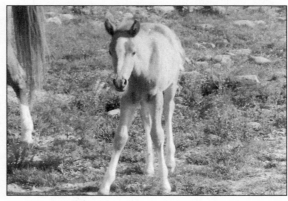

Photo by Ruth Saada.

nosis for survival, even with aggressive treatment, is poor. (*See* Chapter 25, "The Respiratory System and Various Disorders," and Appendix B, "Vaccinations and Infectious Disease Control.")

Diseases of the Lungs

Newborn foals with septicemia or infection with equine herpesvirus 1 may exhibit signs of pneumonia, including an increased respiratory rate and labored breathing. A cough may or may not be present, especially in very young foals. Pneumonia can also be caused by a bacterial infection localized only to the lungs. In older foals infection with the bacterium *Rhodococcus equi* can cause pneumonia and lung abscesses. (*See* Chapter 25, "The Respiratory System and Various Disorders.") During a difficult birth, the foal may defecate the meconium into the fetal fluids and then *aspirate* (breathe in) these fluids into the lungs during delivery, causing pneumonia. Pneumonia may also be seen in foals that aspirate milk into the lungs while nursing the mare or drinking too quickly from a bottle.

In addition to a physical examination, the diagnostic workup for a foal with pneumonia often includes a complete blood count and bacterial culture of fluid from the lungs. A *radiograph* (X-ray study) of the chest may also aid in the diagnosis. Based on the culture results and determination of the most effective antibiotic, the foal may require antibiotic therapy for a few to several weeks before the pneumonia is resolved.

Management practices that help prevent respiratory disease in foals include:

- Vaccination of mares with equine herpesvirus vaccine during pregnancy
- Ensuring that foals receive adequate colostrum at birth
- Provision of a clean and well-ventilated environment

Recently it has been shown that the administration of 1 liter of plasma, rich in antibodies against *Rhodococcus equi*, to foals less than 2 months of age is useful in preventing pneumonia caused by this particular bacterium.

Diseases of the Stomach and Intestines

During the first 24 hours after birth, the foal normally passes the meconium. If the meconium is not passed the large intestine can become impacted, causing the foal to exhibit signs of **colic** (abdominal pain). Therapy for meconium impaction may include mineral oil given by stomach tube, administration of one to several enemas, and occasionally, intravenous fluids. If after extensive efforts the meconium cannot be passed by the foal, surgery may be needed to relieve the impaction. Foals may also develop colic caused by twisting or displacement of the small or large intestine, a condition that requires surgery.

For reasons that are not completely understood, foals are susceptible to the development of ulcers in the stomach and upper portion of the small intestine. Ulcers may be seen in foals that have no other signs or in those that are stressed because of a concurrent illness, especially diarrhea. Signs of ulcers in foals include teeth-grinding, colic, diarrhea, fever, and lying on the back. Treatment includes management changes to minimize stress, and the administration of anti-ulcer medications similar to those used in people. (*See* Chapter 26, "The Digestive System and Various Disorders.")

Newborn foals may develop diarrhea in association with bacterial, viral, or nutritional problems. Depending on the severity of the diarrhea and the presence of other signs such as fever, lethargy, and dehydration, the diagnostic workup may include a complete blood count, bacterial culture of the feces, and examination of the feces for viruses. Treatment may include antibiotic therapy, intravenous fluid therapy, and administration of intestinal protectants such as Pepto-Bismol. It is common for foals to develop a mild diarrhea at 6–10 days of age in association with the mare's foal heat. The cause of this diarrhea is not completely understood and fortunately usually requires no treatment. (*See* Chapter 26, "The Digestive System and Various Disorders.")

Diseases of the Urinary Tract and Umbilical Stump

As a result of the powerful forces of birth, the bladder of the foal may be damaged or ruptured. This is more commonly seen in male foals. After birth, foals with a ruptured bladder become progressively lethargic and develop abdominal distension. They may dribble urine or strain to urinate, or may appear to pass normal quantities of urine. Diagnosis of a ruptured bladder involves collection of abdominal fluid and examining it for the smell of urine, and comparison of the biochemical parameters of serum and abdominal fluid. In uncomplicated cases the prognosis for recovery is good following surgical correction of the rupture.

The umbilical stump of the foal may serve as a portal of entry for disease agents into the foal's body by becoming infected after birth. The practice of dipping the foal's navel in a disinfecting solution one to several times after birth will decrease the incidence of umbilical stump infection. Infection may not be apparent during a visual inspection of the external umbilical stump, necessitating an ultrasound examination to detect enlargement of umbilical structures in the foal's abdomen. Medical therapy with antibiotics may be sufficient for treating foals that do not exhibit outward signs of infection. Surgical removal of the infected umbilical stump is indicated in foals that are ill or have evidence of abscess formation on ultrasound examination.

During fetal life the urine produced by the foal passes into the placental fluids through the *urachus*, a part of the umbilical cord. After birth the urachus normally closes off and the foal urinates out of the penis or vulva. In some cases, however, the urachus does not close or may reopen when the foal is a few days old. This open, or **patent**, urachus, may be treated medically with **cauterizing agents** (caustic substances that destroy tissue). A foal with a patent urachus should be examined closely for concurrent disease, such as septicemia or an umbilical abscess. If medical treatment is not effective in closing the urachus, or if an abscess is detected, surgical correction of the problem is indicated.

Diseases of the Nervous System
Neonatal maladjustment syndrome (NMS) is a disease, or group of diseases, characterized by progressive neurologic dysfunction. Affected foals may appear normal at birth, then develop clinical signs of illness within the first 3 days of life. Early signs include loss of bonding to the mare, discontinuation of nursing, and disorientation. Affected foals are sometimes called "dummies." The disease may progress to inability to stand, convulsions, and abnormal vocalization known as "barking." The cause has not been determined but is thought to be related to inadequate oxygen delivery to the foal during birth, resulting in damage to the brain.

In the evaluation of a foal suspected to have NMS, other problems such as septicemia and failure to receive sufficient colostrum should be investigated. Treatment often involves prolonged medical and nursing care to control convulsions, maintaining salt and water balance, providing adequate nutrition (usually via stomach tube), and keeping the foal quiet and comfortable. The prognosis for foals with NMS not complicated by infection is fair, but poor if the foal has concurrent infection or does not exhibit a good response to treatment within 4 days.

Foals may experience seizures caused by metabolic problems, especially low blood sugar. Also, infection associated with septicemia may lodge in the central nervous system and cause seizures. In addition, seizures may be caused by trauma during or after birth. As with NMS, the foal should receive a complete diagnostic workup. Therapy includes anticonvulsive medication and intensive supportive care.

Diseases of the Immune System
In certain cases the red blood cells of the foal may be attacked by antibodies of the mare. In foals this is called **neonatal isoerythrolysis (NI),** or **hemolytic disease of the newborn.** It is caused when the mare's immune system becomes sensitized to the foal's red blood cell type. When the foal ingests a sensitized mare's antibody-rich colostrum, it unwittingly consumes antibodies that destroy its own red blood cells. (*See* Chapter 29, "The Immune System and Various Disorders.") Affected foals appear normal for a day or two after birth, then become progressively more lethargic. An examination of the **sclera** (the whites of the eyes) reveals a moderate to severe yellowing (**jaundice**). Treatment includes blood transfusions if the foal has become severely anemic.

It is important that measures be taken to *prevent* the disease in subsequent foals. This includes screening the mare in future pregnancies for increased levels of antibodies directed against red blood cells. If these are detected, the delivery of the foal from that mare must be closely observed and the foal muzzled to prevent it from nursing colostrum from its dam. The foal may be fed colostrum from an alternate mare, one that was similarly screened for antibodies against red blood cells and found negative. A blood sample should be drawn from the foal to see that it has received adequate colostrum. The foal's dam should be hand milked several times to deplete the colostrum in her udder. After about 24 to 48 hours, when the foal can no longer absorb antibodies through the digestive tract, nursing from the dam may be allowed.

Diseases of the Legs and Muscles

Foals may be born with tendons that are too weak or lax, a condition most commonly affecting the hindlimbs. The problem may be mild or severe, resulting in the fetlocks of the hindlimbs resting on the ground. Lax tendons are most often observed in foals that seem a little immature in their development. In all cases exercise should be limited until the tendons strengthen.

Mild cases of tendon laxity usually improve in a few days. In severe cases the legs can be *loosely* bandaged to prevent sores from forming on the fetlocks. Special shoes can be constructed to support the hindlegs. Severely affected foals may require 1 to 2 weeks of treatment.

The tendons of some newborn foals may also appear contracted at birth, possibly a consequence of positioning while in the uterus. The severity of this problem can vary from mild contracture, where the heels do not touch the ground, to severe contracture, which is especially harmful if both forelimbs are affected. In these cases the foal may not be able to rise, walk, or nurse from the mare. Treatment for contracted tendons includes bandaging or splinting of the affected limb(s) and physical therapy to promote tendon relaxation and lengthening. (*See* Chapter 8,

"Diseases of Dietary Origin," and Chapter 22, "The Musculoskeletal System and Various Disorders.")

After birth a foal may be observed to have crooked legs, a condition known as **angular limb deformity.** Such deformities may occur in the front or hind limbs, and often involve laxity of the ligaments of the knee or hock, underdevelopment of the *carpal* or *tarsal bones*, or uneven growth. If this problem is observed, the foal should be confined to a stall and a veterinarian consulted. Radiographs may be taken to assess bone development and determine the extent of the deformity. In mild cases stall confinement with controlled exercise, combined with hoof trimming, may correct the problem. In severe cases the affected legs may need to be placed in splints or casts. In very severe cases, surgery may be indicated. (*See* Chapter 22, "The Musculoskeletal System and Various Disorders.")

Foals may be born with or develop muscle disease in association with an inadequate intake of selenium or vitamin E. This condition, called **white muscle disease,** is particularly prevalent in foals born to mares that consumed selenium-deficient diets during pregnancy. Foals with white muscle disease may exhibit muscle weakness, muscle trembling, stiffness, and difficulty rising. The diagnosis can be confirmed by measuring blood levels of selenium. Treatment involves the administration of selenium, initially by injection and then as a dietary supplement. Mares maintained in selenium-deficient areas should receive dietary supplementation with selenium during pregnancy.

Physitis is seen in fast-growing, well-fed foals and weanlings about 4 to 8 months of age. It is characterized by enlargement of the growth plates of certain long bones and of the vertebrae of the neck. Clinical signs include lameness and painful swellings just above the fetlocks, knees, and/or hocks. If this condition is identified, the foal's ration should be reevaluated and checked closely for proper mineral balance, especially copper, calcium and phosphorus. (*See* Chapter 22, "The Musculoskeletal System and Various Disorders.")

CHAPTER 12

Reproductive Disorders

by Marcelo A. Couto

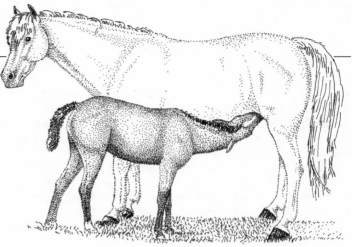

The aim of any breeding program is the pro- duction of viable offspring. The key to repro- ductive efficiency lies in early recognition and treatment of reproductive disorders and in mini- mizing preventable problems through sound management.

Reproductive Problems of Mares

Infertility (diminished ability to produce off- spring) in the mare can be caused by infectious conditions, anatomical defects or trauma, ovarian tumors, or developmental defects. Depending on the cause, common indicators of reproductive dis- ease in the mare include one or more of the fol- lowing:

- Discharge of abnormal fluid (e.g., pus) from the vulva
- Abnormal behavior (irregular, passive, or stallionlike) during estrus
- Repeated failure to conceive or to main- tain pregnancy after mating to a fertile stallion

INFECTIOUS CAUSES OF INFERTILITY

Uterine Infection Infection with inflammation of the uterus (**endometritis**) is the leading cause of infertility in broodmares and is caused chiefly by bacteria (a small proportion of cases are caused by yeasts or other fungi). Bacteria commonly caus- ing endometritis include "**streps**" (*Streptococcus zooepidemicus*), "**coliforms**" (*Escherichia coli* and *Klebsiella pneumoniae*), and "**pseudomonads**" (*Pseudomonas aeruginosa*). Yeast infections, usu- ally caused by Candida organisms similar to those causing vaginal infections in women, are next in order of frequency, while infections caused by other fungi such as *Aspergillus* are relatively rare.

Microorganisms can gain access to the **cervix** (oval-shaped mass whose opening connects the uterus with the vagina) and uterus in a variety of ways. Because normal mares can harbor large numbers of potentially **pathogenic** (able to cause disease) organisms on the vulva, on the clitoral area, or in the vagina, spontaneous con- tamination of the genital tract can occur. Poor vulvar and **perineal** (referring to the area between the thighs, encompassing the anus and genitalia) conformation often contributes to the development of uterine infection by leading to **pneumovagina** (the aspiration of air and debris into the vagina; "wind-sucking") or **urovagina** (urine "pooling" in the vagina).

Potentially pathogenic microorganisms can also be introduced into the genital tract during natural cover by the stallion, during **parturition** (act of giving birth), and during veterinary gynecological procedures. Thus mares are exposed to bacterial contamination almost on a daily basis. Resistant mares are capable of neutralizing this contamination while susceptible mares are not. No matter how pathogenic they are, microorganisms may be unable to establish themselves in a normal healthy uterus. In order for a mare to develop a **chronic** (persistent) endometritis, some breakdown in the normal uterine defense mechanisms must occur.

The uterus protects itself against infection by means of physical barriers (a mechanical response), by an army of white blood cells called **neutrophils** (cellular response), and by antibodies and related molecules (humoral response). An inadequate mechanical response is currently thought to be critical in the development of chronic uterine infections. The ability of the mare to produce uterine contractions and to relax the cervix are important for eliminating pus and contaminating microbes from the uterine environment. While neutrophils also play an important role by ingesting and killing invading microorganisms, the role of antibodies in uterine defense remains less clear.

Although a uterine infection is relatively easy to diagnose by a skilled veterinarian, it is sometimes difficult to treat. The presence of endometritis can be suspected on the basis of irregular estrous cycles (shortened diestrus); appearance of an abnormal fluid (e.g., pus) on the vulvar lips, tail hairs, thighs, and hocks; and failure to conceive after mating to a fertile stallion. To confirm the diagnosis it is necessary to perform a complete clinical evaluation of the reproductive tract—**palpation** (examining with the hands) and **ultrasonography** (technique for visualizing internal structures by means of sound [echo]

reflections; diagnostic ultrasound) of the uterus, **vaginoscopic** exam (visual examination of the vagina using an instrument called a *speculum*), uterine **cytology** (microscopic examination of cells obtained from the uterine wall), and uterine **culture** (laboratory growth of microorganisms obtained from the uterus). These procedures are usually sufficient to diagnose a case of **acute** (rapid-onset) endometritis. Detection of chronic endometritis, on the other hand, often requires a *biopsy* sample of the **endometrium** (uterine wall). A biopsy can reveal uterine **fibrosis** (scarring), the most damaging change leading to infertility. In addition to providing a diagnosis, a uterine biopsy yields important prognostic information regarding the mare's fertility potential. Based on the degree of uterine damage present, biopsies are classified as grade 1 (essentially normal), grade 2 (moderate changes, usually reversible), or grade 3 (severe changes, usually irreversible).

The general approach to treating infectious endometritis consists of the administration of a hormone, **prostaglandin F_{2a} (PGF),** to the mare in order to bring her back into estrus, the time of the estrous cycle during which uterine defenses are at their height. The next step is to eliminate the infection with antibiotic or antiseptic preparations. Once the infection has been removed, reinfection (a common occurrence in susceptible mares) must be prevented.

Although treatment of infectious endometritis is seemingly straightforward, it sometimes fails for a variety of reasons. Present evidence indicates that reinfection of the uterus following treatment is a major cause of persistent endometritis. The uterus of a susceptible mare can become contaminated by very small numbers of bacteria introduced during routine gynecological procedures. The choice of antibiotic, as well as its route of administration, may also play a role in the treatment outcome. The two main routes for administering antibiotics are **local** (direct infusion into the uterus) and **systemic** (either orally or by injection) administration. Most veterinarians favor local treatment by flushing the uterus with large volumes of **saline** (physiological salt solution), often followed by intramuscular injection of oxytocin which causes contraction of uterine muscles and emptying of the uterine contents, followed by infusion of antibiotics or antiseptics directly into the uterus. Flushing the uterus aids in the mechanical elimination of microbes, pus, and debris, which in turn assists the effectiveness of the antibiotic. This approach greatly reduces the antibiotic dose required, since high concentrations can be attained within the uterus.

The primary drawback of local therapy is the risk of introducing contaminating bacteria and reinfecting the uterus at the time of infusion. To avoid this problem, some veterinarians have advocated the use of systemic therapy, i.e., the intramuscular, intravenous, or oral administration of antibiotics. Although this form of therapy is easy to administer and avoids reinfection of the uterus, it presents serious disadvantages. Because abnormal fluids and debris are not flushed from the uterus, their mechanical elimination must rely entirely on the mare's ability to relax the cervix and produce powerful uterine contractions, a mechanism that may already be compromised in susceptible animals. The rate and efficiency of absorption of antibiotics from the digestive tract (when given orally) or from muscle tissue (when delivered by injection) are quite unpredictable, so that the concentration of antibiotic finally delivered to the uterus can vary dramatically.

As indicated earlier, eliminating the original infection is only half the battle; preventing reinfection is just as important. Many times the veterinarian is able to "clean up" the infected mare only to find her reinfected on a subsequent visit to the farm—a very frustrating experience for both owner and veterinarian.

To decrease the numbers of bacteria entering the genital tract, a Caslick's operation should be performed as soon as possible after uterine infection is detected. This procedure involves **suturing** (stitching) together the top of the vulvar lips. The clitoral **sinuses** (cavities or channels), a potential source of pathogenic organisms, should be thoroughly scrubbed in all chronic, stubborn infections. Under special circumstances the clitoral sinuses may need to be surgically removed to eliminate a source of reinfection.

Pyometra Pyometra is the collection of large volumes of pus inside the uterus. It is usually the result of a long-standing, untreated case of endometritis, but can also be caused by the presence of a foreign body in the uterus (such as the detached tip of a bacteriological culture swab). Up to 60 liters (15 gallons) of pus can accumulate in the uterus in a *closed-cervix* pyometra without producing clinical signs of illness. Because of the associated vulvar discharge of pus, an *open-cervix* pyometra is generally easier to diagnose than its closed-cervix counterpart. The accumulation of pus results in damage to the uterine lining and provides an excellent culture medium for the growth of bacteria and yeasts. This condition often leads to permanent infertility secondary to scarring (fibrosis) of the endometrium. In the initial stages of a pyometra, local irritation causes the release of PGF from the uterine lining. Since PGF signals to the ovaries when a new estrous cycle is to begin, its premature release causes the mare to return to estrus before the expected time. As the condition worsens, though, the severe endometrial damage may completely block the release of PGF, causing the mare to skip cycles.

The diagnosis of pyometra can be confirmed by palpation of the uterus and by ultrasound examination. Treatment is almost invariably ineffective and, in most cases, unwarranted unless the vulvar discharge interferes with the mare's athletic activities or the uterus becomes excessively large due to the accumulated pus. The prognosis for pyometra is extremely poor with regard to the mare's fertility potential.

Vaginitis Inflammation and/or infection of the vagina (**vaginitis**) is often associated with windsucking or urine pooling. In itself vaginitis is not a serious condition and usually disappears after the primary cause has been treated.

Cervicitis Inflammation and/or infection of the cervix (**cervicitis**) are generally associated with endometritis or vaginitis and usually have the same cause. Cervicitis can also result from the intrauterine infusion of irritants such as antibiotics or antiseptic solutions. Treatment consists of resolving the primary cause. A special case of cervicitis accompanied by the vulvar discharge of mucus occurs occasionally in pregnant mares.

Generally this condition does not threaten pregnancy unless it spreads to the uterus, causing endometritis and placentitis (inflammation of the *placenta*, the physical connection between the uterus and the developing fetus).

Genital Herpesvirus Infection *See* "Venereal Diseases," below.

Anatomical Defects and Trauma

Abnormalities of the Perineum and Vulva The perineum is the body wall comprising the outlet of the pelvis, the vaginal passage, and the anus. An abnormal anatomical conformation in this area can lead to pneumovagina (wind-sucking), inflammation of the cervix and uterus, and infertility. The mare's vulva consists of the clitoris and the vulvar lips (the **labia**). The shape and tone of the vulvar lips are under hormonal control, *progesterone* causing a shortening and contraction of the labia and *estrogens* causing relaxation and lengthening of the vulva. The right and left vulvar lips should meet evenly and form a firm seal to protect the uterus from the external environment. Subtle damage to the perineum and/or vulva may accumulate from repeated cycles of breeding and foaling. More severe trauma can lead to pneumovagina, perineal lacerations or tears, rectovaginal fistulas, or vesicovaginal reflux (urovagina).

Pneumovagina, the aspiration of air and fecal material into the vagina, can result from faulty perineal conformation, direct trauma, or poor body condition. Older mares are more prone to develop pneumovagina as the fat deposits around the perineum recede with age and the vulvar lips lose tone, i.e., fail to seal properly. The constant aspiration of air and feces, accompanied by microbes, may lead to chronic inflammation of the vagina, cervix, and uterus, ultimately resulting in infertility. Some mares aspirate air only during estrus, when the vulvar lips relax in response to estrogen. Unfortunately, this is the time when the cervix also relaxes and when mating occurs. To evaluate vulvar conformation, one must observe the length, tilt, and tone of the vulvar lips and the distance between the top of the vulva and the pelvis. Mares having a long, tilted vulva with poor tone are more prone to aspirate air, especially if the length of the vulvar opening above the pelvic bone is greater than that below the pelvic bone. Once detected, pneumovagina should be corrected by suturing together the vulvar lips above the pelvic bone (Caslick's operation). Pneumovagina can also lead to the accumulation of air inside the uterus (pneumouterus), another cause of endometritis and infertility.

Perineal lacerations. Most *lacerations* or tears occur at the time of foaling, owing to fetal malpositioning and/or to excessive manipulation during assisted delivery. Based on their extent, perineal lacerations have been divided into first, second, and third-degree lacerations. *First-degree* lacerations involve only the lining of the vulva and the skin at the top of the lips. *Second-degree* lacerations penetrate more deeply into the vulvar wall and affect the muscles that control vulvar closure. *Third-degree* lacerations involve the full thickness of the vulvar and rectal walls and can irreversibly damage the **anal sphincter,** the circular band or ring of muscle that controls the release of feces from the anus. While only minor corrective surgery is usually required for first-degree lacerations, moderate to extensive surgical intervention is necessary for second- and third-degree tears. Scarring of the perineum often occurs after surgery, resulting in pneumovagina (which must be corrected at a later time).

Rectovaginal fistula is a tear from the top of the **vestibule** (entrance to the vagina) to the floor of the rectum. It is almost always a foaling injury but may occur during natural breeding. It is usually recognized by the presence of feces in the vagina. The constant passage of feces into the genital tract can give rise to endometritis and infertility. Surgical correction of the problem is indicated.

Vesicovaginal reflux (VVR, urovagina, urine pooling) is the retention of incompletely voided urine in the forward portion of the vagina, next to the cervix. This condition results from an abnormal downward slope of the vagina from the vulva toward the cervix. It is more often observed in older mares with defective genital conformation (such as pneumovagina and/or a heavy, pendulous uterus with poor tone). Pneumovagina can cause VVR because the aspiration of air inflates the vagina, creating a space for urine to collect. The accumulated urine and secretions in the vagina then flow directly into the uterus when the mare relaxes the cervix at estrus. The presence of urine causes not only chronic irritation of the uterus but also changes the vaginal **pH** (acid-base balance), affecting the viability of the **spermatozoa** (sperm; the male reproductive cells) and reducing conception rates. The treatment is surgical except in cases caused by poor body condition. If VVR occurs as a result of pneumovagina, the Caslick's operation performed for pneumovagina will often solve the VVR as well. Other surgical techniques for correction of VVR are also available. The objective of all of these procedures is to divert the flow of urine outward toward the vulva, rather than inward toward the cervix and uterus.

Cervical Lacerations Lacerations or tears of the cervix can occur during **dystocia** (difficult birth), forced extraction of the fetus, or even after a seemingly normal delivery. Because a cervical tear can easily be missed on a visual vaginoscopic exam, it is essential to perform a manual examination of the cervix in order to make a diagnosis. The degree of cervical closure must be assessed during **diestrus** (the quiescent period between one heat period and the next) when the mare is under the influence of the hormone progesterone. The correction is surgical but not always successful. The use of a breeding roll to limit the penetration of the stallion's penis (*see* CHAPTER 10, "BREEDING MANAGEMENT") is highly recommended after surgery. As an alternative, surgical correction can be postponed until after breeding and ovulation. Cervical tears usually recur at the subsequent parturition, again requiring surgery.

A common complication to cervical lacerations is the development of cervical **adhesions**— bands of scar tissue that develop as a part of the healing process. This excessive tissue can physically block the cervical opening, interfering with the evacuation of uterine secretions and with transport of the sperm to the **oviducts** (uterine or fallopian tubes, connecting the uterus with the ovaries) during natural breeding. Cervical adhesions are usually discovered when manually examining the cervix. Provided that the **lumen** (interior space) of the cervix is not completely blocked, the uterine secretions can be drained out and the mare inseminated artificially.

Ovarian Hematomas These are a form of internal trauma to the ovaries caused by excessive bleeding (**hemorrhage**) into an ovary following ovulation. Hemorrhage results in increased pressure inside the ovary and may lead to distortion or even total obliteration of the normal ovarian architecture. Ovarian hematomas usually resolve spontaneously after one or two estrous cycles. It is important to distinguish ovarian hematomas from ovarian tumors (*see* below).

OVARIAN TUMORS
Most tumors of the ovaries are **benign**, i.e., they do not spread. The most prevalent types are the granulosa cell tumor, cystadenoma, teratoma, and dysgerminoma. Of these, only granulosa cell tumors affect the normal estrous cycle.

Granulosa cell tumor *Granulosa cells* are the cells that surround the developing ovarian **follicle** (the egg and its associated protective layers). Granulosa cell tumors account for about 2.5 percent of all equine tumors. Although they can occur in mares of all breeds and ages, granulosa cell tumors develop more frequently in mares between 5 and 9 years of age. The reproductive behavior of affected mares varies depending on the relative production of sex hormones by the tumor. Affected mares can exhibit stallionlike behavior (caused by production of high levels of the male sex hormone **testosterone**), may be in continuous or intermittent heat, or may cease cycling altogether. Levels of the female hormone **estrogen** are not particularly useful in predicting behavioral abnormalities. Occasionally mares with granulosa cell tumors will cycle normally. Almost invariably this tumor causes enlargement of only one ovary while inducing **atrophy** (reduction in size and function) of the other ovary.

Diagnosis of a granulosa cell tumor is suspected on the basis of the behavioral changes and the size of the ovaries as determined by palpation. Further diagnostic aids include ultrasound and hormone levels. Confirmation of the diagnosis requires microscopic examination of ovarian tissue after surgical removal of the tumor. Granulosa cell tumors can be mistaken for ovarian hematomas (*see* above) and other ovarian tumors, especially cystadenoma (*see* below). After surgical removal of the affected ovary, normal estrous cycling will usually resume within 3 to 12 months.

Cystadenoma This is the second most common ovarian tumor of mares. It is a benign tumor that arises from the lining of the ovary and, unlike granulosa cell tumors, does not affect the opposite ovary or the sexual behavior of the mare. Palpation of the affected ovary will reveal the presence of **cystic** (saclike, fluid-filled) structures on its surface. Some mares with cystadenomas may have higher blood levels of testosterone, but this is not a consistent finding. Most affected mares are presented for veterinary examination because of infertility.

Teratoma Teratoma is an ovarian tumor that often is found accidentally during a routine reproductive examination. Mares with a teratoma usually exhibit normal estrous cycles and the opposite ovary remains unaffected. No hormonal imbalances are observed. The affected ovary may contain **cysts** (fluid-filled sacs) as well as a bizarre combination of different embryonic tissues such as bone, cartilage, teeth, and hair.

Dysgerminoma This is a malignant but fortunately extremely rare tumor in mares. It originates in the ovaries and can spread (**metastasize**) to the abdominal and chest cavities. Affected mares may exhibit weight loss and abdominal discomfort. The prognosis for recovery is poor.

DEVELOPMENTAL DEFECTS

Ovarian Hypoplasia Ovarian **hypoplasia** (underdevelopment or incomplete development), resulting in small, firm ovaries, is a normal finding in sexually **immature** (prepubertal) mares. Many mature mares' ovaries become inactive during the winter. Ovarian hypoplasia may be associated with chromosomal defects such as Turner's syndrome (see below), severe malnutrition, or use of anabolic steroids during training. If ovarian hypoplasia is observed in an adult mare during the breeding season, especially in conjunction with a small uterus, a definitive diagnosis should be based on genetic (**chromosomal**) analysis, i.e., a **karyotype** (magnified photographic array of the chromosomes derived from an individual cell). Examination of the ovaries by ultrasound will help to assess the presence of developing ovarian follicles.

Turner's Syndrome This is the most common chromosomal abnormality of mares and is characterized by a missing X chromosome (normal mares have a pair of X chromosomes, while normal stallions have one X and one Y chromosome; *see* CHAPTER 13, "GENETICS"). Affected animals are usually small for their age and lack normal estrous cycles. Anatomically this syndrome is characterized by small, smooth, firm ovaries (**ovarian hypoplasia**). The uterus and cervix are small and flaccid as a result of the lack of ovarian hormones. Affected mares are irreversibly infertile. (*See* CHAPTER 14, "CONGENITAL AND INHERITED DISORDERS.")

Miscellaneous Developmental Defects *Absence of a cervix and/or uterus, double cervix,* and *enlargement of the clitoris (***hermaphroditism***)* can also result from chromosomal abnormalities. Some developmental defects, however, are not caused by chromosomal aberrations. The two more common among these are:

Persistence of the hymen is caused by the presence of a thick, imperforate **hymen** (membranous tissue partially or completely covering the external opening of the vagina in virgin mares). In the absence of complications, this condition is not serious and does not interfere with fertility. On occasion, however, a persistent hymen may impede the normal evacuation of uterine secretions, which then accumulate in the uterus and can become contaminated. In such cases infertility can result from uterine infection.

Endometrial cysts are a frequent finding during a reproductive examination in older mares. The uterine glands become distended with fluid and secretions, forming cysts that vary in size from microscopic to clearly palpable structures several inches in diameter. Unless the cysts are many in number or are situated at the base of the **uterine horns** (paired branchings of the uterus leading from the body of the uterus to the uterine or fallopian tubes), they tend not to interfere with pregnancy. Endometrial cysts can be confused with an early pregnancy on palpation and ultrasound examination.

Reproductive Problems of Stallions

In general, equine male reproductive physiology is less well-characterized than its female counterpart (*see* CHAPTER 9, "REPRODUCTIVE PHYSIOLOGY.") Nevertheless a variety of conditions that can affect a stallion's breeding performance have been recognized. Because these conditions bear little resemblance to those affecting mares, this section of the chapter is structured differently and will focus on four main areas that may compromise male fertility: abnormalities of the sperm, diseases of the testicles, abnormalities of the penis and sheath, and sexually-transmitted (**venereal**) diseases.

ABNORMALITIES OF THE SPERM
An acceptable ejaculate contains at least 1 to 2 billion **spermatozoa** (sperm; mature male reproductive cells) that are of normal **morphology** (size and shape) and are progressively motile (i.e., can swim forward). Abnormalities of the sperm that may lead to infertility include:

Insufficient Sperm Numbers The primary factors that regulate sperm output are season of the year, testicular size, age of the stallion, and frequency of ejaculation.

Effect of season
Since stallions, like mares, are seasonal breeders, they exhibit a peak of sperm production around June and July in the northern hemisphere, coincidental with the increase in day length and with mares' peak fertility. They will, however, breed at any time of the year in contrast to most mares.

Effect of testicular size
The number of sperm produced is directly related to the amount of functional tissue in the **testicles** (also called the **testes**, the paired male reproductive organs wherein the sperm are produced). Thus, measurement of the testicular diameter can be used to estimate the number of sperm produced per day (**daily sperm production, or DSP**). Even after ejaculation a considerable number of sperm remain stored in the tail of the **epididymis**, the tubelike structure that receives newly produced sperm from the testicles and is responsible for their transport, maturation, and storage. This additional mass of sperm is referred to as the **extragonadal** (outside the testes) reserves. The **daily sperm output (DSO)** is the number of sperm collected per day, after depleting the extragonadal reserves. Both DSP and DSO are important for predicting how many mares can be bred to a particular stallion.

Effect of age
Age of the stallion significantly affects DSP, DSO, and the number of mares a particular stallion can breed. Although stallions can be successfully bred at an early age, the sperm reserves and total number of sperm per ejaculate do not reach their peak until a stallion is 8–10 years old.

Effect of frequency of ejaculation
How often a particular stallion should be used depends on his sex drive (**libido**) and sperm output. Normal mature stallions of average libido participating in a well-managed breeding program can safely breed one or two mares per day during the normal breeding season. In one study, no difference in stallion fertility was found

following a single or multiple (up to three) covers per day. In fact, those mares mated on the stallions' third (evening) cover exhibited higher conception rates—possibly because more mares ovulate at night. Overuse of stallions, however, may lead to behavior and fertility problems. A practical ejaculation frequency for stallions in an artificial insemination (**AI**) program is one ejaculation every other day.

Poor Motility Progressive (forward) motility of spermatozoa is important for fertility. Abnormal motility can be indicative of other defects (metabolic, genetic) and should be seriously investigated.

Abnormal Morphology Defective sperm morphology can be divided into primary and secondary abnormalities. Primary abnormalities are those occurring during sperm development; they affect primarily the head and "neck" (midpiece) of the sperm cell. These types of changes are therefore more serious than are secondary abnormalities that occur during sperm maturation in the epididymis, affecting the tail of the spermatozoa. Having primary abnormalities in up to 10 percent of sperm is considered acceptable and normal, while secondary defects in up to 30 percent of sperm can occur without any appreciable decline in fertility.

Presence of Blood or Urine in the Ejaculate
Hemospermia (blood in the semen) and **urospermia** (urination during ejaculation) occur infrequently but can severely affect fertility.

Hemospermia is easily detected during semen collection by the pink or reddish color imparted to the semen. Under natural breeding conditions, however, this problem can go undetected. A small amount of blood in the ejaculate is compatible with fertility provided that the semen is diluted immediately with a seminal **extender** (fluid added to increase or "extend" the volume). If a significant amount of blood is present the ejaculate should be discarded. Hemospermia occurs most often in heavily booked stallions as a result of bacterial **urethritis** (inflammation of the **urethra**, the membranous tube that trans-

ports urine from the urinary bladder to the exterior of the body). Bleeding into the urethra likely occurs upon erection and ejaculation. Less commonly, bleeding into the ejaculate can result from lesions on the skin of the penis, such as "**summer sores**" (*habronemiasis*), tumors, lacerations, or from infection or inflammation of the **seminal vesicles** (paired pouches near the urinary bladder). When discovered, the primary condition causing hemospermia should be treated and the stallion given adequate sexual rest.

Urospermia probably results from a disturbance of the nerves that are responsible for ejaculation. Nerve stimulation upon ejaculation can contract (squeeze) the urinary bladder at the same time. Diagnosis of the condition can be confirmed by microscopic identification of urinary crystals in the ejaculate. Stallions that urinate into the ejaculate tend to repeat this behavior. Urospermia may be corrected by allowing the stallion to urinate before service. This is accomplished by replacing the stallion's stall bedding with fresh straw which may encourage him to urinate or by administration of a diuretic (drug that promotes urination).

ABNORMALITIES OF THE TESTICLES

Testicular Degeneration Testicular degeneration is a major cause of infertility in stallions and is an acquired condition. Testicular degeneration is usually the result of a thermal injury, i.e., a temperature increase (local or general) that affects the normal development of the sperm. An invading tumor, a localized infection, general illness accompanied by fever, and malnutrition all can result in testicular degeneration. The diagnosis is established by palpation of the testicle and by semen evaluation.

Testicular Tumors Testicular tumors occur only rarely in horses, although their true incidence is difficult to estimate because most male horses are castrated at an early age. Diagnosis is based on palpation and ultrasound examination of the affected testicle(s). If a tumor is diagnosed, the entire testicle should be removed.

DISEASES OF THE PENIS AND SHEATH

Inflammation and infection of the penis (**balanitis**), of the **sheath** (the fold of skin enclosing the penis) (**posthitis**), or both (**balanoposthitis**) are relatively uncommon in stallions. They can result from disturbances of the normal bacterial population (e.g., after washing the penis with strong antiseptics). Tumors of the penis, sheath, and **scrotum** (dependent pouch of skin containing the testicles) can also occur (*see* CHAPTER 34, "CANCER"). Tumor types include papillomas, squamous cell carcinomas, melanomas (more common in old gray horses), and sarcoids.

Venereal Diseases

Sexual transmission of genital infections can lead to infertility due to endometritis, early embryonic death, abortion, or birth of weak, sick foals that die during the neonatal period. Certain **sexually-transmitted diseases (STDs)** cause clinical illness among mares and stallions. In addition, certain sexually transmitted diseases restrict the export of breeding stock from countries in which these diseases are prevalent. Most equine STDs are caused by bacteria and viruses, and their incidence is higher in pasture-breeding or hand-breeding operations utilizing natural service. The overall prevalence of bacterial STDs could be reduced or eliminated altogether by the use of artificial insemination with antibiotic-containing seminal extenders.

BACTERIAL INFECTIONS

Bacterial infections of the female genital tract can be transmitted during breeding. Most of these infections (if not all) may also be spread by mechanical means, e.g., contaminated instruments and supplies. The most significant bacteria in this group are *Streptococcus zooepidemicus,* *Klebsiella pneumoniae, Pseudomonas aeruginosa, Escherichia coli,* and *Taylorella equigenitallium.* The latter organism is the cause of contagious equine metritis. (*See* CHAPTER 31, "BACTERIAL DISEASES.")

VIRAL INFECTIONS

Viral infections vary in their clinical manifestations. While signs of equine coital exanthema (equine herpesvirus type 3 infection) are readily noticeable in both mares and stallions, equine viral arteritis can be sexually transmitted by carrier stallions exhibiting no clinical signs of illness. (*See* CHAPTER 30, "VIRAL DISEASES.")

Equine Viral Arteritis (EVA) Equine viral arteritis is a contagious viral disease of horses causing fever, ocular and respiratory signs, fluid distension or swelling (edema) of the limbs, and abortion. Intriguingly, EVA in the United States affects a higher proportion of Standardbreds than any other breed. The disease is rarely fatal and tends to occur in epizootic (outbreak) form, usually attributable to the movement of horses on racetracks or stud farms. Venereal transmission occurs through the contaminated semen of carrier stallions.

Equine Coital Exanthema Equine coital exanthema is a mild disease affecting both sexes, caused by equine herpesvirus–3. Its primary mode of transmission is venereal, although it can also be spread by contaminated supplies and instruments. Clinical signs consist of multiple, painful, wartlike lesions on the skin of the vulva and perineum or on the shaft of the penis. These lesions usually heal within 2–3 weeks, leaving discolored areas. Mating of affected animals should be postponed until the lesions have completely dried.

CHAPTER 13
Genetics

by Ann T. Bowling

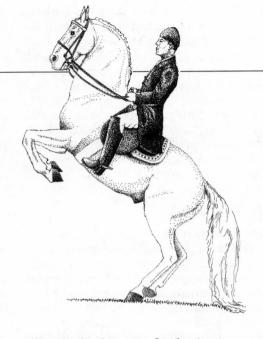

To breed healthy, beautiful horses an understanding of the general principles of genetics can be of great value. Many physical and behavioral attributes of horses have an inherited basis, while others are due primarily to environmental influences. To make effective breeding decisions for or against a selected trait, it is important to know whether the trait is inherited. Most responsible breeders are familiar with the basics of equine genetics, particularly with information pertaining to their chosen breeds. Interest in equine genetics is not limited to people with a breeding program, however. Many owners are fascinated to learn how a favorite horse comes to differ in color, size, shape, or ability from the horse in the neighboring stall. Using horses as an example, this chapter will discuss the general principles of genetics to illustrate the physical basis of inheritance, which was first clearly defined by the Austrian monk and naturalist Gregor Mendel (1822–1884) in his famous studies of garden peas.

The Physical Basis of Inheritance

Genes, the individual units of inheritance, occur as components of the very large and complex molecules of **DNA** (deoxyribonucleic acid) known as **chromosomes** that are found in the nucleus of every living cell. Genes encode information that directs the manufacture of **proteins**, the molecules that control the developmental stages from egg and sperm through foal to adult. Proteins also are needed to maintain all normal body functions. It is estimated that 50,000 to 100,000 genes, each coding for different proteins, are required to direct the incredibly complex processes of life.

The DNA of equine genes is packaged in 64 chromosomes within the cell nucleus. It is impossible to observe or photograph chromosomes without the aid of a microscope and special cellular dyes that stain the normally colorless genetic material. The 64 chromosomes can be arranged as a series of 32 pairs in a photographic print. The array of paired chromosomes prepared from such a print is known as a **karyotype**.

Although the different breeds generally can be distinguished from one another by visual comparison, horses of all breeds have the same number, sizes, and shapes of chromosomes within their cells because the genetic information of all horses is nearly identical. The fact that crosses between breeds of horses widely differing in appearance will produce fertile offspring is evidence of this basic similarity. The only distinguishing feature found in most equine karyotypes is the difference between males and females, which is manifested in a single pair of chromosomes (the X and Y) whose inheritance will be discussed below.

The genes arrayed along the chromosomes are so minute that they cannot be "seen" by any direct process, even microscopy. Classically speaking, genes are only recognized by their end-effects (e.g., black hair versus red hair). The emerging era of biotechnology now is making it possible to delineate the precise molecular sequence of the DNA of many specific genes. Few equine genes have yet been sequenced, but it probably is only a matter of time before the basic information gleaned from genetic research on mice and human beings can be applied effectively to horses as well.

Mendelian Genetics

THE BEHAVIOR OF CHROMOSOMES

An understanding of inheritance patterns can be obtained by a thorough knowledge of the behavior of chromosomes—although Mendel made his discoveries before chromosomal processes were known. Two division processes are characteristic of cells and their chromosomes. The first process, known as mitosis, occurs in all cells of the body. When a body cell divides into two, the cell's chromosomes precisely duplicate themselves, each daughter cell receiving an exact replica of the chromosomes of the original cell. The second division process, known as meiosis, is directly involved in the formation of **gametes** (the reproductive cells—the sperm and **ova** [eggs]) and occurs only in the reproductive organs. Gametes of the horse contain only 32 chromosomes,

exactly half the number found in the other cells of the body. Each pair of chromosomes in the parent cell contributes only a single chromosome to a gamete. When sperm (containing 32 chromosomes) and egg (also containing 32 chromosomes) combine during fertilization, the chromosome number of the resulting fertilized cell or zygote is 64, thus reconstituting the normal chromosomal composition of equine body cells.

THE INHERITANCE OF SEX

The sex of a foal is determined by the genetic contribution of its sire alone. As mentioned earlier, a clear difference exists between the chromosomes of stallions and mares and can be visually observed in a karyotype. For one particular pair of chromosomes, the sex chromosomes, the pair members are distinctly different from each other in the stallion, whereas in the mare the paired chromosomes are essentially identical. The two sex chromosomes of the stallion are designated X and Y. The two sex chromosomes of the mare are designated X. As indicated above, the members of every chromosome pair are split up as the gametes form during meiosis. All gametes of the mare (the ova) have only a single X chromosome, while the male gametes (the sperm) represent an equally divided mixture of X- and Y-bearing cells. An ovum fertilized by an X-bearing sperm will develop into a filly, while an ovum fertilized by a Y-bearing sperm will develop into a colt.

Geneticists often employ a simple diagrammatic tool called a Punnett square (*see* below) to predict the expected outcome of individual matings. On the top of the diagram are listed the alternative traits (in this case, chromosomes symbolized X and Y) that can be contributed by one parent; at the left are listed the alternatives contributed by the other parent (in this case the mare, which can only contribute an X chromosome). In the squares formed by the intersection of the columns and rows of the parental contributions are listed the possible combinations that can be produced in the offspring. For sex, only two outcomes are normally possible: XX (female) and XY (male):

Male Contribution (Sperm)

		X	Y
Female Contribution (Ovum)	X	XX Female	XY Male
	X	XX Female	XY Male

From an understanding of the chromosomal basis of sex determination, it is clear why the YY alternative has never been found. The X chromosome contains genes for many essential functions, the absence of which would be incompatible with life. By contrast, relatively few genes other than those for the determination of maleness are found on the Y chromosome.

Probably the most important genetics lesson to be learned from the study of sex determination is that the inheritance of traits follows the inheritance pattern of the chromosomes. Because chromosomes occur in pairs, only one of two trait alternatives may be contributed by each parent to its offspring. Equal ratios of the trait alternatives (in this case, sex) are expected among the offspring. Thus, genetic differences among siblings may be determined solely by a difference in the contribution of one parent (for traits other than sex, this will not always be the stallion).

DOMINANT GENES AND RECESSIVE GENES
Occasionally matings are observed in which an offspring is distinctly different from both parents. For example, a pair of black Morgans may produce a red (chestnut) foal as well as the anticipated black ones. The inheritance of coat color patterns provides some wonderful examples for an understanding of basic concepts of genetics.

Many studies have verified that the chestnut coat of Morgans and other breeds results from the action of a gene whose alternative form produces black pigment in the hair. The alternative forms of a particular gene are known as **alleles**. If the DNA sequences of the different alleles of a gene are compared, they characteristically are found to differ in only a single **nucleotide** (an individual unit of DNA) out of the thousands of nucleotides of which they are composed. The nucleotides of the DNA code for the production of specific sequences of **amino acids,** the building blocks of protein molecules. A change in a single amino acid (resulting, for example, from a single nucleotide change in the corresponding gene) may destroy the activity of a protein or cause it to produce an altered product.

In the coat-color example illustrated above, red color factors were carried by the black Morgan parents without being physically apparent. The red allele is said to be **recessive** to the black, and the black allele is said to be **dominant** to the red. A dominant allele is one that is expressed even when carried by only one member of a chromosome pair. In this example the presence of just one dominant allele (coding for the production of a black hair coat) will drive the production of black hair pigment, resulting in a black coat, even if the red allele is present as the other member of the chromosome pair. Only when both members of a chromosome pair contain the recessive red allele will the coat color be red.

To provide a simplified notation, geneticists assign letters to genes and their different alleles. In the coat-color example, the responsible gene is called **extension** (the name is assigned due to its similarity to a previously designated gene of mice) and symbolized by the letter E. The dominant allele is assigned a capital letter with a superscript, i.e., E^E, which can be simplified for discussion to E. The recessive allele is referred to as E^e, or more simply, e. Three possible combinations of these alleles are thus possible for individual animals: EE, Ee, and ee.

Because the chromosomes bearing the genes occur in pairs, the coat color will be determined by the interaction of the pair of alleles of the E gene. The term **genotype** is used for the letter symbols describing a gene pair, while the term **phenotype** is used to describe the external attributes resulting from a gene's action. Thus the genotype of black horses (they may be black, bay, or buckskin; the distribution pattern of black hair is caused by genes that will be discussed below) is either EE or Ee, while the genotype of red (chestnut) horses is always ee. Conversely, the phenotype of EE and Ee horses is black, while the phenotype of ee horses is red. When both alleles in a pair are the same (here, EE or ee), the horse is said to be **homozygous** for that trait. When each of the two alleles is different (Ee), the horse is said to be **heterozygous**. Because the black allele E is dominant to the red allele e, for black horses the genotype (either EE or Ee) is not always readily apparent from the phenotype (black). Thus, a red foal can be produced from the mating of black horses if both parents are heterozygous for the color trait, as shown in this Punnett square diagram:

Heterozygous Stallion

		E	e
		E	e
Hetero- zygous Mare	E	EE Black	Ee Black
	e	Ee Black	ee Red

The diagram provides additional information about the foals resulting from the mating of these two horses. The ratios expected for a cross between heterozygotes is 3:1 (in this case, 3 black foals:1 red foal), although the genotypic ratio underlying the colors is 1 homozygous black foal:2 heterozygous black foals:1 homozygous red foal. Among the black foals, the EE horses can never have red foals even if bred to a red mate, while Ee horses in combination with either Ee or ee mates will produce both red and black foals.

The only way to determine which black horses are EE and which are Ee is through a test cross to an ee (red) mate, since no direct laboratory test for the e allele is available. A **test cross** is a mating between a homozygous recessive (here, ee) and an animal with the phenotype of the dominant allele. Sometimes pedigrees or family studies can help determine genotypes that may not always be obvious from phenotypes. For example, a black mare with a chestnut sire, and any black horse that produces a chestnut foal,

will necessarily be Ee. A useful characteristic of a recessive trait such as e is that it will always "breed true," i.e., chestnut bred to chestnut will always produce chestnut, since no E factor is present in the cross to contribute the ability to manufacture black hair pigment.

Occasionally it may be possible to differentiate homozygous and heterozygous genotypes by observation of the phenotype. Another coat-color trait can provide an example of this. The palomino gene (C^{cr}) causes a distinctive golden hair color by dilution of red pigment to yellow, and is highly prized by many breeders. Homozygotes ($C^{cr}C^{cr}$) for the gene exhibit a "dosage effect" in that the coat is diluted to a very pale cream (cremello), which is usually considered undesirable. Since a cremello can be expected to produce all dilute colored foals when bred to a nondilute mate (e.g., black, bay, or chestnut), such a horse could be a valuable asset for a breeder of palominos (or buckskins).

GENE INTERACTIONS

Because the genetic makeup of every horse is composed of thousands of genes, it is important to develop a working understanding of the results expected from the complex interaction of the products of more than a single gene. Using already familiar examples, one can predict the outcome of a mating when two traits are considered simultaneously, such as sex and black/red coat color (both parents being heterozygous for coat color):

Heterozygous Stallion

		XE	Xe	YE	Ye
Hetero- zygous Mare	XE	XX EE Black female	XX Ee Black female	XY EE Black male	XY Ee Black male
	Xe	XX Ee Black female	XX ee Red female	XY Ee Black male	XY ee Red male

The four different parental types of sperm can combine with the two different types of egg to generate eight potential genotypic classes of offspring. Each class is equally likely to occur, owing to the random processes that determine whether a sperm will be XE, Xe, YE, or Ye, and whether it will combine with an XE ovum or an Xe ovum. Based on the dominance interaction between alleles of the E locus, these eight genotypic classes will appear as four possible phenotypes of foals (black males, black females, red males, and red females). Due to chance, however, any particular mating of this type may never produce any red females or red males. If offspring data from many matings between parental combinations of these same genotypes are combined and evaluated by statistical tests, then the frequencies of the hypothesized outcomes diagrammed in the Punnett square will become evident.

Sometimes the actions of alleles of one gene may obscure the actions of alleles of another gene. **Dominance** refers to the interaction of alleles of a single gene; the masking of one gene's activity by another gene is more properly called **epistasis**. The gene that is masked by epistasis is said to be **hypostatic**. (Often this terminology is considered cumbersome and abandoned by lay geneticists, but misuse of the term "dominance" is also a fundamental source of confusion when determining the relationship between alleles of different genes). We can consider an example with a mating between parents heterozygous for genes at two chromosomal locations or **loci** (singular = **locus**). In this case, we can use the familiar E gene in combination with the progressive graying gene G. In the presence of the dominant allele G the horse is gray, **epistatically** suppressing the expression of any E gene alleles. The following Punnett square representation provides an illustration of the interactions of the allelic combinations of these two genes. (See next column.)

The complex interactions of several genes can produce phenotypic ratios that at first glance seem unrelated to those expected by the simple random assortment of genes on chromosomes. In the above example, three colors of foals could be produced by gray parents: gray, black, and red, in an expected proportion of 12:3:1. Even more complicated examples could be constructed, but the point to be made is that a basic understanding of the allelic actions of genes when considered in isolation from each other

Heterozygous Stallion

		GE	Ge	gE	ge
Hetero-zygous Mare	GE	GG EE Gray	GG Ee Gray	Gg EE Gray	Gg Ee Gray
	Ge	GG Ee Gray	GG ee Gray	Gg Ee Gray	Gg ee Gray
	gE	Gg EE Gray	Gg Ee Gray	gg EE Black	gg Ee Black
	ge	Gg Ee Gray	Gg ee Gray	gg Ee Black	gg ee Red

can help predict the outcome of more complex interactions.

Gene Linkage

Each individual gene is located on one particular chromosome and at a specified place (or locus) on that chromosome. Most genes chosen for study are by chance located on different chromosomes. Occasionally, traits of interest are located on the same chromosome and tend to be inherited together more often than they are split apart, a phenomenon referred to as **gene linkage.** Linked genes can be separated from one another as part of the normal process of chromosomal recombination that occurs during meiosis. The proportion of offspring in which linked traits occur in different combinations from those of the parents is related to the physical distance between the genes on the chromosome.

Information concerning the linkage groups distributed on the 32 pairs of equine chromosomes is meager at present, but gene-mapping efforts underway for several mammalian species undoubtedly will contribute added knowledge that will benefit the study of equine gene linkages as well. One useful linkage group in the horse involves several coat-color genes, including E and two dominantly inherited pattern genes, roan (Rn) (basic black, brown, or chestnut with a sprinkling of white) and tobiano (TO) (white spotting). An attentive owner may discover that a black stallion heterozygous for tobiano spotting sires chestnut foals that are seldom spotted (approximately 8 percent). This observation can be explained by linkage of the genes for tobiano and E. For the black stallion, one of his chromosomes has T and E, while the other must have to (solid color, no spotting) and e. For other stallions, the linkage phase of tobiano may be T with e.

One of the ways for an undesirable trait to become widespread in a breed is through close linkage with another trait that is highly prized. It is important to understand just how many off-spring and how much careful testing may be required to produce a foal possessing the valued gene without the linked defective trait, if the genes are closely situated on the same chromosome.

A special case of linkage is related to the genes on the X chromosome (the female sex chromosome), particularly several that produce factors necessary for normal blood clotting. Males, it will be recalled, have only one X chromosome per cell. Some may inherit from their mothers an X chromosome with a defective gene whose expression in females usually is masked by the normal gene on the other X chromosome. The inheritance of so-called **X-linked** disease-causing genes has a pattern of expression that follows the pattern of transmission of the sex chromosomes. Typically, males inherit the defective gene from mothers that are heterozygous (i.e., carriers) for the abnormal gene. On average, half the male offspring of a carrier mother will be affected, but none of the female offspring will be affected, although half will be carriers like the mother. Male offspring of affected fathers never receive the defective gene from the father. Female offspring of affected fathers are usually free of the disease but may transmit the problem to half of their male offspring. X-linked inheritance can be demonstrated with a Punnett square where X* is used to symbolize the X chromosome with the disease-associated gene:

Normal Stallion

		X	Y
Carrier Mare	X*	XX* Carrier female	X*Y Affected male
	X	XX Normal female	XY Normal male

X-linked genes are often called sex-linked genes, to contrast them with autosomal genes, which are the genes located on the other 31 pairs of chromosomes.

POLYGENIC (MULTIPLE-GENE) TRAITS

In general most traits are influenced by more than a single gene, but for many we can only discern the action of a so-called "major gene," which appears to produce most of the genetic variation in the trait of interest. Particularly for traits that can be measured (quantitative traits), the phenotype can be produced by the additive effects of several genes at different loci (and can also typically be influenced by environmental components as well). In traditional animal science, breeding programs concentrating on production traits (milk, meat, eggs) can be assisted by mathematical analyses of production records among related animals, in order to choose the best individuals for breeding stock.

Progress in selecting for or against a trait can be frustratingly slow when the several genes affecting the trait cannot be readily identified. Moreover, quantitative traits may exhibit a "threshold effect," so that breeders may not be aware of the accumulation of useful or problem genes until a critical mass of additive alleles has been attained, producing a phenotypic abnormality. For the future, DNA biotechnology to identify marker genes holds promise for selecting desirable production traits and seemingly could be used to select against deleterious multiple-gene traits as well.

Determination of Inheritance Patterns

To apply genetics to a breeding program requires an understanding of how traits are inherited. How can one determine whether a trait is inherited (or due to environmental effects such as diet or microorganisms), and if inherited, whether it is dominant, recessive, sex-linked, autosomal, multiple allelic, or polygenic? Several years of genetic research may be necessary to provide definitive answers. The components of such research may include:

- Searching the scientific literature for similar conditions in horses of other breeds or in other mammalian species
- Collecting pedigrees of horses expressing the trait to search for relationships
- Collecting breeding data to determine the pattern of transmission in a lineage
- Designing test matings

Among the above projects pedigree collection is ultimately the least informative, since purebred horses are likely to be related to each other and to be produced from matings between stock that are at least distantly related. Test matings, on the other hand, are likely to provide a good deal of information. Characteristic inheritance patterns of different classes of genes can be recognized and matings designed to investigate trait transmission. Characteristics of autosomal dominant genes include:

- Transmission from an affected parent (except in the unlikely event that the trait has just appeared as a new mutation)
- Approximately 50 percent of offspring of both sexes will have the trait.

Recessive traits will probably be seen first in both males and females as a result of matings between normal parents, but when affected animals are mated together, the offspring (inheriting two recessive alleles) will all exhibit the trait. Generally, X-linked traits are obvious from their apparent association with males. Several examples exist in the scientific literature wherein an erroneous conclusion about the inheritance of a trait was reached before a thorough genetic study was completed, so it is important not to rush to conclusions before test matings have been performed.

Inbreeding, Linebreeding, Outcrossing

To produce horses with desirable traits, most breeders work with purebred animals of known pedigree. Many studbook regulations prevent the use of animals outside the registry, effectively creating a closed genetic pool. The aim of this restriction is to encourage the breeding of

stock of a consistent type, with excellence for a selected set of breed characteristics.

Owners generally see no more than five- or six-generation pedigrees of their animals, owing perhaps to constraints as trivial as paper size for printing pedigrees, but also to the time necessary to research and compile the more distant generations (which seldom seem to be available readily in computer databases). If distant generations could be viewed as easily on paper as the more immediate ones, breeders might be surprised to learn how few founders their purebred animals trace. Of course, this will vary widely from breed to breed, but nonetheless purebred animals are by definition more inbred than are animals outside a closed studbook format.

Inbreeding is a breeding technique that pairs closely related animals, such as father–daughter, brother–sister, or cousins. However, the strict scientific definition of inbreeding counts all relationships that are duplicated on both sides of a pedigree, no matter how distant. Animal breeders by tradition consider distantly related crosses to be linebreeding rather than inbreeding, but the scientific basis of this concept is not obvious. It is also traditional that purebred livestock breeders in general consider that their breeding philosophy encompasses linebreeding, while inbreeding is the breeding program practiced only by rivals.

The theoretical purpose of inbreeding (or linebreeding) is to produce stock of consistent excellence through creation of a homozygous type. Inbreeding increases the probability that any gene will be homozygous by descent. Of course, inbreeding favors homozygosity for genes of excellence as well as deleterious genes, so a thorough understanding of the process is vital for a sound breeding program. Among some animal stocks, inbreeding may lead to reproductive problems (ultimately infertility) and reduced disease resistance. Breeders are continually warned of these possibilities, although documented examples in many animal species are difficult to find.

The general premise of inbreeding (linebreeding) is that "homozygosity is good." It is well known that at times the optimal type actually is obtained in heterozygotes (e.g., the palomino coat-color gene) rather than in homozygotes. Even though heterozygosity does not produce a consistent breeding animal, it should not be considered as an inappropriate breeding tool. In fact, so little is known about the genetics of desirable conformation traits that it is probably premature to state that inbreeding as a general technique for structuring pedigrees produces either good or bad stock.

The best approach for responsible horse breeding includes an awareness of pedigree structure but focuses on breeding for quality, while not ignoring real or potential problems of defective genes. It would be irresponsible to assume that any animal is devoid of deleterious genes; the task is to minimize the risk of producing a defective foal while at the same time producing an example of true excellence for the particular breed of concern.

Additional Examples of Equine Genes

BASIC COLORS

In mammals, **melanin** is the most important pigment of coat color. Melanin occurs as granules of pigment in the hair, skin, and **iris** (the circular, pigmented tissue behind the cornea of the eye) in two basic forms: **eumelanin** (black or brown in color) and **pheomelanin** (red or yellow). Genes of coat color produce their effects by influencing the switch between eumelanin and pheomelanin production, or by altering the presence, shape, number, or arrangement of pigment granules.

The basic coat colors of horses are produced by the interactions of alleles for at least 11 different gene loci. A breed may not have recognizable genetic variation at all the loci, and indeed some breeds (e.g., Friesian, Cleveland Bay) have been selected to be invariant for the recognized coat-color genes. A comprehensive understanding of the interactions of so many gene loci requires a review of the basic effects of each gene.

The major color-producing genes of horses are agouti (A) and, as has already been described, extension (E). Alleles at the E locus either extend (E) or diminish (e) the amount of eumelanin (black) in the coat, with the opposite effect on

the extent of pheomelanin (red or yellow). This gene is responsible for producing the difference between black-coated horses and red/yellow-coated horses. Suffolk draft horses are an example of a breed in which all animals are ee.

The agouti gene also influences the distribution pattern of eumelanin. The black points pattern known as bay is produced by the dominant allele A, which causes eumelanin (in an EE or Ee horse) to be restricted to hairs of the mane, tail, and lower legs, in contrast to the rest of the body which is some shade of red. The recessive allele of the A locus produces a uniformly black horse in the presence of EE or Ee.

Color dilution is produced by three independent genes. The golden color of palominos and buckskins is produced by c^{cr}, as discussed previously. The dominant allele at the D (dun) locus affects the clumping of pigment granules in hair. Its combination with other genes produces diluted colors with dun markings (darker markings), such as mouse dun (grullo) and claybank dun (red dun). Horses homozygous for dun are not noticeably more diluted than are heterozygotes. The third dilution gene is the dominantly inherited silver dapple, mostly associated with ponies. Its most favored combination is with black, which produces the classic dappled chocolate with flaxen mane and tail. In association with the bay genotype, the resulting diluted color comes very close to a flaxen chestnut, often contributing to confusion about coat-color inheritance in ponies.

A dominant gene for progressive graying (G) causes the hair of most Lippizans and Andalusians to become white or nearly white with age, although foals may be born in a variety of black, brown, and red colors. Horse registries may use gray color inheritance as a tool to identify an incorrectly assigned parentage, e.g., every gray foal must have a gray parent.

Roan is a pattern of interspersed white and dark hairs produced by a dominant gene (Rn). Dark-eyed white horses are produced by a dominant gene (W), which is lethal in the homozygous condition. Appaloosa spotting patterns are generally thought to be produced by one or more dominant genes, and there is some evidence to indicate that the desirable blanket pattern may occur only in heterozygotes. The leopard spotting pattern may be the phenotype produced by homozygosity for an(other) Appaloosa gene.

Tobiano and overo are two white spotting patterns produced by unlinked genes (T and O) that behave as dominant traits in Paint horses and other breeds with spotting patterns. More than one gene may be responsible for overo, thus confusing a complete understanding of the inheritance pattern. Horses may be homozygous for tobiano, in which case all their offspring will be spotted, but the classic overo gene is lethal in homozygotes.

BLOOD GROUPS, PROTEIN POLYMORPHISMS, AND DNA MARKERS

Although horses do not have the same ABO and Rh blood groups that people have, they do possess their own systems of red blood cell antigens, which vary from individual to individual and from breed to breed. Determination of blood groups is important in horses, as it is in human beings, for selecting a compatible blood donor when a whole-blood transfusion is required.

Blood is composed of a complex mixture of proteins that can be sorted out by **electrophoresis** (separation of components of a mixture by their differing migration in an electric field) and visualized with protein-specific dyes or stains. The resultant banding patterns represent the protein products of genes. The genetic basis of band pattern variation for a specific protein can be studied using blood samples from members of family groups. Inheritance of variants is due to **codominant** alleles, wherein both members of an allelic pair are fully expressed.

The high degree of **polymorphism** (genetic variation) for blood group, protein, and DNA marker systems (identification of DNA banding patterns in individual animals) combined with the codominant pattern of inheritance of variants, makes such markers useful for identification, parentage testing, and gene mapping. Genetic tests may exclude a parent because it fails to share genetic factors with its alleged offspring. Alternatively, an offspring may be excluded because it possesses a factor not present in at least one of the parents. Any system of genetic markers can be employed in parentage testing, provided that a solid foundation of published research supports interpretation of the results so that any legal challenge can be successfully met.

Establishment of a genetic map for the horse will require the identification of hundreds of genetic markers. When an extensive equine gene map is available it may allow breeders to design matings that are more certain to meet specific production goals than is possible with the empirical techniques now available. Identification of markers closely linked to a disease for which no biochemical test is available could allow selection of proper mating pairs to avoid mating inapparent carriers. In the future special performance abilities, seldom the result of a single gene, may be more effectively selected using assayable linked marker genes, rather than by relying on the performance records of parental stock.

CHAPTER 14

Congenital and Inherited Disorders

by Ann T. Bowling

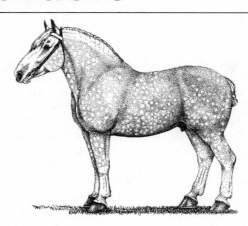

A **congenital** abnormality is a defect of structure or function that is present at birth. The incidence of congenital defects in foals has been estimated at about 3–4 percent. Defects can be caused by environmental factors that interfere with normal developmental processes or by abnormal genes. Environmental factors to consider include nutritional deficiencies or excesses, inhaled or ingested chemicals, drugs, and toxins. Inherited diseases can be congenital, but many do not become evident for several months or even years after birth. To prevent the recurrence of a congenital problem in subsequent foals, it is important to discover the underlying basis of the problem. Unfortunately, many defects have no known cause.

This chapter will focus on inherited defects in horses, and will summarize the varieties of evidence available that allow scientists to determine whether a condition has a genetic basis. A discussion of carrier testing and selective breeding schemes will be presented to guide horse owners and breeders. For definitions and explanations of the genetic terms that are used extensively in this chapter, readers are urged to

review CHAPTER 13, "GENETICS," as a prelude.

Normal development of the equine fetus requires approximately 48–49 weeks, which represents the normal **gestation period**. The fertilized ovum, or **zygote**, representing the union of egg from the mare and sperm from the stallion, proceeds by way of cell division through a series of developmental stages on its way to becoming a newborn foal. By approximately 8 weeks the developing **embryo** attaches to the uterine wall, and survives by receiving nourishment from the mare through a specialized tissue known as the **placenta**, which serves as the physical connection between mother and offspring. During the second half of the gestation period rapid development occurs, as the future foal grows larger and larger and the different organ systems within it take on recognizable shapes and begin to function. During any of these stages of development, genetic or environmental influences may interfere with one or more of the normal developmental events and so produce a birth abnormality. (For additional information on the reproductive and birth processes of horses, *see* CHAPTER 9, "REPRODUCTIVE PHYSIOLOGY," and CHAPTER 11, "PREGNANCY, PARTURITION, AND THE YOUNG FOAL.")

Characteristics of Genetic Problems

In general, genetic diseases can be broadly categorized as belonging to one of three groups:

- Chromosomal defects
- Single-gene defects
- Polygenic (multiple-gene) defects

Abnormalities in the first two categories are ultimately the easiest to document and understand but are rarely seen. Polygenic traits, produced by the interaction of several genes, are more likely to be the source of commonly observed defects such as those of conformation. However, polygenes producing undesirable traits have not been definitively documented in horses, so this category of equine defects must remain hypothetical at present.

Usually the first evidence of a problem is the birth, in repeated matings, of foals exhibiting similar defects of structure or function. It is unlikely in the extreme that all offspring of a given mating or an entire foal crop would be affected by a genetic disease, so such a situation would be presumptive evidence of a nongenetic (i.e., environmental) cause. Another clue that an abnormality may have a genetic basis is an association with a particular breed. Breed association is more indicative of a genetic disease than is a **familial** (within family lines) or herd association because families, coexisting in the same environment, would be more likely to be exposed to any problem peculiar to that environment than would an entire breed, whose members are spread out over many families in many different environments.

Disruption of normal development during the early stages is usually incompatible with life, resulting either in immediate death of the embryo or in failure of the embryo to implant in the uterine wall. Dominantly inherited defects often exert extreme effects on the organism, and animals with such genes seldom survive to breeding age (although there are rare exceptions, such as hyperkalemic periodic paralysis in Quarter

Horses; *see* below). The majority of identified genetic anomalies are inherited as recessive genes, meaning that the parents are heterozygote carriers and are unlikely to be clinically affected. Recessive genes are masked in heterozygotes by the dominant normal gene and so may be more widespread within a breed than is generally acknowledged. Those mutations that survive are usually chance "hitchhikers" in highly successful breeding lines, otherwise the homozygous genotype producing the problem condition would be so rarely encountered as to be overlooked.

Pedigree studies of affected animals can provide tentative evidence for the heritability of some diseases. However, because most purebred animals tend to be related to varying degrees, pedigree relationships alone cannot be used to substantiate the inheritance of a defect. Clinical and other studies may relate the abnormality to an analogous, proven genetic disease in another species. Verification of the inheritance of a trait in horses usually requires data documenting the number of affected and unaffected foals produced from selected, informative matings. To determine whether a genetic basis exists for problems in which the affected animals survive to reproductive age, it is possible to design matings (**test crosses**) between affected and normal animals. If the defect in question is produced by a lethal gene, however, matings can only be designed between animals that have sired or produced an affected foal (i.e., presumptive heterozygotes), and many more offspring will be needed than in a test cross of a nonlethal gene.

Chromosomal Defects

Most chromosomal abnormalities are eliminated before they can be observed or studied because they are associated with the loss or rearrangement of a large number of genes—a situation incompatible with life. Although rarely seen, the most common viable chromosome problems involve the sex chromosomes, X and Y. For certain problems of **infertility** (diminished ability to produce offspring), karyotyping may be an important diagnostic tool for identifying the basis of the abnormality (*see* CHAPTER 13, "GENETICS"). Unfortunately, karyotyping for domestic animals is only available at a few veterinary research hospitals, and relatively few veterinary clinicians are fully familiar with the presenting signs that may be linked to chromosomal abnormalities.

63,X GONADAL DYSGENESIS (TURNER'S SYNDROME)

A rare few infertile mares have been identified that are missing one of the pair of X chromosomes. The karyotype is analogous to that described for human female gonadal dysgenesis, also known as Turner's syndrome. Affected mares are small in stature, are chronically infertile, and fail to cycle regularly (if at all). The condition appears to occur sporadically, probably from failure of the sex chromosome pair to separate during meiosis. No compelling evidence has been found to indicate that the condition is inherited. Because affected mares are infertile, the condition is essentially self-limiting and will not be transmitted to the next generation.

64,XY SEX REVERSAL

Also a rare condition, the second most common chromosomal abnormality found among infertile mares is a male karyotype. Race winners and show champion mares are among the cases that have been identified in the Shetland Pony, Arabian, Quarter Horse, Appaloosa, Morgan, Thoroughbred, and Standardbred breeds. The phenotype is similar to that for 63,X gonadal dysgenesis (*see* above) except that affected mares may be taller than normal. The condition *may* be inherited as a single-gene defect, but there is probably more than one genetic type involved. As a result the precise inheritance pattern will need to be determined for each family situation.

Autosomal Abnormalities An extra autosomal chromosome has been identified in each of four cases of yearlings, described as being small for their age, with an abnormal gait and poor conformation. At least two of these cases were foals produced by older mares—a condition reminiscent of human *autosomal trisomy (Down's syndrome),* whose incidence is highly correlated with increased maternal age.

Single-Gene Defects

Generally, single-gene defects are confined to one breed or to breeds with similar origins. Once the necessary research has been completed conclusively proving the single-gene origin of a defect, the breeder's work has just begun. If a laboratory test for carriers of the defective gene is available, breeders may choose to breed only from non-carriers or, alternatively, to select breeding stock in subsequent generations that are free of the problem gene. If no carrier test is available, avoidance of breeding with carriers will, unfortunately, be an imperfectly lofty goal. While every effort may be made to avoid breeding from carriers, a large number of carriers will by chance remain undetected. Development of a laboratory test thus is a highly desirable goal for the management of any single-gene defect.

SKELETAL DISORDERS

Fore- and hindlimb bony defects that interfere with gait occur in Shetland Pony foals of both sexes and are caused by an autosomal recessive gene. The disorder has also been documented in Miniature Horses. Unfortunately a candidate gene has not been identified, so at present there is no laboratory test for detecting carriers.

MUSCULAR DISORDERS

Sporadic episodes of generalized muscle tremors and stiffness not associated with exercise, accompanied by elevated serum levels of potassium, have been reported in Quarter Horses and derived breeds (Paints, Appaloosas). This condition, known as *hyperkalemic periodic paralysis (HYPP),* is caused by a defective gene that is involved in the movement of sodium across muscle-cell membranes, and is inherited in an autosomal dominant manner. A laboratory test is available for identifying animals with this trait. For many affected animals the disease can be controlled by regular exercise and a diet low in potassium. The effects of the gene are usually not seen in foals, except in those inheriting two copies of the gene (i.e., homozygotes), who may die from paralysis of the breathing muscles.

CENTRAL NERVOUS SYSTEM DISORDERS

Cerebellar Abiotrophy Progressive loss of function in the **cerebellum** (the portion of the brain concerned with motor function, balance, and coordination of movement) in the horse is characterized by **ataxia** (incoordination), lack of balance equilibrium, and head tremors. The disorder has been documented in young Arabians of both sexes, while a similar condition has been reported in Oldenburgs and Gotland Ponies. No genetic test is available. The conditions are most likely inherited as autosomal recessive traits.

Overo White Lethal In breedings between overo-marked Paint horses, blue-eyed white foals may be produced that appear normal at birth but within a few hours develop signs of **colic** (abdominal pain). The consistent abnormality in these foals is the absence of **ganglia** (nerve connections) throughout the large intestine and portions of the small intestine. Breeding records suggest that this lethal trait is associated with homozygosity for a gene which, when inherited singly, produces the desirable overo pattern of white spotting.

SKIN DISORDERS

Collagen Defect A skin disorder has been reported in related Quarter Horses. It is characterized by hyperextensibility and extreme fragility of the skin, probably due to a defect of **collagen** (a protein constituent of connective tissue). The skin is usually of normal thickness but may be stretched well beyond what is possible in a normal horse. As a consequence wounds occur readily and heal very slowly. Additional studies of the equine disorder are needed to identify the involved gene and its mode of inheritance.

Epitheliogenesis Imperfecta This is a rare, lethal skin defect and is inherited as an autosomal recessive. Affected foals are missing skin and hair on at least one limb below the knee or hock, and in some cases hand-size or larger

patches of hair are missing on the head, shoulder, back, or croup. Hooves of affected limbs lack normal horn material. The foals usually succumb to overwhelming infections within a few hours of birth. This problem has been reported in draft and saddle-horse breeds.

CIRCULATORY/IMMUNE SYSTEM DISORDERS

Neonatal Isoerythrolysis (NI); Hemolytic Disease of the Newborn An otherwise healthy newborn foal may develop signs of lethargy, elevated pulse and respiration rates, and clinical evidence of an acute **hemolytic** (characterized by red blood cell destruction) anemia within 2–5 days of birth. Antibodies to surface components of the foal's red blood cells are present in the **colostrum** ("first milk," milk produced by the mare during the first day or two after birth of the foal) and are the cause of the anemia. Affected foals are usually from the second or later pregnancies of the mare. Recovery may be spontaneous or the disease may progress to severe anemia and death. NI is a genetic disease only in that the red blood cell components involved in the immunologic reactions are inherited (*see* CHAPTER 29, "THE IMMUNE SYSTEM AND VARIOUS DISORDERS," and CHAPTER 11, "PREGNANCY, PARTURITION, AND THE YOUNG FOAL"). The presence of strongly reactive antibodies to those components in the mare is the result of prior sensitization, either through blood transfusions, traumatic birthing, or immunization with vaccines contaminated with red blood cells. No data are available to suggest a familial susceptibility to sensitization. With this disease horse owners need not assume that sires or dams of affected foals possess a transmissible liability that would ethically dictate their removal from the breeding pool.

Hemophilia A (Factor VIII Deficiency) This recessive, X-linked disease is the most common bleeding disorder of horses and has been reported in the Thoroughbred, Standardbred, and Quarter Horse breeds. Signs of hemophilia include recurrent episodes of **subcutaneous hematoma** (localized pockets of blood under the skin), **hemarthrosis** (bleeding into joints), and internal hemorrhage with anemia, the last commonly being the cause of death. Affected individuals lack a factor (factor VIII) essential to the blood-clotting process. Owing to the severity of the disease, it is unlikely that affected stallions will be used for breeding, but mares and (on average) half of the sisters of affected males will pass the disease to their offspring if they are allowed to breed.

Severe Combined Immune Deficiency (SCID, CID) This well-described, lethal disease of Arabian foals is inherited as an autosomal recessive. Lacking the *T-* and *B-lymphocytes* essential for a competent immune system (*see* CHAPTER 29, "THE IMMUNE SYSTEM AND VARIOUS DISORDERS"), CID foals usually succumb before they are 5 months of age to massive infections, primarily of the respiratory tract. The specific gene defect involved has not been identified, so no carrier test is available; however, the birth of an affected foal provides solid evidence of the carrier status of both its parents. As with any recessive trait for which only progeny testing is available, it is virtually impossible to prove, through unselected matings, that any given stallion is *not* a carrier; mating the stallion to known carrier mares is needed to provide the appropriate progeny data.

Polygenic (Multiple-Gene) Defects

Most physical traits are influenced by more than a single gene. This is particularly evident when considering the multifaceted aspects of conformation. Progress in selection against an undesirable trait can be frustratingly slow when several genes affect the trait and cannot be readily identified. Moreover, polygenic traits may exhibit a "threshold effect," so that breeders may not be aware of the accumulation of problem genes in the selected breeding stock until a critical mass of additive alleles has been attained, producing a phenotypic abnormality. As mentioned earlier, polygenes producing undesirable traits have not been definitively documented in the horse, so this category of equine defects must remain hypothetical at present.

Carrier Testing

To avoid producing foals with an inherited defect resulting from the action of a dominantly inherited gene, it is sufficient to avoid breeding from an affected parent. To avoid producing foals with defects resulting from the actions of recessive genes, matings between two carriers (heterozygotes) must not occur (matings involving only one carrier will of course not produce an affected foal). Practically speaking, identifying carriers is an extremely difficult problem. In the absence of a specific biochemical or DNA test for the defective gene, carriers can be recognized only by having sired or given birth to an affected foal. Many carriers will of course go undetected with such a screening method. Providing lists of known carriers serves to establish "guilt by association," because 50 percent (on average) of the offspring of a carrier will *not* inherit the defective gene, and these offspring (as well as the carrier) may represent a source of valued genes at other chromosomal loci.

The requirements of progeny testing to ascertain carrier status involve a certain level of statistical assurance. For example, to determine whether a young stallion carries a specific recessive lethal gene requires breeding to mares known to be carriers of the gene. If no affected foals are produced in 12 matings, then the stallion is considered at the 97 percent level of certainty not to be a carrier for that gene. Progeny testing is slightly easier for recessive traits that are deleterious but not lethal, e.g., no affected foals in five matings with a carrier mare would strongly suggest that the stallion is not a carrier. If a greater degree of certainty were required, more matings would be necessary. Of course, birth of even one affected foal would immediately prove that the stallion being tested is a carrier for the trait of concern. With the increasing interest in gene sequencing in mammals, it is quite likely that within a decade DNA-based diagnostic tests (such as the one currently available for HYPP) could be developed for certain inherited equine diseases, so that for these diseases at least costly and time-consuming progeny tests will become a relic of the past.

CHAPTER 15

Birth Control

by Irwin K.M. Liu

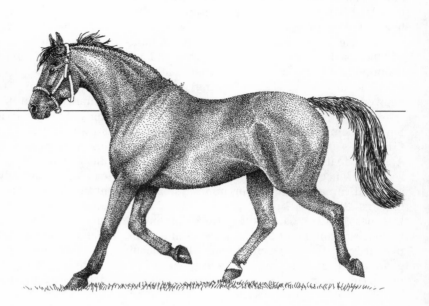

Attempts to control equine populations are aimed chiefly at the free-roaming *feral* (wild) horse. Feral horses have been increasing in numbers in recent years and have been the subject of discussion among public and government interest groups, particularly with regard to the horses' effects upon the forage of public and private lands. Much of the debate and controversy has focused on the means by which populations of wild horses ought to be controlled. In domestic horses surgical removal of the reproductive organs by *castration* or *spaying* is standard practice throughout the world. However, the social life of feral horses is determined by their reproductive patterns. Castration and spaying are not acceptable procedures for use in feral horses because these procedures produce sterility rather than temporary infertility, making other approaches necessary.

Population control methods for feral horses are limited by government regulations and by public interest and humane groups, whose primary intentions are to ensure that the contraceptive methods used are safe, effective, reversible, and do not require capture and/or surgical inter-

vention. In addition, maintenance of horses' social behavior and band integrity following contraception are considered absolutely essential.

Contraception in the Stallion

Several hormones have been used to control sperm numbers in dominant stallions of a herd. These compounds ultimately have long-term adverse effects because the manipulation of hormonal rhythms eventually disturbs normal behavioral patterns. **Testosterone, gonadotropin-releasing hormone (GNRH)**, and related hormones have been used with success in several pilot studies in feral stallions. Long-term behavioral changes were not monitored, however, and the logistics of delivering the hormones to the animals were such that the method had to be discontinued. Other means of contraception, such as **vasectomy** (sterilization by tying off the tubes through which the sperm travel during ejaculation), have been attempted, but the immobilization procedures and surgical intervention required are cost prohibitive. Additional concerns for the safety of the stallions during immobilization, particularly when it is intended that a stallion later undergo vasectomy reversal, have led to disapproval of this method.

Contraception in the Mare

The rationale for focusing attention on the mare rather than the stallion as a means for controlling population levels is twofold. First, band infidelity is common among feral horses, where bachelor stallions often breed mares within a band herded by a dominant stallion. Second, difficulties arise in contracepting all stallions within a given population in an area. Such factors as these have made the mare a much more attractive target for contraceptive efforts.

In the past, attempts were made to contracept mares by manipulation of their hormonal cycles using the female sex hormones **progesterone, estrogen,** or their various synthetic derivatives. The hormones were delivered in the form of implants, which allow for a slow, steady release of the hormone into the bloodstream over a designated period of time. Although this form of contraception has been successful in preventing pregnancy, it has a major disadvantage in that the injected hormones alter the estrous cycling of the mares, thus disrupting normal social behavior within the herd. The use of hormones and/or their synthetic derivatives also carries the risk of producing undesirable effects on predators and scavengers, should the mare die or be killed and the hormone-laden carcass be consumed.

Newer strategies based on the use of antibodies for blocking cyclicity or the fertilization process are now being tested. One concept is to block GNRH, which is responsible for the production and secretion of secondary hormones (**follicle-stimulating hormone [FSH]** and **luteinizing hormone [LH]**) which, in turn, affect the development, maturation, and release of the eggs. This can be accomplished by injecting natural or synthetic, *but foreign*, forms of GNRH into the mare, causing her to produce cross-reacting antibodies against her own GNRH, which block its action. Although this strategy has been successful in preventing pregnancy, long-term side-effects on normal behavioral patterns and cyclicity are inevitable and have met with disapproval from some governmental agencies and public interest groups.

Recently a new form of contraception has been tested in a field setting (feral horse populations in Nevada and California) with unequivocal success. In this technique, vaccines made from the outer membrane (**zona pellucida**) of eggs obtained from pig ovaries are injected into mares. The mares subsequently develop antibodies against the membrane particles. The antibodies circulate through the bloodstream and enter the fluid portion of the ovary, where they bind to the eggs. When the antibody-bound eggs are released into the **fallopian tube** (the site of fertilization) during ovulation, the antibody prevents sperm from attaching and penetrating, thus blocking fertilization. Such zona pellucida vaccines have additional advantages as well:

- They can be delivered from a distance by a darting gun
- Fertility is regained once the antibody levels drop sufficiently
- There is no interference with normal social behavior or band integrity

This method of contraception represents the most ideal form of contraception in horses to date. One major disadvantage, as in many other forms of immunization, is that two inoculations are required (a primary plus a booster) in order to evoke an antibody response adequate to prevent pregnancy for one entire breeding season. This necessitates capture of each mare twice in order to achieve contraception. Researchers are currently developing a single-shot inoculation designed to last for at least *two* breeding seasons. This latter technique incorporates **microspheres** (tiny beads) into the vaccine. The microspheres are designed so that they will release the vaccine only when it is needed (e.g., a month or a year after the injection).

Zona pellucida vaccines have also been used successfully in equids in zoos (zebras, Przewalski horses). Contraception in zoo animals is useful for preventing the inheritance of undesirable traits, and is useful as well in other equids for which a surplus of animals exists.

PART V

Equine Body Systems and Various Disorders

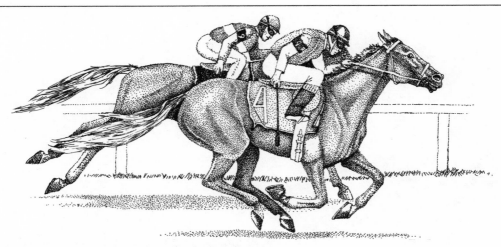

Half the failures in life arise from pulling in
one's horse as he is leaping.

—AUGUSTUS WILLIAM HARE
GUESSES AT TRUTH

CHAPTER 16

Anatomy

by Charles G. Plopper and Jeffrey Lakritz

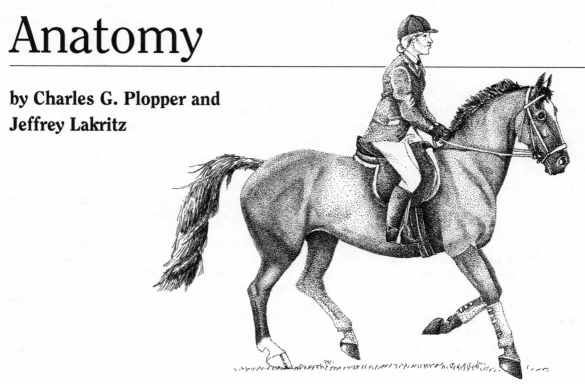

The **anatomy**, or structure, of the body is the framework for the functions of the body, or **physiology**, and is responsible for the overall conformation of the animal. The anatomical organization of an individual animal results from the combination of different organ systems of the body. These include the **integument** (skin), the skeleton, and the musculature. There are a number of other organ systems, most of which function internally, that also show a close relationship between their structure and their functional capabilities. These include the circulatory and immune systems, the digestive tract, respiratory tract, urinary tract, the reproductive system, and the **endocrine** (hormonal) and nervous systems. The components of these systems, the organs, interact to provide the basic functions for each system. The systems together interact to produce the living animal.

This chapter is intended to provide a broad overview of the anatomical structure of the horse, including the external conformation (**topographical anatomy**) and the organization of each of the organ systems. The material presented here does not represent an exhaustive review of the subject; more detailed information on some of the individual body components can be found in other relevant chapters.

Topographical Anatomy

The basic anatomical makeup of the horse produces what is known as the *conformation*. (*See* FIGURE 1.) To understand how different conformations result in defects, or **unsoundness**, one must have a general understanding of the nomenclature of the areas of the body, or landmarks, for evaluation of a horse. Once a general knowledge of the conformation and basic equine anatomy has been acquired, one can utilize this information to develop a logical procedure for examining a horse as a part of its daily care or before purchase.

The *muzzle* (1) of the horse is composed of the upper lip and nostrils. The muzzle is used to prehend food, and has large appendages known as **vibrissae** (whiskers) for sensation. The *bridge of the nose* (2) is continuous with the *forehead* (4) and muzzle. The coloration of hairs in this area is often used to describe an animal for official identification. The **forelock** (5) is the area where hair of the mane falls between the ears.

The eyes are set on either side of the head and should be clear, without evidence of scars or opacity. When examining the horse's head from the front, the two eyes and the muzzle should form a triangle, which maximizes the animal's field of vision. The nostrils are located on either side of the muzzle and are capable of opening widely for inhalation and exhalation of air. The **nasolacrimal** (tear) *duct* openings are located inside each nostril, at the junction of the darker pigmented skin of the muzzle and the pinkish nasal **mucosa** (inner surface lining). These ducts periodically become clogged and require flushing in order to prevent tears or ocular secretions from draining down a horse's face.

The *cheeks* or *jowls* (6) of the horse's head are comprised mainly of large muscles (the *masseter* muscles) for closing the mouth and grinding food. Forward of the cheeks is the *facial crest* (3). The large *facial nerve* runs beneath the skin over each masseter muscle and is responsible for movement of the face and lips. The jaws meet at the tip of the lower lip and hold the lower *incisor* teeth in place.

In younger horses (2–4 years of age), small lumps may be found protruding from beneath the jaw bones. These are the erupting lower *premolar* teeth, which can produce a mild bony inflammation and swelling that usually resolves with time.

The head is attached to the *neck* (37) and forms a depression called the **throatlatch** (39), where the *windpipe* or **trachea** (38), gut tube (**esophagus**), and large *jugular veins* meet at the back of the throat. The throatlatch is important because many horses with an abnormal structure or function in this area produce excessive respiratory noise (a condition known as *roaring*) when worked and so cannot perform optimally. The skin over the throatlatch should be soft. When the throatlatch is **palpated** (felt with the hands), hard lumps should not be present, nor should the horse resent gentle massage of the area.

On the back of the head, between the ears, lies a large bony protuberance called the **poll** (7), a flat region of the skull where large muscles of the neck are attached. The **crest** (8) runs down the back of the neck to the *withers* (9), or region above the shoulders. The **back** (10) and **loin** (11) represent the region of muscles surrounding the vertebral column, supporting the weight of the body and head. The **croup** (12) and **dock** (13) are the regions just behind the *hip* (16) and in front of the tail-base. The large muscles of the **buttock** (14) and **haunch** (15) form smooth, rounded surfaces attaching the powerful rear limbs to the body. These muscles extend forward, covering the *thigh* (17) where the large muscles of this region attach to the *stifle* (18) or knee-cap for straightening the upper leg. These muscles work to advance the leg below the stifle, while those of the buttock work to flex the stifle and move the limb **caudally** (rearward). The underside of the horse is the belly or **abdomen** (28), while the **flank** (27) is the fleshy region between the ribs and the hip.

The muscles that flex the stifle attach to the back of the leg at the *quarter* (19). The portion of the hindlimb below the stifle is known as the **gaskin** (20). The **hock** (21) is the joint formed by the lower part of the *tibia* bone and the hock bones (*tarsals*) between the lower part of the leg and the extension of the toes. The long bones extending below the gaskin form the **cannon** (22). The lower part of the foot attaches to the cannon at the *ankle* (23). The bones, tendons, and ligaments below the ankle form the **pastern**

(24). The *hoof* (26) is joined to the pastern at the **coronet** (25).

The front limb of the horse is attached to the **barrel** (29) and is composed of the *shoulder* (30), *arm* (31), *forearm* (33), and foot. The arm joins the forearm at the *elbow* (32). The area between the two forelimbs is termed the *chest* (34). The most forward part of the shoulder is termed the *point* (35), which is formed by the junction of the arm and the bone of the shoulder, or *scapula*. The forearm joins the **cannon** (22) at the *knee* (36) joint.

The Muscles

(*See* FIGURE 2.) The muscles of the head and neck include the muscles of facial expression, muscles of **mastication** (chewing), and the muscles responsible for raising and lowering the head. The muscles of facial expression include the *buccinator* (2), *caninus* (3), *levator nasolabialis* (4), *scutularis* (5), and *parotidoauricularis* (6). Each performs individual functions, but together they narrow or widen the diameter of the mouth or eyes, move the ears forward or backward, and raise or lower the lips. The muscles responsible for chewing include those that open the mouth and those that close it. The most powerful of these muscles is the *masseter* (1), which closes the jaws, effectively crushing any material between the large flat molar and premolar teeth.

The wings of the **atlas** (7) protrude on either side of the neck, just behind the base of the skull, and represent the lateral extensions of the first vertebra. This structure acts as an anchor to promote side-to-side movement of the head and to stabilize its movement. The *rhomboideus* (8), *splenius* (9), *serratus cervicis* (10), *serratus ventralis thoracis* (24), *trapezius* (11), and *latissimus dorsi* (12) form a sling that stabilizes the front limb and supports the weight of the horse's head, neck, and body. The splenius also provides support for the head and neck, keeping them upright when contracted. The latissimus dorsi also acts to pull the forelimb backward because of its attachment on the inner surface of the shoulder region.

The *superficial pectorals* (28) and *deep pectorals* (25) form the muscle mass lying between the front legs and under the chest. These two muscles provide lower support for the front limbs and advance the front limb in conjunction with the shoulder muscles, i.e., the *brachiocephalicus* (32), *deltoideus* (31), and *biceps brachii* (29). The *external abdominal oblique* (23) is a large, superficial muscle that forms part of the abdominal wall.

The *lumbodorsal fascia* (13) is a thick layer of connective tissue that covers the rear of the neck and back, protecting and supporting the muscles of this region. The *gluteal fascia* (14) lies over the *gluteal* muscles (18) and hip region, providing protection and support for these large muscles. The *sacrococcygeus* (15) acts at the base of the tail to raise or lower it. The *semitendinosus* (16), *semimembranosus*, and *biceps femoris* (17) are the large muscle masses comprising the rear and lateral rump region and are responsible for flexing the stifle and moving the hind limb rearward (extension of the hip). The biceps femoris also provides stability for the stifle region.

The gluteal muscles and the *tensor fascia latae* (19) run from the hip into the region of the *femur* (thigh bone), pulling the rear limb forward and flexing the hip. The *soleus* is a small, powerful muscle that lies behind the tibia and flexes the stifle. The *lateral digital extensor* (21) and *long digital extensor* (22) act to flex the hock and extend the digits (cannon, ankle, pastern, hoof).

The rear aspect of the limb is composed of large, powerful tendons known as the *superficial* and *deep digital flexors* (20) and the *suspensory ligament*. These structures provide support for the lower legs, maintaining the elevation of the fetlock and the angles of the feet with the upper limb.

In the fore limb the *extensor carpi radialis* (27) extends the carpus by pulling on the front of the cannon. In addition, the *common digital extensor* (26) extends the carpus and the digits because it runs across the front of all the joints of the limb below the knee. The *triceps brachii* (30) helps extend the elbow.

The Skeleton

(*See* FIGURE 3.) The bones of the head support the brain and special senses such as sight and sound, and the openings to the respiratory and digestive tracts. The *premaxilla* and *maxilla* (1) are the bones of the upper jaw that support the upper incisor and cheek teeth (molars). The *nasal* bone (2) forms the roof of the nasal cavity and the upper portion of the nostril. The paired *mandibles* (3) join at the front of the skull to form the lower jaw. They support the lower teeth and anchor the base of the tongue. The rear aspect of each mandible anchors the lower jaw to the base of the skull and supports chewing through the attachment of the masseter muscles. The *frontal* (4), *parietal* (5), and *occipital* (6) are the bones of the front, back, and sides of the skull. They surround and protect the brain and nasal sinuses.

The vertebral column is divided into five different regions. The *cervical vertebrae* (8) constitute the neck of the horse. There are seven cervical vertebrae in most horses, with the first two—the *atlas* (7) and *axis*—having specialized functions for movement of the head from side to side and up and down. The *thoracic vertebrae* (9) begin at the point of the shoulder and run as far back as the attachment of the last rib to the vertebral column. There are 18 thoracic vertebrae; extending from each are the *ribs* (31), which support and protect the *thorax* (chest) and abdomen. The ribs from either side curve underneath and attach either to the *xiphoid process* or to each other through the *costal cartilages* (30). The thoracic vertebrae closest to the neck have prominent *dorsal spinous processes* for the attachment of muscles that support the front limbs, head, and neck. The *lumbar vertebrae* (10) and *sacrum* (11) have five vertebrae each. The vertebrae of the sacrum help support the hind limbs, their associated sacral ligaments forming broad attachments to the pelvic bones and muscles. In most

horses there are 14 *coccygeal* (12) or tail vertebrae, which support the muscles that move the tail.

The pelvis of the horse is a cagelike structure that is responsible for attachment of the hind limbs and passage of manure and urinary wastes from the body. In addition the pelvis is crucially important for the normal release of the newborn foal from the mare's uterus. The *ischium* (14; plural: *ischia*) and *ilium* (13; plural: *ilia*) are the bones that form the sides, front, and back of the pelvic cage. The ilium attaches to the vertebral column by means of strong *sacroiliac ligaments*. The paired ischia form the rear projection of the cage and serve as attachments of the powerful muscles of the rump. The floor of the pelvic cage consists of paired *pubis* bones, which fuse along the midline to form a rigid bony structure. The distance between the pubis and sacroiliac region defines the height of the pelvic canal, while the distance between the paired ilia defines the width of the pelvic canal. Injury or inadequate development of these bones in the mare can produce a narrowing of the pelvic canal and subsequent difficulty in birthing.

The hind limb consists of an upper bone, the *femur* (15), which is attached to the pelvis by a ball-and-socket joint; the *patella* (kneecap) (16); and two lower bones, the *tibia* (18) and *fibula* (17). Technically, the bones of the hind foot include the *tarsus* or *hock* (20), which contains six bones, including the *calcaneus* (19), and corresponds to the human ankle and heel; the *metatarsus* or *cannon* (21), and the *phalanges* (22).

The muscles holding the fore limb to the barrel and chest are attached to the *scapula* (32), more commonly known as the shoulder blade.

The upper end of the scapula is lined by a large sheet of cartilage (34) for added muscle attachment. The lateral edge of the scapula includes a long *spine* (33) which also adds area for muscle attachment. The large bone of the upper arm, the *humerus* (29) extends down from the scapula. It joins the two bones of the forearm, the *radius* (26) and *ulna* (27) at the

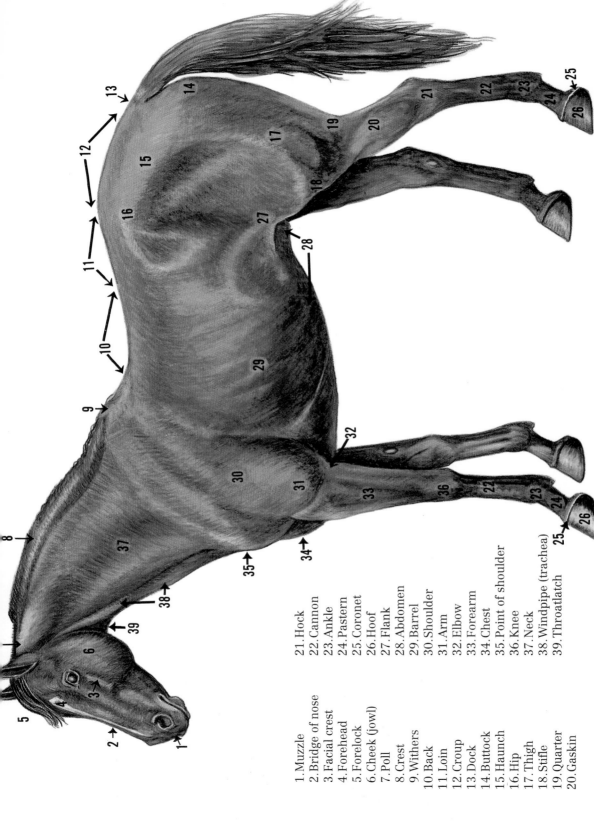

1. Muzzle
2. Bridge of nose
3. Facial crest
4. Forehead
5. Forelock
6. Cheek (jowl)
7. Poll
8. Crest
9. Withers
10. Back
11. Loin
12. Croup
13. Dock
14. Buttock
15. Haunch
16. Hip
17. Thigh
18. Stifle
19. Quarter
20. Gaskin
21. Hock
22. Cannon
23. Ankle
24. Pastern
25. Coronet
26. Hoof
27. Flank
28. Abdomen
29. Barrel
30. Shoulder
31. Arm
32. Elbow
33. Forearm
34. Chest
35. Point of shoulder
36. Knee
37. Neck
38. Windpipe (trachea)
39. Throatlatch

Figure 1.

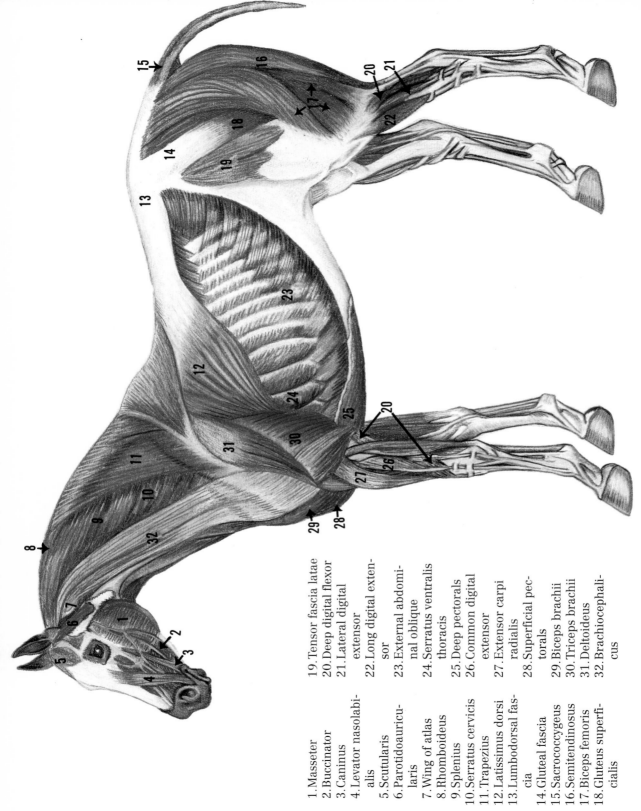

1. Masseter
2. Buccinator
3. Caninus
4. Levator nasolabi-
   alis
5. Scutularis
6. Parotidoauricu-
   laris
7. Wing of atlas
8. Rhomboideus
9. Splenius
10. Serratus cervicis
11. Trapezius
12. Latissimus dorsi
13. Lumbodorsal fas-
    cia
14. Gluteal fascia
15. Sacrococcygeus
16. Semitendinosus
17. Biceps femoris
18. Gluteus superfi-
    cialis
19. Tensor fascia latae
20. Deep digital flexor
21. Lateral digital
    extensor
22. Long digital exten-
    sor
23. External abdomi-
    nal oblique
24. Serratus ventralis
    thoracis
25. Deep pectorals
26. Common digital
    extensor
27. Extensor carpi
    radialis
28. Superficial pec-
    torals
29. Biceps brachii
30. Triceps brachii
31. Deltoideus
32. Brachiocephali-
    cus

Figure 2. The muscles.

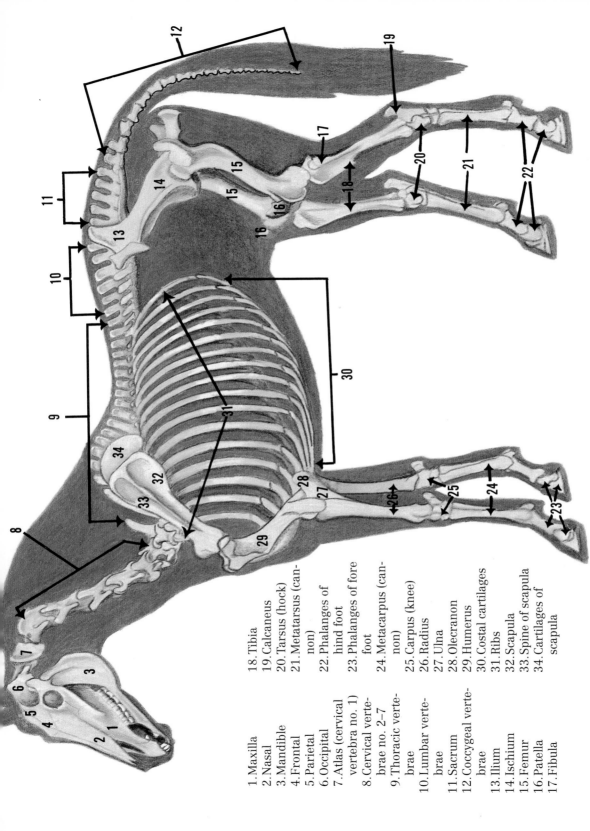

1. Maxilla
2. Nasal
3. Mandible
4. Frontal
5. Parietal
6. Occipital
7. Atlas (cervical vertebra no. 1)
8. Cervical vertebrae no. 2–7
9. Thoracic vertebrae
10. Lumbar vertebrae
11. Sacrum
12. Coccygeal vertebrae
13. Ilium
14. Ischium
15. Femur
16. Patella
17. Fibula
18. Tibia
19. Calcaneus
20. Tarsus (hock)
21. Metatarsus (cannon)
22. Phalanges of hind foot
23. Phalanges of fore foot
24. Metacarpus (cannon)
25. Carpus (knee)
26. Radius
27. Ulna
28. Olecranon
29. Humerus
30. Costal cartilages
31. Ribs
32. Scapula
33. Spine of scapula
34. Cartilages of scapula

Figure 3. The skeleton.

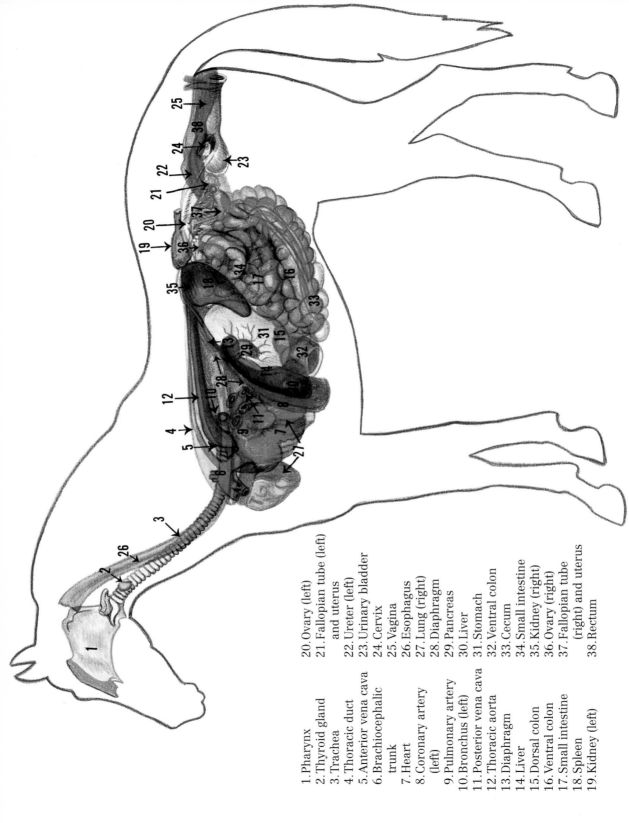

1. Pharynx
2. Thyroid gland
3. Trachea
4. Thoracic duct
5. Anterior vena cava
6. Brachiocephalic trunk
7. Heart
8. Coronary artery (left)
9. Pulmonary artery
10. Bronchus (left)
11. Posterior vena cava
12. Thoracic aorta
13. Diaphragm
14. Liver
15. Dorsal colon
16. Ventral colon
17. Small intestine
18. Spleen
19. Kidney (left)
20. Ovary (left)
21. Fallopian tube (left) and uterus
22. Ureter (left)
23. Urinary bladder
24. Cervix
25. Vagina
26. Esophagus
27. Lung (right)
28. Diaphragm
29. Pancreas
30. Liver
31. Stomach
32. Ventral colon
33. Cecum
34. Small intestine
35. Kidney (right)
36. Ovary (right)
37. Fallopian tube (right) and uterus
38. Rectum

Figure 4. The thoracic and abdominal organs (viscera).

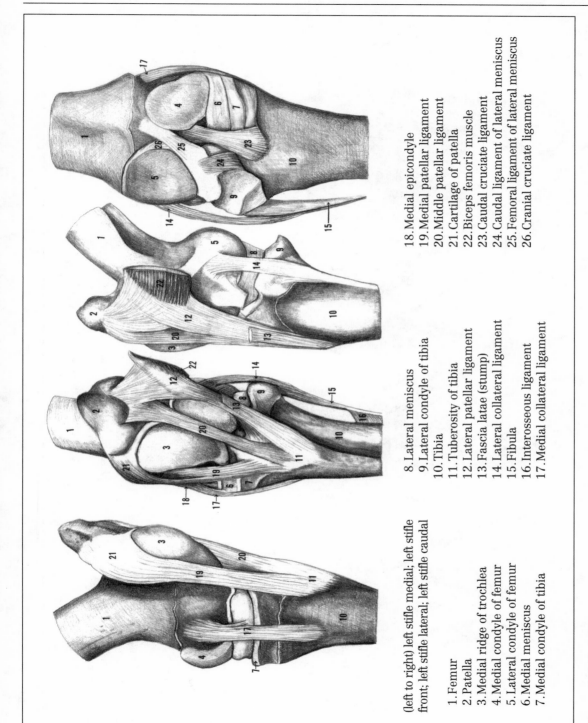

(left to right) left stifle medial; left stifle
front; left stifle lateral; left stifle caudal

1. Femur
2. Patella
3. Medial ridge of trochlea
4. Medial condyle of femur
5. Lateral condyle of femur
6. Medial meniscus
7. Medial condyle of tibia

8. Lateral meniscus
9. Lateral condyle of tibia
10. Tibia
11. Tuberosity of tibia
12. Lateral patellar ligament
13. Fascia latae (stump)
14. Lateral collateral ligament
15. Fibula
16. Interosseous ligament
17. Medial collateral ligament

18. Medial epicondyle
19. Medial patellar ligament
20. Middle patellar ligament
21. Cartilage of patella
22. Biceps femoris muscle
23. Caudal cruciate ligament
24. Caudal ligament of lateral meniscus
25. Femoral ligament of lateral meniscus
26. Cranial cruciate ligament

Figure 5. Stifle joint.

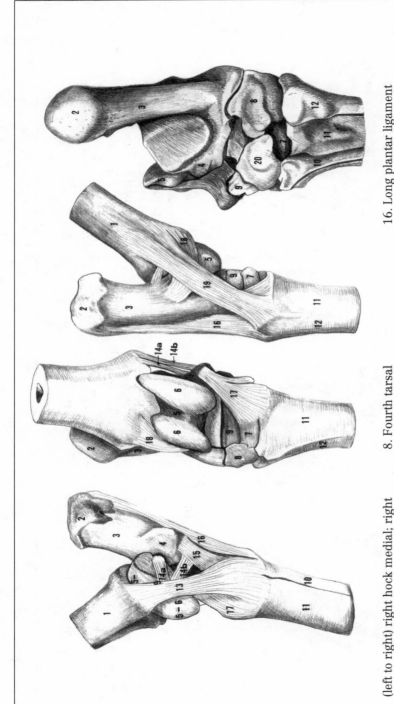

(left to right) right hock medial; right
hock front; right hock lateral; right hock
caudal

1. Tibia
2. Tuber calcanei
3. Calcaneus
4. Sustentaculum
5. Talus
6. Trochlea of talus
7. Third tarsal
8. Fourth tarsal
9. Central tarsal
10. Second metatarsal
11. Third metatarsal
12. Fourth metatarsal
13. Long medial collateral ligament
14a. Short medial collateral ligament
     (branch)
14b. Short medial collateral ligament
     (branch)
15. Plantar tarsometatarsal ligament
16. Long plantar ligament
17. Dorsal tarsal ligament
18. Short lateral collateral ligament
19. Long lateral collateral ligament
20. First tarsal

Figure 6. Hock joint.

elbow. The *olecranon* (28) is the part of the ulna that forms around the elbow joint and serves as an attachment for large muscles that extend the forearm. The eight small bones that attach the radius and ulna to the lower part of the limb are known collectively as the *carpus* or *knee* (25), which corresponds to the human wrist. The *metacarpus* (24) is also known as the *cannon*. The small bones in the foot are the *phalanges* (23).

The Thoracic and Abdominal Organs (Viscera)

(*See* FIGURE 4.) The respiratory, or gas-exchange, system opens into a large cavity in the head, the *pharynx* (1),which is connected to both the mouth and nose. A long tube, the *trachea* or *windpipe* (3), connects the pharynx to the rest of the respiratory system, which is located in the chest. In the chest the trachea divides into two branches or *bronchi* (10), which connect to the lungs on the right and left sides. The majority of the chest cavity is filled by the *lungs* (27), which press against the ribs and *diaphragm* (13, 28). The diaphragm is a large muscle that controls the inhalation and exhalation of air.

The digestive, or gastrointestinal, system also opens into the pharynx. Food in the mouth passes through the pharynx when it is swallowed and is then carried to the *stomach* (31) by the *esophagus* (26). The esophagus runs down the lower part of the neck alongside the trachea, passes through the diaphragm and connects to the stomach. Food is carried from the stomach to the *small intestine* (17, 34), where enzymes from the exocrine portion of the *pancreas* (29) and bile from the *liver* (14, 30) digest the food. The small intestine is a long curved tube in which food is digested and the digested contents are then absorbed. Farther on the small intestine joins the *large intestine* or *colon* (15, 16, 32). The colon forms a U-shaped loop that includes tubes on the bottom (*ventral colon*; 16, 32) and top (*dorsal colon*; 15) of the abdominal cavity. In the horse a large additional digestive chamber

with a blind sac, the *cecum* (33), lies in the bottom part of the abdomen. The cecum opens into the rest of the digestive system at the junction of the small intestine and colon. The final waste product (feces, manure) is excreted through the *rectum* (38).

The urinary system filters metabolic waste products from the bloodstream and excretes them through the urine. The filtering organs are the *kidneys* (19, 35), which are found in the upper part of the abdominal cavity. The filtrate from the kidneys drains into the *urinary bladder* (23) through two tubes, the *ureters* (22). The urine of horses normally contains large amounts of protein, mucus, and salts, making it appear very cloudy and thick at times.

The circulatory system consists of the *heart* (7) and the blood vessels. The heart is located in the chest cavity between the two lungs. Large blood vessels enter and leave the heart carrying blood to and from various parts of the body. The large arteries that supply oxygenated blood to the rest of the body exit the heart by means of the *aorta* (12). Blood carried to the head from the aorta travels through the *brachiocephalic trunk* (6). Oxygenated blood for the heart muscle itself is transported by the *coronary arteries* (8). Deoxygenated blood returns from the body through the *vena cava*. Blood from the head, neck, and fore limb returns to the heart through the *anterior vena cava* (5), while blood from the abdomen, pelvis, and hind limb returns through the *posterior vena cava* (11). Deoxygenated blood is carried to the lungs for oxygenation by the *pulmonary artery* (9). Excess fluid that leaks from capillary beds is carried back to the circulatory system by the *thoracic duct* (4), which empties into the anterior vena cava. Extra blood, and also white blood cells that fight infection, is stored in the *spleen* (18), a large organ that sits in the upper left part of the abdomen behind the stomach.

The reproductive tract of the mare is composed of four parts. New eggs are produced in the *ovaries* (20, 36), which are located in the rear portion of the abdomen. The ovaries are situated beside the *fallopian tubes* (21, 37), which carry the eggs from the ovaries. The fallopian tubes open into the *uterus* (21, 37) where the fertilized egg matures. The newborn foal passes from the uterus into the *vagina* (25) through a muscular opening known as the *cervix* (24). The external reproductive tract of the stallion includes the *scrotum*, which contains the *testicles*, as well as the *penis* and *prepuce* (or *sheath*).

A number of glands in the body release chemicals, called *hormones*, which circulate in the blood to produce changes in other organs. Among these glands is the *thyroid* (2), which is found alongside the upper trachea. Another gland, the *pancreas* (29), is the source of *insulin*, a hormone important in the absorption of nutrients; this hormone is lacking or deficient in many animals and humans with *diabetes mellitus*. In the mare the ovaries release a number of hormones that regulate secondary sex characteristics and control the reproductive cycle.

Stifle Joint

(*See* Figure 5.) The *stifle joint* is the equivalent of the knee in humans. It is located where the large bone of the upper hind limb, the *femur* (1), joins the *tibia* (10). The muscles that extend the hind limb at the stifle operate through attachments to a small bone, the *patella* or *knee-cap* (2), which is located at the knee joint. The *trochlea* (3) is a modification of the femur that forms a groove between two ridges for the movement of the patella.

The femur moves on the tibia through two modifications at the end of the femur, the *medial* (4) and *lateral condyles* (5). Separating each condyle is a small plate of cartilage called a *meniscus*. There is one on the *medial* (6) and one on the *lateral* (8) side below each condyle. The lateral meniscus is held to the tibia by the *caudal ligament of the lateral meniscus* (24) and is held to the femur by the *femoral ligament* (25). The condyles of the tibia are in the same position on the end of the tibia as are the condyles of the femur, on the *medial* (7) and *lateral* (9) sides. The narrow *fibula* (15) runs

alongside the tibia and is connected to it by means of an *interosseous ligament* (16).

On the front of the tibia is a ridge called the *tuberosity* (11). The patella is attached to the tibia by three ligaments that join the tibia at the tuberosity; these are the *medial* (19), *middle* (20), and *lateral patellar ligaments* (12). Some muscles that move the upper part of the hind limb, such as the *biceps femoris* (22), attach directly to the patella and its ligaments.

Two pairs of ligaments attach the femur to the tibia. The *collateral ligaments* (14, 17) run down the medial and lateral sides of the joint outside the condyles. The other two ligaments run between the femur and the tibia in the center of the joint; these ligaments cross and are known as the *cranial* (26) and *caudal cruciate ligaments* (23).

Hock Joint

(*See* Figure 6.) The *hock* is the position in the hind limb where the *tibia* (1) joins the tarsus. There are six tarsal bones in the hock of the horse and they are arranged in two rows. The two nearest the tibia are the *calcaneus* (3) in back and the *talus* (5) in front. The calcaneus has a long *tuberosity* (2) and a *sustentaculum* (4), while the talus has a large *trochlea* (6). The tibia articulates with the tarsal bones through the trochlea of the talus.

Beside the talus is the *central tarsal* bone (9), which occupies most of the space in front, and the *first tarsal* (20) and *fourth tarsal* (8) bones, which are found on the sides and back. The *third tarsal* (7) articulates with the other tarsal bones and the long *metatarsal* bones (10, 11, 12).

The tibia, tarsals, and metatarsals are joined by a number of ligaments. The *long medial collateral ligament* (13) extends from the medial side of the tibia to the second and third metatarsal bones. In front of this ligament is a shorter ligament, the *dorsal tarsal ligament* (17), which joins parts of the talus and central and third tarsal bones to the third metatarsal. The branches of the *short medial collateral liga-*

ment (14a, 14b) join the tibia to the calcaneus and talus.

On the lateral side the *long lateral collateral ligament* (19) joins the tibia to the second metatarsal bone. The *short lateral collateral lig-* *ament* (18) joins the tibia to the talus and calcaneus. The *long plantar ligament* (16) and the *plantar tarsometatarsal ligament* (15) join the calcaneus and the other tarsal bones to the metatarsus.

CHAPTER 17

The Skin and Various Disorders

by Anthony A. Stannard and
Jeffrey E. Barlough

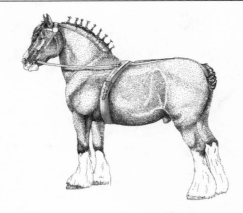

The skin is the outer covering of the body and represents the primary interface between the body and the environment. Anatomically the skin is composed of three major layers, known as the *epidermis*, *dermis*, and *subcutis*.

The Three Major Layers of the Skin

EPIDERMIS

The outermost major layer of the skin is called the **epidermis**. It is an **avascular** (lacking blood vessels), multilayered structure, the exact number of layers varying from species to species and from body area to body area. In general, in any given area an inverse relationship exists between the thickness of the epidermis and the amount of hair present. In haired skin the epidermis is quite thin, consisting of only one to four layers of viable cells, but in nonhaired skin it is much thicker. Both the hair and hooves of the horse represent extensions of the epidermis, as do the **chestnuts** (masses of horn on the inner side of each front leg above the knee, and inner side of each rear leg below the hock) and **ergots** (small masses of horn found in the fetlock hair).

Three major cell types occupy the epidermis. The majority of cells in the epidermis are **keratinocytes**. These are the cells that manufacture **keratin**, an insoluble, sulfur-rich protein that represents the principal structural component of skin, hair, nails, and horn. The other major cell types in the epidermis are the **melanocytes** (cells that produce the skin pigment **melanin**) and **Langerhans cells** (which are important for generating immune responses in the skin).

Keratinocytes

The keratinocytes are arranged in multiple layers. The lowermost layer is referred to as the **basal cell layer**. The basal cells are generally cuboidal in shape and rest on a basement membranelike structure that separates the epidermis from the underlying **dermis** (the middle major layer of the skin). It is through the multiplication of the basal cells and the subsequent maturation of their daughter cells that the upper layers of keratinocytes are formed. The next several layers above the basal cell layer are referred to collectively as the **prickle cell layer** or **squamous cell layer.** The prickle cells are **polyhedral** (having many faces or sides) in shape. Above the prickle cell layer is the **granular cell layer,** composed of flattened cells containing many **basophilic** (staining dark-blue) granules. The outermost layer is the **horny layer,** which is composed entirely of tightly adherent, dead keratinocytes containing abundant quantities of keratin.

The keratinocytes of the epidermis are not in a static condition but instead are constantly replacing themselves. As keratinocytes are generated and mature, they progress upward through the several epidermal cell layers, gradually changing from the cuboidal basal cell form to the prickle cell form to the granular cell form, finally transforming into the horny cells constituting the very outermost layer of the epidermis. This entire process whereby keratinocytes mature to form the horny layer is referred to as *keratinization.*

Melanocytes

Melanin is the major pigment of the skin. Two types of cells are important in melanin production. **Melanoblasts** are the immature melanin-forming cells that originate early in fetal life. During fetal development, the melanoblasts migrate from their point of origin to their point of maturation in the basal cell layer of the epidermis. One out of every 5 to 10 cells in the basal cell layer is a mature melanin-forming cell, or **melanocyte**. In addition to migrating to the epidermis, some melanoblasts migrate to the roots of the hairs, where they will provide color for the future developing hairs. A few of the melanoblasts do not complete their migration and instead remain in the connective tissue portion of the skin (the **dermis**).

The ability of melanocytes to produce melanin depends on their ability to synthesize a key enzyme, **tyrosinase**. Through the action of this enzyme, the amino acid **tyrosine** is converted to melanin. Pigmentation of the epidermis is accomplished by the melanocytes' transfer of melanin to the surrounding basal cells (i.e., the keratinocytes). The exact mechanism by which this occurs is not fully understood. The melanin is then dispersed throughout the epidermis by the multiplication and maturation of the keratinocytes.

Langerhans Cells

Langerhans cells are part of the immune system and serve the important function of processing **antigens** (substances against which an immune response can be raised) in certain hypersensitivity states, such as allergic contact dermatitis.

DERMIS

The **dermis** is the middle and thickest major layer of the skin and provides the skin with most of its bulk. It is made up of connective tissue fibers and a ground substance composed of acid mucopolysacchrides. The connective tissue fibers are about 90% **collagen** (the major protein constituent of the dermis) and 10% **elastin** (which provides the skin with its suppleness and elasticity). The connective tissue fibers are large and densely packed throughout most of the dermis. The fibers are smaller and more loosely arrayed directly under the epidermis and surrounding the **epidermal appendages** (i.e., the hair follicles and skin glands).

A variety of cell types can normally be found in the dermis. The most common cell type is the **fibrocyte** or **fibroblast**, which resembles similar cells found in other areas of the body. The next most common cell type is the **mast cell**. Mast cells are round to spindle-shaped cells and contain large numbers of granules. Within the granules are a variety of noxious chemical substances, including **histamine** and **serotonin**—important mediators of inflammation that are also involved in the production of allergic disorders. Mast cells tend to concentrate around capillary beds; thus, most mast cells are present in the more superficial dermis and surrounding the epidermal appendages. The final cell type present in the dermis under normal conditions is the **histiocyte**. Histiocytes are tissue **macrophages** (specialized white blood cells that ingest cellular debris and foreign material) originating in the bone marrow. They exist in the dermis in very small numbers.

SUBCUTIS

The innermost major layer of the skin is the **subcutis** (also called the **hypodermis**). It is composed of fat cells and thin strands of collagen-containing connective tissue. The nerves and blood vessels supplying the skin weave their way through the strands of connective tissue to reach the overlying dermis.

The Epidermal Appendages

The major epidermal appendages include the hair and hair follicles, sebaceous glands, and sweat glands. Despite their name, epidermal appendages extend down to the dermis.

Hair and Hair Follicles

Hair has become a rudimentary, vestigial structure in human beings, for whom it now has little value as a form of protection but instead serves primarily as ornament. The haircoat of horses and all animals, by contrast, is of great practical importance to their daily existence. Because of its fibrous and bulky nature, hair is an efficient filter and insulator and affords considerable defense against cuts, abrasions, heat, sunlight, and chemical irritants. Physical trauma also is greatly blunted by the haircoat before it can reach the sensitive surface of the skin.

The basic unit of hair production is the **hair follicle.** Each hair follicle consists of two major components, the **follicular sheath** and the **hair bulb.** The follicular sheath is a long tubelike structure through which the hair passes and exits to the skin surface. The hair bulb is the deepest portion of the hair follicle. The cells of the hair bulb (the **hair matrix cells**) and the associated **dermal papilla** are responsible for the actual production of hair.

The hair follicles are placed in the skin at an oblique angle. Bundles of smooth muscle known as **arrector pili** muscles are present in haired areas of skin. These tiny muscles stretch from the dermis to the hair follicles; when they contract, they cause the hairs to "stand up." These muscles may be called into action in response to a perceived threat, fear, a cold environment, or emotional stress.

Hair and hair growth Hair, like the horny layer of the epidermis, is in actuality a lifeless, keratinized structure. Each hair consists of an upper, free portion known as the **hair shaft** and a lower, anchoring structure known as the **hair root.**

The hair shaft is composed of three layers. Working from the outside in, the three layers are known as the *cuticle*, *cortex*, and *medulla*. All hairs have a cuticle and a cortex. The degree of development of the inner layer, the medulla, varies according to the animal species and the type of hair.

Hair does not grow continuously, but instead is periodically shed and renewed in a rhythmic fashion. Hair follicles actively produce hair during the **anagen** phase of hair growth. In this phase the hair matrix cells in the hair bulb divide, the resulting daughter cells **differentiating** (becoming increasingly specialized) to produce the hair shaft. This phase of growth normally alternates with a resting phase known as **telogen**. In telogen the hair matrix cells become inactive. The root of the hair detaches from the matrix cells in the hair bulb, although the hair itself is still retained within the follicular sheath by a structure known as the **internal root sheath.** After a variable period of time the dormant hair matrix cells reactivate and a new hair begins to form. As the new hair grows and moves up the follicular sheath, the old hair is finally pushed out of the follicle and lost.

In human beings the average period of growth of each individual hair is approximately 1,000 days, with a range of 2 to 6 or more years. The duration of hair growth is genetically determined in each individual. The resting phase of growth lasts approximately 100 days. Thus, at any given time, about 90% of human hair follicles are in anagen and about 10% are in telogen. Adjacent hair follicles tend to be in different phases of the growth cycle, so that no obvious "shedding" is observed.

In animals, there is a distinct tendency for hair-follicle growth to become synchronized, resulting in seasonal shedding of hair. This is most apparent in wild animals living in colder climates. Horses living outdoors in cold climates grow a much thicker winter coat. The most important factor regulating synchronization of hair-follicle activity is the length of daylight; environmental temperature plays a much lesser role. In horses, the body hair normally is shed twice a year, once in the spring and again in the fall.

Sebaceous Glands

Sebaceous glands are simple, **lobulated** (divided into small branched lobes, or **lobules**) glands associated with the hair follicles. Each gland is connected to the **lumen** (interior space) of the upper part of its associated follicle by a short **duct** (small tube or passageway). Sebaceous gland cells secrete their product by a **holocrine** type of secretion, i.e., each entire cell of the central cells of the gland disintegrates with the cell contents becoming the secretion. The peripheral cells remain and continue to reproduce, serving as the source for new glands. The product or secretion of sebaceous glands is known as **sebum**, a complex fatty substance whose composition varies from species to species. Its primary functions appear to involve insulation, lubrication of the skin, and protection of the hair against overwetting. Sebum also has some inherent **antimicrobial** (killing or suppressing the growth of microorganisms) activity as well.

Sweat Glands

There are two types of sweat glands: **apocrine** and **eccrine**. Strictly speaking, the sweat glands of the horse are apocrine. Apocrine sweat glands are coiled structures with a large lumen; they empty their contents into an associated hair follicle. Apocrine sweat glands are found throughout the body and produce a scented, fluid secretion that may play a role as a sexual attractant. Eccrine sweat glands also have a coiled structure, but the lumen is much smaller and the glands empty their contents directly onto the skin surface. Eccrine sweat glands are found in the footpads and nasal pad of carnivores. In animals the majority of sweat glands are of the apocrine type. In human beings, by contrast, most sweat glands are of the eccrine type, with apocrine sweat glands being limited to the armpits and the anal and genital regions.

Although domestic animals are abundantly supplied with sweat glands, significant functional differences exist among different species. In horses, sweat glands are found over most of the body except the legs and are highly functional, assisting in the regulation of body temperature through sweat evaporation. In dogs and cats, by contrast, sweat glands appear to exist only as rudimentary structures and are essentially non-functional.

Definition of Terms

In addition to the anatomic and physiologic terms described in CHAPTER 16, "ANATOMY," a number of common medical terms must be defined as a prelude to discussing the individual skin diseases of the horse. These are terms that veterinary dermatologists use to describe the pathologic changes produced in the skin by different disease processes. Accurate description and identification of such changes are a necessary prerequisite to making a diagnosis.

ALOPECIA. Absence or loss of hair.

CRUSTS. Residue of dried serum, blood, pus, epidermal, keratinous, and bacterial debris.

DEPIGMENTATION. Localized loss of normal skin color.

DERMATITIS. Any inflammatory skin disease.

DERMATOSIS. Any skin disease, particularly one *without* an inflammatory component.

EROSION. A superficial denudation of the skin involving only the epidermis.

ERYTHEMA. Reddening of the skin, due to congestion of the underlying capillaries.

EXCORIATION. Erosions and ulcerations produced by self-trauma.

FISSURES. Cracks in the skin secondary to loss of normal skin tone associated with inflammatory processes.

LESION. Any disease-induced abnormality of tissue structure or function.

NODULE. A large papule; a small lump.

PAPULE. A minute, firm, well-demarcated elevation of the skin.

PLAQUE. A flat area in the skin.

PRURITUS. Itchiness.

PUSTULE. A vesicle containing *pus* (fluid produced by an inflammatory process, containing many white blood cells).

SCALE(S). Accumulated fragments of the horny layer of the epidermis.

TUMOR. A large nodule, or obvious cancerous mass.

ULCER, ULCERATION. A severe sloughing of the skin surface, extending at least into the dermis.

VESICLE. A circumscribed elevation of the epidermis, filled with *serum* (fluid component of blood); a *blister*.

WHEAL. A hive: a discrete, well-circumscribed, reddened swelling with a flat top and steep-walled margins, produced by *edema* (excessive fluid in the intercellular tissue spaces) in the dermis; often associated with allergic reactions (i.e., urticaria).

Disorders of the Skin

BACTERIAL SKIN DISEASES

Pyoderma (Pastern Folliculitis)

Pyoderma is a general term for any skin disease in which pus is formed. The most commonly encountered form of pyoderma in horses is *pastern folliculitis*, caused by *Staphylococcus aureus*. There is no recognized age, breed, or sex predilection. One or more legs may be involved, but lesions are usually limited to the back of the pastern and fetlock. The initial lesions consist of papules, which if left untreated coalesce to form large areas of ulceration and pus formation. The disease is not associated with **systemic** (bodywide) illness; i.e., the general health of the horse is unaffected.

Diagnosis is made on the basis of the history and physical examination. If available, papule contents may be obtained for identification and isolation of bacteria and for antibiotic sensitivity testing (*see* APPENDIX C, "DIAGNOSTIC TESTS"). The affected area(s) should be clipped and washed well with a mild soap. (Because the lesions can be quite painful, it may be necessary to sedate or even anesthetize the horse for this initial procedure). An appropriate antimicrobial ointment should then be applied twice daily until the condition has resolved.

Dermatophilosis

Dermatophilosis is a relatively common disease found throughout the world. Also known as *streptothricosis* and **rain-scald,** it primarily affects horses, cattle, and sheep, and is caused by an unusual **filamentous** (threadlike) bacterium, *Dermatophilus congolensis*. The disease in horses is usually of sporadic occurrence. The lesions consist of numerous crusts that can spread over a large portion of the body, primarily along the back. Chronically affected animals represent the primary source of infection. When the lesions are wetted, motile **zoospores**, the infective stage of the bacterium, are released. Normal healthy skin is quite impervious to infection; instead, some predisposing factor is needed that decreases the skin's normal resistance (e.g., prolonged wetting of the skin by rain). Mechanical transmission of the organism can be effected by both biting and nonbiting flies.

The disease is usually seen during the fall and winter months. In the early stages the lesions can be felt before they can be seen; i.e., the thick crusts can be **palpated** (felt with the hands or fingers) beneath the hair coat. When the crusts are removed the overlying hair comes off as well, exposing the pink, moist skin surface beneath. Occasionally the lesions involve the lower extremities, when animals are kept in "wet" pastures ("dew poisoning").

Diagnosis is made on the basis of the history, clinical signs, and identification of the causative organism in crust material. Occasionally it may be necessary to culture the organism in the laboratory if it cannot be readily visualized by direct microscopic examination.

Affected animals should be protected from exposure to rainfall. Vigorous grooming will remove many of the crusts and is encouraged.

In severely affected animals, systemic antibiotic therapy may be required. Most cases of dermatophilosis regress spontaneously with the advent of dry weather.

Cutaneous Actinomycosis

Bacteria of the genus *Actinomyces* are thread-like organisms that cause pus-forming infections in human beings and a number of animal species. *Actinomyces* bacteria are present throughout the environment but are also part of the normal bacterial population of the oral cavity. Trauma and puncture wounds, and occasionally inhalation or ingestion, can allow these bacteria access to normally sterile tissues of the body.

Cutaneous actinomyosis is a rarely encountered disease of horses. In essence it is a **lymphadenitis** (inflammation of one or more lymph nodes) and/or **lymphangitis** (inflammation of a lymphatic channel) in the region of the lower jaw. A variety of species of *Actinomyces* can be responsible. Usually, a break in the surface of the skin inside the mouth is needed for the organism to gain entrance; trauma resulting from the chewing of exceptionally sharp roughage or foreign material in the feed (pieces of wood, wire, etc.) is suspected. As the disease develops, the lymph nodes in the **mandibular** (pertaining to the lower jaw) region become firm and enlarged, and draining tracts (**fistulas**) may be found opening onto the skin surface of the lower jaw, throat, or neck. The consistency of the discharge from these tracts varies from **serous** (thin, resembling **serum**, the clear fluid portion of the blood) to **purulent** (composed of thick pus).

Diagnosis is made by culturing the organism from samples of the discharge. Appropriate antimicrobial medications are available for treatment.

VIRAL SKIN DISEASES

Aural Flat Warts (Aural Plaques)

These skin warts are common in horses greater than a year of age and are caused by an equine *papillomavirus*. There is no recognized breed or sex predilection. The lesions consist of one to several, gray or white plaques involving the inner surface of the **pinna** (the external portion or flap of the ear). The individual plaques are sharply **demarcated** (have sharp borders) and vary from less than 1 millimeter to more than 2 centimeters in diameter. When large plaques are present, there is a tendency for them to coalesce; in severe cases up to 50% of the inner surface of the pinna may be involved. During the summer, black flies (*Simulium* spp. [multiple species], of the family Simuliidae) can be found feeding on the inner surface of horses' ears, and it is possible that they may serve as a **vector** (organism that carries a disease agent from one animal to another) of the causative virus. The plaques appear to cause the affected horse no discomfort. Once they have developed, they usually persist indefinitely. Identical lesions have occasionally been observed around the anus, vulva, and groin region.

Diagnosis is usually straightforward and is based on the history and physical appearance of the lesions. Horses exhibiting additional signs such as itching or head-shaking should be examined for other causes of ear irritation, such as ticks or foreign bodies. Aside from their unsightly appearance, the lesions are of little health consequence to the horse.

FUNGAL SKIN DISEASES

Ringworm

Ringworm (*dermatophytosis*) is a common skin disorder affecting many domestic animal species. It is caused by fungi known as *ringworm fungi* or *dermatophytes*, which invade the outer, superficial layers of the skin, hair, and nails (**horn**). Ringworm fungi feed on keratin shed from the dead cells of the horny layer of the epidermis (as a rule ringworm fungi cannot survive in living tissue). Some ringworm fungi inhabit the soil, while others are strictly parasitic.

Equine ringworm is caused most frequently by *Trichophyton equinum. Trichophyton mentagrophytes, Trichophyton verrucosum*, and *Microsporum equinum* are found less commonly. Younger horses are particularly at risk. Transmission of ringworm fungi occurs by direct contact with infected animals or with objects (grooming instruments, blankets, tack) carrying contaminated hair or scale. Ringworm fungi that are well adapted to their host species usually induce little or no host response, but infected horses may become inapparent carriers, i.e., they harbor the fungi and serve as a source of infection but exhibit no clinical signs themselves. By contrast, infection with poorly host-adapted dermatophytes usually elicits a greater inflammatory reaction in the host. Soluble substances produced by the fungi must reach the underlying dermis in order for an inflammatory response to occur. These substances can either be **toxins** (i.e., irritants) or **allergens** (substances inducing an allergic response). Reactions to toxins often are milder than reactions to allergens.

Normal, unbroken equine skin is resistant to invasion by dermatophytes; a disruption of this natural resistance is necessary for clinical disease to develop. Abrasions of the skin (particularly in the saddle area), warm temperatures, high humidity, overcrowded stable conditions, and poor grooming practices represent ideal predisposing factors for dermatophyte infections. Affected horses often exhibit circular, expanding patches of hair loss, with reddened margins, scaling, crusting, variable amounts of itching, and an area of central clearing (hence the term "ringworm"). Any remaining hairs usually are thickened and broken. In some cases there may be extensive flaking and crusting with little or no hair loss. The withers and saddle area are common sites for initial ringworm lesions to develop. From there they may spread to the neck, chest, flanks, croup, or head. The lesions may persist for 1–2 months before the immune system of the horse finally brings the disease under control. Occasionally the disease may involve one or more extremities and be limited to the back of the pastern.

Diagnosis relies on the history, clinical signs, and microscopic examination of hair or scale for the presence of ringworm fungi. Scale and hair are collected by scraping the suspected lesions. In some cases a fungal culture, the most definitive means for diagnosing ringworm, may be necessary to identify the fungi.

Treatment is aimed at eliminating the fungus from the horse and its environment. Because the disease in most horses is essentially self-limiting, little or no therapy may be necessary. The affected areas can be clipped clean with scissors to remove hair and crusts, and a topical antifungal medication may be applied. In resistant cases oral antifungal medication may be necessary. For treating the environment, pressure hosing should be employed to attack woodwork that may be contaminated with the fungi. Tack, blankets, brushes, combs, and other objects that have come into contact with an affected horse should be thoroughly scrubbed and disinfected.

Certain ringworm fungi can be transmitted from affected horses to people. Thus horses with ringworm should be handled with care, keeping this aspect of the disease in mind. A physician should be consulted if suspicious lesions develop on any individuals in close contact with an affected horse.

Subcutaneous and Systemic Mycoses

The *subcutaneous mycoses* are a group of relatively rare fungal diseases affecting the skin and underlying (**subcutaneous**) tissues. Occasionally they may spread to involve other regions of the body, including one or more organ systems. By and large, however, they are pathogens of more superficial body surfaces. Among the subcutaneous mycoses affecting the skin of horses are *sporotrichosis*, *phycomycosis*, and *phaeohyphomycosis*. The *systemic mycoses* are rare fungal diseases in which inhalation (usually) of the causative organism is followed by widespread dissemination to internal organs and other tissues, including in some cases the skin. Of the systemic mycoses, *coccidioidomycosis* and *epizootic lymphangitis* are of importance in horses. (For pertinent information on these diseases, *see* CHAPTER 32, "FUNGAL DISEASES.")

PARASITIC SKIN DISEASES

Scabies (Mange)
See CHAPTER 18, "EXTERNAL PARASITES."

Focal Ventral Midline Dermatitis
This is a frequently encountered disease of horses kept in close proximity to cattle. It is found in areas with warm climates and has a seasonal pattern, appearing in the spring and regressing in the fall. This seasonality, together with the observation of horn flies (*Haematobia*

irritans, a major cattle pest) feeding in the area of the lesions, suggests that horn-fly bites are a major causative factor.

The lesions are limited to the **ventral midline** (central underside) of the belly and chest and consist of one to several, sharply demarcated areas of scaling, alopecia, ulceration, crust formation, and skin thickening, varying from 1 to 10 inches in diameter.

Diagnosis is based on the history and clinical picture. For treatment, the affected areas should be thoroughly cleansed with a mild soap and any crusts removed. A combination antibiotic/corticosteroid ointment should be applied twice daily for several days, after which the frequent application of a fly repellent is recommended. A thick coat of vaseline over the lesions will provide protection against fly bites.

Cutaneous Habronemiasis (Summer Sores)
This is a specific skin disease of horses caused by stomach worms (*Habronema* spp.). The adult worms reside in the stomach, where they are generally of little concern (*see* CHAPTER 33, "INTERNAL PARASITES"). The larvae are passed in the feces and are ingested by fly maggots, in which they undergo further development. The normal life cycle is completed when infective larvae are deposited by the adult flies around the horse's lips, where they are subsequently swallowed.

Cutaneous habronemiasis is a form of aberrant parasitism wherein the larvae gain access to the deeper layers of the skin in a presumably hypersensitive host. The infective larvae cannot penetrate normal, healthy skin; for cutaneous habronemiasis to develop, the larvae must be deposited on previously damaged skin or mucous membranes. The occurrence of the disease is seasonal, first appearing in the spring and (in most cases) spontaneously regressing in the fall. The incidence is sporadic, only a few horses in any given area being affected at a time. Once the disease develops in a horse, it usually will recur each succeeding summer unless stringent preventive measures are taken. Common sites for the lesions are the inner angle of the eye, **conjunctiva** (mucous membranes lining the inner surface of the eyelids), male genitalia, and the lower extremities. The lesions themselves consist of areas of ulceration, usually containing small, gritty, yellow nodules.

Diagnosis is based on the history and physical appearance of the lesions. Corticosteroids are used to reduce the inflammation and an **anthelmintic** (deworming medication) often is given to kill the worm larvae. Strict attention to fly control is also essential. The overall prognosis is favorable.

Cutaneous Onchocerciasis
Onchocerca cervicalis, a threadworm, lives in the **nuchal ligament**, a large, strong band of connective tissue that provides support for the neck (*see* CHAPTER 33, "INTERNAL PARASITES"). A fairly high percentage of horses in most parts of the United States are infected with this parasite. The females produce large numbers of minute, prelarval forms called **microfilariae**, which travel through the bloodstream and localize in the skin of the head, neck, withers, chest, and underside of the belly (95 percent of the microfilariae migrating to this last location). Biting **midges** (tiny two-winged flies) of the genus *Culicoides* pick up the microfilariae as they feed. Inside the midge the microfilariae transform into larvae, find their way to the mouthparts, and then are transmitted to another horse when the midge feeds again.

The presence of even extremely large numbers of microfilariae in the skin will not necessarily produce lesions; rather, circumstantial evidence suggests that a hypersensitivity to dead microfilariae is involved. Two disease syndromes have been described:

- Inflammatory lesions involving the face and **periocular** (around the eye) region. Inflammatory lesions occurring in the center of the forehead are nearly always caused by *Onchocerca*
- A diffuse inflammatory disease involving most of the underside of the body

Most cases occur in horses older than 3–4 years. Diagnosis is based on the history, clinical findings, demonstration of microfilariae in skin scrapings taken from the lesions, and/or response to therapy. Treatment with an anthelmintic will kill the microfilariae but not the adults; thus, treatment must be repeated in 3–12 months to kill new microfilariae that have repopulated the skin during the interim.

Dermatoses Associated with Simuliid Flies

The family Simuliidae contains several species of blood-sucking flies that attack animals as well as people. They occur in most areas of the world but are particularly troublesome in regions with warm climates. The flies are dark-colored and vary in length from 1–5 millimeters. They have a rather characteristic appearance, with the **thorax** (midsection) humped over the head. They are often referred to as "black flies" or "buffalo gnats." (*See* Chapter 18, "External Parasites.")

The flies are most active in the morning and late afternoon and cause considerable annoyance and irritation. Dark-colored animals are selected for attack by the females (the males do not feed on blood). In addition to damaging the skin, the flies secrete a potent toxin that can cause heart and lung problems and even death (such severe signs occur only when large numbers of flies attack an animal). It is not known if a hypersensitivity reaction plays a role in the development of the skin lesions.

Cutaneous manifestations The bites produce small skin wounds that are quickly covered with droplets of dried blood. The usual sites include the udder, male genitalia, inner surface of the thigh and upper forelimbs, throat, ears, chest, underside of the belly, and body orifices. It is likely that each species of black fly has its favored site to feed. For example, *Simulium vittatum* and *Simulium argus* feed almost exclusively on the inner surface of horses' ears, and may serve as vectors for aural flat warts (*see* above). Urticaria and **angioedema** (recurrent wheals caused by dilation and/or increased permeability of capillaries in the skin) may be prominent signs when large numbers of flies attack an animal. Considerable pruritis leading to excoriations may be evident.

Systemic manifestations Generalized clinical signs occur when large numbers of flies are involved and are usually evident either immedi-

ately or within a few hours of the attack. Affected horses appear weak and listless and exhibit a rapid pulse and respiratory rate. The body temperature is normal or below normal, rising only in cases that are advanced or terminal. Pregnant mares may abort. In severe cases, death many occur within a few hours to a few days.

Diagnosis is usually based on the history, clinical signs, and observation of black flies feeding on the patient. Treatment is entirely supportive. The lesions should be gently cleansed to remove crusts. If they are confined to a small area, a topical corticosteroid preparation may be applied twice daily. If large areas of skin are involved or if the itching is intense, a short course of oral corticosteroid therapy may be indicated. Stringent fly control measures should be instituted. Horses should be stabled during the day, preferably in screened stalls. Insect repellents must be applied at least two or three times a day to be effective.

Hypoderma *Infestation (Warbles)*

Infestation of horses with the larvae of warble flies (*Hypoderma* spp., major cattle pests) is an example of an aberrant parasitism and is usually observed in horses kept in close proximity to cattle. The adult flies are active in the hottest part of the summer and attach their eggs to hairs of the animal. After hatching, the **larvae (grubs)** penetrate the skin and migrate through the tissues toward the skin of the back. By spring some of the larvae will have reached this location, where they are visible as small nodular swellings in the skin, each with a "breathing pore" opening to the exterior. (In horses, an abnormal host, most of the larvae do not reach normal size and fail to complete their life cycle. Most affected horses usually have only one or two grubs.)

Diagnosis is based on the history and the location of the lesion(s), and the presence of a breathing pore in the nodule(s). In most situations simply enlarging the breathing pore with a scalpel and extracting the grub is curative.

Allergic Skin Diseases

Urticaria (Hives)

Urticaria or "hives" is an acute, usually localized swelling of the skin caused by an increase in the permeability (leakiness) of capillaries. The result is an outpouring of clear fluid from the blood into the tissue spaces and a characteristic skin wheal. The overlying hair may stand erect when wheals are present in haired areas. Wheals vary in size from small circular spots to lesions many centimeters in diameter. Individual lesions may expand by coalescing with adjacent wheals. The degree of itchiness of the lesions varies dramatically. It should be stressed that urticaria is not a single, specific disease entity but a specific skin lesion with many different causes.

Horses are affected with urticaria more often than are any of the other domestic animal species. Urticaria may be instigated by immunologic or nonimmunologic factors. The most common *immunologic causes* involve a **hypersensitivity** (exaggerated sensitivity) reaction to some substance that has been introduced into the body. In almost all such cases of *allergic urticaria* the inciting substance or **allergen** is thought to reach the skin by the systemic route, i.e., it has been either ingested, inhaled, or injected into the body. Drug reactions, food allergies, and allergies to inhaled pollens or molds (*atopy*) are included among the possible causes. *Nonimmunologic* or *physical causes* of urticaria include cold, exercise, and **dermatographism** ("pressure" urticaria, caused by scratching or rubbing at a site).

The diagnosis is usually quite obvious, based on the history and the physical appearance. The initial episode may be treated with a short course of anti-inflammatory medication. If the urticaria recurs, therapy may need to be repeated several times. After several recurrences, further diagnostic and management measures are indicated.

Therapy also involves eliminating the underlying cause, if it can be identified. Of great importance in this effort is the medical history. Is this the first episode of urticaria? If not, how many episodes have occurred in the past? Are they seasonally related? A complete drug history of the horse should be obtained, especially focusing on medications given in the preceding two weeks. In addition, other factors such as exercise or cold weather should be considered as possibly associated with the onset of urticaria.

The possible involvement of dermatographism can be easily investigated by "writing" on the animal with a blunt instrument such as a capped ball-point pen, putting a fair degree of pressure on the skin. The development of a line of urticaria along the pressure line within 15 minutes would represent a positive reaction. Likewise the possibility of cold urticaria can be investigated by placing an ice cube on the horse's skin for several minutes and watching for the development of urticaria at the site.

Food allergies can be evaluated by using elimination diets. First, a complete feed change is instituted, i.e., if the horse is on oat hay then it is switched to alfalfa hay, or vice versa. If no improvement occurs within 3 weeks, the feed is changed again for another 3 weeks. If no visible improvement occurs after two such feed changes, food allergy can probably be ruled out as the cause of the urticaria.

Immunologic testing for **atopy** (genetic allergic sensitivities) would be the next step if a diagnosis still has not been reached. If all attempts at identifying an underlying cause prove fruitless, long-term antihistamine therapy may be necessary.

Culicoides *Hypersensitivity (Queensland Itch, Sweet Itch)*

This is a commonly encountered skin disease of horses, resulting from an allergic reaction to the bites of tiny insects belonging to the genus *Culicoides* (midges or "no-see-ums"). There is evidence to support an underlying hereditary predisposition. *Culicoides* hypersensitivity is rare or nonexistent in horses under a year of age. The initial onset usually occurs between 2 and 4 years of age. Seasonal at first, it appears in the spring, worsens during the summer, and regresses in the fall, in concert with the activities of the *Culicoides*. The disease is recurrent, however, and with each succeeding year becomes more protracted and severe. There is no apparent breed or sex predilection.

Because *Culicoides* hypersensitivity is allergic in nature its occurrence is sporadic, i.e., it usually develops in only one animal in a group at any time. Two major patterns of disease are seen. One affects primarily the base of the tail, rump, back, withers, crest, poll, and ears, while the other involves the entire lower body surface.

Different species of *Culicoides* are responsible for each pattern. The first sign observed is pruritis; all other lesions result from this. In mild cases there is only partial alopecia. Severe lesions are characterized by total alopecia, thickening of the skin, and excoriations.

Diagnosis is based on the history and physical findings. Treatment is aimed at preventing attack by *Culicoides* and at reducing the inflammation resulting from the hypersensitivity reaction. *Culicoides* feed at dusk and during the early evening, so efforts at control should be directed at these times. As a minimum, affected animals should be stabled from early afternoon until dawn. Outside openings of the stall should be screened. Owing to the very small size of *Culicoides*, ordinary window screens will not suffice. Instead, an extremely fine mesh will be required. The effectiveness of standard window screening may be improved, however, by "painting" the screen with an insecticide having good **residual** (long-lasting) activity. Box fans in front of nonscreened openings to create a wind stream away from the stall are also helpful.

Corticosteroid drugs given orally are used to reduce the inflammation (antihistamines appear to be of little value). Except in very mild climates it is usually possible to stop medicating during the winter months. Owing to the underlying hereditary predisposition, owners of affected horses are strongly encouraged to remove affected animals from breeding programs.

Equine Collagenolytic Granuloma (Nodular Necrobiosis)

This is the most common equine **nodular** (characterized by nodules) skin disease and is seen throughout the United States. There is no apparent age, breed, or sex predilection. Although the exact cause is a mystery, a hypersensitivity reaction to insect bites (mosquitoes in particular) may be involved. The most prominent feature of the disease is **collagenolysis**, or **necrobiosis** (degeneration of collagen in the skin).

There is a tendency for the disease to appear during the warmer months of the year. The lesions consist of single or multiple firm nodules, 0.5 to 5 centimeters in diameter, situated in the dermis. Occasionally, very large lesions are pre-

sent. The nodules can be found anywhere but are particularly common on the withers, back, and sides of the neck. Unless they have been traumatized, the skin and hair overlying the nodules are usually normal in appearance. There is no associated pruritis and usually no pain.

Diagnosis is made on the basis of the history, clinical findings, and (preferably) biopsy. Therapy consists of corticosteroids and/or surgical removal.

Autoimmune Skin Diseases

A number of skin diseases exist whose origins lie in an inappropriate or exaggerated response on the part of the immune system. When this response is directed against the body's own cells and tissues, it is referred to as an **autoimmune disease**. The underlying cause of such misguided attacks is often unknown. Many different hypotheses have been proposed to account for the development of autoimmune diseases. It is likely that a combination of factors, including genetic predisposition and reactions against foreign substances, initiate and maintain these diseases. Some autoimmune diseases are characterized, at least in part, by clinical signs of skin disease. (*See* Chapter 29, "The Immune System and Various Disorders.")

Cutaneous Lupus Erythematosus

Cutaneous lupus erythematosus is a relatively rare, incompletely defined autoimmune disorder. Lupus erythematosus ("lupus"), as it occurs in human beings and some animal species, is considered to be the prototypic autoimmune disease. It is presently classified into two forms, **discoid lupus erythematosus** (involving the skin and occasionally the mucous membranes) and **systemic lupus erythematosus** (involving many organ systems and frequently the skin). The disease described here as equine cutaneous lupus erythematosus shares some features of both the discoid and systemic forms.

The condition occurs in adult horses and has no recognized breed or sex predilection. The major clinical sign is a rapid or gradual loss of skin pigment around the eyes, lips, and nostrils. The skin around the anus, vulva, and male genitalia may also be affected. The areas of depigmentation are usually well demarcated from the surrounding normal skin. Varying degrees of scaling and erythema may also be present. In long-standing cases the affected skin may take on the appearance of "wrinkled parchment paper." Involvement of haired skin usually results in localized alopecia, which may be permanent. There may also be a photosensitive component to the disease, with exacerbation of the lesions following exposure to sunlight.

Diagnosis is made on the basis of the history, clinical signs, and results of supportive laboratory tests, including the **antinuclear antibody (ANA) test** (which detects antibodies directed against DNA) and skin biopsies. As in almost all autoimmune disorders, the practical goal of therapy is control rather than cure. If the case has a photosensitive component, exposure to sunlight should be minimized. Decisions related to additional therapy depend on the severity of the skin lesions and the extent (if any) of systemic involvement. At present the only available medications that are potentially effective and affordable in horses are corticosteroids. If the lesions are small and/or associated with erythema, a topical corticosteroid can be applied. Systemic (oral or injectable) steroid therapy may be required in more severe cases. Lifelong therapy will usually be necessary.

A major goal of therapy is repigmentation of the lesions. Although this will occur to some extent using corticosteroids, the response to therapy is usually not cosmetically rewarding.

Pemphigus Foliaceus

Pemphigus foliaceus is a relatively common autoimmune disease characterized by the presence of "anti-self" antibodies (**autoantibodies**) directed against components of the skin, with subsequent development of vesicles and pustules in the superficial skin layers. The areas most commonly affected include the head and lower extremities. In severe cases the entire body surface may be involved. Appaloosas appear to be predisposed to the development of pemphigus foliaceus. There is no recognizable sex predilection and no apparent seasonality. Age at onset, however, is very important. Most cases occur in mature horses (5 years or older). When it occurs

in younger animals, the disease is usually less severe, responds very well to therapy, and may spontaneously disappear. The inciting event that triggers the production of autoantibodies in affected horses has not been identified.

The earliest lesions usually noticed are crusted papules, best seen in lightly or nonhaired skin adjacent to the nostrils, lips, or eyelids. The lesions quickly coalesce to form larger, more diffuse areas of crusting. The lesions tend to develop in waves; horses may progress rapidly from the total absence of disease to the sudden appearance of dozens of papules. Transient, persistent, or recurrent urticaria may also be seen. **Edema** (swelling) of the extremities (especially the hind limbs) and the lower abdominal region is commonly observed. Pruritis may or may not be present. Severely affected horses may also exhibit fever, depression, inappetence, and malaise.

Diagnosis is based on the history and clinical signs, multiple skin biopsies (three to four are preferred), and selected immunologic testing. Considering the severity of the disease, the prognosis, and the extensive and costly therapy involved, every attempt should be made to arrive at a definitive diagnosis.

Immunosuppressive drug therapy (corticosteroids or other, more potent medications) is the mainstay of treatment. As indicated above, the age of the horse is of major importance in prognosis and response to therapy. Pemphigus foliaceus in horses 1 year of age or younger responds excellently to corticosteroids; once the disease is in remission, it usually requires no additional therapy. Thus it is probably always worthwhile to treat animals in this age group. By contrast, the disease in older horses usually requires lifelong, expensive medication. Gold (in the form of gold salts) may be of value as an adjunct to corticosteroid therapy in these horses. The prognosis for pemphigus foliaceus in older horses is guarded.

OTHER IMMUNOLOGICALLY MEDIATED SKIN DISEASES

Erythema Multiforme, Epidermal Type

Erythema multiforme is an uncommon but highly characteristic equine skin disease with a proposed immunologic basis. In the human form of the disease, the most frequently associated inciting factors include drugs, concurrent infections, and cancer. In several affected horses, there has been a strong association with the use of the rhinopneumonitis (herpesvirus) vaccine. There is no known age, sex, or breed predilection. Single or multiple lesions are located along the back anywhere from the withers to the base of the tail. They consist of crusts approximately 1–5 millimeters in diameter. The most striking clinical sign of the disease, however, is pain: Affected animals react violently if the lesions are touched or even approached. Occasionally, the pain will precede visible development of the lesions. Within a few weeks white hairs appear in the areas of crusting. The disease runs a natural course of 1–3 months, after which the pain subsides and the crusts disappear. The **leukotrichia** (whiteness of the hair), however, persists. Recurrences are uncommon.

Diagnosis is based upon the history and characteristic clinical signs. There is no effective treatment. Corticosteroids, even at high doses, appear to be of only marginal value.

Axillary Nodular Necrosis

This uncommon, sporadic disease is characterized by the development of skin nodules in the **axillary** region (inner aspect of the junction between the forelimbs and the body; "armpit"). It is not seasonal, and no breed or sex predilection has been identified. The disease occurs in both working and non-working horses. The cause is unknown, but is suspected to have an immunologic basis.

Owing to their location, the nodules are often erroneously identified by owners as "girth galls" and attributed to overwork and ill-fitting tack. They occur in the subcutaneous tissue of the axillary region just behind the elbow and are almost invariably **unilateral** (present on only one side of the horse). The nodules range from less than half an inch to over 2 inches in diameter. There may be from one to ten or more of them, with most affected horses having three or fewer. When many nodules are present they tend to be arranged in chains. Occasionally, a thin "cord" of tissue can be felt connecting the nodules. The nodules are not painful to the horse and the overlying skin has a normal appearance. Affected horses may however exhibit discomfort when the cinch is tightened. Little information is available on how long the nodules persist if left untreated.

Diagnosis is made on the basis of the history, physical examination, and sampling of one or more nodules (aspiration smear and/or biopsy). Surgical removal is advised. In horses with many nodules or a very large nodule that would be difficult to excise, corticosteroid therapy may be attempted (the response to corticosteroids is quite variable, however). The corticosteroid can be given orally or injected directly into the area of the lesion(s).

Generalized Granulomatous Disease

Generalized granulomatous disease (GGD) is a recently recognized, uncommon disease characterized by skin lesions and widespread involvement of internal organs. There is no recognized sex or breed predilection. The cause is unknown, but is believed to be related to an abnormal immunologic response to some unidentified substance. The striking similarity between generalized granulomatous disease of horses and a human disorder, *sarcoidosis*, also of unknown cause, suggests that they may have similar origins. The human disease is characterized by an impairment of cellular immune responses and an augmentation of **humoral** (antibody-generating) immune responses.

The onset of clinical signs may be insidious or explosive. The skin lesions may take two forms (which may both coexist in the same animal):

- The more common form consists of scaling and crusting with varying degrees of hair loss
- In the less common form, the lesions consist of nodules or large tumorlike masses

The internal organs are also affected in virtually all cases of GGD. However, except for weight loss, inappetence, and a persistent low-grade fever, clinical signs attributable to systemic involvement are uncommon. When signs do arise they most often involve the lungs, e.g., exercise intolerance, increased resting respiratory rate, mild **dyspnea** (difficult respiration). Occasionally, liver and gastrointestinal lesions may cause diarrhea or **jaundice** (yellow discoloration of the mucous membranes). The clinical course can vary from a chronic, progressive disease to spontaneous regression.

Diagnosis is based on the history, physical examination, and supportive laboratory findings. The diagnosis can be confirmed by biopsies (skin, peripheral lymph nodes). Oral corticosteroids are the treatment of choice. Once initiated, therapy should probably be continued for several months.

SCALING SKIN DISEASES

Seborrhea (Keratinization Disorders)

"**Seborrhea**" is a term used to describe clinical signs of excessive scaling, crusting, and greasiness. Several probably unrelated equine skin diseases characterized by scaling and crust formation are grouped together under this general designation. Most probably represent diseases of abnormal keratinization (contrary to popular belief, there is little evidence that seborrhea is related to excessive sebum production by sebaceous glands). Keratinization, as described earlier, is the series of genetically programmed events by which keratinocytes, the skin cells that manufacture keratin, proceed through an orderly series of developmental stages to produce the outermost layers of the epidermis. Various defects in this complicated process probably lead to the array of disorders known commonly as seborrhea.

In *mane and tail seborrhea* the clinical signs include heavy scaling with little or no pruritis in the mane and tail. In some cases there may be considerable alopecia of the tail. In *cannon keratosis*, a common equine skin condition, the front surface of the rear cannon bone is affected. The lesions consist of scaling and crusting without pruritis and with varying degrees of hair loss.

Treatment involves frequent use of antiseborrheic shampoos. Tar-based shampoos are the most effective and should be used every 2 to 3 days at the outset. During this initial phase of therapy, scaling and crusting may increase.

After the desired improvement has occurred, the frequency can be gradually decreased until the maximum interval between treatments that will keep the condition under control is determined.

INHERITED SKIN DISEASES

Hyperelastosis Cutis

Very little information is available concerning this recently recognized condition in the horse. To date it has been seen only in Quarter Horses. Both sexes are affected. Although good pedigree data are not available, the condition is undoubtedly hereditary in nature. The basic defect involves a lack of subcutaneous attachment of the skin to the underlying tissues; the skin itself appears to be normal.

The condition is probably present at birth but may go unnoticed for several months. Usually only a single area of the skin is involved. The affected area varies in size but is usually five to ten centimeters (several inches) in diameter. It is sharply demarcated and with proper lighting appears as a slight depression. The overlying skin is easily movable, hyperelastic, more easily "torn" than normal skin, and slow to heal. The horse may exhibit pain when traction is applied to the edge of the affected area.

The overall health of horses with hyperelastosis cutis is excellent. Unless the defect is very large or is located in an area subjected to stress (e.g., under the saddle), affected animals may lead a normal life. Owing to the hereditary nature of the condition, however, such animals should not be used in breeding programs.

NEOPLASTIC (CANCEROUS) SKIN DISEASES
See CHAPTER 34, "CANCER."

MISCELLANEOUS SKIN DISEASES

Photosensitization

Photosensitization is a clinical syndrome resulting from excessive exposure to **ultraviolet radiation** (sunlight). Although some features are common to all cases of photosensitization, several different underlying disease mechanisms may be involved. Three features basic to all types of photosensitization are:

- Presence of a **photodynamic agent** (compound activated by light) in the skin
- Concomitant exposure to a sufficient amount of light of certain wavelengths (ultraviolet)
- Absorption of the light into skin containing the photodynamic agent

Most photodynamic agents involved in photosensitization in animals are classified as **phototoxic**, i.e., they produce damage by a nonimmunologic, chemically induced mechanism. (**Photoallergic** agents, only poorly documented in animals, act by an immunologic mechanism and require prior immunologic sensitization). Photodynamic agents can reach the skin either through the blood circulation (*systemic photosensitization*) or by direct absorption (*contact photosensitization*). They act by absorbing light of highly energetic wavelengths and passing the extra energy on to the surrounding cells, causing tissue injury. Superficial blood vessels and the epidermis are the primary targets for damage.

Systemic photosensitization A classic but rare example is seen in horses grazing pastures containing *Hypericum* spp. (St.-John's-wort), which contains the photodynamic agent *hypericin*. In addition to developing skin lesions, affected animals exhibit **photophobia** (visual hypersensitivity to light), squirm in apparent discomfort, and often scratch or rub at the head and ears.

Contact photosensitization Most recognized cases of contact photosensitization occur in horses grazing pastures containing clover. Why clover plants sometimes produce a photodynamic agent is unknown.

Most skin lesions of photosensitization occur in unpigmented skin that lacks hair (lips, eyelids, etc.). Haired regions and areas that are lightly pigmented may be involved to a lesser extent. With contact photosensitization, only the areas of direct contact will be affected; thus lesions will usually be limited to nonpigmented areas of the lower extremities and muzzle. The lesions themselves vary tremendously from an urticarial type to erythema, scaling, and severe **necrosis** (cell death).

Diagnosis is based on the history and physical findings. Treatment involves removing the animal from exposure to sunlight and preventing reexposure to the photodynamic agent. The inflammatory component of the lesions can be treated with corticosteroids (most effective when used *early* in the course of the disease).

Photoaggravated Vasculitis

Photoaggravated vasculitis is a specific disease entity unique to the horse. It is an unusual type of **vasculitis** (inflammation of blood vessels) that appears to be "triggered" and subsequently aggravated by exposure to sunlight. It is relatively common and affects mature horses of either sex. The only breed predilection relates to the amount of nonpigmented skin on the extremities. The disease occurs primarily during the summer months in areas with abundant sunlight. The incidence is sporadic, usually affecting only one animal in a group. The cause is unknown.

The lesions are limited almost exclusively to lower extremities lacking pigment. They are also usually limited to a single leg, even though pigment may be lacking in several legs. (Rarely, lesions may be observed in horses with lightly pigmented extremities). The lesions are multiple and reasonably well demarcated. Favored sites are the inner and outer aspects of the pastern. Erythema, oozing, crusting, erosions, and superficial ulcerations may develop during the initial, acute phase of the disease. An important (but inconsistent) feature is swelling of the affected limb. In chronic cases the lesions usually develop a rough, "warty" surface that resists mechanical removal. The lesions tend to be painful rather than itchy.

Diagnosis is made on the basis of the history, physical examination, and results of selected laboratory tests. Clinical management involves preventing further exposure of the affected area to sunlight and reducing inflammation. The horse should be stalled during the daylight hours or wear leg wraps. Relatively large doses of oral corticosteroids should be given. The majority of cases respond favorably to such treatment. Occasionally, lesions may recur after the medication has been stopped. If so, the treatment regimen should be repeated.

Leukoderma and Leukotrichia

Several skin diseases are characterized by a loss of melanin pigment. The **melanocytes** (cells producing melanin) in the epidermis and the melanocytes in the hair bulbs often are affected independently. When the melanocytes in the hair bulbs are affected and the hairs lose their normal amount of melanin, the condition is referred to as **leukotrichia** (whitening of the hair). When the melanocytes in the epidermis are affected and the skin itself loses its normal amount of melanin, the condition is called **leukoderma** (whitening of the skin). Leukotrichia without a coexistent leukoderma occurs frequently; leukoderma, however, is usually accompanied by leukotrichia. The causes of these conditions in the horse are potentially legion, but most remain speculative at this time. The prognosis varies. In some cases the loss of melanin is permanent, while in others it is temporary. There are no practical methods of therapy.

Reticulated leukotrichia This form of leukotrichia is seen primarily in Quarter Horses. Although an hereditary factor may be involved, the exact cause of the condition is a mystery. Most horses develop the problem as yearlings (although it occasionally develops in older horses). The lesions develop along the back, from the withers to the base of the tail. The initial lesions consist of linear crusts arranged in a characteristic cross-hatched (**reticulated**) pattern. The crusts are shed, but the new hairs that grow into the affected areas are white. If the areas are clipped it will be noted that the skin itself retains its normal pigmentation. The color change in the hair is permanent. Owing to the possible involvement of an hereditary factor, affected animals probably should not be used for breeding programs.

Juvenile Arabian leukoderma Also known as *Arabian fading syndrome* and *pinky syndrome*, this is a characteristic depigmenting syndrome seen in young Arabian horses. It may also occur in some Quarter Horses. The predilection for Arabians and the occurrence of the syndrome in certain lines of Arabians would suggest that some hereditary factor is at work. There is no

evidence to implicate an infectious agent or nutritional factors. The underlying mechanism seems to involve a malfunctioning of previously normal melanocytes. (A similar pattern of leukoderma is occasionally seen in mature Arabian horses, and rarely in mature horses of other breeds. The exact relationship between the syndrome in young Arabians and that in mature horses is unknown).

Clinical signs usually appear at 1–2 years of age. The lesions are limited to the eyelids and the periocular skin, muzzle, nostrils, genitalia, anus, perineum, groin, and undersurface of the tail base. Initially, a few minute areas of slate-gray skin are seen to develop. Over the next several months they gradually increase in size and continue to lose pigment. Signs of inflammation (erythema, scaling, crusting, pruritis) are completely absent. Once the lesions are fully developed, the syndrome will evolve in one of three different ways:

- Pigment spontaneously reappears in the affected areas and the horse remains normal for the rest of its life (the most common outcome).
- The affected areas remain permanently depigmented.
- The degree of pigmentation waxes and wanes, e.g., the affected areas may repigment and then subsequently lose pigment and possibly repigment again later.

There is no way to predict which of the above patterns will develop in an individual horse. Aside from the depigmentation, affected animals are normal in every respect. Owing to the possible involvement of an hereditary factor, affected animals probably should not be used in breeding programs.

Cutaneous Mastocytosis

The term *cutaneous mastocytosis* is used to refer to an infiltration of (noncancerous) mast cells into the skin. The cause is unknown. Although there is no strong breed predilection for cutaneous mastocytosis in the horse, Arabians may have a higher incidence, while Thoroughbreds are known to have a much lower incidence. The mean age of affected animals is 7 years, and males are affected much more frequently than females. Two distinct forms of cutaneous mastocytosis have been observed:

- The most common form consists of a single nodule, 2 to over 20 centimeters of diameter, which frequently is located on the head. The surface of the nodule may be normal, hairless, or ulcerated. The nodule is composed of aggregates of mast cells and, later, **eosinophils** (white blood cells active in allergic reaction).
- A less common form consists of a diffuse swelling of a lower extremity, usually below the carpus or hock. The swelling is very firm and the overlying skin is normal in appearance. Most often there is no associated lameness. **Radiographs** (X-ray studies) of the affected limb reveal areas of soft-tissue mineralization.

Diagnosis is based on the history, physical findings, and sampling of the affected tissue (aspiration smear and/or biopsy). Growth of the lesion appears to be self-limiting. Surgical removal is the usual treatment. Recurrence of the lesion after surgery is very rare.

Unilateral Papular Dermatosis

Unilateral papular dermatosis is a poorly understood disease of unknown cause, seen only in Quarter Horses. Both sexes are affected. The striking unilateral (present on only one side) nature of the disorder might suggest an underlying peripheral nerve problem. There is no evidence that an infectious agent is involved.

The clinical picture is that of a horse with *many* (30 to 300+) papules on one side of its body. Most of these are concentrated on the side of the chest, with some lesions occasionally found on the shoulder, neck, or abdomen. The papules vary in size from $\frac{1}{3}$ to $1\frac{1}{2}$ centimeters ($\frac{1}{8}$ to $\frac{1}{2}$ inches) in diameter and are not itchy. In most cases they develop in the spring and early summer. Spontaneous regression in 2 weeks

to 2 months is the rule, although horses may develop the disease again in succeeding years.

Diagnosis is based on the history and clinical signs. Therapy is usually not necessary, although oral corticosteroids may in some cases shorten the natural course of the disease.

Grease Heel

The term "grease heel" is commonly used by veterinarians and horse owners alike in reference to a variety of inflammatory skin conditions affecting the pastern region. Grease heel is not a single, specific disease entity, but a collection of conditions with different underlying causes and a similar clinical picture. This partially explains the present confusion regarding the mechanism of disease development as well as the inconsistency of response to any given form of therapy.

Frequently only a single extremity is involved, usually a hind limb. There is a distinct tendency for extremities with white socks to be affected. The initial lesions involve the back of the pastern. With time the lesions extend up the leg and around to the sides and occasionally the front of the pastern and fetlock. The nature of the lesions depends on the underlying cause, duration, and past therapy. Erythema, oozing, and alopecia are common early signs, usually followed by crusting. Ulceration frequently develops in conditions characterized by blood-vessel inflammation (**vasculitis**). As time progresses the skin becomes thickened, and fissures may develop owing to the constant, repeated flexion in the affected region. The lesions often are painful and may result in lameness.

To formulate an appropriate therapy, it is important to identify the specific disease entity involved. The possible causes of grease heel are legion; they include: contact dermatitis, pastern folliculitis, dermatophilosis, ringworm, chorioptic mange, photosensitization, photoaggravated vasculitis, and immune-complex vasculitis ("**purpura**"). In many cases of grease heel, however, the cause cannot be determined; under such circumstances, symptomatic therapy (treating the clinical signs without addressing the underlying cause) is all that can be provided.

CHAPTER 18

External Parasites

by David G. Baker

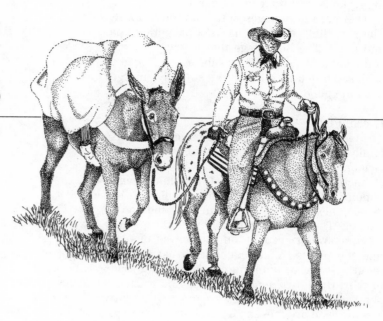

Horses have their external parasites (**ectoparasites**) just like any other species. The most common are flies, **midges** (gnats), mosquitoes, lice, mites, and ticks. In general external parasites are said to "infest" a host where internal parasites "infect". Ectoparasites live on the skin; **endoparasites** (internal parasites) live chiefly in the gastrointestinal tract.

External parasites affect horses in many ways. Some may annoy or "worry" a horse, causing it to forgo feeding, which results in a loss of condition. Severe annoyance may cause a horse to injure itself in its attempts to escape from the pests. External parasites may cause a blood-loss **anemia** (abnormal decrease in the red blood cell count), local or generalized skin irritation, trauma, inflammation, or secondary infection. Many external parasites also transmit other, very significant disease-causing agents, including viruses, bacteria, and internal parasites.

This chapter will focus on parasite biology and the clinical signs of external parasite infestation. Awareness of the biological needs and signs of infestation will allow concerned horse owners to lessen the negative impact of these

pests on their horses. The parasites to be discussed are those that most commonly affect horses in the United States. Horse owners are encouraged to consult a veterinarian for confirmation of any diagnosis of an infestation and for appropriate drug therapy.

Flies

This group of ectoparasites contains some of the most important pests of horses. Fly infestation is associated with skin damage, allergic reactions, annoyance, transmission of other disease agents, and blood loss.

It is common to classify flies as either *biting* or *nonbiting*. Actually, no flies "bite" as we typically understand it. So-called biting flies feed by piercing the skin with a tubelike structure called a **proboscis**, through which they suck blood, or by slashing the skin with knifelike structures and then lapping up the blood as it flows from the wound. Among the biting flies, usually only the female parasitizes animals, the males generally feeding on plant juices. Nonbiting flies feed on body secretions, lapping up fluids with a spongelike structure; they are incapable of inflicting wounds with their mouthparts.

There are four stages in the life cycle of a fly. These include the egg, **larva** (maggot), **pupa**, and adult. The only stage that actually "grows" is the larva, which has four substages or *instars*, each separated by a molt. The adult fly emerges from the pupa.

HORSE FLIES

The term "horse fly" refers to a large and diverse family of flies. *Tabanus americanus* is a large, vicious black fly reaching up to 2½ centimeters (1 inch) in length (Figure 1a). Adult females obtain a blood meal, which they require for egg development, by a "slash and lap" method of feeding. They normally lay 500 to 600 eggs near standing water, usually on the leaves of overhanging plants. After hatching the larvae drop into the water or onto mud, where they develop further. Up to two generations may be produced per year. Most horse flies appear in the early summer and are most active on hot, sunny days.

Horse flies are of tremendous annoyance to horses and are painful biters (as many trail riders can attest). They tend to feed repeatedly on the legs, belly, neck, and shoulders, and can be responsible for a significant amount of blood loss. Swellings often develop at the sites of feeding. Oozing lesions left by horse flies often attract other, nonbiting fly species, some of which may carry and transmit agents of disease. In this regard horse flies themselves may on occasion transmit many disease agents, including equine infectious anemia virus and the bacterium that causes anthrax. (*See* CHAPTER 30, "VIRAL DISEASES," and CHAPTER 31, "BACTERIAL DISEASES.")

Horse flies are very difficult to control, owing to the wide diversity of habitat in which they can breed. However, because they tend to remain near their breeding places, drainage of wetlands, where possible, can greatly limit the local horse-fly population. Adult horse flies are reluctant to enter barns and are more commonly found near wooded areas. Therefore, large open pastures and readily accessible barns can provide horses with a refuge from fly attacks.

In addition, insecticides are available that are effective repellents of horse flies. In particular,

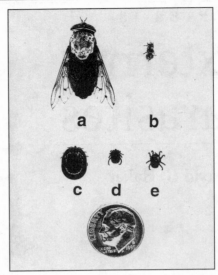

Figure 1. Selected external parasites of the horse. a) Horse fly; b) Stable fly; c) Engorged adult female hard tick; d) Adult male hard tick; e) Nymph of *Otobius megnini* (spinous ear tick). A dime is included for size comparison.

the *synthetic pyrethroids* exhibit some degree of residual activity, and when applied to the horse's legs, belly, neck and shoulders as a spray or wipe-on formulation, may offer significant protection against these pests.

STABLE FLIES AND HOUSE FLIES

Other flies feeding on horses include the stable fly (*Stomoxys calcitrans*) and the house fly (*Musca domestica*). Both flies are roughly the same size, approximately ³⁄₅ centimeters (¼ inch) in length (FIGURE 1b).

The stable fly is a biting fly, both sexes feeding by a painful "pierce and suck" method. If given the opportunity, stable flies will also feed on people, inflicting an equally painful bite. The house fly is a nonbiting fly that feeds on body fluids, including serum or blood oozing from wounds (some of which may have been inflicted by horse flies or stable flies) and fluids around the nostrils, mouth, and eyes. Both stable flies and house flies lay their eggs in a wide variety of decaying organic matter. The stable fly prefers a mixture of hay, water, manure, and urine. The house fly prefers fresh manure but will readily deposit eggs in piles of grass clippings or weeds, leftover feed in feed troughs, or vegetable-garden wastes.

Stable flies and house flies are most abundant in summer. Stable flies feed primarily in the morning and evening, commonly attacking the legs and belly of the horse, while house flies are active throughout the day. Both flies may transmit several disease agents, including viruses, bacteria, and parasites, such as the worms that cause *cutaneous habronemiasis* (*see* CHAPTER 33, "INTERNAL PARASITES.") In addition house flies readily enter homes, feeding on almost anything moist, including milk, sugary food, meat, and garbage. In this way house flies can also transmit disease agents to people.

Significant control of these pests can be achieved through a reduction in the number of breeding sites. Prompt disposal of manure, hay, and other organic debris is absolutely essential. While the composting of manure will kill maggots in the center of a pile, the sides of the compost pile require rigorous treatment with insecticides. Therefore, disposal of manure and other organic wastes is preferable to composting.

Horses can be treated by applying insecticides to the face, neck, legs, and belly. In addition, face nets can be used to reduce fly-feeding on ocular secretions. It must be emphasized, however, that these measures used alone, without the concomitant, prompt disposal of organic wastes, will be ineffective.

HORN FLIES AND FACE FLIES

The horn fly (*Haematobia irritans*) and the face fly (*Musca autumnalis*) are smaller flies (about $\frac{1}{2}$ centimeter or $\frac{3}{16}$ inches in length) and are primarily parasites of cattle.

The horn fly spends virtually its entire adult life on cattle. Eggs are laid in fresh cattle manure, where the larvae emerge and undergo further developmental changes. Blood-sucking adults appear in the early spring and are present until late fall. Populations are heaviest in hot, humid regions. When populations are high the horn fly will feed on horses. Favored feeding sites include the neck, withers, shoulders, and sparsely haired regions such as the belly.

Though horn flies are not considered to be significant carriers of disease, they can inflict painful bites that result in ulcers and crusted, scabby wounds in the horse's skin. These lesions can then attract other types of flies that may be capable of transmitting disease agents.

Face flies are nonbiting flies. Like horn flies they lay their eggs in fresh cow manure. When populations become excessively dense, face flies will attack horses, feeding on secretions of the eyes, mouth, and nostrils, and causing extreme anxiety to the animals. Face flies transmit eyeworms (*see* CHAPTER 33, "INTERNAL PARASITES") and bacterial disease agents.

Cattle should be treated to remove horn flies and face flies. If horses cannot be separated from cattle, the application of insecticide sprays and wipe-ons can provide a high degree of protection. Unfortunately, resistance to insecticides is an increasing problem among some horn-fly populations. Face flies do not like to be indoors, so stabling horses during hours of peak fly activity in the given area may provide additional relief.

BITING MIDGES

Biting midges ("no-see-ums," "punkies," or gnats) of the genus *Culicoides* are very small flies (about $\frac{1}{6}$ centimeter or $\frac{1}{16}$ inch in length) that can cause considerable hardship despite their diminutive size. Adult females lay eggs in standing water or in moist places, such as rotting vegetation, tree holes, and wet manure (the exact location of the egg-laying depends on the species of midge). Multiple generations can be produced in a year, with greatest activity from late spring through early fall. Time of feeding (day, early evening, night) is species-dependent. Most species feed in the evening or at night.

Because of their small size and potential for night feeding, biting midges, even in large numbers, are often overlooked by horse owners— that is, unless the offending species also happens to feed on people! Depending on the species of midge, horses may develop severe allergic reactions to the secretions deposited by the midges as they feed—a condition known commonly as *Queensland itch* or *sweet itch*. (*See* CHAPTER 17, "THE SKIN AND VARIOUS DISORDERS.")

Because the midges tend to bite most commonly along the backline, withers, base of the tail, and occasionally on the face, these are the areas that itch the most. The subsequent scratching by the horse may cause localized loss of hair and occasionally skin, leaving serum crusts and scabs. One aid to diagnosis is the seasonality of the problem. Skin lesions may completely disappear during the winter, only to return with greater severity each subsequent spring. In addition to causing incessant itching, midges may transmit several equine disease agents, including Venezuelan equine encephalomyelitis virus and a parasite, *Onchocerca cervicalis*. (*See* CHAPTER 30, "VIRAL DISEASES," and CHAPTER 33, "INTERNAL PARASITES.")

Control of biting midges is difficult. Measures for reducing exposure to midges include the use of synthetic pyrethroid sprays or wipe-on formulations, insecticide misters, stabling of horses during hours of peak midge activity (e.g., 4:00 P.M. to 7:00 A.M. during warm months), and screening stable windows. The midges' small size allows them to fly through standard mosquito screening. As an added precaution screens can be treated with insecticides having residual activity.

BLACK FLIES

In many ways black flies are similar to biting midges. Like the midges, black flies are small (about ³/₁₀ centimeter or ⅛ inch in length), dark flies that feed on horses and people. They are known commonly as "buffalo gnats" because of their hump-backed appearance. Black flies deposit eggs on objects such as rocks and plants, just below the surface of fast-moving water. The larvae remain attached and submerged while they feed and develop. The emerging adults float to the surface in a bubble of air and may spread out over several miles in search of a blood meal. Fly activity is greatest in the summer months. Unlike most of the biting midges, feeding takes place during the daylight hours.

Black-fly bites, like midge bites, cause intense itching in horses and people. Horses are frequently bitten about the ears, head, neck, and belly. Allergic reactions tend to be quite severe,

occasionally to the point of causing death. The bite wounds may swell and appear as bloody crusts. Horses may rub the hair and skin off affected areas.

Prevention or reduction of black-fly attacks is difficult because the adult flies can travel up to three miles. Some control may be attained by the use of insecticide sprays, wipe-ons, or smears, especially when applied to the head, neck, and belly line, and by treating the inner surface of the ears with insecticide dust or petroleum jelly. Ear or face nets can also be quite helpful. Because black flies feed outdoors during the daytime, stabling horses when they are not being ridden can provide some protection.

Mosquitoes

Mosquitoes are often considered pests primarily of people and smaller animals. However, mosquitoes also feed on large animals, including horses. In fact, mosquitoes are quite important as **vectors** (transmitters) of the viruses causing western, eastern, and Venezuelan equine encephalomyelitis. (*See* CHAPTER 30, "VIRAL DISEASES.") In addition, blood loss can be quite significant when a swarm of reproductive female mosquitoes attacks a horse. (The males and nonreproductive females feed on nectars and plant juices).

Mosquitoes lay their eggs on floating vegetation or standing water. Depending on the species, suitable habitats for egg-laying include bogs, tree holes, drainage or irrigation ditches, rain gutters, old tires, buckets, etc. Where possible, elimination of standing water, or application of insecticides to standing water, can greatly reduce local mosquito populations. The application of pyrethroid sprays or wipe-ons can also provide temporary protection to individual horses.

Lice

Lice are small (usually less than ³/₁₀ centimeters or ⅛ inch in length), wingless, six-legged insects. Two kinds of lice are known to infest horses. *Biting* or *chewing lice* feed on skin debris and secretions, while *sucking lice* feed on blood. The entire life cycle is spent on the horse. The eggs (called **nits**) are attached to the hair shafts and eventually hatch, releasing **nymphs**, which undergo several molts before reaching the adult stage. Since the life cycle can be completed in only 3 weeks, several generations of lice can be produced in a year. However, because lice utilize the hair coat as habitat, populations are greatest in the winter when the coat is thickest and huddling of animals is more likely.

Lice can be found on any haired portion of the body but tend to occur in greatest numbers on the head, neck, mane, and base of the tail. Because lice cannot fly, transmission of an infestation is primarily by horse-to-horse contact. People can unknowingly facilitate this transfer by using grooming instruments, blankets, or other gear on more than one horse. While lice do not transmit diseases to horses, they can cause a modest amount of itching, which induces the horse to rub and lose condition. Rubbing can be persistent to the point of skin loss. Because lice are very host-specific, there is no concern that lice feeding on horses will feed on, or remain on, horse owners.

Lice can be controlled with insecticides. It is often most effective to brush the insecticide into the coat, with a reapplication in 2 weeks. Grooming instruments, which may be contaminated, should be treated at the same time.

Chiggers

Mites and ticks belong to the same class (the *Arachnida*) as spiders and scorpions. All adult arachnids have eight legs. Several kinds of mites, differing from one another biologically, can be found infesting horses; few, however, are common. All mites are small—only up to about one-half the size of lice—and thus can be easily overlooked. In this chapter only the chiggers, or "harvest mites," will be discussed.

Chiggers are tiny (about less than $1/10$ centimeter or $1/32$ inch in length), yellow to orange or red mites that spend the egg, nymph, and adult stages of their life cycle in the environment, feeding on either other invertebrates or plants. The six-legged larval stage is usually parasitic on rodents, but will attack a variety of other animals, including horses and people. The body of a chigger is covered with hairs, giving it a velvety appearance. The larvae feed on host skin, causing the formation of nodules that may be crusty. Horses may be attacked on any area of the body, but chigger attacks tend to be greatest on the head, neck, chest, and legs. The lesions sometimes itch considerably.

Chiggers are most common in the fall and are found in fields, wooded areas, and other prime rodent habitats. Control can be facilitated by applying insecticides to horses before trail rides or other activities that infringe upon rodent territory.

Ticks

A wide variety of ticks infest horses. Ticks are similar to mites in many ways but are much larger. They are not readily visible, however, because they often are buried within the hair coat or are found feeding in the ear canals.

Ticks are classified as either *hard* or *soft* ticks. This refers to the presence of a hard "shield" or **scutum** on the back of hard ticks (and its absence in soft ticks), and to differences in the position of the mouthparts.

Several species of hard ticks feed on horses in the United States (FIGURE 1). The stages (larva, nymph, adult) of the life cycle that feed on horses depend on the individual species of tick involved. While the adult male ticks remain small (less than $3/5$ centimeters or $1/4$ inch in length), adult females can attain sizes of up to 2 centimeters ($3/4$ inch) in length when fully engorged with blood. Up to 18,000 eggs per female are laid in protected places, frequently crevices of barns and fences, and usually just above ground level. The eggs are laid in one batch and are reddish in color. In general, tick populations are greatest during the summer months.

Hard ticks can be found on virtually any part of the body, but most frequently on the chest, chin, mane, base of the tail, and along the folds of skin in front of the legs. Most hard ticks will also feed on people. Hard ticks feed for relatively short periods of time (generally several days) and then drop off the horse. To feed, the tick inserts a feeding apparatus into the skin of the host and "cements" it in.

When removing a hard tick that has become cemented to the skin, it is important to grasp the tick as close as possible to the surface of the skin (tweezers work well for this purpose). The tick should then be removed with firm, steady pressure, taking care not to separate the tick from its embedded mouthparts (which may then remain in the horse and serve as a site for bacterial infection).

Hard ticks affect horses in a variety of ways, none of them good. They may cause anxiety, anemia, pain, or loss of condition, and can transmit the viral, bacterial, and parasitic agents of several important equine diseases. In addition, the feeding sites may become irritated and infected, providing a nidus (nest) for the development and feeding of fly maggots.

The soft tick of greatest importance to horse owners is the spinous ear tick, *Otobius megnini* (FIGURE 1e). As the name implies (**oto** referring to the ear), this tick feeds in the ears of horses. Only the six-legged larval and the eight-legged nymphal stages are parasitic. The larvae suck tissue fluids and when engorged are about $3/10$ centimeters ($1/8$ inch) in length. They are usually yellow-white or pink in color and feed for about a week. The nymphs may feed over a period of months, and when engorged may be $3/5$ centimeters ($1/4$ inch) in length. After feeding, the nymph leaves the horse and finds a crevice in which it molts to the adult stage. Favorite molting sites include barns, fences, and other protected structures. An adult female tick can lay 500 to 600 eggs in soil near these protected spots.

The spinous ear tick causes blood loss, annoyance, and irritation, and its activities can promote secondary bacterial infections of the ear. Heavily parasitized horses appear dull and lose condition. Often the diagnosis can be made by examining the inside of the ears, where the feeding ticks can be observed. *This tick will also feed in the ears of people.*

Control of ticks includes eliminating undergrowth, wooden structures, and other nesting sites. In addition, the use of residual insecticides as spray or wipe-on formulations, or ear dusts for control of the spinous ear tick, can facilitate control. Spraying barns or fences with insecticides may be necessary in heavily infested areas in order to eliminate the egg-laying adults.

CHAPTER 19

The Eye and Various Disorders

by Roy W. Bellhorn

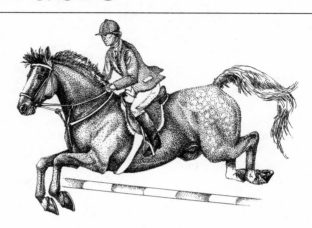

Our mental picture of the members of the equine family, especially those living in the wild, is of elegantly sleek and athletic creatures moving at a rapid rate of speed across the savannah, tails and manes flowing in the wind. What we do not always keep in mind is that it is this swiftness that has helped to assure the survival of these unique animals. Swiftness, coupled with the ability to detect the movement of predators, is a necessary prerequisite for survival in the wild. We must also remember that, unlike many other large prey species, horses possess neither antlers, horns, nor cloven hooves with which to defend themselves. It is obvious that horses must have an exceptional capability to spot the movement of potential predators. It follows that the equine eye must be constructed and placed in the head in a manner that maximizes motion detection over a very broad area.

Looking at a horse, we see that the eyes are placed more to the side of the head than to the front. This lateral placement, combined with the horse's horizontally rectangular **pupil** (the central opening of the iris, through which light penetrates the inner reaches of the eye), provides

the horse with a ready means of visualizing a very broad field of landscape. In fact, horses are capable of seeing almost 360 degrees around; only a small area directly behind is not visible without turning the head. And because the horse's **retina** (the light-sensitive tissue at the back of the eye) is richly endowed with motion-detecting cells known as *rods*, it is evident that the horse's eyes are optimally constructed and positioned for survival of the species. (*See* FIGURES 1 and 2.)

Human beings have, of course, domesticated certain members of the equine species in order to provide services that we deem important; thus we place upon the equine visual system demands not necessarily tantamount to the horse's survival in the wild. It is readily apparent that under unnatural conditions we human beings, in turn, must become partners in the effective use of the equine eye.

The Normal Equine Eye

Just as all cameras have basically similar components, the equine eye is similar to the eye of

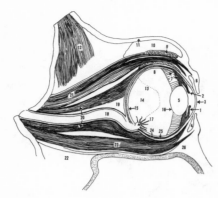

Axial View

1. Iris
2. Anterior chamber
3. Cornea
4. Conjunctiva bulbi
5. Lens

6. Eyelid
7. Ciliary body
8. Obliquus dorsalis muscle
9. Lacrimal gland
10. Supraorbital process
11. Skin
12. Temporalis muscle

13. Cavity
14. Vitreous
15. Tapetum
16. Retina
17. Lens capsule
18. Optic disk
19. Optic nerve
20. Rectrobulbar fat
21. Retractor oculi muscle
22. Rectus dorsalis muscle
23. Extraorbital fat
24. Rectus ventralis muscle
25. Sclera
26. Choroid
27. Obliquus ventralis muscle

Figure 1. Axial view.

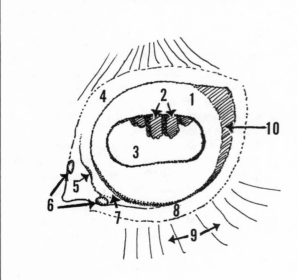

Anterior View

1. Iris
2. Corpora nigra
3. Pupil
4. Corneo scleral junction (limbus)
5. Lacrimal caruncle
6. Lacrimal puncta
7. Third eyelid
8. Eyelid margin
9. Vibrissae
10. Perilimbal pigment

Figure 2. Anterior view.

virtually all other mammalian species. And like all cameras, the primary function of mammalian eyes is to capture images of the outside world. The eye is a wondrously and intricately constructed organ that testifies to the ability of living creatures to cope with a complex environment. In the eye we have essentially a piece of brain tissue (the **retina**) that has been brought "outside" the brain and placed inside a tough, protective structure known as the **globe** (the eyeball). The globe is constructed in such a way that an optically clear and focusable pathway is provided, whereby light rays from the outside world pass into the globe and reach the light-sensitive retina. In turn, the retina transmits its perceived information via the **optic nerve** to the final processing unit, the brain. The brain, of course, is where visual perceptions are converted into images.

The eye has three major layers or **tunics**. The outer layer is the **fibrous** (composed of thickened connective tissue) tunic, the middle layer is the highly **vascular** (supplied with blood vessels) and pigmented *uvea*, and the innermost layer is the **nervous tunic** or retina. The exposed portion of the outer layer consists primarily of a central, circular, transparent window, the **cornea**, and a surrounding white portion called the **sclera**. The middle coat or **uvea** is divided into three sections, the **iris** (in front), the **ciliary body** (centrally), and the **choroid** (in the back). The **tapetum**, a reflective layer in the upper half of the back of the eye, is a modification of the choroid and is responsible for the "glow" of reflected light seen in equine eyes at night. The choroid is composed primarily of blood vessels, pigmented cells (**melanocytes**), fibrous tissue, and the **intraocular muscles**. These muscles, which are inside the eye, control the size of the pupil (primarily in response to light) and the fine focusing of images by the **lens** onto the retina (a feature highly important to human beings, but much less so to horses).

Between the cornea and the iris is the **anterior chamber,** which is filled with a clear fluid known as **aqueous humor.** Behind the iris is the transparent lens. The retina represents the innermost coat and lines the back of the eye. Between the lens and the retina is the **vitreous chamber** which is filled with a transparent, gelatinous material called the *vitreous body* or, more simply, the **vitreous**.

Muscles attached to the outside of the eye (the **extraocular muscles**) control the movement of the eyes. In the horse, there is also a strong muscle attached at the very rear of the eyeball which, when contracted, causes the equine eye to be pulled inward.

Recognizing the Normal

To recognize *abnormalities* of the equine eye it is important to understand first what is *normal*. To recognize the normal requires a detailed study of the horse's **ocular** (pertaining to the eye) and **periocular** (pertaining to the area around the eye) features.

Begin by examining a horse in bright sunlight, or in a shaded area using a focusable flashlight. As noted above, the purpose is to establish in our mind the normal appearance of the head and eyes.

THE HEAD
Notice the erectness of the ears, which should be symmetrical. Are the eyelids symmetrical in appearance and position? The muzzle and other facial features should also be symmetrical.

Orbits (Eye Sockets)
Standing somewhat back, assess the placement of the eyes in the **orbits** (eye sockets). Is the placement symmetrical? Is the positioning also symmetrical? Are the bony aspects of the orbits symmetrical? Is the concave space above and behind the upper rim of the orbits symmetrical?

Eyelids
Lightly touch the eyelids and observe their movement. Do they move (blink) evenly and briskly? Take notice of the eyelashes and the pigmentation pattern of the eyelids. Are the lids symmetrical in appearance?

The horse, like many species of animals, has what is termed a **third eyelid**. It is located in the **medial** (inner) aspect of the lid opening, toward the muzzle, and becomes quite apparent when the horse retracts the eye into the orbit. Many times this will happen if you forcibly hold open the upper and lower eyelids. Make note of the pigmentation of the third eyelid and its normal position, and observe that it moves freely, sweeping upwards toward the center of the cornea.

Conjunctiva

This mucous membrane lines the inner surface of the eyelids and the outer surface of the sclera. Its pinkness is more pronounced on the eyelid surface; small red lines (blood vessels) are readily observed against the background whiteness of the sclera. The surface of the conjunctiva should be moist and shiny.

Cornea

The cornea is the forward portion of the globe and is essentially transparent. Its surface should be moist and shiny. The curvature of each cornea should be symmetrical.

Anterior Chamber

This is the space between the cornea and the colored portion of the eye (the **iris**). It is filled with a clear fluid and therefore is also transparent. Assess the depth of the space between the cornea and iris, as well as the symmetry of the chamber's size in each eye.

Iris, Pupil, and Lens

The iris establishes the color of the eye, be it brown, gray, or so forth. Typically both irises are of the same color; however in those animals with genetically induced multicolored haircoats, it is not unusual to have differently colored irises and/or different colors within the same iris. When exposed to a bright light, the **pupil** of the iris (the horizontally shaped hole in the iris) should decrease in size. This movement of the iris is typically brisk and should occur in both eyes simultaneously and symmetrically—even when only one eye is stimulated. (It is not as brisk as what one observes in a dog or cat, however.) When stimulating pupil movement, it is important that the intensity of the light be comparable each time.

The horse typically has a row of dark protuberances along the upper pupillary border of the iris; they can also be present to a lesser extent along the lower border. These protuberances are called the **corpora nigra** ("black bodies") or the **granula iridica** ("iris granules"). They are believed to shield the lower portion of the retina from the overhead sunlight during grazing. When the pupil is tightly constricted there will still remain a small opening at the margins of the pupil so that peripheral vision remains (for motion detection). Typically the pupil should be devoid of color, i.e., a dark space. A faint grayishness may be seen, especially in older horses, due to a very slight change in clarity of the lens, which sits behind the pupil.

Posterior Portion of the Eye

This part of the eye, called the "**fundus**," is not visible unless instrumentation is used allowing the examiner to view through the pupil and into the back of the eye. Under certain conditions (especially in darkness), light will be reflected from the back of the eye, causing the pupil to "glow." This glow is usually yellowish to greenish-blue; it is caused by the reflection of light by the tapetum. The tapetum lies just beneath the retinal **photoreceptors** (cells sensitive to light) in the upper portion of the fundus and is thought to enhance vision in dim light. By this means the horse is better able to detect movement during the early morning and late evening hours.

Recognizing the Abnormal

Basic Cardinal Signs

Pain

Blepharospasm (squeezing together of the eyelids, caused by spasms of the eyelid musculature) is a primary indication of ocular pain, either inside or outside the globe. **Photophobia** (visual hypersensitivity to light) is primarily a manifestation of pain inside the globe, typically resulting from an intense constriction of the *pupillary sphincter* muscle. An affected horse may remain in a shaded or darkened area in an attempt to ease the intense constriction. **Epiphora** (an overflow of tears) is another manifestation of either intra- or extraocular pain, as is rubbing the ocular area against a foreleg or other object. Owing to the blepharospasm, use of medication to anesthetize the nerve that serves the eyelid musculature may be necessary in order to examine the eye. This is referred to as an **auriculopalpebral nerve block.** It does not block sensation but simply interferes with muscle function. In addition, use of a topical anesthetic agent may be required to block sensation in the cornea and conjunctiva.

Change in Color
Redness may indicate congestion of the conjunctival blood vessels or actual hemorrhage into the tissue. It may also be an indication of bleeding into the anterior chamber (a condition called **hyphema**), or, if the intraocular redness is confined to the pupillary space, an indication of bleeding into the posterior portion (vitreous chamber) of the eye behind the lens.

A milky-white color appearing in the cornea could indicate a localized or diffuse corneal **ulceration** (severe sloughing of the surface). If the milky-white color is localized to the pupillary space, this could be an indication of a developing **cataract** (opacity) of the lens.

Swelling
Swelling, which is essentially an accumulation of fluid in the tissues, may be observed involving the orbit, the eyelids, and/or the conjunctiva.

SIGNS ASSOCIATED WITH
SPECIFIC OCULAR STRUCTURES

Orbit
Sudden onset of puffiness (swelling) of the orbital region could indicate bruising from trauma. While bruising in and of itself may not be particularly harmful, it is important that the region be examined to ascertain if damage to the ocular structures has occurred, or if a foreign body (a piece of wood, for example) may be embedded in the tissues. If the trauma is severe, careful assessment of the orbital bones by **radiography** (X-ray examination) may be indicated. In some instances a foreign body may become embedded in the orbital region, unnoticed, with the subsequent inflammation resulting in orbital

swelling. A slow development of swelling in the orbital space may be an indication of an orbital mass such as a tumor. Surgical removal of some tumors is feasible, although many times the eye may have to be removed as well.

The placement of the eye in the orbit may be abnormal at birth (usually a smaller-than-normal eye sitting deeper in the orbit) or may become abnormal over time. With age and subsequent loss of fatty tissue within the orbit, the eyes may begin to sink deeper into their orbits. If this occurs in only one eye, it could suggest loss of orbital tissue secondary to previous inflammation.

Lacrimal System
Tearing is a normal function, and under normal conditions the tears drain from the eye into the nose via the **nasolacrimal duct.** If the tears begin to spill over the lower lid in the nasal region, it could suggest pain or a blockage of the nasolacrimal duct. Having the duct flushed may remove the blockage; sometimes that does not happen and persistent epiphora may result. If the epiphora is accompanied by blepharospasm, it is another indication of excessive tearing associated with pain.

Eyelids
A turning-in of the eyelids, such that the skin surface contacts the cornea, is known as **entropion**. It can be **congenital** (present at birth) or can develop later in life, usually secondary to scarring. In foals, temporary surgical correction is usually preferred because the condition may be self-correcting with time. If the condition is secondary to inflammation, bruising, or laceration causing a scar, surgical correction may be curative. If it is left untreated, the potential for the skin surface of the lid to cause damage to the cornea is great and can lead to serious complications.

Lacerations of the eyelids should be treated as quickly as possible by careful surgical reapposition of the edges of the wound. This is necessary to minimize or prevent the formation of scar tissue, and is especially critical if the eyelid margin is involved.

Localized pockets of chronic inflammation

can develop in the lids secondary to aberrant migration of parasite larvae, such as *Habronema* (stomach worms). Face masks may be helpful in protecting the eyelid region from the flies that deposit the parasite eggs. (*See* CHAPTER 33, "INTERNAL PARASITES.")

Tumors comprise a large proportion of eyelid problems in the horse. *Sarcoid* and *squamous cell carcinoma* are the two most common types encountered (*see* CHAPTER 34, "CANCER"). **Melanoma** (tumor of pigmented skin cells) is another tumor of importance. When eyelid tumors are noticed, it is important that the possible presence of similar tumors in or on other areas of the body be assessed. Squamous cell carcinoma may involve the conjunctiva, cornea, and/or third eyelid. In many instances it may begin as a small area of roughened eyelid margin (it appears "fleshy" when involving the conjunctiva or cornea). Horses with lightly pigmented eyelids seem to be more susceptible to the development of squamous cell carcinoma. A number of treatment methods may be used, including freezing (**cryosurgery**), burning, surgical excision, radiation therapy, immunotherapy, and chemotherapy. (*See* CHAPTER 34, "CANCER.")

Conjunctiva

A misplaced piece of skin tissue (a **dermoid**) can be present on the conjunctiva as a congenital lesion. It may also involve the cornea. It is not a tumor, but if it irritates the eye or is aesthetically unacceptable it can be surgically removed.

Inflammation of the conjunctiva (**conjunctivitis**) is manifested by redness and swelling. It usually is only irritating rather than painful. If marked pain is also evident, the conjunctivitis may be secondary to a more serious ocular problem. Dirt and other minor foreign materials may be the cause of a pure conjunctivitis, in which case flushing of the conjunctival region with a mild eyewash may be curative. If not relieved within a few hours, further assessment must be made, e.g., searching in the immediate area and behind the third eyelid for a more substantial foreign body. The use of local nerve blocks and topical anesthetic agents is necessary for this procedure.

The most common tumor of the conjunctiva is squamous cell carcinoma, which appears as a fleshy thickening of the tissue or as a flattened plaquelike lesion. Surgical removal is usually the treatment of choice. **Angiosarcoma**, a tumor of blood or lymphatic vessels, appears as a fluctuant swelling. Surgical removal and postsurgical treatment are required, because this tumor has been shown to be highly malignant (i.e., able to spread).

Cornea

A congenital dermoid may involve only the cornea, or both the conjunctiva and the cornea. As noted earlier, surgical removal may be warranted.

Trauma to the eye frequently results in damage to the cornea and subsequent development of a corneal ulcer. Because the cornea does not normally have blood vessels running through it, secondary infections may occur and will complicate corneal healing. A corneal ulcer appears as an opacity on the surface of the cornea accompanied by marked ocular pain. This condition warrants immediate treatment with antibiotics and an intraocular pain reliever. Treatment may require instillation of a medicinal delivery system (e.g., plastic tubing placed into the upper reaches of the conjunctiva, through the eyelid) owing to the strong muscular closure of the eyelids.

If a horse exhibits some ocular irritation that appears to vanish within a day, and then a few days later manifests ocular pain, it is possible that a minor wound to the cornea has occurred. The wound may have quickly healed and relieved the pain, but if an infection was introduced into the deeper layers of the cornea, an **abscess** (walled-off lesion filled with pus) within the cornea itself may have developed. Immediate and thorough treatment by a veterinarian is needed for such a condition.

If the cornea has been punctured the eye will appear partially collapsed. Surgical repair is required immediately if the eye is to be saved. However, the prognosis usually is not good owing to postsurgical complications such as infection, extensive scarring, and/or **glaucoma** (buildup of excessive fluid pressure within the eye).

Squamous cell carcinoma may involve the cornea as an extension of a carcinoma affecting the conjunctiva, or appear in the cornea itself as a primary tumor. Characteristically it develops as a localized opacity that progresses to a fleshy-appearing mass. Surgical removal is the treatment of choice, followed perhaps by ancillary anticancer treatments.

Iris and Ciliary Body

The iris and ciliary body comprise the *anterior uvea*, which is a very important area of the equine eye. The terms **moon blindness, periodic ophthalmia,** and **equine recurrent uveitis** refer to a condition characterized by inflammation primarily of the anterior uvea (in some cases the choroid, or *posterior uvea*, may be involved as well). This is a condition that is very well known to horse owners.

Congenital abnormalities of the iris include **iris cysts,** which cause the overlying iris to bulge forward. In general there is no need to try to "deflate" the cysts because they cause no actual problem. A condition that may resemble iris cysts involves underdevelopment (**hypoplasia**) of the iris tissue, such that the pressure of the aqueous humor behind the iris causes the iris to bulge forward. This condition, too, usually does not require treatment. Cysts can usually be differentiated from hypoplasia by the veterinarian by careful examination with specialized ophthalmological instruments (e.g., a **slit-lamp**).

Inflammation of the iris and ciliary body, referred to as **anterior uveitis,** may result from trauma or, more frequently, from an undetermined cause. The inflammation causes a spasm of the pupillary sphincter muscle so that the pupil contracts down in size (the pupil of the other eye can often be used for comparison) and does not respond well to light. The cornea may be diffusely and mildly **edematous** (swollen) with a hazy appearance, and the blood vessels within the conjunctiva will appear enlarged and congested. Anterior uveitis is a very serious condition that can lead to devastating complications, including cataract, glaucoma, loss of vision, and even loss of the eye. Recurrence of the condition is not uncommon. *A painful eye with a constricted pupil requires veterinary attention as quickly as possible.* The cause of the uveitis in most cases is unknown.

Iris and ciliary body tumors occur and are most frequently melanomas. A mass developing within the iris may appear as an excessively pigmented area, and may cause the shape of the pupil to be distorted. Because melanomas can spread to other areas of the body, removal of the affected eye is usually necessary. X-ray studies of the lungs may be performed to determine if the ocular tumor has spread.

Glaucoma—excessive fluid pressure within the eye—manifests as a painful eye with a (usually) dilated pupil. In the horse, glaucoma is usually encountered as a late-developing complication of anterior uveitis. Equine glaucoma is quite difficult to treat and unfortunately often necessitates removal of the eye.

Lens

The lens is a somewhat flattened, transparent, and malleable "marble" that sits behind the iris and helps focus images on the retina. A diseased lens usually responds by becoming opaque; the opacity may be localized, regional, or diffuse. In horses most such opacities or *cataracts* are late-developing complications of anterior uveitis. If the cataract is diffuse, vision will be reduced. Because many cataracts are progressive in nature, serious visual loss may occur over time. Removal of the affected lens is possible, but in the adult horse it is not frequently successful. This is because the anterior uveitis that results from the surgery causes further complications.

Congenital cataracts may be present in the newborn foal; fortunately, these can be much more readily and successfully removed. Veterinary attention should be sought as soon as congenital cataracts are noticed, i.e., the observance of a milky-appearing pupil, or evidence of abnormal vision (the foal stays very close to the mare, stumbles, or is reluctant to move). Removal is usually accomplished after the foal is halter-broken so that postsurgical treatment is facilitated; however, it should always be performed as soon as possible. Useful vision may well be provided to the foal following successful removal of the cataracts.

Retina/Choroid

Diseases of the innermost region of the eye often go undetected until reduced or lost vision becomes apparent. Appaloosas can develop an hereditary abnormality of the retina known as **congenital stationary night blindness.** As the name implies, it is present at birth and represents a nonprogressive malfunction of the motion-detecting retinal cells (the **rods**), which function best in dim light conditions. Hence, day vision is usually normal (and remains so), but in the evening vision is seriously impaired. In young foals it may not be readily evident that the foal stays close to the mare when it is dark. There is no effective therapy for this condition; however it is important to obtain professional advice regarding the genetic implications of the breeding history.

Inflammation of the retina (**retinitis**) may be associated with a *posterior uveitis* or *choroiditis*, which might also be a manifestation of equine recurrent uveitis. Retinal detachment or scarring may ensue with permanent blindness, either partial or total, of the affected eye. Trauma to an eye can result in a posterior uveitis and retinal detachment. Surgical reattachment of the retina in the horse is not a realistic possibility, as it is in human beings. In some instances medical treatment for the uveitis may result in subsequent reattachment of the retina, provided that the treatment is effective in stopping the inflammatory component of the disorder within 7–10 days. Unfortunately, this is a rarity.

Cosmetic Ocular Devices

Enucleation (removal of the eye) unfortunately may be the treatment of choice when an ocular disease process has, in spite of the best efforts, left the horse with a blind and painful eye. Enucleation may also be the option of choice in the case of intraocular tumors. Following removal of the eye, the eyelids are **sutured** (stitched) together so that the orbit is now covered with skin. Over time the scarring process within the orbit may, in some instances, draw the skin into the orbital cavity and give the area a "sunken" appearance. This may be an aesthetically unacceptable outcome for some horse owners. Alternative surgical procedures exist that may avoid or minimize this complication.

Placement of a silicone ball into the orbit after removal of the eye and before the skin is sutured is one method for avoiding the development of a sunken appearance. In some cases, however, the ball may slowly migrate downward or be "rejected" by the tissues and extruded. Placement of a silicone ball *within the eye* after removal of the intraocular contents is also feasible, unless it is known or becomes known during the surgery that an intraocular tumor exists. The cornea and sclera remain and provide some semblance of an eye (although the cornea will lose its transparency). However, for simple cosmetic purposes this can be quite acceptable.

Fashioning a glass eye may be an acceptable procedure to restore a relatively normal appearance after enucleation. This is done through the service of specialists who work within the human ophthalmologic community. After the enucleation site has healed (the lids are left intact for this situation), a mold is made and it along with a picture of the remaining eye is submitted to the specialist. The glass eye is made to resemble the fellow eye closely in appearance. Appropriate use and care of the implant need to be fully understood by the owner, in the event that subsequent complications develop.

CHAPTER 20

The Cardiovascular System and Various Disorders

by William P. Thomas

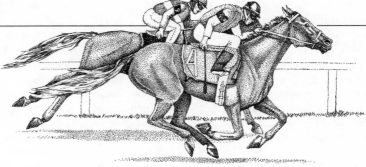

The cardiovascular system of the horse, consisting of a pump (the heart), a distributing system (the *arteries*), exchange areas (the *capillary beds*), and a collection and return system (the *veins*), is quite remarkable. It must supply blood to all parts of one of the largest domesticated land mammals (weighing 1,000 pounds or more), not only at rest and during routine activities, but also during periods of extreme physical stress, such as strenuous training or racing. That it is able to do so attests to the cardiovascular system's remarkable efficiency and adaptability. Cardiovascular health and fitness thus plays an important role in determining the athletic prowess of performance and working horses.

Normal Anatomy and Function

The heart of a 1,000-pound adult horse is about the size of a large melon and constitutes about 1% of the total body weight, or about 10 pounds. As in all mammals, it consists of left and right atrial chambers or **atria** (singular = **atrium**), left (**mitral**) and right (**tricuspid**) **atrioventricular**

valves, left and right **ventricles**, and **aortic** and **pulmonic semilunar outflow valves,** plus attached inflow veins and outflow arteries. The left side of the heart, or **left heart**, collects blood returning from the lungs via the **pulmonary veins** and pumps it out into the body through a large vessel called the **aorta**. The right side of the heart, or **right heart,** collects blood returning from the body through the large veins (the **cranial vena cava** and **caudal vena cava**) and directs it to the lungs via the **pulmonary artery**.

The output of each ventricle in an adult horse is about 25–40 liters per minute, compared to about 4–5 liters per minute for an average adult human being (1 liter is approximately equal to 1.05 quart). Because the resistance to flow through the lungs is only about one-fifth that of the rest of the body, the pressure in the right ventricle and the thickness of the right ventricular walls are much less than in the left ventricle.

From the standpoint of the ventricles, the cardiac cycle consists of a contraction/ejection phase called **systole** and a relaxation/filling phase called **diastole**. The output of the heart is the product of the heart rate times the **cardiac out-**

put of each individual systole (the **stroke volume**). The stroke volume, in turn, is influenced by:

- The structural integrity of the various anatomic components of the heart
- The strength of muscular contraction of the ventricles (**myocardial contractility**)
- The resistance to flow faced by the ventricles during systolic ejection (**ventricular afterload**)
- The ability of the ventricles to fill adequately during diastolic relaxation (**ventricular preload**)

Structural or functional abnormalities of any of these factors can adversely affect the overall functioning of the cardiovascular system, resulting in reduced cardiac output either during periods of increased demand (e.g., exercise), or, in severe cases, while at rest.

Detection of Cardiac Disorders

The principal observable signs of **cardiac insufficiency** (heart failure) in horses include:

- Loss of condition
- Increased exertional fatigue
- Shortness of breath
- Increased rate or effort of breathing
- Weakness, occasionally resulting in collapse or fainting
- Signs of fluid accumulation in the abdomen or beneath the skin of the lower **thorax** (chest)

Depending on the severity of the problem, such signs may initially appear only when the horse is subjected to moderate or strenuous exercise. With a severe cardiac disorder, clinical signs may develop during normal, nonstrenuous activities or even while at rest. Physical examination of a horse with cardiac disease will usually reveal an abnormality in the audible heart sounds (most commonly the presence of a heart **murmur** and/or a **"gallop" rhythm** at rest) or in the heart rate and rhythm (most commonly an increased resting heart rate, or abnormal irregularity caused by electrical disorders in the heart known as **arrhythmias**). When the physical examination suggests an abnormality, further examination may include an **electrocardiogram** (**ECG**) to identify arrhythmias and an **echocardiogram** (*two-dimensional echocardiography*; imaging of the anatomy and motion of the internal structures of the heart by means of reflected ultrasonic sound waves) to identify more precisely the nature and severity of the disorder. Chest **radiographs** (X-ray studies) may occasionally be used to help determine the size of the heart and identify abnormalities within the lungs and chest cavity. However, radiographs of sufficient quality are often difficult to obtain with conventional equipment in adult horses because of the animals' large size.

Fortunately for the species, cardiovascular disease accounts for a distinct but relatively small percentage of illnesses and deaths in horses, when compared to human beings, dogs, and cats. However, because most horses are not kept as companion pets but are expected to perform work or athletic feats with a rider, the implications of cardiovascular disease in a horse may be greater than for animals not routinely expected to "earn their keep." In addition to the effect on performance (which may have significant economic implications for the owner), the safety of the rider must also be considered in any discussion of the prognosis and future use of an affected horse.

Congenital Heart Defects

Congenital heart disorders are those present at birth. They are most often discovered within the first few weeks to months of life, when a heart murmur is detected during an examination of the chest and heart. A wide variety of simple or complex defects may occur, but only a few have been recognized often enough to have been reported in more than a few individual horses. The most accurate technique for identifying specific defects and evaluating their severity is two-dimensional echocardiography, supplemented by **Doppler echocardiography** (direct imaging of the direction and velocity of blood flow within the heart and associated blood vessels). Detection of congenital heart defects usually allows only for removal of an individual horse from the pool of potential athletes, since few surgical procedures are available to correct these conditions.

VENTRICULAR SEPTAL DEFECT (VSD)

Ventricular septal defect (VSD), a hole in the muscular wall between the two ventricles, is the most commonly recognized congenital heart defect of horses. It can occur alone or as one of several more complex defects that may be present concurrently. In uncomplicated cases the hole results in the passage or **shunting** of oxygen-rich blood from the higher-pressure left ventricle to the lower-pressure right ventricle and pulmonary artery, primarily during ventricular systole. A systolic heart murmur is usually heard on the right side of the chest over the forward portion of the heart. Depending on the size of the defect and the amount of blood shunting through it, the pulmonary arteries and veins and the left atrium and ventricle are all subjected to an increased workload because of the extra volume of blood (a phenomenon known as **volume overloading**). If the defect and the resulting shunt are small, the adverse effect on cardiac function may be minimal and the horse may be fully capable of engaging safely in moderate physical activities without evidence of fatigue or shortness of breath. If the defect is larger and the shunting is greater, signs of cardiac insufficiency may be present on minimal exertion and the horse may become very limited in its athletic ability. Confirmation of the defect can usually be accomplished using two-dimensional and Doppler echocardiography.

PATENT DUCTUS ARTERIOSUS (PDA)

The **ductus arteriosus** is a large blood vessel present in the developing fetus that connects the pulmonary artery to the aorta, allowing blood from the right ventricle to bypass the lungs, which are nonfunctional during fetal life. In mammals, the ductus normally constricts at or very shortly after birth, eliminating this temporary connection and allowing for the normal development of the **vasculature** (blood vessel supply) in the lungs.

Unlike most other domestic animal species, however, complete closure of the ductus arteriosus is commonly delayed in newborn foals. Because the pressure in the aorta is higher than that in the pulmonary artery throughout the cardiac cycle, in newborns some blood will flow "backward" through the **patent** (open) ductus from the aorta to the pulmonary artery, resulting in the presence of a "continuous" heart murmur over the pulmonary artery on the left side of the chest. Natural closure of the ductus and disappearance of the murmur usually occur within the first week of life. If the ductus remains open beyond the first week, it is referred to as a **persistent** or **patent ductus arteriosus (PDA)**. The resulting shunt may cause blood-volume overload in the pulmonary arteries and veins and left atrium and ventricle. Fortunately, PDA is a rare condition in horses.

TRICUSPID VALVE DYSPLASIA OR ATRESIA

Defective development (**dysplasia**) of the valve lying between the right atrium and right ventricle is more common in horses than in most other species. The Arabian breed is predisposed to tricuspid valve defects, suggesting that there may be a heritable, genetic basis in some cases. The defect may cause the valve to leak during ventricular systole, a condition known as **tricuspid regurgitation** or **insufficiency,** resulting in a systolic murmur on the right side of the chest. Rarely, a narrowing (**stenosis**) of the valve may cause obstruction to inflow from the right atrium to the right ventricle during ventricular diastole. In extreme cases the entire valve may be absent or only minimally developed, a severe condition referred to as **atresia** which requires the concurrent presence of atrial and ventricular septal defects in order for the foal to survive. Mild tricuspid regurgitation may be well tolerated in young horses, while more severe defects usually cause severe exertional fatigue and other signs during the first few weeks or months of life.

COMPLEX DEFECTS

Overall, congenital heart defects are uncommon in horses, but when they do occur, those involving several individual, concurrent defects appear to be more common among horses than in some other species, especially dogs and cats. Such complex or multiple defects may develop in combinations of unrelated defects or in a recognized combination such as **tetralogy of Fallot** (consisting of a VSD, pulmonic stenosis, rightward malpositioning of the origin of the aorta, and right ventricular thickening [**hypertrophy**]) or **truncus arteriosus** (consisting of a VSD and a single large arterial trunk exiting both ventricles). In the most severe cases, there may be shunting of oxygen-poor, venous blood from the right heart chambers to the left heart, bypassing the lungs and causing **cyanosis** (a bluish coloration of the mucous membranes of the mouth and eyes) at rest or during exertion. These defects can be accurately diagnosed only by means of specialized X-ray studies or, more recently, by two-dimensional and Doppler echocardiography.

Acquired Diseases of the Cardiovascular System

Acquired heart problems are not present at birth but develop later. Overall, acquired heart problems are considered to be much more common than congenital defects. Although acquired heart disease is occasionally encountered in horses between 2 and 4 years of age, it most often occurs in horses over 5 years of age. Degenerative changes affecting the heart valves, heart muscle or **myocardium**, and lungs are associated with aging in horses, as in many other species, so that the frequency of acquired degenerative heart disease (though still relatively uncommon in all age groups) increases with age. The most common clinical signs include a reduction in exercise capacity (exertional fatigue), shortness of breath (especially following exertion), or development of a heart murmur, irregular heart beat, or other audible abnormality without other signs of illness.

ATRIAL FIBRILLATION
Serious electrical disorders of the heart rhythm (**arrhythmias**) overall are not very common in horses. The most frequently recognized arrhythmia associated with diminished athletic performance or more serious signs of cardiac insuffi-

ciency is *atrial fibrillation*. The normally regular, organized waves of electrical activity across the atria become irregular, disorganized, and chaotic, such that the atria fail to contract normally. This results in a very unpredictable, irregular heart beat. Although atrial fibrillation often develops in horses with advanced structural heart disease and atrial **dilatation** (expansion), because of the comparatively large size of the equine atria horses most often develop this arrhythmia with few or no additional signs of heart disease. In such cases signs of cardiac insufficiency are usually not recognized at rest or with mild to moderate exertion, but become apparent at moderate to severe levels of exercise.

Accurate diagnosis of this arrhythmia (and others) requires evaluation by ECG, where the absence of normal atrial waves and the very irregular ventricular waves can be readily identified. Further evaluation of the structure and mechanical function of the heart by echocardiography is also recommended because the prognosis for treatment, recovery, and return to previous activity levels is directly related to the presence or absence of underlying mechanical cardiac dysfunction.

If serious cardiac disease with atrial dilatation is present, the prognosis for functional recovery is poor. Treatment of the signs of cardiac insufficiency with drugs such as digitalis and **diuretics** (drugs that promote fluid loss) may be considered in selected cases where little physical activity is expected. If there is little or no evidence of underlying cardiac dysfunction, administration of oral or injectable medications, especially quinidine, is often successful in converting the arrhythmia to a normal rhythm. In most such cases, horses are able to return to their previous levels of activity and performance, although some may experience one or more recurrences of the arrhythmia, necessitating retreatment or possibly retirement from strenuous activity.

VALVULAR HEART DISEASE
The most commonly recognized acquired structural heart disorders in horses are degenerative valvular deformities. Such disorders result in incompetence and insufficiency of one or more

heart valves, producing associated heart murmurs and dilation of the cardiac chambers that must handle the extra blood regurgitating on either side of the incompetent valve. If the valvular leak is severe enough, the pressure in the veins leading to the affected side of the heart increases to the point where fluid accumulation (**edema**) occurs.

In horses the valves most commonly affected by degenerative changes sufficiently severe to cause valvular incompetence are the mitral, aortic, and tricuspid valves, in that order. The pulmonic valve is rarely affected. As a result the most commonly recognized pathologic heart murmurs in adult horses are those of mitral regurgitation (systolic murmur over the left rear portion of the heart), aortic regurgitation (diastolic murmur, often with a buzzing or musical quality, over the left forward portion of the heart), or tricuspid regurgitation (systolic murmur over the right side of the heart).

Degenerative changes in heart valves usually occur slowly and progressively over many years, resulting in gradual thickening and irregular deformation of the valve surfaces. Sudden or more rapid worsening of mitral or tricuspid insufficiency and signs of illness may also result from the rupture of one or more of the valves' supporting structures, the **chordae tendineae**.

Valvular disease is initially diagnosed by the detection of a heart murmur on physical examination. It is very important, however, to recognize that soft, innocent ("normal") murmurs are often heard in normal foals and adult horses. To advise an owner or rider about the significance of any heart murmur, it is critical to distinguish between a normal murmur (which is usually more variable and inconsistent as the heart rate changes) and a pathological murmur of valvular regurgitation, and to assess the severity of any suspected valve leaks. Two-dimensional and Doppler echocardiography are the most accurate and least invasive methods for making such determinations. In general, mild to moderate valvular insufficiency in a horse without reported signs of illness is compatible with continued use of the horse for mild to moderate physical activity. More severe valvular disease, especially when accompanied by obvious signs of cardiac

insufficiency, atrial fibrillation, or severe cardiac enlargement, is cause for a poor prognosis and a strong recommendation against any riding or forced physical activity.

MYOCARDIAL DISEASE

Although **necropsy** (animal autopsy) studies have shown that small areas of muscle death and scarring are commonly found in the atrial and ventricular muscle of horses dying of many different causes, most of these cardiac lesions have been considered to be "incidental" findings. Such lesions appear unlikely to have affected the overall function of the heart muscle; however, it has been proposed that they may contribute to the tendency for some horses to develop abnormal cardiac electrical activity. **Myocarditis** (inflammation of the heart muscle) is occasionally suspected (but rarely proved) in horses that develop arrhythmias or other electrical disorders following an infectious disease such as strangles, equine influenza, or an internal abscess. Toxic damage to the heart muscle may occur rarely as a result of a severe dietary deficiency of vitamin E and selenium, or from ingestion of the chemical **monensin** in cattle feed. Diseases that originate within and affect primarily the heart muscle have not been clearly proved to occur in horses.

PERICARDIAL DISEASE

The **pericardium** is a thin, fibrous sac that surrounds the heart, stabilizing its position and protecting it from disease affecting nearby structures. Inflammation or infection of the pericardium (**pericarditis**), as well as cancerous involvement of the pericardium, are quite rare in horses. The most common result of pericardial disease is the accumulation of excess fluid within the pericardial sac. Since the pericardium is limited in its ability to expand to accommodate this fluid, the pressure within the sac restricts and compresses the heart chambers, preventing adequate filling of the ventricles and limiting cardiac output.

COR PULMONALE

The term *"cor pulmonale"* refers to right-heart disease caused by increased pressure within the pulmonary artery. The increased pressure is the result of markedly increased resistance to blood flow through the lungs, either because of obstruction or destruction of a large portion of the pulmonary vascular bed, or because of intense constriction of these vessels. Horses are well known for developing recurrent allergic and/or infectious chronic obstructive lung disease and associated physical signs (*see* Chapter 25, "Respiratory System and Various Disorders.") In a few advanced cases the destruction of lung tissue and the resulting increased resistance to pulmonary blood flow cause dilatation and muscular hypertrophy of the right ventricle, secondary insufficiency of the tricuspid valve, and ultimately right-heart failure. Increased pulmonary artery pressure and enlargement of the right ventricle may also occur in some young horses with complex congenital heart defects, and in older horses with moderate to severe mitral valve regurgitation and increased left atrial pressure. In most cases the presence of cor pulmonale is a poor prognostic sign because of the severity of the underlying condition.

Vascular Disease

Horses are known to develop some disorders that affect primarily the blood vessels (arteries and/or veins). **Atherosclerosis**, the vascular disease associated with high blood pressure and high cholesterol and fats in people, is exceptionally rare in domestic animals, including horses. Thus the consequences of this condition, including **myocardial infarction** ("heart attack"), stroke, and other arterial diseases, are also very uncommon in horses.

The only common condition affecting the veins of horses is **thrombophlebitis** of the jugular vein, caused by repeated jugular vein puncture (as to obtain a blood sample), accidental injection of material outside the vein, or use of a jugular vein **catheter** (flexible tubular instrument for insertion into a blood vessel). The resulting chemical or physical irritation or infection in or around the vein causes inflammation (**phlebitis**), swelling, and tenderness, followed by **thrombosis** (formation of a firm clot) in a segment of the vein. Treatment involves removing the cause and applying symptomatic treatment for discomfort and any associated infection.

Several conditions may affect the systemic arteries in horses. The most common is parasitic **arteritis** (arterial inflammation) caused by vascular migration of the larval forms of the intestinal parasite *Strongylus vulgaris* (*see* Chapter 33, "Internal Parasites"). The resulting dilatation and thrombosis (and potential obstruction) usually occur at the origin of the large arteries to the intestines (sometimes causing colic), although other arteries may be affected. Fortunately this condition can usually be treated or prevented by an appropriate antiparasitic drug treatment program.

Another recognized arterial disorder is **aorto-iliac thrombosis.** In this condition a **thrombus** (clot) develops at the point where the aorta branches toward the hind legs. The resulting restriction of blood flow to the hind limbs can cause signs of lameness, stiffness, weakness, and abnormal gait, which usually develop during exercise and disappear following rest. Unfortunately this condition is often progressive and rarely reversible, markedly limiting the athletic use of an affected horse.

Degenerative changes in the walls of large arteries may occur that weaken a vessel and predispose it to rupture and **hemorrhage** (bleeding). The most commonly reported sites of such ruptures are the base of the aorta in stallions and the uterine artery in mares.

CHAPTER 21

The Urinary System and Various Disorders

by Lais R.R. Costa and
John E. Madigan

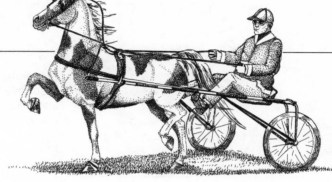

The Urinary System

The urinary system consists of the two *kidneys*, two *ureters*, the *urinary bladder*, and the *urethra* (FIGURE 1). The urinary system is responsible for regulating the volume and composition of the body fluids. It maintains the balance of water and **electrolytes** (elements such as sodium and potassium) and eliminates metabolic by-products from the body. Two important by-products of body metabolism are the nitrogen-containing compounds **urea** and **creatinine**, both of which must be continually excreted so that they do not reach toxic levels. In addition, many chemical compounds such as hormones, antibiotics, and anti-inflammatory medications are eliminated through the urinary system.

The kidneys of the horse are heart-shaped, and each is divided into an outer **cortex** and an inner **medulla** (FIGURE 2). The functional unit of the kidney is the microscopic *nephron*. Each kidney has literally hundreds of thousands of nephrons. The blood enters the kidney through the **renal artery** and flows through a network of progressively smaller vessels, ultimately reaching

an individual **glomerulus** (microscopic network of tiny blood vessels) in each nephron, where the cellular components of the blood (red cells, white cells, platelets) are filtered out. The filtrate then moves through the nephron—down the **proximal tubules,** the **loop of Henle,** and the **distal tubules**—during which time it is progressively modified. As the filtrate passes through the proximal tubules, reusable constituents such as glucose (**blood sugar**), protein, amino acids, sodium, and phosphorus are reabsorbed and cycled back into the bloodstream. The filtrate is then concentrated, water and electrolytes being reabsorbed during passage through the loop of Henle, the distal tubules, and collecting ducts. The end-product is the **urine**, which collects in each **renal pelvis** (central portion of the kidney) and flows through a ureter into the urinary bladder, where it is stored until it is eliminated.

The bladder is composed of two parts: the body, which stores the urine, and the neck, which is funnel-shaped and connects with the urethra. In the mare, the urethra is short and opens into the **external meatus** located on the floor of the **vagina**, about 10 cm (4 inches) from

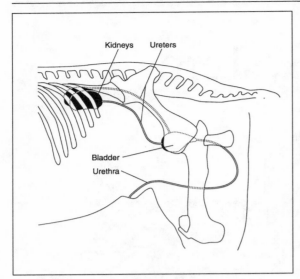

Figure 1. Anatomy of the urinary tract of the horse.

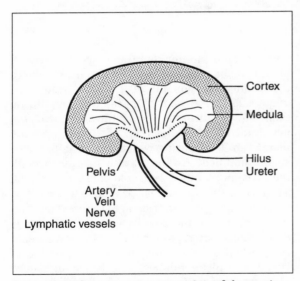

Figure 2. Schematic representation of the equine kidney. The renal artery, renal vein, lymphatic vessels, nerves, and ureter pass through an indentation in the kidney called the **hilus**.

the opening of the **vulva**. In males, the urethra extends from the bladder throughout the length of the **penis**.

The kidneys have many additional functions,

including the production of **erythropoietin** (a hormone responsible for regulating the production of red blood cells) and **renin** and **angiotensin**, which function in regulating the cardiovascular system. Diseases that involve the **upper urinary tract** (the kidneys) are associated with disturbances of many or all of the renal regulatory and excretory functions. By contrast, diseases of the **lower urinary tract** (the ureters, bladder, and urethra) are characterized largely by disturbances in urine flow.

Signs of Urinary Tract Disease

Normally, male and female horses spread their hindlimbs before urinating, lowering the rump and exerting pressure by contracting the abdominal muscles. Males usually extend the penis from its sheath. Horses generally do not urinate on hard surfaces. They urinate only while resting and not while feeding, and they may emit groans during the process. An adult horse may urinate 4 to 6 times a day, with a total daily urine volume ranging from 4 to 15 liters. The amount of water consumed is important in this regard: daily water consumption of horses can vary from 19 to 66 liters, depending upon the diet, climate, and working conditions.

A disorder of the urinary system should be suspected when a horse exhibits signs of abnormal urination, which can include one or more of the following:

- Frequent passage of small quantities of urine
- Straining or pain associated with urination, manifested by grunting at completion or by remaining in a crouched posture
- Urine soiling or scalding (burn caused by a liquid) of the **perineum** (region between the thighs encompassing the anus and genitalia), tail, and hindlimbs

An affected horse may exhibit signs of colic (acute abdominal pain), which must be differentiated from abdominal discomfort of gastrointestinal origin. Horses with kidney disease may consume large amounts of water (a condition referred to as **polydipsia**) and pass unusually large volumes of urine (**polyuria**). Discoloration of the urine by blood or blood pigment (**hematuria** or **hemoglobinuria**, respectively) or by the red pigment of skeletal muscle known as **myoglobin** (**myoglobinuria**) may occur in certain diseases of the urinary tract. Blood may be seen throughout urination, indicating **hemorrhage** (bleeding) in one or both kidneys; at the end of urination (hemorrhage in the bladder); or at the beginning of urination (hemorrhage in the urethra). Chronic diseases of the urinary system are often accompanied by chronic weight loss, decreased appetite, and weakness.

Diagnostic Aids for Evaluating the Urinary Tract

A **urinalysis** (examination of the urine) can provide important information about the presence and type of urinary disease (*see* APPENDIX C, "DIAGNOSTIC TESTS"). Urine samples may be collected by "free-catch" or by the passing of a **catheter** (a flexible tube) through the urethra and into the bladder. Normally, male horses will require sedation in order to catheterize the bladder; mares usually will not. The urine sample can be sent to a laboratory for urinalysis and for the culture of microorganisms (in cases where an infection is suspected).

The urinalysis provides information on the horse's ability to concentrate its urine (a test known as **urine specific gravity**), its ability to reabsorb glucose and proteins (which are normally absent in the urine), and on the pH of the urine (equine urine normally is alkaline, a reflection of the horse's diet). Horse urine varies in appearance from pale yellow to light brown and can be very cloudy owing to its high mucus content. Horses consuming diets rich in calcium (e.g., alfalfa) often have high quantities of calcium carbonate in the urine, which imparts a cloudy appearance to the urine. The presence of high numbers of red and white blood cells or other cell types (e.g., tumor cells) in the urine are often indicative of abnormalities of the urinary tract.

Blood chemistry tests are also important in an examination of the urinary tract (*see* APPENDIX C, "DIAGNOSTIC TESTS"). The **blood urea nitrogen** (**BUN**) and **creatinine** levels in the blood are widely used indicators of the blood-filtering capacity of the kidneys. A severe decrease in filtering caused by dehydration or kidney disease will culminate in an elevation of BUN and creatinine levels in the blood, a condition referred to as **azotemia**. Azotemia develops when approximately 75% of the horse's nephrons have been damaged. Electrolyte disturbances also occur in kidney disease, with blood levels of sodium generally falling as levels of potassium and calcium rise. Clearance tests such as the **inulin** and **sodium sulfanilate** tests are also available for evaluating the filtering capacity of the kidneys.

An **endoscopic examination** of the urethra and bladder can also provide valuable diagnostic information. In this procedure a small flexible tube (an **endoscope**) equipped with a video camera at its tip is inserted through the urethra and possibly as far up as the bladder. Lower urinary tract abnormalities, such as an obstruction, hemorrhage, or tumor, can often be identified in this way. **Biopsies** (samples of tissue) can also be obtained from any part of the lower urinary tract. The endoscope can be used to guide a small catheter into one ureter, so that urine can be collected from only one kidney.

Ultrasonography (a noninvasive procedure for visualizing internal structures of the body by means of sound [echo] reflections; **diagnostic ultrasound**) has been used to assess the size, shape, and structure of the kidneys and bladder. Kidney biopsies are also an excellent diagnostic aid, and can be obtained with or without ultrasonography guidance.

Disorders of the Upper Urinary Tract

Kidney disease can be either **congenital** (present at birth) or acquired. Congenital kidney diseases are very rare in the horse. Examples include **renal hypoplasia** (a subnormal number of functioning nephrons) and **polycystic kidneys** (kidneys containing many **cysts** [fluid-filled pockets or sacs]). In both conditions the horse will usually develop signs of chronic renal failure.

Horses with kidney disease often exhibit some of the following clinical signs, depending upon the underlying cause and the progression of the illness:

- Increased water consumption and increased urine volume
- Decreased appetite and weight loss
- Weakness, lethargy
- Diarrhea
- Dull haircoat
- Sores in the mouth
- Discolored urine or abnormal urination
- Intermittent abdominal pain
- Fever
- Swelling (**edema**) of the lower limbs

ACUTE RENAL FAILURE

Horses with acute renal failure develop a sudden, rapid, and severe reduction in kidney function. The potential causes can be divided into (1) **vascular** or **perfusion injuries,** in which impairment of blood flow through the kidneys is followed by a deterioration of function, and (2) **nephrotoxic** injuries, in which the cause is direct damage to the kidney cells themselves.

Vascular or perfusion injuries can be caused by:
- Severe dehydration
- Hemorrhage
- Hypotension (low blood pressure)
- Hypovolemia (decreased circulatory blood volume)
- Generalized infection
- General anesthesia
- Blockage of renal blood vessels

Nephrotoxic injuries can be caused by:
- Heavy metals
- Insecticides
- Blister beetle poisoning
- Nonsteroidal anti-inflammatory medications
- Certain antibiotics (gentamicin, kanamycin, sulfonamide)
- Hemoglobin (from destruction of red blood cells, as in equine infectious anemia)
- Myoglobin (from muscle destruction, e.g., "tying-up")
- Endotoxemia (infections by bacteria that possess a potent endotoxin [a toxin within the bacterial cell])

Treatment involves identifying and treating (when possible) the underlying cause, and supporting blood flow through the kidneys with intravenous fluid therapy and other appropriate measures. The prognosis is dependent on the nature of the underlying disorder.

CHRONIC RENAL FAILURE

Chronic renal failure usually results from damage to the glomeruli or the kidney tubules. It most often affects older horses (except in the case of congenital disorders). The major presenting clinical sign is unexplained weight loss. There are many possible causes of chronic renal failure, some of which are listed below:

- **Glomerulonephritis** (inflammatory disease resulting in damage to the glomeruli by an immunological reaction)
- **Nephritis** (inflammation of the nephrons, often associated with bacterial infections in foals)
- **Pyelonephritis** (infection of cells of the renal pelvis, usually as a result of an ascending infection from the lower urinary tract)
- **Leptospirosis** (a bacterial infection)
- **Amyloidosis** (deposition of insoluble protein substances [*amyloid*] in the glomeruli)

Treatment involves identifying and treating (if possible) the underlying cause, and supporting kidney function through the use of intravenous fluid therapy and other measures. Unless the underlying cause is amenable to therapy, the prognosis for long-term survival is usually poor.

RENAL TUBULAR ACIDOSIS

Renal tubular acidosis is a disorder of the kidney tubules and is characterized by **acidosis** (abnormally acid blood) and an elevation of chloride levels in the bloodstream. These metabolic disturbances are caused by an inability of the kidneys to control the amount of bicarbonate and acids excreted in the urine. Possible clinical signs include weakness, depression, incoordination, and weight loss. Treatment involves correction of the acidosis by means of intravenous or oral fluid therapy. Some horses may recover, but the prognosis is guarded.

KIDNEY TUMORS

Primary tumors of the kidney are rare. *Renal cell carcinoma* occurs in middle-aged or older horses; it generally involves only one kidney. The signs of a kidney tumor are similar to those seen in other kidney diseases; however, blood in the urine and abdominal pain are often more common. **Metastasis** (spread of tumor cells beyond the primary tumor site) to the lungs and lymph nodes may occur; the prognosis for most such tumors is poor.

KIDNEY STONES

Kidney stones occur only rarely in horses. (The formation of stones in the urinary tract is discussed in "DISORDERS OF THE LOWER URINARY TRACT," below). Horses with kidney stones may exhibit signs of weight loss, inappetence, and moderate to severe abdominal pain. The diagnosis can be made by an ultrasonographic examination of the kidneys. Surgical treatment may be required.

Disorders of the Lower Urinary Tract

URINARY STONES (UROLITHIASIS)

Urinary stones or *calculi* can form in any part of the urinary tract, and depending upon their location are referred to by different names:

Kidney stone = **nephrolith**
Stone in the ureter = **ureterolith**
Stone in the urinary bladder = **cystolith**
Stone in the urethra = **urethrolith**

The formation of urinary stones, a condition referred to as **urolithiasis**, is uncommon in horses. When stones do occur they are usually found in the bladder. Male horses may be more affected by urethral stones because the urethra of males is much longer.

Urinary stones are formed by the deposition of various forms of calcium carbonate, predominantly calcite. Several factors can facilitate this deposition. The alkaline pH of horse urine favors the formation of carbonate and mixed-phosphate stones. The excessive concentration of urine solutes, which occurs following water deprivation or excessive water loss, also favors deposition. Ingestion of high-concentrate and low-roughage diets may play a role as well.

Affected horses exhibit abnormal, painful urination (small amounts of urine voided frequently), signs of colic and straining, urine scalding, and blood in the urine after exercise. Treatment requires the insertion of a catheter into the urethra to flush the urinary bladder. Surgery to remove particularly large stones or to correct an obstruction may be necessary.

Horses developing urolithiasis should receive special care to prevent recurrence of the problem. Such care involves supplementation of the diet with ammonium chloride (to alter urine pH), changes in the diet (decreasing the intake of concentrates and calcium), and assurance of an abundant supply of fresh drinking water to prevent dehydration.

CYSTITIS

Inflammation of the bladder (**cystitis**) often occurs secondary to diseases causing incomplete emptying of the bladder, such as bladder paralysis or urolithiasis. Paralysis of the bladder musculature is caused by interference with the neurologic functioning of the bladder. Affected horses develop **urinary incontinence** (loss of voluntary control over urination) and signs of other neurologic problems, such as paralysis of the anus and tail.

In mares, cystitis may also be a result of chronic **vaginitis** (inflammation of the vagina). Bacteria can also be introduced into the urinary bladder through urinary catheterization. The bacteria most often involved in equine cystitis include *Escherichia coli*, *Staphylococcus*, *Corynebacterium*, and *Pseudomonas*.

Clinical signs of cystitis include frequent urination, straining to urinate, urine dribbling, and urine scalding. Treatment of any underlying cause of the cystitis is imperative. Antibiotic therapy should be based on culture and sensitivity testing of bacteria recovered from the urine.

PROLAPSE OF THE BLADDER (DISPLACED BLADDER)

Prolapse (bulging) of the urinary bladder through the vulvar opening of the female is very uncommon, and is usually a complication of foaling. The relaxation of the pelvic muscles and ligaments, together with straining, may predispose the mare to prolapse. Treatment includes control of straining, edema, and hemorrhage, and careful replacement of the bladder in the pelvic cavity with the mare under sedation. Postoperative antibiotic therapy is usually recommended.

Bladder Tumors

Tumors of the bladder are extremely uncommon in the horse, and usually found in older horses. Tumor types that have been reported include the *squamous cell carcinoma* and *transitional cell carcinoma*. The major clinical sign of a bladder tumor is blood in the urine. Unfortunately, most bladder tumors in the horse are malignant and essentially untreatable.

Rupture of the Bladder

Rupture of the urinary bladder is very rare in mature horses. When it does occur it is usually associated with the birthing process, paralysis of the bladder, or urinary obstruction. Rupture of the bladder is much more common in newborn foals, most often colts. Surgical correction is usually required. Surgery should be performed as soon as possible after a diagnosis is made; a delay in seeking treatment may result in death of the foal.

Disorders of the Urethra

Urethral obstruction is uncommon in horses. It may be caused by urethral stones, tumors such as *squamous cell carcinoma*, and certain diseases of the penis or urethral process. The accumulation of **smegma** (a thick, cheesy secretion that collects beneath the sheath of the penis) can form a solidifed mass in the urethra known as a **urethral diverticular concretion,** or "**bean**," resulting in inflammation and urethral obstruction. The bean can be removed manually with the horse under sedation. Male horses may require periodic cleaning of the penile sheath to remove accumulated smegma.

Urethral stones are also rare. Surgical treatment is required if passage of a catheter fails to dislodge the stone.

Trauma may cause an obstruction or laceration, with resultant rupture of the urethra. This generally occurs in male horses, often following a kick to the penis. In severe cases of trauma or obstruction by tumors or other processes, amputation of the penis may be necessary.

Patent Urachus

A condition referred to as *patent urachus* occurs in foals. While the foal is in the uterus, a hollow tube called the *urachus* drains the urine from the bladder of the fetus to the **allantoic fluid** (fluid stored in one of the "bags" that surrounds and protects the fetus). At birth, when the umbilical cord ruptures, the urachus begins to degenerate; no urine should then pass through it. Detection of moisture or fluid coming from the umbilical structure of a foal indicates that the urachus is still **patent** (open and functioning) and that urine is passing through it from the bladder.

There are three situations wherein patent urachus may be observed. The first is in foals that are under intensive care and have been restrained very frequently. In this situation pressure from the straining may drive the urine from the bladder into the urachus, forcing it open. The second situation occurs within 14 days of birth and without any prior history of illness; surgical correction is often required. The third situation is found in foals with infected umbilical structures, in which case cystitis and **uroperitoneum** (accumulation of urine in the abdominal cavity) may develop.

Many cases of patent urachus resolve spontaneously without treatment. Should infection occur, surgical correction is indicated to remove the infected umbilical tissue.

CHAPTER 22

The Musculoskeletal System and Various Disorders

by Mark D. Markel

The Musculoskeletal System

The musculoskeletal system participates in many essential functions, including protection of the internal organs, facilitation of muscle action and body movement, and storage of the vital minerals calcium and phosphorus. As its name implies, the musculoskeletal system is composed of the *skeleton* and the *muscles*.

THE SKELETON
The skeleton is the rigid frame upon which the soft tissues depend for support. **Bone**, the principal component of the skeleton, is living connective tissue made rigid by the orderly deposition of minerals. Bone possesses unique structural characteristics that allow it to carry out many of the musculoskeletal system's important duties. It is one of the toughest substances in the body, rivaling only the teeth for hardness. Bone's intricate structural organization and its high **metabolic** (pertaining to life-sustaining biochemical processes) activity together allow it to respond rapidly to the many physical and biological demands that are made upon it.

Bone is a highly **vascularized** (supplied with blood vessels) tissue with an excellent capacity for self-repair. Bone surfaces are covered by many different types of cells that regulate the continual turnover of bone through its periodic formation and **resorption** (biochemical dissolution). In addition bone cells called **osteocytes**, in response to certain hormones, are responsible for maintaining normal calcium and phosphorus levels in the bloodstream. These and other cells help bone tissue respond quickly to mechanical and metabolic needs.

It is frequently convenient to divide the skeletal system into two major components: the **appendicular skeleton,** composed of the bones of the limbs and the pelvis; and the **axial skeleton,** consisting of the vertebrae, skull, ribs, and sternum.

Bones of the appendicular skeleton in general are long, tubular structures with expanded ends called **epiphyses**. Each end of a long bone is covered by a substance called **articular cartilage,** which is responsible for the smooth, almost frictionless gliding of the joint surfaces against one another (*see* below). The narrow mid-portion of a long bone is known as the **dia-physis**. In immature long bones, a **growth plate** or **physis** is present at one or both ends of the bone. The growth plate is responsible for the majority of long-bone growth in young horses. As a horse matures the growth plate is gradually obliterated. The region immediately beneath the growth plate is called the **metaphysis**. The dia-physis of a long bone contains the bone's major blood supply as well as the **bone marrow**—the soft center of the bone which contains the blood-forming elements (precursor cells of the red and white blood cells) of the circulatory system.

The entire long bone, except in regions cov-ered by articular cartilage or where ligaments, tendons, or joint capsules are attached (*see* below), is covered by a thin sheath of connective tissue called the **periosteum.** The highly sensitive perios-teum contains a rich blood and nerve supply and provides for the nutrition, growth, repair, and protection of the underlying bone.

The complex structures known as **joints** are major components of the musculoskeletal system and one of the principal components responsible for body motion. A typical joint is located at the apposition of two bone ends, each end being covered by a sheath of articular cartilage. Articular cartilage has two major functions:

- To distribute over a wide area the forces to which a limb is subjected, thus decreasing the stresses within the cartilage
- To provide relatively frictionless movement between opposing joint surfaces

Articular cartilage is specially designed to withstand the repeated and rigorous forces it is subjected to throughout a horse's lifetime. Articular cartilage is virtually isolated from the rest of the body, being devoid of blood vessels, lymphatic channels, and nerves. In addition, articular cartilage has a very low cellular den-sity, containing fewer cells than any other tissue in the body. Articular cartilage is notoriously poor in its ability to respond to injury without permanent scarring and secondary **arthritis** (joint degeneration).

The three principal structures that surround, stabilize, and connect the joints of the skeletal system are the *tendons*, *ligaments*, and *joint capsules*. Although none of these structures pro-duces motion by itself, each plays an important role in movement.

Both **ligaments** and **joint capsules** connect bone to bone. Their function is to augment the stability of joints, to guide motion in the appro-priate direction, and to prevent excessive motion. Tendons attach muscle to bone and transmit the muscular forces responsible for motion to bone. Tendons and ligaments are made of dense con-nective tissues composed primarily of **collagen**, a fibrous protein constituting approximately one-third of the total protein in the body. Collagen has a unique mechanical supportive function in other connective tissues as well, including carti-lage, blood vessel walls, the heart, kidneys, skin, and liver. The exceptional mechanical stability of collagen gives tendons and ligaments their flexibility and strength. Similar to articular carti-lage, tendons and ligaments contain relatively few cells, occupying approximately 20 percent of the total tissue volume. The joint capsule is a thin, saclike structure that envelopes the joint and contains within it all the elements of the joint, such as the articular cartilage, **synovial membrane** (lining membrane of the joint), and **synovial fluid** (joint fluid).

THE MUSCLES

The muscular component of the musculoskeletal system consists of three muscle types:

- **Cardiac muscle,** which composes the heart
- **Smooth** or **involuntary muscle,** which lines the hollow internal organs
- **Skeletal** or **voluntary muscle,** which attaches to bones via tendons and causes the bones to move

Skeletal muscle is the most abundant tissue in the body, accounting for approximately 40 to 45 percent of total body weight. In addition to causing movement, muscles provide strength and protection to the skeleton by distributing forces and absorbing shock. Unlike connective tissues such as cartilage, tendons, and ligaments, muscles are well-supplied with blood vessels and contain an abundance of cells that are responsible for providing the energy needed for muscular contraction.

EQUINE ANATOMY

To understand the many musculoskeletal disorders occurring in the horse, it is important to have a fundamental knowledge of equine anatomy as it pertains to the musculoskeletal system. (*Readers are strongly urged to consult* CHAPTER 16: "ANATOMY," *before proceeding on with the remainder of this chapter*).

Horses are **quadrupeds,** meaning that they walk on all four limbs. These limbs can be divided into two **forelimbs** and two **hindlimbs**:

THE FORELIMB

Starting at the foot, the equine forelimb begins with a **hoof wall** which incorporates the **distal third phalanx** (also called **coffin bone** and **pedal bone**), the **navicular bone** (distal sesamoid bone), and the **coffin joint.** Progressing up the limb, the *middle (second) phalanx* (**short pastern bone**) joins with the coffin joint at its lower end and with the **pastern joint** at its upper end. The *proximal (first) phalanx* (**long pastern bone**), the next bone up the limb, joins with the pastern joint at its lower end and with the *fetlock joint* at its upper end. Above the fetlock joint is the *third metacarpal bone* (**cannon bone**). Above the cannon bone is the **carpus** (knee), which is composed of three **carpal joints.** Above the carpus is the **radius**, which along with the **ulna** comprises the long forearm of the horse. The radius and ulna meet the **humerus** (upper forearm) at the elbow joint. The humerus then joins the shoulder joint.

THE HINDLIMB

Starting at the foot, the hindlimb is similar to the forelimb up to the level of the cannon bone. In contrast to the forelimb, the cannon bone is joined with the **tarsal joints,** known collectively as the **hock.** Above the hock are the **tibia** (equivalent of the shin bone) and its smaller accompanying **fibula**, which join with the **stifle joint** (equivalent of the knee joint). Above the stifle joint is the **femur** (thigh bone), which at its ball-and-socket upper end joins with the **hip joint** of the pelvis.

Musculoskeletal Disorders of Young Horses

ANGULAR LIMB DEFORMITIES

Angular limb deformities include some of the most common musculoskeletal disorders of the growing foal. Angular limb deformities most often result from an imbalance of growth at the ends of the long bones. If one side of a growth plate grows more rapidly than the other, the limb will begin to deviate from its normal axis. The carpus of the forelimb is the area most frequently involved, with the lower part of the limb usually deviating **laterally** (to the outside), resulting in a knock-kneed individual. Less frequently, the limb may deviate **medially** (to the inside), resulting in a bow-legged horse. Other (relatively rare) sites for angular deviation include the fetlocks and the hocks.

The diagnosis of an angular limb deformity must be made early if treatment is to be successful. Often, newborn foals will exhibit a mild to moderate angular limb deformity that is present at birth and results simply from joint **laxity** (looseness). This type of deformity often resolves on its own within the first few weeks of life. By contrast, angular limb deformities that develop after birth usually do not resolve spontaneously and require corrective treatment.

Treatment of angular limb deformities is dependent on the age of the foal and the severity of the deviation. For very mild deformities, corrective trimming of the hoof walls on a weekly basis may be all that is necessary. If the deformity worsens or is more severe, surgical correction may be required. Surgical correction relies on either of two strategies: speeding up growth on the side of the bone that is growing more slowly, or retarding growth on the side of the bone that is growing faster. Today the most common surgery for angular limb deformities is **periosteal stripping** of the portion of the growth plate that has slowed. Periosteal stripping effectually "releases" the growth plate and allows it to grow more rapidly, thereby straightening the limb. Retardation of growth of the side of the bone that is growing faster may be accomplished by placing screws and wires across the growth plate, thus preventing its continued growth. In horses in which bone growth has ceased, or which have little growth remaining in the growth plate, the surgeon's only option is to perform a series of bone cuts (osteotomies) to help straighten the limbs, followed by stabilization of the cuts with one or two plates and screws.

The prognosis for horses with angular limb deformities is good to excellent if the condition is treated early and the deviation is relatively small. If affected horses are not treated, or are treated too late, the persistent angular deviation may result in chronic lameness and arthritis of the joints of the affected limb. Depending on which joint is involved, treatment must be initiated when the horse is between 2 and 4 months of age if a successful outcome is to be achieved.

PHYSITIS

Physitis is an extremely important, generalized bone disease of young growing horses. It is characterized by enlargement of the growth plates of certain long bones and of the vertebrae of the neck. Two syndromes have been described. One affects rapidly growing horses such as foals and weanlings, with a peak occurrence at 4 to 8 months of age. The other syndrome is seen in young horses that have begun training between 1.5 and 2 years of age. The term "physitis" is actually a misnomer, since there is no active inflammation of the growth plate of the bone.

Physitis is usually seen in horses on a high plane of nutrition, particularly those being fed high-grain rations that have been formulated without regard to mineral balance. The condition also occurs in horses on high-protein diets. Physitis is often compounded by the fact that sires and dams frequently are selected to produce rapidly growing offspring that will perform better in the show-ring or on the track.

Physitis is manifested clinically as a flaring of the ends of long bones, giving a characteristic "hourglass" shape to the bones. Particularly affected are the lower ends of the radius, tibia, and cannon bones. All limbs may be involved and the condition is associated with a variable degree of lameness. In severe cases the flared regions of bone may be warm and cause pain if touched. Physitis can affect a single individual in a herd, or several members of a herd at the same time.

The cause of physitis is unknown, but nutrition, rapid growth rate, trauma, and genetic predisposition appear to be involved in its development. In general, diets low in calcium and high in phosphorus are responsible for the condition. Other trace minerals in the diet may play a role.

The first step in treating physitis is to evaluate the diet of the affected individual(s). If abnormalities are detected in the ration they should be corrected. Affected horses should also be examined for other musculoskeletal disorders associated with the feeding of high-grain diets that are low in calcium and high in phosphorus. Such disorders include osteochondrosis and flexural deformities (*see* below). If the horse is obese, a general weight-reduction program should be instituted. Weight reduction will help by decreasing trauma to the affected growth plates. Anti-inflammatory medication may be indicated if the horse is stiff or lame on a particular limb. The prognosis for recovery is good to excellent, with the disease usually resolving spontaneously as the horse matures. In severe cases, however, affected horses may be left with a residual problem that can limit future athletic soundness.

WEAKNESS OF THE FLEXOR TENDONS

This is a common condition of newborn foals that frequently affects only the hindlimbs; occasionally, all four limbs will be involved. The condition usually resolves spontaneously within the first few days of life. Affected foals tend to walk on their heels and do not bear weight on their toes. In cases that do not spontaneously resolve, corrective trimming and exercise may be required. The heels should be trimmed to provide a flat surface for the foal to walk on; the toes should not be trimmed. Protective bandages or casts usually are not indicated because they may exacerbate the tendon weakness.

CONGENITAL FLEXURAL DEFORMITIES

Congenital (present at birth) flexural deformities are often thought to occur secondary to malpositioning of the fetus within the uterus. Other predisposing factors may include genetics and damage to the fetus during the embryonic stage of pregnancy. Congenital flexural deformities may affect one or more limbs, and most commonly involve the fetlock or carpus. Affected foals are unable to extend fully the involved joint.

Foals with mild flexural deformity may improve on their own without treatment. This is most often the case with deformities occurring secondary to fetal malpositioning. In cases that do not resolve spontaneously, forced extension of the affected joint to lengthen the flexor tendons of the limb is required. The most effective method of achieving this is through the use of polyvinyl chloride (PVC) tubing cut in half long-ways and used as a splint. It is imperative that the limb and PVC splint be thoroughly padded to prevent pressure sores from developing on the affected limb. Splints should be checked twice daily to guard against this complication.

A more recently described treatment involves the intravenous administration of the antibiotic oxytetracycline. Complete resolution of early cases has been documented with a single dose of this medication, although occasionally a second dose is required. If exercise, splinting, or oxytetracycline do not correct the deformity, then more aggressive therapy must be applied. Such therapy might include the application of a cast or corrective shoes, or surgical cutting of the affected tendons (**tenotomy**). The prognosis for horses responding to conservative therapy is good to excellent. Horses requiring more aggressive treatment often have a poor to guarded prognosis for future soundness.

ACQUIRED FLEXURAL DEFORMITIES

Acquired flexural deformities occurring in foals usually involve one or both forelimbs and are most often centered at the fetlock or coffin joints. The causes of these disorders are multifactorial, often involving chronic pain in a limb, poor nutritional management, and a genetic predisposition for rapid growth. Chronic pain in a limb results in decreased weight-bearing on the limb and is accompanied by flexor muscle contraction. The result is an altered joint angle. The pain can be the result of physitis, osteochondritis dissecans (OCD) (*see* below), **septic** (caused by an infectious agent) arthritis, soft-tissue wounds, or hoof infections.

Poor nutritional management may also influ-

ence the development of flexural deformities. Both overfeeding and poorly balanced rations have been implicated, for reasons similar to those described for physitis. One possible explanation may be that the acquired flexural deformity is secondary to rapid bone growth, with failure of the flexor tendons and ligaments to develop at the same rate as bone lengthening.

Clinically, there are two distinct forms of acquired flexural deformities:

- Flexural deformity of the coffin joint, resulting in a raised heel (commonly called *club foot*)
- Flexural deformity of the fetlock, with normal hoof-wall alignment.

Horses with disease involving the fetlock joint frequently knuckle over at the fetlock and exhibit a very upright fetlock-joint angle. Flexural deformities of the coffin joint occur most commonly in foals and weanlings, while fetlock deformities typically occur in 1- to 2-year-old horses.

Treatment is dependent on the severity of the disorder. Conservative methods of treatment such as dietary changes, exercise, and hoof-trimming are often effective in mild or early cases. Dietary changes should be designed to reduce feed intake in order to slow growth and minimize obesity. Concurrent with dietary management, affected horses should be exercised and anti-inflammatory medication administered if it is considered necessary.

Horses with coffin joint deformities should have their heels trimmed so that tension is placed on the flexor tendons to help stretch them. Use of corrective trimming for fetlock deformities is more controversial, although raising of the heels does appear to produce a positive clinical response.

Surgical intervention is indicated in cases that prove unresponsive to conservative therapy.

RUPTURE OF THE COMMON DIGITAL EXTENSOR TENDON

Rupture of the *common digital extensor tendon* is generally present at birth or develops soon after. The characteristic feature of this problem is the presence of a swelling over the front of the carpus. Affected foals often have an accompanying carpal flexural deformity, although fetlock angles are usually normal. Frequently the ruptured extensor tendon is not recognized, the horse being presented to the veterinarian for flexural deformity of the carpus instead.

Treatment depends on the severity of the disease. In foals without contraction of the tendon, stall rest is indicated. If the foal has a flexural deformity of the carpus or fetlock, PVC splints should be used (as described above). The prognosis for rupture of the common digital extensor tendon, if unaccompanied by flexural contraction, is good to excellent for soundness, although a small bump may always be present over the front of the limb. When flexural deformity of the carpus or fetlock is also present, the prognosis for soundness is fair to guarded.

PHYSEAL INJURIES

Injury to the growth plate or physis is a common occurrence in foals. When a severe force is applied to a joint, a growth-plate injury is likely to occur because the cartilage-containing portion of the growth plate is weaker than the bone. Thus a traumatic incident that would cause a fracture in an adult horse might result in a growth-plate injury in a foal. In fact, approximately 20 percent of all injuries to the bones of foals involve the physis. Physeal injuries are frequently categorized according to whether or not they involve the articular surface of the joint, and whether the fracture courses through the metaphysis of the bone.

Treatment involves stabilization of the injured joint through cast immobilization, bandaging, or **internal fixation** (setting of a fracture through surgical intervention) with plates or screws. Often physeal injuries occur in very young horses, and the affected limb can be adequately stabilized with a cast for 3 to 4 weeks. The injured limb is stabilized for as short a period of time as possible in order to avoid cast sores and weakening of the flexor tendons, and because the growth plate heals rapidly in young individuals.

The prognosis for horses with physeal injuries ranges from guarded to good and is dependent on the severity of the injury and the degree of trauma to the growth plate. Growth cessation of a portion or all of the growth plate will result in permanent limb deformity and chronic lameness. It is important, therefore, that these injuries be identified and treated as soon as possible after they occur.

INFECTIOUS ARTHRITIS/PHYSITIS

Infectious arthritis is a term describing bacterial infection of one or more joints. In foals this condition arises secondary to spread of bacteria from the umbilical cord into the bloodstream or because of inadequate transfer of immunity (**antibodies**) from the mare to the foal in the **colostrum** (first milk). Successful transfer of immunity requires adequate production of colostrum by the mare and ingestion of the colostrum by the foal within its first 24 hours of life. Without colostrum the foal is unable to fight off many important infectious disease agents. (*See* CHAPTER 29, "THE IMMUNE SYSTEM AND VARIOUS DISORDERS.") **Systemic** (bodywide) bacterial infection of the lungs, joints, and abdomen are frequent complications of inadequate delivery of colostrum.

In foals with infection derived from the bloodstream, the arthritis characteristically involves many joints. The joints most commonly affected are the hock, stifle, carpus, and fetlock. Clinical signs include fever, lameness on one or more limbs, and swelling and heat around the involved joint(s). Diagnosis is based on the history and clinical signs, sampling of the affected joint(s) for laboratory examination and bacterial culture, and X-ray evaluation. X rays are often helpful for grading the severity of the disease. In addition, X rays may be able to identify extension of the infection into the adjacent bone or growth plate.

Treatment involves elimination of the causative bacteria through the use of appropriate antibiotics. Removal of infected joint fluid and flushing of the joints with a balanced salt solution will aid in removing harmful enzymes that can further damage the articular cartilage of the joint. If the foal did not receive adequate colostrum from the mare, the administration of **plasma** (the fluid portion of blood) will provide needed antibodies.

In general the prognosis for recovery is guarded. It is imperative that foals be treated immediately after clinical signs develop. If the infection is allowed to progress without therapy, the causative organisms will invade the cartilage and bone around the joint, causing secondary complications. It is important to emphasize that even when the problem has apparently resolved, horses should be given a prolonged period of rest before exercise is begun in order to restore the affected joints to normalcy.

OSTEOCHONDROSIS

Osteochondrosis refers to a disorder of growing cartilage that may affect either the growth plate or the articular cartilage. Progressive breakdown of the cartilage can lead to the development of **osteochondritis dissecans (OCD)** or **subchondral bone cysts.** Osteochondritis dissecans is characterized by the presence of large flaps of cartilage or loose cartilaginous bodies within the joint, most frequently the tarsus, stifle, or shoulder joint. Subchondral bone cysts may occur in any bone, but most often are found in the lower end of the femur, within the stifle joint. The causes of OCD and subchondral bone cysts in horses are unknown, but are probably similar to the nutritional factors that result in physitis.

In OCD, lameness and distension of the affected joint usually develop between 6 months and 2 years of age. While some horses will be visibly affected before 1 year of age, others will not exhibit clinical signs until they are placed in heavy training. X-ray studies typically reveal separation of one or many fragments from the affected joint surface. Horses usually develop subchondral bone cysts within this same timeframe, although there are many cases that do not become evident until the horse is 3 to 5 years of age. Horses with subchondral bone cysts often present with only mild lameness and not the joint swelling seen in OCD. This may account for the older average age at presentation for subchondral bone cysts, as compared to that for OCD. X-ray studies of subchondral bone cysts usually reveals cystlike lesions beneath the articular cartilage of affected joints. These cysts may be as small as a few millimeters in diameter,

or as large as 3 to 4 centimeters in diameter.

Treatment of OCD involves **arthroscopic surgery** (surgery using a tubular instrument [**arthroscope**] for examining and carrying out surgical procedures within the joint, without the need for an extensive incision). Following surgery, horses with OCD of the stifle and tarsus have a good to excellent prognosis for return to soundness as performance horses. Horses with OCD of the shoulder joint, however, have a poor to guarded prognosis for athletic soundness.

Treatment of subchondral bone cysts remains a controversial matter. Some authorities have advocated conservative treatment in the form of stall rest or mild exercise. Horses with small cysts have a better prognosis for return to soundness with conservative treatment than do horses with larger cysts. For those individuals not responding to conservative treatment, surgical methods for removing the cyst contents have been described, with modest success reported for lesions affecting the lower end of the femur. Subchondral cysts involving the radius and metacarpus have a more guarded prognosis.

INCOMPLETE OSSIFICATION OF THE CARPAL OR TARSAL BONES

Incomplete **ossification** (bone formation) of the carpal or tarsal bones is manifested by an angular deformity of the carpus or a flexural deformity of the tarsus. The underdeveloped bones become deformed because they are weaker than normally ossified bones. Typically, carpal and tarsal bones assume their normal mature shape within the first 30 days of life, during which time they become fully ossified. In horses born prematurely or those exhibiting incomplete ossification for unknown reasons, ossification may not occur for many months. This predisposes the underdeveloped bones to injury, deformation, and the resultant angular or flexural deformity.

Foals with incomplete ossification of the carpal bones typically present with an angular deformity that has been present since birth or that developed soon after birth. X rays usually reveal one or more small or misshapen carpal bones. With collapse of the tarsal bones, there is increased flexion of the hock ("sickle-hocked"), with accompanying pain and swelling.

Treatment is dependent on the severity and stage of the condition. If treated early, prior to the onset of arthritis, horses with carpal bone collapse may respond to straightening of the limb, followed by placement of a tube-cast to prevent further deformity. The cast usually is changed every 1 to 2 weeks, for a period of 3 to 4 weeks. At this time, ossification of the affected carpal bones should have occurred.

For foals with tarsal bone collapse, tube-casting may be beneficial if the lesion is diagnosed within the first 2 to 4 weeks of life. In horses that are not treated and allowed to develop chronic angular or flexural deformities, the prognosis is poor to guarded for long-term soundness.

Hereditary Multiple Exostosis

Hereditary multiple exostosis is characterized by the development of numerous small projections along the bones, resulting in an abnormal bony contour. The condition affects the ribs, pelvis, and extremities. As the name implies, this is an hereditary condition and affects approximately 50 percent of an individual's progeny. The characteristic swellings of this disorder are usually present at birth and are probably initiated during fetal development within the uterus. They are frequently similar in each limb and are firmly attached to the bone. Lameness associated with the condition is usually mild and is caused by impingement of the bony projections on various tendons and muscles. Diagnosis is based on the history and typical clinical signs. There is no known treatment. Affected individuals should not be bred in order to avoid propagating the defect.

Musculoskeletal Disorders of Horses of Any Age

Osteitis, Osteomyelitis, and Sequestrum

Osteitis and *osteomyelitis* are terms used to describe inflammatory conditions of bone. Osteitis occurs in the lower extremities, with the cannon bone affected most often (probably because it is only poorly protected by overlying soft tissue). Osteitis is frequently seen secondary to trauma, a kick being the most common cause. Bacteria enter through the broken skin and set up a localized infection of the bone. Often the blood supply to the outer surface of the bone is disrupted, causing a small dead piece of bone (a **sequestrum**) to form. Typically the wound will continue to drain until the dead piece of bone is removed. X-ray studies are helpful in diagnosing sequestrum formation.

Treatment of osteitis involves removal of any infected or dead bone and **lavage** (irrigation, washing out) of the surrounding soft tissue. If the limb is not swollen and there is no evidence of systemic infection, antibiotics are often not necessary. Protective bandaging of the affected site will limit further contamination and trauma.

Osteomyelitis begins within the inner medullary cavity of the bone and results from bacterial contamination of open fractures, penetrating wounds, or internal fixation devices such as screws and plates. Osteomyelitis in general is a much more serious condition than osteitis. Often the blood supply to a major portion of bone has been affected, allowing bacteria to grow within the dead tissue inside the bone. Clinical signs include increased lameness on the affected limb, swelling of the skin over the bone, and fever. If osteomyelitis is suspected, X rays and bacterial cultures will help confirm the diagnosis.

Treatment of osteomyelitis includes drainage of the infected material, administration of antibiotics and an appropriate anti-inflammatory medication, and removal of any infected or dead tissue. The prognosis for recovery is guarded to poor, depending on the bone involved and the organism causing the infection.

Bran Disease (Osteodystrophia Fibrosa)

Bran disease is a generalized disorder caused primarily by a deficiency of calcium in the diet in the face of a phosphorus excess. Although common in the past, bran disease is rare today owing to improved feeding practices. It occurs in horses that are fed predominantly cereal and cereal byproducts such as bran. It may also occur in horses that are fed high-grain or grain-only diets. The cause of the disorder is defective mineralization of bone secondary to low calcium levels in the blood. The "classic" clinical signs include enlargement of the lower jaw and facial bones. The teeth may also eventually loosen secondary to bone resorption. If bran disease is suspected, an analysis of the feed should be performed and the calcium/phosphorus ratio corrected through calcium supplementation.

FRACTURES

Fractures are probably the most common bone disorder in horses. Generally, fractures cause lameness and swelling of the affected limb. Diagnosis is based on **palpation** (feeling with the hands) of the limb and X-ray studies of the affected bone.

There is a popular misconception among the general public that fractures in horses cannot be treated. In reality, most fractures in foals and many of the fractures in adult horses can be treated quite successfully, depending on the fracture configuration and joint involvement, with horses returning to full performance or to breeding. Successful treatment results rely on:

- Early diagnosis of the fracture
- Successful prevention of secondary infection
- Adequate stabilization of the fracture
- Successful maintenance of stabilization until the broken bone heals

Factors that improve the prognosis include the age of the horse (younger horses have a better prognosis), lack of infection and/or joint involvement, and attitude (quiet horses have a better prognosis than excitable horses). Specific fractures and their individual prognoses will be discussed in detail in the sections that follow.

Joint Disorders

Joint disorders can be detected and evaluated by a number of means, including clinical examination for pain and gross physical changes of the joint, measurement of skin temperature, X-ray studies, **arthroscopy** (inspection of the joint using an arthroscope), and analysis of joint fluid. Horses with joint disorders typically exhibit one or more of the following clinical signs:

- Joint swelling or enlargement
- Pain upon joint **flexion** (bending)

- Localized or diffuse tenderness around the joint
- Changes in skin temperature or color
- Decreased motion and/or **crepitus** (sensation or sound of grating or scraping) during motion
- Joint deformity

BOG SPAVIN AND ARTICULAR WINDPUFFS

Bog spavin of the hock and *windpuffs* of the fetlock are chronic swellings of the affected joints. The cause is unknown. The swellings are not associated with lameness, tenderness, heat, or tissue changes observable on X rays. Horses with bog spavin have a chronic, low-grade **synovitis** (inflammation of the joint capsule), with minimal changes in joint fluid. Bog spavin is most often seen in horses with faulty tarsal conformation (straight hocks, sickle-hocked, cowhocked), suggesting that abnormal stresses on the tissues around the joint cause the disorder. Other causes include lameness of the opposite limb, heavy training, and poor shoeing.

Windpuffs often occur in horses with straight fetlocks that are under a heavy training schedule.

Diagnosis of these two conditions is based on observation of the typical swelling and ruling out of other potential causes. The best treatment often is to do nothing. In young horses with one or more involved joints, the condition may disappear as the horse matures. In persistent cases of bog spavin, drainage of the joint combined with administration of anti-inflammatory medication may reduce the distention. Irradiation of the affected joint has also been used successfully. For horses with windpuffs, treatment is generally limited to the application of pressure bandages. The prognosis for bog spavin and windpuffs is guarded. Since affected horses are not lame, however, both conditions can be thought of as cosmetic blemishes rather than as limiting factors for performance.

TRAUMATIC SYNOVITIS

Synovitis (inflammation of the lining membrane of a joint) may occur following trauma to a joint. Although the problem can occur in any joint, the most common ones affected are the carpal and fetlock joints of young racehorses. Repeated trauma to these joints rather than a single traumatic episode is the cause of this condition.

With acute synovitis of the carpus, horses tend to hold their limbs in slight flexion in the standing position. In chronic cases, lameness may only be evident at fast gaits. A hard, thickened swelling over the front of the carpus may also be present. X-ray studies of the carpus reveal bone production on the front of the carpal bones, resulting from joint capsule tearing at the attachments to these bones.

With synovitis of the fetlock joint, the horse moves with a choppy gait if both front limbs are affected. Pain, heat, and swelling may be present in the affected limbs. Swelling is most prominent on the front of the fetlock and may extend approximately half the way around the joint.

The diagnosis of these conditions is based on the history and clinical signs. X rays of the affected joints must be performed to eliminate other possible causes of synovitis within a joint, such as a fracture. Analysis of joint fluid is useful for determining the degree of inflammation within the joint, and to evaluate the potential response of the joint to therapy.

Treatment depends on the severity of the condition and the number of joints involved. Rest is helpful in resolving the acute inflammatory phase of the disorder. Bandage support may also assist in healing. Prolonged immobilization is probably not indicated, since it may lead to muscle wasting and cartilage degeneration. Physical therapy in the form of **hydrotherapy** (treatment involving the use of water, externally applied) may be useful immediately after the injury. Cold hydrotherapy is indicated in the first 24 to 48 hours after a joint injury to limit the inflammatory process within the joint. As the synovitis becomes chronic, warm hydrotherapy may be employed to relieve pain. If available, swimming helps maintain a horse's cardiovascular condition and joint and muscle tone. Other forms of therapy include:

- Flushing the affected joints with a balanced salt solution
- Application of dimethylsulfoxide (DMSO) onto the skin over the joints

- Administration of anti-inflammatory agents systematically or other medications into the joints

All of these treatments are aimed at reducing the inflammation within the joint and normalizing both joint fluid and cartilage properties.

SPRAINS AND LUXATIONS

A **sprain** is defined as a stretching or tearing of the ligaments supporting a joint. In simple sprains there is only minimal disruption of the ligamentous fibers following injury, with little if any joint swelling. With severe sprains there may be total disruption of the ligaments with distension and instability of the joint. For mild sprains rest and a support bandage are the appropriate therapy. If the sprain is more severe, and particularly if the ligamentous structures within the joint have been disrupted, surgical intervention may be necessary to repair the damage.

Luxation (dislocation) of a joint may be classified as either **complete** or **partial**. Luxations usually are associated with severe sprains as well as damage to other surrounding joint structures. Complete luxations most commonly occur in the pastern, fetlock, and hock joints. Depending upon the severity of the luxation, various treatments have been proposed. For mild **subluxation** (partial dislocation), a heavy support bandage or cast may be sufficient to allow healing of the joint. For more severe luxations with complete disruption of ligamentous and joint capsule structures, surgical intervention may be required, followed by the application of a cast postsurgically.

The prognosis is dependent upon the severity of the condition and the joint involved. For joints with limited motion, such as the lower joints of the hock, treatment may result in the return of complete soundness. By contrast, in high-motion joints such as the fetlock, even mild arthritis secondary to a sprain or luxation may cause permanent lameness.

INTRA-ARTICULAR (JOINT) FRACTURES

Joint fractures can occur in any joint in the horse, although the carpus and fetlock are more frequently affected. These injuries are most common in racehorses and are the result of repeated trauma to the joint. Intra-articular fractures produce clinical signs that are identical to those of traumatic synovitis (*see* above). Swelling, heat, and pain are usually present. The fracture itself usually cannot be felt through the skin; a definitive diagnosis must rely on X-ray studies.

Treatment is dependent on the joint involved, the size and nature of the fracture, and the intended use of the horse after surgery. For small intra-articular fractures, arthroscopy is the treatment of choice for removing the fractured fragment and evaluating the joint. For larger fractures, reduction of the fragment into its original position and stabilization with a screw is indicated. Conservative therapy usually results in moderate to severe degenerative arthritis in the affected joint. Thus horses may be useful for breeding after conservative therapy, but will probably not return to performance.

The prognosis for small joint fractures that are treated by arthroscopy is dependent on the joint involved and the severity of the damage. In mild cases horses can be expected to return to full performance. In severe cases with multiple fragments and degenerative changes in the joint cartilage, horses may remain lame following surgery. Generally horses do return to performance following removal of small intra-articular fragments, although possibly at a lower level of performance than before the injury.

DEGENERATIVE JOINT DISEASE

Degenerative joint disease or *degenerative arthritis* represents a group of disorders resulting in progressive deterioration of the articular cartilage of a joint, accompanied by bone proliferation around the joint margins and thickening of the soft tissues of the joint. Degenerative joint disease can occur secondary to any of the previously discussed conditions causing trauma to a joint, including intra-articular fractures, luxations, infectious arthritis, OCD, and wounds. Degenerative arthritis can also develop as a complication of repeated, low-grade trauma as might occur in a performance horse that has competed for a number of years.

The essential component of degenerative joint disease is destruction of the articular cartilage. Characteristically the cartilage loses its normal resiliency and becomes soft and yellow. Thinning and wearing of the cartilage progress gradually over time, resulting eventually in overt exposure of regions of underlying bone. Affected joints become less flexible owing to pain, joint capsule thickening, and the production of new bone around the joint.

Treatment is dependent upon the severity of the disease. For horses with only minimal signs, mild to moderate exercise may be all that is needed to maintain muscular condition, thereby cushioning the joints and limiting the pain. With more severe arthritis, treatment can be divided into three distinct areas:

- Treatment or prevention of the primary cause of the arthritis. In cases of intra-articular fractures, OCD, or infectious arthritis, proper treatment of these conditions should be instituted
- Resolution of the soft-tissue inflammation causing articular cartilage degeneration. Therapy includes rest, anti-inflammatory medication, physical therapy, joint flushing, and surgical removal of synovial tissue
- Treatment or prevention of cartilage degeneration. This may include surgical removal of affected or traumatized cartilage and bony protuberances around the joint

The prognosis for horses with degenerative joint disease is dependent on the joint or joints involved and on the severity of the condition. In low-motion joints such as the lower joints of the hock, mild to moderate degenerative joint disease may not limit performance. By contrast, moderate to severe degenerative joint disease may result in chronic and persistent lameness in high-motion joints such as the carpus, fetlock, the upper hock joint, shoulder, and stifle. Thus every effort should be made to limit progression of the degenerative changes in the early stages of the disease.

Muscle Disorders

Muscle tissue may respond to injury in a number of ways:

- It may degenerate
- It may regenerate following degeneration, so long as the supporting structures around the muscle remain intact
- It may become inflamed
- It may **atrophy** (shrink or become wasted) because of poor nutrition, lack of usage, or lack of nerve supply secondary to nerve damage
- It may **ossify** (develop bone within it) or **calcify** (develop calcium deposits) because of degeneration or inflammation

MYOSITIS

The term **myositis** is used to describe inflammation of muscle tissue. There are many causes of myositis, including trauma and infection. Horses with myositis typically demonstrate pain upon palpation of the affected muscle. The muscle itself is usually swollen and firm. Fever may be an accompanying feature. The degree of lameness evident will be dependent on the muscle involved. Horses with **clostridial myositis** caused by bacteria of the genus *Clostridium* tend to be severely lame (*see* CHAPTER 31, "BACTERIAL DISEASES.")

One of the most common causes of clostridial myositis is the intramuscular injection of anti-inflammatory medication or vitamin preparations. The use of aseptic practices and proper preparation of the skin prior to injection will limit the incidence of clostridial contamination of injection sites. If a horse develops a swelling over an injection site, a veterinarian should be called immediately to evaluate the lesion and institute appropriate treatment if necessary.

PHYSICAL TRAUMA TO MUSCLE

Lacerations (tears in the skin and underlying muscle) occur commonly in horses and are usually secondary to wire cuts, kicks, or encounters with automobiles. Following injury, the wound should be thoroughly cleansed and any dead or infected tissue removed. If possible, the wound should be closed to limit further bacterial contamination. Often the lower edge of the wound is left open to drain (sometimes a plastic drain may be placed within the wound to augment seepage). In some cases a laceration may be bandaged to limit and reduce swelling and to protect the site. Horses should be stall-rested with only mild exercise until the wound has healed.

Muscle ruptures (**hernias**) or tears represent another common problem in horses. Such injuries are usually caused by overexertion or the violent contraction of a muscle. Violent contractions can produce an injury wherein the body of the affected muscle herniates through the **fascia** (sheath of connective tissue) that encloses it. If the muscle has not been completely disrupted, such tears or ruptures will normally fill with scar tissue, which may ossify as the muscle heals. The prognosis for future soundness is fair to good so long as the muscle or tendon has not been severed.

EXERTIONAL MYOPATHIES

Exertional myopathies (muscle diseases caused by exertion) are seen most frequently in performance horses. These disorders are usually the result of exercise following a period of inactivity during which the horse was maintained on a full ration high in carbohydrate (i.e., grain). A similar condition is seen in unfit horses that have received inadequate conditioning for the exercise attempted. This latter problem is also seen occasionally in endurance athletes. Nervous or excitable horses and heavily muscled horses may on occasion develop exertional myopathy.

The myopathies can be divided into three broad categories:

Azoturia

This may occur in the more severe forms of the disorder. **Azoturia** (presence of excessive quantities of nitrogen waste products in the urine) is caused by the excessive breakdown of muscle tissue, which sends large amounts of nitrogen waste to the kidneys for elimination in the urine. It is seen in heavier breeds and occurs shortly after the horse is put to work. Profuse sweating, increased heart and respiratory rates, fever, muscle stiffness, and muscle spasms are the most common clinical signs. Often it is difficult to distinguish azoturia from severe colic. Urine color will vary from a red-brown to black, depending upon the degree of muscle breakdown.

Kidney failure may develop if proper treatment is not instituted.

"Tying-Up"

This is a mild form of azoturia. Affected horses may or may not have discolored urine. The condition commonly occurs at the start of, or when the horse has cooled down after, vigorous exercise. The muscles are hard on palpation and the horse is often reluctant to move.

Endurance-Related Myopathy

This disease is similar to tying-up, but occurs in adequately conditioned horses that have been ridden for long distances (e.g., endurance events, long trail rides). Affected horses may be severely dehydrated with salt and water imbalances in the blood.

Treatment of horses with exertional myopathies is primarily supportive. Affected animals should not be allowed to exercise after exhibiting clinical signs. Tranquilizers are frequently administered to relieve the horse's anxiety. Tranquilizers may also increase blood flow to the muscles. Aggressive intravenous fluid therapy is indicated in severe cases, particularly if the horse has discolored urine. Fluid therapy will alleviate dehydration and metabolic imbalances, maintain urine output, and help prevent kidney failure. Anti-inflammatory medication may be useful for limiting inflammation and pain. In severe cases, muscle relaxants may be indicated.

The prognosis is good to excellent for return to performance in the less severe cases. Severe and recurring cases of azoturia have a more guarded prognosis. Some horses appear susceptible to the condition. For horses that have not been conditioned appropriately, improved conditioning will reduce the possibility of a recurrence. For horses that frequently tie-up, feed and exercise management is indicated.

GENERALIZED MYOPATHIES SECONDARY TO PROLONGED RECUMBENCY

Local or generalized myopathy may occur in horses following an extended period of recumbency. This most often occurs in horses that have been under general anesthesia for more than 2 or 3 hours or that have been positioned on hard surfaces during surgery. It can also be seen in animals that have experienced low blood pressure during anesthesia. The myopathy is thought to be caused by decreased blood flow to the affected muscles during the time the horse is immobilized. Typically horses recover from anesthesia without complication, then very shortly thereafter become agitated and unable to bear weight on the affected limb. The muscles become hard and swollen, and the horse usually resents manipulation of the limb.

Treatment of this condition is similar to that for exertional myopathy. Mild cases involving isolated muscles may only require temporary supervision or observation. Horses with more generalized disease or lameness may require anti-inflammatory medication and intravenous administration of a balanced salt solution. Prevention is centered around maintaining adequate blood pressure during anesthesia, limiting total surgery time, and providing adequate padding for the horse.

The prognosis is good to excellent for horses with only localized swelling, but guarded for horses with generalized myopathy. Many horses with generalized myopathy cannot rise despite intensive nursing care and may ultimately develop kidney or heart failure.

Tendon Disorders

A tendon is a dense band of fibrous connective tissue that attaches muscle to bone. Tendons possess great strength and are designed to transmit the muscle forces to the bone that cause motion of the limb. In general tendons possess a good blood supply at their muscle origin, but it decreases through the body of the tendon. The result is a relatively poor ability for the middle portion of a tendon to heal without significant scarring.

TENDINITIS

Tendinitis (inflammation of a tendon or tendon muscle attachment) is a frequent occurrence in horses, secondary to either exercise or trauma. The most frequent tendon affected by tendinitis is the *superficial digital flexor tendon* in racing

Thoroughbreds and Quarter Horses. The tendinitis is usually caused by repeated forces placed on the tendon. It occurs most frequently in the mid-portion of the tendon over the central region of the third metacarpus. Predisposing causes for tendinitis in the superficial digital flexor tendon include:

- Inadequate training and muscle fatigue at the end of a race
- Abnormal angulation of the fetlock, secondary to either muscle weakness or poor conformation
- Uneven or slippery track surfaces, which cause excessive loading of a limb
- Long toes, which may place extra stresses on the tendon
- Muddy tracks, which may increase the workload on the tendon

The degree of tendinitis can range from a mild condition that is not detectable clinically, to complete rupture of the tendon. Typically horses with acute tendinitis demonstrate pain on the affected limb and have evidence of swelling, heat, and tenderness upon palpation of the inflamed tendon (**bowed tendon**). **Ultrasonography** (diagnostic ultrasound; noninvasive technique for visualizing internal structures of the body by means of sound [echo] reflections) is useful for diagnosing this condition, as well as for determining the prognosis.

Initial therapy includes cold hydrotherapy, ice packs, support bandaging, and anti-inflammatory medication. These treatments are designed to minimize the heat, pain, and swelling associated with the condition. Horses should not be placed back in performance until all available evidence indicates that the inflamed tendon has healed. Unfortunately an affected tendon never regains the strength it had initially. Horses may also be predisposed to recurrence of the condition.

Horses with only mild swelling within the tendon tissue and no evidence of blood clots or holes in the tendon have a fairly good prognosis for return to performance. By contrast, horses with large **cavitary lesions** (holes) within the tendon have a poor prognosis.

TENOSYNOVITIS

Tenosynovitis is a term describing inflammation of the lining membrane that surrounds the tendon sheath, resulting in swelling of the sheath. Tenosynovitis can be divided into four distinct categories:

Idiopathic Tenosynovitis

Idiopathic tenosynovitis is defined as tenosynovitis with swelling of the tendon sheath in the absence of pain, inflammation, or lameness. As implied by the term **idiopathic,** the cause of the condition is unknown, although low-grade trauma is felt to be the inciting factor in many cases. Poor conformation may be the underlying cause leading to trauma in many horses. Diagnosis is based on the history and physical examination. The fluid within the tendon sheath is generally normal, although it may be somewhat thin. Infectious and traumatic causes of tenosynovitis must be ruled out in order to arrive at a diagnosis of idiopathic tenosynovitis.

Idiopathic tenosynovitis is a cosmetic blemish and does not warrant treatment.

Acute Tenosynovitis

Acute tenosynovitis is a rapidly developing swelling accompanied by heat, pain, and some degree of lameness. Acute tenosynovitis is usually the result of trauma, either from overwork or a more direct cause such as a fall or kick. Diagnosis is based on the history and physical examination, with a finding of heat and pain together with tendon sheath swelling. Treatment includes the application of ice, cold hydrotherapy, and rest. Support bandages will also assist in elimination of the fluid. The prognosis for recovery is good to excellent, so long as therapy is instituted immediately after an injury. If the horse is not treated appropriately and continues to be exercised, chronic tenosynovitis may be the result.

Chronic Tenosynovitis

Chronic tenosynovitis is a persistent swelling of the tendon sheath, with an associated thickening of the sheath. The condition is often accompanied by **stricture** (narrowing, contraction) of the tendon sheath and by **adhesions** (fusion or sticking together of surfaces), both of which limit tendon motion and cause pain. Chronic tenosynovitis often occurs secondary to an acute tenosynovitis that has not been resolved satisfactorily. Diagnosis is based on the history and physical examination. In all cases, chronic tenosynovitis is accompanied by lameness and decreased function of the affected limb. Chronic tenosynovitis is best treated by removal of the fluid and administration of anti-inflammatory medication. If a horse does not respond to this treatment, radiation therapy may be indicated. For completely unresponsive cases, surgical exploration of the tendon sheath may reveal an underlying cause of the persistent swelling.

Infectious Tenosynovitis

Infectious tenosynovitis is characterized by tendon-sheath swelling, heat, pain, severe lameness, fever, and infection within the tendon sheath. Infectious tenosynovitis can result from direct trauma or be secondary to spread of microorganisms through the bloodstream, as was described for infectious arthritis in foals. The septic process may rapidly cause the formation of adhesions limiting tendon motion within the sheath and result in destruction of the tendon. Diagnosis is based on the history, physical examination, and analysis of the fluid within the tendon sheath. The principles of treatment are similar to those described for the treatment of infectious arthritis. The prognosis is poor to guarded unless the horse responds quickly after the initiation of therapy.

TENDON SHEATH LACERATION

Management for tendon sheath lacerations is identical to that for tendon lacerations. The sheath should be flushed with large quantities of a balanced salt solution and the sheath **sutured** (stitched together). Often, the application of a cast for 2 or 3 weeks after surgery will be helpful in limiting motion and preventing breakdown of the suture site. Antibiotics and anti-inflammatory medication are indicated to prevent infectious tenosynovitis from developing and to limit the formation of adhesions within the tendon sheath. The prognosis is good to excellent if the horse responds to treatment and does not develop infectious tenosynovitis. In contrast, horses that develop a secondary infectious tenosynovitis have a poor to guarded prognosis.

TENDON LUXATION

Dislocation of the superficial digital flexor tendon of the hindlimb is a periodic occurrence in horses. The luxation is often secondary to direct trauma over the point of the hock. Physical examination usually reveals excessive side-to-side motion of the tendon and flexion of the hock joint. Surgical management is required to treat the condition. A long limb cast up to the stifle is usually applied for 3 to 4 weeks after surgery to allow for soft-tissue healing. The prognosis is good to excellent in horses responding to surgical management.

TRAUMATIC TENDON RUPTURE

Spontaneous tendon rupture caused by trauma usually occurs only if there has been previous infection or degeneration of the tendon. The tendons of the *peroneus tertius*, *gastrocnemius*, and superficial digital flexor muscles of the hindlimb are the most common tendons affected. (*See* CHAPTER 16, "ANATOMY.") The peroneus tertius runs along the front side of the hindlimb, causing the hock and stifle to flex simultaneously. The peroneus tertius may rupture when a horse is attempting to free a trapped hindlimb or following a traumatic injury. The gastrocnemius and superficial digital flexor tendons of the hindlimb on the back of the limb enable the horse to stand. Ruptures of these tendons may occur secondary to a fall with the hindlimbs flexed and underneath the body.

Diagnosis of peroneus tertius rupture is made by extending the hock and demonstrating that the stifle can be flexed at the same time. Normally when the hock is extended the peroneus tertius causes the stifle to extend. With gastrocnemius rupture, the hock is dropped so that there is excessive angulation of the hock joint. If the superficial digital flexor tendon is ruptured, the fetlock drops lower to the ground, and there is excessive angulation to the fetlock joint.

Horses with a ruptured peroneus tertius should be treated by stall rest for 4 to 6 weeks. Most cases have a good prognosis for return to soundness. In contrast, horses with ruptured gastrocnemius tendons or ruptured superficial digital flexor tendons have a much more guarded prognosis. An attempt may be made surgically to reconnect the tendon and stabilize the limb in a cast. Unfortunately, this treatment is often unsuccessful in achieving healing of the tendon.

Degenerative Rupture of Tendons

Tendons may rupture owing to any of a number of degenerative conditions including septic tendinitis, degeneration of the deep digital flexor tendon caused by *navicular disease* (*see* below), or as a complication to the repair of severed tendons. Rupture of the deep digital flexor tendon secondary to navicular disease is a relatively common condition in horses with severe navicular-bone changes. The condition occurs most frequently in horses that have had a **neurectomy** (severing of a nerve) to relieve the pain of navicular disease and that have then been worked. Unfortunately, alleviation of the pain allows the horse to place more force on the limb and on the degenerating navicular bone and deep digital flexor tendon. Both navicular bone-fracture and deep digital flexor-tendon rupture can occur in such cases.

Diagnosis of ruptured degenerative tendons is easily made upon palpation of the limb and evaluation of the horse's gait. In most circumstances treatment is unsuccessful, however. The prognosis is poor to guarded.

Severed Tendons

Owing to the lack of muscular covering in the distal limb of the horse, severed tendons are a common occurrence. Trauma—with wire cuts accounting for the majority of cases—is always the cause. The clinical signs depend on the tendon involved. For extensor tendons on the front side of the limb, horses may knuckle over or drag their toe (although they are often able to stand on the limb normally). By contrast, horses with severed flexor tendons are often unable to bear weight normally on the limb. There is usually excessive flexion of the fetlock, and the toe may turn up when weight is placed on the hoof.

Treatment is dependent on the degree of trauma delivered to the tendon, the length of time from injury to repair, and whether the tendon involved is an extensor tendon or a flexor tendon. With extensor tendons, the wound is cleaned, any infected or dead material is removed, and an attempt is made to suture the ends of the severed tendons. Cast application may be necessary for the first 4 to 6 weeks after injury to prevent knuckling over at the fetlock. Often stall rest is all that is necessary to achieve adequate healing of the tendon site. The prognosis is good to excellent for return to performance.

In marked contrast, horses with severed flexor tendons have a poor prognosis for soundness. Because of the large weight-bearing stresses that are placed on the flexor tendons, it is imperative that the tendon be immobilized by a cast following surgical repair.

It is important in all cases of severed tendons that the horse be evaluated and surgery performed very soon after the injury has occurred. Ideally, tendons should be sutured back together within 4 to 6 hours after injury. If a longer period of time passes, the tendon becomes contaminated with bacteria and successful repair (particularly in flexor tendon lacerations) becomes much more difficult.

Ligament Disorders

Ligaments are dense bands of fibrous connective tissue that attach bone to bone. Ligaments function to maintain normal joint alignment and allow normal joint motion. Ligaments have an even poorer blood supply than do tendons, and are notorious for their inability to heal well following traumatic injury.

Desmitis of the Suspensory Ligament

The *suspensory ligament* originates in the upper portion of the cannon bone and inserts on the **sesamoid bones.** Suspensory ligament **desmitis** (ligament inflammation) is seen most commonly in Standardbred racehorses. It occurs secondary to excessive stress placed on the ligament during training or racing. The condition can also be caused by direct trauma, or irritation secondary to a fracture.

Diagnosis is based on the history and physical examination. Ultrasonography may assist in determining the severity of the condition.

Treatment is identical to that described for tendinitis (*see* above). One additional form of therapy that has been successful in treating this condition is *ligament splitting*, which involves the making of small puncture holes in the suspensory ligament to increase its blood supply and help strengthen the ligament.

The prognosis for Standardbreds with suspensory ligament desmitis is fair for racing. Thoroughbreds with the condition have a poor prognosis for return to performance.

CURB

Curb describes inflammation and thickening of the *plantar ligament*, the ligament that courses along the back of the *calcaneus* bone in the hock. (*See* CHAPTER 16, "ANATOMY."). Horses with sickle-hocked or cow-hocked conformation are predisposed to the condition. Other causes of the condition include direct trauma, such as would occur by receiving a kick or as a result of a horse's kicking a solid structure.

Clinical signs associated include enlargement of the back side of the calcaneus, which in the acute stages may be accompanied by heat, swelling, and lameness. Horses tend to stand with the heel elevated when the affected limb is at rest. If acute cases are allowed to become chronic, new bone formation may occur on the back portion of the calcaneus as a result of the inflammation.

Treatment of acute cases of curb include the application of ice, cold hydrotherapy, and anti-inflammatory medication. Chronic cases are much more difficult to manage because of scarring at the site. The overall prognosis is good so long as the horse has normal hindlimb conformation and the curb is managed successfully as described. For horses with poor conformation and/or chronic cases of curb, a cosmetic defect will probably always be present. In horses with good hock conformation, chronic cases of curb usually are not associated with lameness.

RUPTURE OF THE SUSPENSORY APPARATUS

Rupture of the suspensory apparatus is a severe traumatic syndrome and is also known as a *breakdown injury*. Breakdown injuries occur due to the loss of one or more supporting structures of the fetlock. The condition occurs in racehorses and occasionally in jumping horses.

Diagnosis relies on the history and physical examination. Severe lameness, swelling, and an inability to bear weight on the affected limb are always associated with breakdown injuries. In addition, the fetlock sinks when weight is placed on the limb. Irreparable damage to the blood supply of the tissues around the fetlock may occur in conjunction with this condition. It is imperative that injured horses be placed *immediately* in a support brace even while still on the track. This will prevent further trauma to the blood and nerve supply and help protect the soft tissues around the site.

Treatment is based solely on salvage of the animal for breeding purposes. The treatment of choice is surgical fusion of the fetlock through the application of bone plates and screws. The prognosis for horses with breakdown injuries is poor to guarded even if surgical fusion of the fetlock is attempted.

DISTAL SESAMOIDIAN LIGAMENT DESMITIS

The *distal sesamoidian ligaments* serve an important function in limb support. Inflammation of these ligaments can occur due to a sprain or secondary to fractures. The clinical picture is one of acute lameness. Often there is a mild swelling on the back of the pastern. As the condition becomes chronic, bone proliferation may occur at the site and be visible on X rays.

Ice, cold hydrotherapy, bandage support, and rest are indicated for acute cases. If severe, casting for 2 to 3 weeks may minimize further trauma. Affected horses should be slowly returned to work after 6 to 8 weeks of stall rest. The administration of anti-inflammatory medication may be helpful in reducing swelling and pain. As is the case for any ligament disorder, prolonged convalescence (sometimes as long as a year) may be required before the horse can return to performance. In severe cases with rupture of the distal sesamoidian ligaments, complete breakdown of the limb will occur. The prognosis for return to soundness is guarded because of the high incidence of recurrence of the condition.

Disorders of the Foot

LAMINITIS

Laminitis ("**founder**") is an inflammation of the **laminae** of the foot, which serve to attach the coffin bone to the hoof wall. Laminitis can be caused by any number of factors, including overeating (grain or lush green pasture), trauma, systemic infection, ingestion of cold water, and certain anti-inflammatory drug treatments.

Clinical signs are dependent on the severity of the disease. In mild cases, horses will alternately lift one or the other foot. Lameness may not be evident at a walk, but the horse will have a short stilted gait at a trot. As the condition becomes progressively more severe, horses will be more reluctant to move and will resist lifting a foot. Although laminitis most frequently affects the forefeet, all feet may be affected in horses whose laminitis is secondary to systemic disorders such as a uterine infection or diarrhea. Horses with laminitis are palpably hot over the hoof wall and **coronary band** (ring of vascular tissue along the upper edge of the hoof wall), with "bounding" pulses in the arteries supplying the feet. Owing to the painfulness of the condition, affected horses exhibit increased respiratory rates, trembling, and anxiety. Horses with laminitis affecting only the forefeet have a tendency to stand with the hindlimbs carried well up underneath the body.

Chronic laminitis is defined as laminitis of greater than 48 hours' duration, or laminitis of any duration in which the coffin bone has rotated within the hoof wall. As the coffin bone rotates, separation of the lamina at the toe may occur and result in what is called "seedy toe." Separation in this region may allow bacteria to invade the hoof wall. Horses with chronic laminitis typically have a "dished" hoof wall with visible rings across the front of the hoof.

Diagnosis of laminitis is easily made by a physical examination and X rays of the affected feet. X rays should be taken every 3 to 5 days during the acute stages of laminitis to determine if rotation of the coffin bone is occurring. *Acute laminitis is a medical emergency and treatment should be initiated immediately to prevent rotation of the coffin bone.*

Treatment is centered first around eliminating any obvious cause of the laminitis. For example, a horse with grain overload should have its stomach flushed to remove as much grain as possible, while a mare with a retained placenta or an infected uterus should be treated appropriately. Treatment of the laminitis itself often involves the administration of antibiotics and anti-inflammatory medications. Some advocate the use of one or more of the following additional drugs:

- Heparin, to prevent blood clotting in the affected area
- Phenoxybenzamine, to prevent constriction of the blood supply to the laminae of the feet
- Acepromazine, to keep the blood vessels supplying the laminae dilated

External support to take weight-bearing forces off the toe and help return blood flow from the foot to the limb is recommended in most cases. Placing a horse in soft sand in the acute stages of laminitis is also useful by providing good physiologic support for the sole. Grain should be eliminated from the diet, particularly in overweight ponies or horses.

Treatment of chronic laminitis involves preventing or eliminating any known causes of the laminitis, in addition to addressing coffin bone rotation. Infection within the hoof must be opened and drained. Attempts to return the coffin bone to its normal orientation through corrective trimming should be made slowly. Often, removal of the toe helps to minimize stress on the laminae and makes the horse more comfortable. In severe cases, cutting the deep digital flexor tendon may help prevent rotation and minimize stress. Horses should not be exercised, and owners should realize that the toe region of the hoof wall takes approximately *one year* to regrow. Even in cases that have apparently resolved, care should be taken during this time to prevent recurrence of the condition.

The prognosis for horses with laminitis is always guarded. If the source of the laminitis can be quickly eliminated and cannon-bone rotation does not occur, horses may ultimately return to their previous performance without complications. By contrast, horses with chronic laminitis tend to experience episodic recurrences of the condition, resulting in further rotation, disability, and pain. One of the best prognostic indicators for future soundness is the degree of coffin bone rotation that has occurred. Horses with less than 5° of rotation have a favorable prognosis, while horses with greater than 10° of rotation usually do not return to athletic performance.

NAVICULAR DISEASE

Navicular disease is one of the most common causes of intermittent forelimb lameness in the horse. Quarter Horses and Thoroughbreds, particularly geldings, seem to be at greatest risk. The condition occurs only rarely in ponies and Arabian horses. There appears to be an hereditary predisposition for navicular disease that most likely is related to upright conformation. Concussive effects on the foot also play an important role, since horses working on hard surfaces have a greater likelihood of developing navicular disease. Small feet in relation to body size, a condition that has been promoted by selective breeding programs in certain breeds, increases concussion of the navicular bone during work and thus predisposes to navicular disease. Improper trimming of the feet may increase the pressure of the deep digital flexor tendon across the navicular bone and thereby increase the forces across the navicular bone.

Horses with navicular disease exhibit intermittent lameness of one or both forefeet. The lameness is usually worse the day after heavy work. In mild cases, horses may respond to periods of rest by appearing sound, but as soon as they are returned to work lameness recurs. Both forefeet are almost always involved in navicular disease, although one foot may be more severely affected than the other. Horses with navicular disease tend to land on their toes to avoid concussion of the heel region. This gives a characteristic appearance of "walking on eggshells." They have a tendency to stumble as they attempt to land on their toes. When the horse is circled (moved in a circle), increased lameness of the inside limb becomes apparent. It is relatively common for horses with navicular disease to be presented for shoulder lameness because the shortened stride characteristic of navicular disease resembles the gait of horses with shoulder pain.

Diagnosis of navicular disease is based on the history and a thorough lameness examination. X-ray studies will confirm the diagnosis. Treatment is dependent largely on the severity of the clinical signs and the magnitude of the degenerative changes that have occurred within the navicular bone. Conservative approaches are most applicable to young horses having minimal changes as seen on X ray. In mild cases corrective shoeing and the administration of anti-inflammatory medication often result in prolonged improvement. As the severity of the disease increases, conservative methods of therapy become less successful in ameliorating a horse's pain. In the most severe cases of navicular disease, **neurectomy** (cutting of a nerve) of the nerves supplying sensation to the heels of the foot may be indicated. There are many potential complications of this surgical procedure, however, including **neuroma** (tumor arising from a nerve) formation, secondary rupture of the deep digital flexor tendon (as described in above in the section on degenerative tendon disorders), loss of the hoof wall, regeneration of the severed nerves, and incomplete desensitization of the heel. In horses with severe degenerative changes of the navicular bone, surgical intervention may not be a wise choice because these horses are predisposed to navicular bone fracture and deep digital flexor tendon rupture.

The prognosis for horses with navicular disease is guarded in all cases. It is difficult if not impossible to predict which horses will only slowly progress to disability and remain useful for a number of years, and which will exhibit such rapid progression that they become chronically lame at a young age.

NAVICULAR BONE FRACTURES

Navicular bone fractures occur rarely and usually are the result of navicular disease or trauma. Small **avulsion** (pulling or tearing away) fractures or chip fractures of the border of the navicular bone are most often associated with navicular disease. Such fractures have a poor prognosis for future soundness. There is no surgical treatment, and if the horse is persistently lame a neurectomy or retirement of the horse may be indicated. Simple longitudinal fractures of the navicular bone usually are the result of the horse's stepping on a sharp object. The condition may also occur in horses with severe navicular disease that have had a neurectomy performed on the affected limb.

The diagnosis of navicular bone fracture is difficult because of the number of lines crossing the navicular bone on a normal X ray. The fracture must be evident on more than one X-ray view to be certain that it is a real finding.

The navicular bone has only a poor capacity for healing after a fracture. Generally, both a **simple fracture** (one in which the bone is broken in two pieces) and a **comminuted fracture** (one in which the bone is crushed) of the navicular bone is treated by stall rest and the application of bar shoes. For some simple fractures, a single bone screw may be sufficient for stabilization. Nevertheless, many navicular bone fractures do not heal. A neurectomy may improve some horses sufficiently to allow them to return to work. The overall prognosis is poor to guarded.

SHEARED HEELS

Sheared heels describes breakdown of the tissue between the bulbs of the heel, caused by the hoof walls being out of balance. Sheared heels are the result of improper trimming and/or shoeing that leaves one heel longer than the other. This creates an abnormal shearing force between the heel bulbs, leading to structural breakdown of the tissue.

Diagnosis is made by physical examination. Palpation of the heel bulb region usually reveals a loss of structural integrity between the heel bulbs. The heel bulbs can be easily separated and displaced in opposite directions. Often horses resent this manipulation. Horses with sheared heels exhibit clinical signs similar to those seen in navicular disease. X rays should be taken to rule out any other bony abnormalities that could cause heel pain.

Treatment is aimed at balancing the foot. Corrective trimming and application of a bar

shoe are usually sufficient to alleviate the condition. The prognosis is good to excellent.

PEDAL OSTEITIS

Pedal osteitis refers to increased **vascularization** (formation of blood vessels) and **demineralization** (removal of bone) affecting the coffin bone, usually secondary to inflammation resulting from repeated, excessive concussion on the sole. Other conditions that can cause pedal osteitis include persistent corns, laminitis, puncture wounds, and navicular disease.

Diagnosis is made upon physical examination. Affected horses are lame at all gaits and very sore to hoof testers placed across the soles. X-ray studies of the feet reveal the demineralization and increased vascularization of the coffin bone. In addition the outer margin of the coffin bone is roughened.

Treatment is dependent upon the underlying cause. Shoeing with a full pad or rim pad may alleviate lameness in some horses. If pedal osteitis affects only the wings of the coffin bone, a neurectomy may improve the horse's gait. Ideally the underlying cause should be eliminated to optimize chances for recovery. The prognosis overall is poor to guarded, particularly if the disease is chronic and secondary to an incurable ailment such as navicular disease.

COFFIN BONE FRACTURES

Fractures of the coffin bone are rare and usually the result of exercise on hard tracks. Approximately 90 percent of these fractures occur in the forelimbs. Thoroughbred and Standardbred racehorses are most commonly affected. The fractures are thought to result from a twisting action as the foot lands on a hard surface. Affected horses are moderately to severely lame on the affected limb; some will not place the affected limb on the ground. X rays are necessary to confirm the diagnosis.

Treatment is aimed at immobilizing the fracture. Stabilization of the hoof with a full bar shoe and quarter clips will help achieve this. The foot should be managed in this fashion for 6 to 8 months, until there is evidence of fracture healing. The horse should not be worked for 8 to 12 months after the injury. For fractures through the center of the bone, screw fixation of the fracture has been described. Because the screw must be placed through a hole in the hoof wall, diligent efforts must be made to sanitize the hoof wall prior to the surgery. Infection is the most common complication of this procedure.

The prognosis for coffin bone fractures not involving the joint is good to excellent if sufficient stall rest is provided. Affected horses often must have a neurectomy performed on the affected side of the hoof wall to achieve soundness. Horses with central fractures of the coffin bone have a more guarded prognosis for soundness. Degenerative arthritis of the coffin joint is a frequent complication of these fractures.

EXTENSOR PROCESS FRACTURES OF THE COFFIN BONE

Fractures of the *extensor process* of the coffin bone most frequently occur in the forelimbs, affecting either one or both forefeet. The fractures are caused by excessive tension of the common digital extensor tendon at its attachment site on the coffin bone. Affected horses exhibit a variable degree of lameness, often only a shortened stride.

The diagnosis is confirmed using nerve blocks and X-ray studies. Treatment involves removal of the fracture fragment, or screw fixation of the fragment to the parent bone if the fragment is large enough. There have been reports of successful conservative management of affected horses, although only approximately one-third of cases managed in this way returned to soundness. The overall prognosis is poor to guarded, depending on the duration of the fracture and the size of the fragment(s). If degenerative arthritis sets in the prognosis becomes less favorable.

BUTTRESS FOOT

This disorder represents an advanced form of degenerative arthritis and is caused by new bone growth in the region of the extensor process of the coffin bone. The new bone formation may be secondary to a fracture of long duration, or inflammation over the surface of the bone caused by direct trauma. Horses with mild buttress foot exhibit variable degrees of lameness and have a tendency to point the affected

foot. They also may land heavily on their heels, which is in direct contrast to horses with navicular disease which land on their toes.

The diagnosis in advanced cases is not difficult, as the front of the coronary band can be seen bulging where the new bone formation has occurred. In milder cases the diagnosis may not be as readily apparent. There is no specific therapy. If the disorder is secondary to a fracture of the extensor process of the coffin bone, surgical removal of the fracture fragment may prove beneficial. Radiation therapy has been used to limit the production of new bone over the surface of the coffin joint. Neurectomy and corrective shoeing may limit some of the lameness. The prognosis is guarded to poor for long-term soundness.

PUNCTURE WOUNDS OF THE FOOT

Puncture wounds of the foot are a common occurrence in horses. In their simplest form, puncture wounds may penetrate only the sole and create a small sole **abscess** (walled-off lesion filled with pus). In its severest form, a puncture wound to the foot may penetrate the navicular **bursa** (a fluid-filled sac) and result in infectious **bursitis** (inflammation of a bursa), infectious arthritis of the coffin joint, and infectious tenosynovitis of the tendon sheath of the deep digital flexor tendon.

The clinical signs may range from no lameness at all to severe, non–weight-bearing lameness. Rarely the penetrating foreign body (such as a nail) is still in the foot, making the diagnosis relatively simple. More commonly the foreign body has dropped out of the foot and is no longer present. The horse's gait will reflect the location of the puncture wound, e.g., horses with puncture wounds in the toe will place more weight on the heel. If the puncture wound goes undiagnosed because the horse initially exhibited no lameness, an infection may develop in the foot which may then result in lameness.

The diagnosis is made by performing a thorough lameness examination. Treatment involves establishing drainage of the lesion, keeping the wound clean and protected until healing occurs, and preventing **tetanus** (*see* CHAPTER 31, "BACTERIAL DISEASES.")

The entire sole should be thoroughly cleaned and trimmed. Any dark areas should be explored. If a puncture wound is discovered, a sterile probe should be inserted into the site to determine the direction and depth of the puncture.

If the puncture is in the toe, removal of any separated sole and protection of the foot may be all that is necessary to achieve healing. If the wound has penetrated into the coffin bone, X-ray studies should be performed to determine the degree of bone destruction. Systemic antimicrobial agents are indicated if the coffin or navicular bones, navicular bursa, coffin joint, or deep digital flexor tendon sheath are infected. The infected tissue should be cultured for bacteria and the appropriate antibiotic selected based on antibiotic sensitivity testing. If the coffin joint is involved, a thorough flush of the coffin joint should be performed, usually with the horse under general anesthesia.

The prognosis is good to excellent if deeper structures of the foot are not involved. For horses with coffin bone infection, the prognosis is fair to good if drainage can be established and dead bone removed. For those that have developed an infection of the navicular bone or bursa, coffin joint, or tendon sheath of the deep digital flexor tendon, the prognosis for return to soundness is poor to guarded.

QUITTOR

Quittor is a chronic inflammatory process of the *collateral cartilage* of the coffin bone. The condition can be secondary to an abscess in the coronary band, or a penetrating wound to the sole that has become infected and gained access to the collateral cartilage. Diagnosis is made by physical examination. Affected horses exhibit swelling, heat, and pain over the coronary band, along with a draining sinus from the affected site. Lameness is usually present in the acute stages of the disease but may lessen as the disease becomes chronic. X-ray studies are helpful in ruling out infection of the underlying bone.

Because cartilage is a cell-poor structure and does not heal readily on its own, it is necessary to remove any dead or infected cartilage in order to achieve successful resolution of the condition. Following removal of the diseased carti-

lage and the establishment of drainage through the hoof wall, the site is bandaged and the foot protected until the lesion has completely healed. The prognosis for horses is good to excellent for future soundness. In chronic cases, however, there may be a permanent deformity of the foot.

GRAVEL

"Gravel" is a common term describing drainage at the coronary band. It is often thought to result from migration of a piece of gravel that has penetrated the sole, but in fact this is not what happens. Instead, an infection that has migrated up the hoof wall breaks out as an abscess at the coronary band. Gravel may also occur secondary to "seedy toe" in horses with laminitis (*see* above).

The diagnosis is difficult before the lesion has broken out at the coronary band. Horses may be variably and intermittently lame. The sole should be thoroughly checked for any evidence of penetration. Treatment consists of establishing drainage. The prognosis is good to excellent unless the condition occurs secondary to chronic laminitis, in which case the prognosis is much less favorable.

SIDEBONES

The term "sidebones" is used to describe ossification of the collateral cartilages of the foot. The condition usually occurs in the forefeet of horses with poor conformation. It is caused by concussion to the quarters of the foot, causing trauma and secondary ossification of the cartilages. Horses with a base-narrow stance tend to traumatize the outside of the foot and have **lateral sidebones** (occurring on the outside portion of the foot), while horses with a base-wide stance experience trauma to the inside of the foot and have **medial sidebones** (occurring on the inside portion of the foot).

Sidebones are considered a cosmetic blemish and only rarely cause lameness. When lameness does occur, the region over the collateral cartilage will be warm and painful. In such horses grooving or thinning the hoof walls to release pressure across the heels and allow expansion of the foot may alleviate the pain. The horse should be shod with full roller-motion shoes to decrease coffin joint action.

CORNS AND BRUISED SOLES

Corns are found in the sole at the angle formed by the wall and the bar of the sole. They occur most frequently on the inside of the front feet, and develop when the shoes are left on the feet for too long a period. As a result the feet overgrow the shoes and the heels of the shoes impinge on the angle of the wall and bar. Because farriers commonly bend the inside branch of the shoe to prevent the horse from stepping on the shoe and removing it, the inside angle is more frequently affected than the outside angle.

Sole bruising occurs in horses with thin soles or flat feet. The lesions are similar to those of corns except that the toe or quarter regions of the sole are involved rather than the angle of the wall and the bar. For either sole bruising or corns, lameness will be variably present depending on the severity of the lesion. Horses tend to favor the affected site, e.g., a horse with a corn on the inside angle would place more weight on the outside of the foot.

Treatment involves regular and timely shoeing. Shoes should extend well back on the buttresses of the foot and should fit full on the wall at the quarters and heels of the foot. If the corn is infected, drainage should be established and an antiseptic/astringent solution applied to help clean and dry the site. The region should be correctively trimmed so that weight-bearing forces are not placed on the angle. Affected horses should not be worked on hard, rocky surfaces. Often the application of full pads will provide temporary relief, although the sole tends to become softer with their use. Rim pads may be more beneficial in that they provide some cushioning effect but do not completely cover the sole.

The prognosis for corns and sole bruising is fair to good if the underlying lesion can be corrected. Chronic sole bruising may occur in horses with flat feet or thin soles, resulting in inflammation of the coffin bone and persistent lameness.

CANKER

Canker is a chronic overgrowth of the horn-producing tissues of the foot and may involve one or more feet. The disorder appears to occur most commonly in horses housed in unsanitary conditions, and that are required to stand for prolonged periods in mud or bedding soaked with urine and feces. Lameness is usually present and is associated with a foul-smelling **exudate** (high-protein fluid derived from blood and deposited in tissues or on tissue surfaces, usually as a result of inflammation) underneath the horn.

Diagnosis is based upon physical examination and the presence of a foul-smelling exudate within the foot. Several treatment methods have been described, with varying results. First and foremost housing conditions must be improved, with horses placed on clean, dry bedding. Topical application of **metronidazole** (a medication effective against certain bacteria and protozoa) appears to be the most effective means of therapy. The prognosis for canker, if caught early and housing conditions are improved, is fair to good. For chronic cases the prognosis is guarded.

THRUSH

Thrush is a degenerative condition of the **frog** (thickened, horny area in the middle of the sole) characterized by infection and blackening of the affected area. The infection may penetrate the horny tissue into the underlying sensitive structures of the foot. As for canker, the predisposing cause of thrush is housing a horse under unsanitary conditions.

Physical examination reveals increased moisture of the frog and a variable quantity of black, odorous fluid underneath or adjacent to the frog. Large areas of the frog may be easily removed. In severe cases swelling of the limb may occur. Treatment is based on:

- Improvement of housing conditions
- Removal of dead or infected tissue from the affected area
- Application of a topical antiseptic such as iodine or 10% formalin

The prognosis is good to excellent, so long as housing conditions are satisfactorily upgraded.

KERATOMA

A *keratoma* is a slowly growing tumor of the underlying hoof wall structures that causes lameness by putting pressure on the sensitive laminae of the hoof. Diagnosis can be made by physical examination and X-ray studies (on X ray, evidence of bone destruction beneath the keratoma may be present). Treatment involves surgical removal of the keratoma and protective shoeing of the foot until the affected area is fully healed. The prognosis is fair to good for future soundness.

HEEL AVULSION

Avulsion of the heel is a common injury and may seriously limit the athletic activity of a horse. The most common cause is trauma (kicking or stepping on sharp objects, imbalanced feet, improper removal of shoes such that the nails tear out the heel). Infection with subsequent separation of the heel may also produce this condition. Lameness is variably associated with heel avulsion and ranges in intensity from mild to severe. The diagnosis is readily made by physical examination, wherein separation of the hoof wall from the sensitive laminae can be visualized.

Treatment involves removal of the separated hoof wall. The sensitive tissue is then bandaged after administration of a topical antiseptic such as iodine. A full bar shoe is usually applied to stabilize the heel region. If possible, a prosthetic hoof-repair material should be applied over the site after the wound has dried. The overall prognosis is good to excellent for normal hoof wall growth. The only factor that may limit future soundness is damage to the coronary band; if this occurs it can result in a permanent hoof wall deformity.

HOOF WALL CRACKS

Hoof wall cracks most commonly originate at the weight-bearing surface of the hoof wall and progress up the wall towards the coronary band. On occasion coronary band defects may produce a hoof wall crack that progresses down the wall. These cracks are classified according to the region affected, i.e., toe cracks, quarter cracks, or heel cracks.

The most common cause is an excessively dry foot. Dry hoof walls are more brittle and more susceptible to cracking. Horses with thin hoof walls, and barefoot horses whose feet are trimmed inadequately or infrequently, are predisposed to the condition. For hoof wall cracks originating at the coronary band, the predisposing factor is injury to the coronary band. Affected horses exhibit variable degrees of lameness, depending on the extent of involvement of the sensitive underlying tissue. If an infection develops beneath the crack, horses will be lame on the affected limb.

Treatment of hoof cracks is dependent on the length of the crack and whether or not infection has set in. For small cracks without infection, stabilization of the hoof wall with a bar shoe may be all that is necessary to prevent the crack from progressing. For toe cracks, lowering the hoof wall immediately beneath the crack will limit the forces placed on the toe and help prevent further expansion of the crack. For long cracks in any region, the crack can be enlarged with a cast cutter or motorized burr, and synthetic patch material placed over the crack. This treatment method should be combined with a bar shoe to stabilize the hoof wall. Clips applied to the shoe also help stabilize these cracks.

The prognosis is good to excellent for cracks originating on the bearing surface. For cracks secondary to coronary band injury, surgical repair of the coronary band defect often is necessary. Even with successful surgical repair of the coronary band defect, however, the hoof wall, although improved, may have a permanent cosmetic defect.

Disorders of the Pastern

RINGBONE

Ringbone is characterized by new bone growth adjacent to the pastern or coffin joints. **High ringbone** describes bone growth around the pastern joint while **low ringbone** describes bone growth around the coffin joint. The disorder may or may not involve the actual articulating surface of these joints (when the joints are involved degenerative arthritis develops as well).

The new bone production occurs because of tearing of the collateral ligaments stabilizing the joint. Trauma (such as wire cuts) may cause high ringbone without joint involvement. Ringbone involving the joint surface, particularly high ringbone, occurs most commonly in horses used at high speed for other than racing, such as western performance horses, polo ponies, and some show horses. Ringbone may also develop as a complication of subchondral bone cyst formation (see above) in the bones adjacent to the pastern or coffin joints.

In general the forelimbs are more frequently affected than the hindlimbs. Ringbone involving the joint usually causes a lameness that is present at all gaits and upon turning. In high ringbone, enlargement of the pastern region may be palpable. Low ringbone may be associated with a buttress foot, as was described for horses with avulsion fractures of the extensor process of the distal phalanx (see above).

Affected horses may exhibit few or no clinical signs when ringbone occurs without joint involvement; consequently, the diagnosis must be made by X-ray examination. In acute cases of ringbone, heat and swelling are often palpable over the affected area. The swelling (but not the warmth) will persist as the condition becomes chronic.

Treatment is dependent on the site of the injury and whether the bony proliferation involves the joint. For ringbone without joint involvement, medical or surgical management is probably not required. If the swelling is acute, application of cold hydrotherapy or ice packs accompanied by oral administration of anti-inflammatory medication may be indicated.

For mild cases of ringbone involving a joint, corrective shoeing and anti-inflammatory medication are usually recommended. In high ringbone, as the condition progresses and becomes more severe, surgical fusion of the pastern joint may be indicated. Fusion is accomplished by removing the cartilage within the joint and applying a series of screws to compress the joint surface. The prognosis following fusion is fair to good; the majority of horses can return to their previous level of performance.

By contrast, horses with low ringbone involv-ing the joint surface have a poor to guarded prognosis for future soundness. Surgical fusion of the joint, although possible, will not result in a sound horse. For a horse with severe lameness, however, surgical fusion may improve the condition enough to keep the horse useful for breeding. Neurectomy may also improve a horse's gait by eliminating sensation on the back side of the coffin joint.

FRACTURES OF THE MIDDLE PHALANX

Middle phalanx fractures occur most frequently in the hindlimbs of western performance horses such as Quarter Horses. The more common major fractures are probably caused by a compressive, twisting type of motion that occurs during sudden stops, starts, or short turns. Horses that have been shod with heel calks have a higher propensity to develop this fracture. Heel calks prevent rotation of the foot after it contacts the ground, increasing the forces on the middle phalanx.

Horses with fractures of the middle phalanx exhibit an acute onset of lameness, with **crepitus** (crackling sound) and swelling above the coronary band in the more severe fractures. Horses with lesser fractures may be more difficult to diagnose because they are correspondingly less lame.

A definitive diagnosis is made with X-ray studies. Treatment is dependent on the configuration of the fracture and future intended use of the horse. Lesser fractures can be removed by means of **arthroscopy** (through an instrument inserted into the joint space). Major fractures of the middle phalanx that are in only two or three pieces can sometimes be repaired with bone screws. Fractures with multiple fragments (**comminuted fractures**) are much more difficult to repair and need to be managed with a cast.

Despite successful surgical repair horses frequently develop ringbone, depending on the joint surface that the fracture affects. If a horse has involvement of the pastern joint, surgical fusion of the joint may eliminate the lameness and allow the horse to return to work. For horses with involvement of the coffin joint and secondary arthritis, the prognosis for return to performance is guarded. Horses with lesser fractures have a fair to good prognosis for return to performance.

Disorders of the Fetlock

PROXIMAL PHALANX FRACTURES

Fractures of the proximal phalanx are a relatively common occurrence, with Thoroughbreds, Standardbreds, and hunter/jumpers most frequently affected. Severe, comminuted fractures can also occur in western performance horses. Proximal phalanx fractures usually occur secondary to a combined compressive and twisting motion (as for fractures of the middle phalanx, above). Clinical signs are dependent on the severity of the fracture and its exact location. Horses with minor fractures may exhibit no lameness at all, while those with complete and/or comminuted fractures are usually severely lame.

Definitive diagnosis requires X-ray studies. Treatment is dependent on the location, size, and degree of comminution of the fracture. For lesser fractures, arthroscopic removal is usually indicated. All other fractures should be repaired using screw fixation. Occasionally, horses shatter the bone so severely that it comes to resemble "a bag of ice" on X rays. Such severe fractures may not be surgically repairable; cast application may be the only beneficial treatment.

In general, the prognosis for horses with proximal phalanx fractures is fair to good for return to soundness so long as the fracture fragments can be pieced together with bone screws. By contrast, horses with severely comminuted fractures that cannot be repaired surgically have a poor to guarded prognosis. Often such horses become so lame that they must be humanely destroyed.

PROXIMAL SESAMOID BONE FRACTURES

Proximal sesamoid bone fractures are a frequent occurrence in racehorses. Thoroughbreds and Quarter Horses are affected more commonly in the forelimbs, Standardbreds more often in the hindlimbs. Fractures of the proximal sesamoid bones are classified according to the region of bone that is fractured. Fractures at the top of the bone are termed **apical** sesamoid fractures;

these fractures are the most common. The less common fractures of the base of the proximal sesamoid bone, termed **basilar** sesamoid fractures, are caused by an avulsion or tearing off of the distal sesamoidian ligament from its attachment on the proximal sesamoid bone. Fractures of the outside (or **abaxial**) portion of the proximal sesamoid bone are the least common fractures. The abaxial portion of the proximal sesamoid bone serves as the site of attachment for the suspensory ligament. Fractures of the mid-portion or mid-body of the proximal sesamoid bone occur most frequently in young foals under 2 months of age and may affect one or both proximal sesamoid bones of a limb. If both bones are fractured, the result is a breakdown injury (as previously described above).

With the exception of mid-body fractures in young foals, proximal sesamoid bone fractures can be thought of primarily as racehorse injuries. Cyclical forces placed on the proximal sesamoid bones during heavy work cause a structural weakening of the bones and predispose them to fracture. Muscular fatigue is also felt to play an important role in the development of these fractures. As the muscles tire during a race, the suspensory apparatus takes more and more of the horse's weight. The fetlock hyperextends to a greater extent, placing greater force on the proximal sesamoid bones. Two other suspected causes include unequal tension applied across the proximal sesamoid bones, as when a foot strikes the ground in an unbalanced position, and direct trauma as might occur to the medial sesamoid bone when a horse interferes with itself.

The typical signs associated with proximal sesamoid bone fractures include severe lameness during the acute stages of the injury. Swelling, heat, and pain will be evident over the affected site. Inflammation of the suspensory ligament and/or the distal sesamoidian ligaments may occur concurrently. In young foals, a history of galloping to exhaustion to keep up with the mare is a common finding.

Diagnosis is based on the history, physical examination, and X-ray studies. X-ray films will reveal the location, size, and severity of the fracture. Therapy will be dependent on the type of fracture and its severity. Treatments include application of a cast, screw fixation, bone grafting, or surgical removal. Generally, horses that will be retired for breeding can be managed conservatively, either with support bandaging and/or cast application. For horses continuing an athletic career after the injury, surgical removal or fixation of the fracture is the treatment of choice.

Apical sesamoid fractures and basilar sesamoid fractures are often best treated by surgical removal using arthroscopy. Abaxial sesamoid fractures not involving the joint can be left in place. If the fracture involves the joint, however, the fracture fragment should be removed to prevent degenerative arthritis from developing. A mid-body fracture of a single proximal sesamoid bone is best treated by screw fixation, either alone or in combination with bone grafting. When both proximal sesamoid bones are affected by mid-body fractures, the condition is termed a breakdown injury. Because the suspensory apparatus of the limb is lost there is no support to the fetlock. As described for disruption of the suspensory ligament, surgical fusion of the fetlock is the treatment of choice in such cases.

The prognosis is fair to good for apical sesamoid bone fractures involving less than one-third the length of the bone. One of the limiting factors for return to athletic soundness in these horses is the trauma that has occurred to the suspensory ligament. Often, despite successful removal of the fracture fragment, progressive and/or severe suspensory ligament inflammation will prevent a return to performance. For the three remaining types of fractures the prognosis for return to racing performance is guarded. In horses with mid-body proximal sesamoid bone fractures of both bones of a limb, the prognosis is poor because the surgical procedure used to fuse the fetlock in these horses has a high complication rate.

SESAMOIDITIS

Sesamoiditis refers to inflammation of the proximal sesamoid bones, sometimes involving the suspensory ligament and distal sesamoidian ligaments as well. Sesamoiditis may also occur secondarily in association with degenerative arthritis of the fetlock joint.

Sesamoiditis is seen most commonly in young Thoroughbred racehorses and in hunter/jumpers between 2 and 5 years of age and occurs because of increased stress placed on the fetlock joint. Most often it results from disruption of the attachment of the ligaments of the suspensory apparatus onto the proximal sesamoid bone. As the structures tear, increased vascularization and/or bone production may develop and cause a weakening of the proximal sesamoid bone.

Clinical signs associated with this condition resemble those of proximal sesamoid bone fractures except that they are milder in nature. Initially there may be a small bit of swelling over the site, with heat over the abaxial surface (outside) of the proximal sesamoid bone. As the disorder becomes more chronic, soft-tissue swelling over the outside of the bone becomes a prominent feature. Horses with this disease have a variable degree of lameness, being most lame at the start of exercise or when they are exercised on hard surfaces, and often will be reluctant to extend the fetlock completely. Pain is elicited upon palpation of the inside or outside surface of the proximal sesamoid bone, while flexion of the fetlock often exacerbates the lameness.

The diagnosis of sesamoiditis is based on the history, physical examination, and X-ray studies. X-ray changes usually are not evident until about 3 or 4 weeks after the onset of inflammation. The changes include an increase in the number and irregularity of blood vessels supplying the proximal sesamoid bone. In addition, new bone production may occur on any surface of the bone.

Treatment is aimed at eliminating the inflammation within the bone. Cold hydrotherapy or ice are useful in the acute stages of the disease. The application of a cast for 2 to 3 weeks may also be helpful. Corrective shoeing may help eliminate or decrease some of the stress being placed on the fetlock joint. The prognosis is guarded. It is imperative that horses be treated in the acute stages before progression of the disease causes increased vascularity of the proximal sesamoid bones. In chronic sesamoiditis, horses are predisposed to develop proximal sesamoid bone fractures due to the decreased mineralization of the bone. In addition, the athletic careers of horses with sesamoiditis are limited by the severity of the horse's distal sesamoidian ligament **desmitis** (ligament inflammation).

FETLOCK LUXATION

Luxation (dislocation) of the fetlock is an uncommon occurrence and can be seen in any breed of horse. Rupture of one or both **collateral ligaments,** which help stabilize the joint, often occurs concurrently with this injury. The injury usually is secondary to a horse's stepping in a hole or getting its foot caught in a fence. The clinical signs of the disorder are apparent upon physical examination. The lower part of the limb is seen to deviate markedly either to the inside or outside, centered at the fetlock joint. The diagnosis is confirmed by X-ray studies which also will reveal any associated fractures.

Treatment of fetlock luxation is a relatively straightforward procedure so long as fractures are not present. The application of a cast for 6 to 8 weeks will usually resolve the problem. If the luxation is **open** (i.e., the bone has broken through the skin), it will be necessary to flush the joint and remove any dead or infected tissue.

The prognosis is fair to good for horses intended for breeding, but guarded so far as a horse's future athletic abilities are concerned. Often degenerative arthritis develops 2 to 3 months after repair of the luxation, probably secondary to the soft-tissue injuries that occurred at the time of the luxation.

ANNULAR LIGAMENT CONSTRICTION

Annular ligaments function to maintain tendon alignment as the tendons cross a joint. If an annular ligament becomes inflamed or a tendon swells within an annular ligament, constriction of the tendon by the annular ligament may ensue. A classic example of such constriction occurs over the back side of the fetlock in a horse with tendinitis of the superficial digital flexor tendon. Annular ligament constriction can also occur on the back side of the carpus, a condition termed **carpal canal syndrome.** Affected horses usually are lame.

The diagnosis of annular ligament constric-

tion can be difficult to make because the constriction may not be palpable. Often, clipping the hair over the site will aid in visualizing the constriction, which may be accompanied by tenosynovitis of the affected tendon sheath.

Surgical treatment involves **sectioning** (cutting) of the constricting ligament. This releases the constricted tendon and frequently eliminates the lameness. The overall prognosis is usually good. Although a similar surgery is often performed for relieving constriction of the carpal annular ligament, the prognosis for such cases is less favorable.

Disorders of the Metacarpus and Metatarsus

BUCKED SHINS AND STRESS FRACTURES

Bucked shins and *stress fractures* of the front of the cannon bone are common injuries in 2- and 3-year-old racehorses. The term "bucked shins" refers to a painful condition caused by inflammation and hemorrhage over the front surface of the bone. Occasionally, small stress fractures along the surface of the bone may also occur.

Bucked shins are the result of repeated, severe weight-bearing on a horse's forelimbs. The forelimbs are more frequently affected because horses that work at a gallop, such as Quarter Horses and Thoroughbreds, place more weight on their forelimbs than on their hindlimbs. The forelimbs are therefore stressed to a greater extent. The affected bone tissue responds to this stress by attempting to give a stronger, more resilient shape to the bone. During this process the bone actually becomes weaker for a period of time, resulting in small microfractures that cause bleeding and inflammation along the bone surface. Occasionally, a larger stress fracture occurs that is visible on X rays.

Bucked shins can be divided into three categories: acute, chronic, and stress fractures. In the acute form of the disease lameness after intense exercise is seen, particularly in young Thoroughbred racehorses less than $1\frac{1}{2}$ years of age. The horses exhibit evidence of pain upon palpation of the front of the cannon bones. X rays at this time are usually negative for any bone proliferation over the surface of the bone. Horses that are not treated appropriately, or that are unresponsive to treatment, may go on to develop the chronic form of bucked shins. In these cases there may only be mild degrees of lameness, and palpation of the front of the cannon bones may or may not elicit a pain response. X-ray examination of the horse's cannon bones at this stage usually reveals **callus** (bony proliferation) production over the surface of the bone.

Horses with stress fractures tend to be older (3 to 5 years of age) than horses with bucked shins. Lameness may not be evident when the horse is at rest, but often develops during strenuous exercise. Palpation of the limb may reveal a painful bump over the surface of the cannon bone. X-ray studies will confirm the diagnosis.

Treatment of bucked shins and stress fractures is dependent on the severity of the disorder. Horses with acute disease often respond to a short period of rest and controlled exercise. Treatment of the chronic form is more difficult, however, with some horses requiring prolonged periods (as long as a year) of controlled exercise and rest to resolve the disorder.

Treatment of stress fractures of the cannon bone is somewhat controversial. Some clinicians recommend a conservative approach with rest until the fracture has healed. More commonly surgical approaches, such as drilling of the fracture site or screw fixation, are used to resolve the problem.

The prognosis for horses with bucked shins is good to guarded, depending on the stage of the disease. For horses with acute disease, the prognosis is good for return to soundness with controlled exercise. For horses with the chronic form the prognosis is more guarded, because some may require lengthy time periods to resolve the condition. Horses with stress fractures should be given a guarded prognosis, although many ultimately return to racing. Occasionally, however, horses will completely fracture the cannon bone right through the stress fracture—an event that may ultimately necessitate humane destruction of the horse.

CONDYLAR FRACTURES

Fractures of the **condyles** (rounded processes at the end of the bone) of the cannon bone occur frequently in Thoroughbred racehorses and less frequently in other racing horses. The fracture is seen in 3- to 4-year-old horses and is 2 to 3 times more common in the forelimbs than in the hindlimbs. Standardbreds, although less frequently affected than Thoroughbreds, tend to fracture their hindlimbs more frequently than their forelimbs. The **lateral** (or outside) condyle is the most common site of the fracture.

Condylar fractures occur secondary to a compressive, twisting action placed on the cannon bone. The clinical signs associated with this fracture are variable and dependent on the severity of the injury. For short, nondisplaced fractures, horses may be mildly lame with very little joint swelling. More commonly, horses exhibit moderate to severe lameness with heat, pain, and swelling of the affected joint. For short fractures that go undiagnosed, horses will be more lame following exercise.

The diagnosis of condylar fractures is made using X-ray studies. If a condylar fracture is suspected and not visualized on the initial X rays, multiple X-ray views should be taken to identify the fracture.

Treatment is dependent on the degree of displacement of the fracture. For nondisplaced fractures, conservative therapy has been recommended by some clinicians. Horses that have been managed conservatively do return to racing, although at a later time than horses treated surgically. For most cases, surgical fixation of the fracture with screws is recommended. Surgical stabilization of the fracture decreases motion at the joint surface and speeds healing of the fracture. This ultimately minimizes the chances for degenerative arthritis and maximizes prolongation of the horse's athletic career.

The prognosis is good following surgical repair of the fracture. For horses managed conservatively or for those with significant **comminution** of the fracture (i.e., the fracture is in multiple fragments), the prognosis is more guarded.

METACARPAL/METATARSAL (CANNON) BONE FRACTURES

Fractures of the cannon bone are common in horses of all ages and breeds. Cannon bone fractures in older horses tend to be fragmented (**comminuted**). Because there is only minimal soft-tissue coverage of the cannon bone, fractures are often **open** (broken through the skin).

There are many causes of cannon bone fractures, including:

- Direct trauma (as from a kick)
- Injury secondary to stress fractures/bucked shins, stepping in a hole, or catching a limb in a fence
- Slipping accidents
- Injuries associated with being hit by a motorized vehicle

Usually, horses with cannon bone fractures are severely lame. Instability of the limb below the fracture is a prominent diagnostic sign. X-ray studies of the affected limb will confirm the diagnosis.

Treatment centers on adequately stabilizing the fracture during transport to a surgical facility, minimizing trauma to the soft tissues over the bone, using appropriate antibiotics and anti-inflammatory medications, protecting the opposite limb with a support bandage, and performing corrective surgery within a short period of time after the injury. All of these are prerequisites for a successful outcome.

The definitive surgical repair procedure is the application of two bone plates with screws on the front and side of the cannon bone, followed by casting of the limb. In the case of foals, the cast is removed immediately after surgery. In adult horses the cast is often left on the limb for 8 to 12 weeks postsurgery. Bone grafting (transplanting additional bone into the fracture site to aid healing) is highly recommended.

The prognosis for horses with complete cannon bone fractures is dependent on the severity of the fracture and whether it is open. In closed fractures in younger horses, the prognosis is fair for successful healing and return to soundness. By contrast, adult horses and horses with open fractures have a poor to guarded prognosis for survival. Often these horses will develop a severe infection (**osteomyelitis**) within the bone and around the implants, requiring humane destruction.

SPLINTS

"Splints" is a term used to describe inflammation of the **interosseous ligament** that attaches the **splint bones** (the second and fourth metacarpal bones) to the cannon bone. The condition most commonly affects the forelimbs of young horses, with the **medial** (inside) splint bone affected more often. Splints may occur after tearing of the interosseous ligament, external trauma in the form of a kick, or healing of a fracture of the splint bone. Although splints may occur in any horse, conformational abnormalities may predispose certain horses to the condition. Horses that are base-narrow with a toed-out conformation place more stress on the inside of the limb, thus predisposing the medial splint bone to the condition.

Splints usually causes lameness in 2-year-old horses undergoing heavy training, although 3- to 4-year-old horses can be affected as well. The resulting lameness is most obvious at a trot, with heat, pain, and swelling developing over the affected splint bone.

Initial diagnosis is made on the basis of the history and physical examination. Because fractures of the splint bone (*see* below) may be confused with splints, X-ray studies should be performed to distinguish between the two conditions and provide a definitive diagnosis.

For horses in the acute phase of the disease, ice, cold hydrotherapy, and support bandaging are helpful for resolving the inflammation. Some practitioners advocate injection of corticosteroids into the site to help reduce inflammation. For horses with splints caused by interfering with themselves, shin guards may help prevent further trauma. If the reason for interference is improper trimming or shoeing, the horse should be correctively shod to eliminate this problem. In horses with large bony protuberances over the splint bone, surgical removal of the excessive bone may be required. It is often helpful to remove both the bone and the periosteum over the bone to help prevent regrowth of the proliferating bone. Unfortunately, some of these horses will regrow the excessive bone despite all efforts to minimize trauma and inflammation at the site after surgery.

The prognosis for horses with splints is good to excellent except in those with large bony proliferation encroaching on the suspensory ligament, which causes lameness secondary to suspensory ligament inflammation.

SPLINT BONE FRACTURES

Fractures of the splint bone are common and can occur anywhere along the bone's length, although the lower third of the bone is the usual site. These fractures occur in older horses (5 to 7 years of age) and are thought to result from forces placed on the bone by the interosseous ligament. Thus young 2- to 4-year-old horses tend to develop splints (as described above), while older horses tend to fracture the splint bone.

Splint bone fractures develop most frequently in the outside left splint bone and the inside right splint bone in horses racing in North America. This predisposition is probably the result of racing in the counterclockwise direction, which puts greater stress on the splint bones facing the inside of the track. The forelimbs are affected more frequently than the hindlimbs, with the left forelimb fractured more often than the right.

Splint bone fractures may result from stresses delivered by the interosseous ligament; external trauma, as from a kick; a direct blow from hitting another object; a horse's interfering with itself; or a puncture. Clinical signs include heat, pain, and swelling over the affected site. Horses exhibit a variable degree of lameness, although in the acute stage they tend to point the affected foot. The diagnosis is confirmed by means of an X-ray examination.

Treatment is dependent on the location of the fracture. For lower splint bone fractures, surgical removal of the end of the splint bone is recommended. If these fractures are treated conservatively without surgery, the callus that forms to heal the fracture may impinge on the suspensory ligament and result in lameness. Surgical removal of the fracture prevents this complication. In upper splint bone fractures, surgical stabilization of the fracture is often necessary. Stabilization can be achieved by the application of a small reconstructive bone plate.

The prognosis is dependent on the degree of involvement of the suspensory ligament. If suspensory desmitis is not present, horses have a fair to good prognosis for return to racing soundness. For horses with suspensory desmitis, the prognosis for return to performance is dependent on the degree and severity of the desmitis. The splint bone fracture itself rarely limits a horse's return to performance.

Disorders of the Carpus

HYGROMA OF THE CARPUS

Carpal *hygroma* is a swelling over the front of the carpus, most often caused by trauma. Horses that get up and down on hard surfaces are the most commonly affected. The diagnosis is based on physical examination and needle drainage of the swollen site, with submission of the drainage fluid for laboratory analysis. X-ray studies of the carpus should be performed to rule out any underlying bony abnormalities.

The most effective treatment is drainage of the fluid, injection of anti-inflammatory medication, and application of a pressure bandage over the site. Injections may be repeated at weekly intervals for 3 to 5 treatments. If a horse does not respond to anti-inflammatory injections, the site can be drained through a skin incision and the inner surface cleansed with iodine.

The prognosis is fair to good for acute cases. In chronic cases with thickening over the carpus, a permanent cosmetic defect may always be present. Carpal hygromas are rarely if ever associated with lameness.

CARPAL FRACTURES

Fractures of the carpus are a common injury in racehorses, hunters, jumpers, western performance horses, and many other athletic breeds. Thoroughbred and Quarter Horse racehorses between 2 and 4 years of age have a higher prevalence of the disorder. Simple "chip" fractures off the corner or edge of a carpal bone are the most common type of injury, although larger "slab" fractures and comminuted fractures may also occur. Lesser fractures involving only one joint surface may be firmly attached to the parent bone or floating freely within the joint. The radial carpal bone, the third carpal bone, the intermediate carpal bone, and the lower end of the radius are the most commonly affected with chip fractures.

In contrast to chip fractures, slab fractures involve both joint surfaces of a carpal bone. The third carpal bone is by far the most commonly affected, although the intermediate and radial carpal bones occasionally suffer slab fractures. Comminuted fractures of the carpus may involve any or all of the carpal bones, but most frequently affect the radial carpal bone, intermediate carpal bone, and fourth carpal bone. Comminution may or may not include slab and chip fractures simultaneously.

Carpal fractures are the result of cyclical forces placed on the carpus during racing or race training. As a forelimb begins to bear the horse's weight during racing, the carpus goes into mild to moderate hyperextension, greatly increasing the force on the front of the carpal bones. Repeated loading in this fashion may either traumatize the bone slowly, causing microfractures, or decrease the vascularity of the bone. Both of these factors may lead to an increased susceptibility of the front surfaces of the carpal bones to fracture.

Horses with chip fractures exhibit variable degrees of lameness. Often a horse will develop a mild swelling of the affected joint accompanied by heat and some lameness. In the more chronic stages the joint swelling may subside while swelling over the site of the fracture continues. In slab fractures, horses are significantly lame on the affected limb. Horses with comminuted fractures of the carpus are usually non–weight-bearing on the affected limb, and will not place the limb on the ground. Flexion of the carpus will exacerbate the lameness. X-ray examination of the carpus is necessary to confirm the diagnosis.

Carpal fractures are best treated by surgical intervention. Chip fractures and any damaged cartilage can be removed by arthroscopy. This should be followed by stall rest for a variable period of time, depending on the magnitude and size of the joint lesion. For small lesions, box stall rest for 3 to 4 weeks and paddock confinement for an additional 6 to 8 weeks may be all that is needed before a return to race training. For larger defects, a total rest period of 6 to 7 months may be required to achieve adequate healing.

For slab fractures, screw fixation of the fractured fragment to the parent bone will achieve the most rapid return to athletic performance. Often this technique can be performed with arthroscopy. As for the larger defects, a total period of rest of 6 to 7 months is recommended.

For horses with comminuted carpal fractures, surgical repair of the fracture should be aimed at salvaging a good breeding horse, since it is highly unlikely that the horse will have any athletic future. Surgical repair is achieved by a screw fixation and/or cast application following surgery.

The prognosis for horses with chip fractures is good to excellent; approximately 80 percent of horses return to racing following arthroscopic removal of the fragment. The prognosis for horses with slab fractures is guarded to poor for return to racing soundness. These horses can and often are sound enough to be useful for pleasure riding or as breeding stock. The prognosis for horses with comminuted fractures of the carpus is poor to guarded for soundness.

ACCESSORY CARPAL BONE FRACTURES

Accessory carpal bone fractures occur less frequently in racehorses and more often in horses that perform in steeplechase events and in hunter/jumpers. The exact origin of these fractures is uncertain, although direct trauma through a kick or by a horse interfering with itself are potential causes. These fractures may also occur when a horse lands on a partially flexed forelimb, catching the ulnar carpal bone between the cannon bone and the radius. Horses with accessory carpal bone fractures are usually only mildly lame on the affected limb, with swelling of the carpal sheath being the most prominent sign of the condition.

Treatment has been universally unsuccessful. Some surgeons advocate conservative therapy in the form of box stall rest for 3 to 6 months, while others recommend screw fixation of the fracture. The prognosis is guarded for return to performance. Horses that will be retired to breeding or to light pleasure riding may not require surgical repair of the fracture, because conservative management often achieves the necessary level of soundness.

CARPAL JOINT LUXATION

Dislocation of the carpal joints is an uncommon occurrence in horses. When it does occur it can involve any of the three carpal joints. Carpal luxation is felt to be the result of external trauma, such as would occur during jumping, falling, or slipping. Affected horses exhibit swelling and angular deviation of the limb, centered at the luxated joint. Horses will usually be lame on the affected limb; palpation will reveal heat, pain, and swelling over the site. The diagnosis is confirmed by X-ray examination.

Treatment consists first in attempting to reduce the luxation under general anesthesia, i.e., by manipulating the joint back into its normal position without making a skin incision. If this is not successful, open reduction using one or more skin incisions may be necessary to achieve reduction of the luxation. Following reduction, a cast should be applied to maintain the limb in normal alignment. Casts are usually left on for 4 to 6 weeks in foals and 6 to 8 weeks in mature horses. As stated in the section on angular limb deformity (see above), foals have a propensity to develop cast sores, so the cast should be changed every 10 to 12 days during the treatment period in young animals.

If carpal luxation is accompanied by comminution of the carpal bones, humane euthanasia should be strongly considered unless the horse is of great sentimental or financial value. Attempted treatment usually consists of screw fixation of all repairable fractures together with reduction of the luxation. Cast application may be necessary for 3 to 4 months until the fractured bones have healed. Unfortunately, screw fixation often breaks down before the fractures have completely healed.

The prognosis for horses with luxation without comminuted carpal bone fractures is good for achieving a useable limb for breeding and mild exercise. The prognosis for return to athletic performance is guarded. The prognosis is poor to guarded for survival for horses with comminuted fractures associated with luxation of the carpus.

Disorders of the Radius

RADIAL FRACTURES

Fractures of the radius are a relatively common occurrence in horses. They can develop anywhere along the length of the radius and may be simple, comminuted, open, or closed. Since the ulna lies in close apposition to the radius, the ulna is frequently fractured at the same time as the radius. The most common cause of such a fracture is high-energy impact, such as a kick or being struck by a motorized vehicle.

The principal clinical sign is non–weight-bearing lameness of the affected limb. Palpation of the limb usually reveals crepitus and excessive motion in the body of the radius. The medial aspect (inside) of the limb should be inspected closely for evidence of protrusion of the fractured bone.

Diagnosis of a radial fracture is based on the history, physical examination, and confirmatory X-ray studies. Radial fractures should usually be repaired using surgical fixation. A full limb cast will not immobilize most radial fractures because the elbow joint cannot be prevented from moving with such a cast. In fact, the application of a cast to a radial fracture may actually *increase* the forces on the fracture, causing additional damage. Most radial fractures are best repaired surgically using a combination of screws and bone plates. Often, two bone plates are required to stabilize the fracture.

The prognosis for fractures of the radius is dependent on the size and age of the horse. Young horses weighing under 600 pounds have a fair prognosis for survival and future athletic soundness. By contrast, adult horses and horses weighing more than 600 pounds have a guarded to poor prognosis.

Disorders of the Elbow

ULNAR FRACTURES

The **olecranon** (upper portion of the ulna) is the most common portion of the ulna to fracture, although fractures of the upper growth plate, fractures occurring in conjunction with luxation of the radius, and lower ulnar fractures, are also seen. Ulnar fractures frequently involve the elbow joint and are almost always the result of direct trauma, usually a kick by another horse. Penetrating wounds, falls, encounters with motorized vehicles, and running into solid objects are other potential causes.

The diagnosis of an ulnar fracture is relatively simple to make, although occasional fractures may prove more difficult. Most affected horses have a "dropped elbow" appearance similar to a radial nerve injury (*see* below). They usually will not bear full weight on the affected limb, carrying the limb in partial flexion. Swelling over the elbow joint and crepitus are other signs that may be noted on physical examination. The diagnosis is confirmed by X-ray studies.

Treatment is dependent on the severity of the fracture, its location, and whether the elbow joint is involved. In young horses with growth plate fractures, a single bone plate attached to the back side of the bone may be sufficient to allow the fracture to heal. More commonly, a combination of pins and wires is used to achieve stabilization of the fracture. In adult horses and in the more severely comminuted fractures, plate and screw fixation is usually required to achieve adequate stabilization.

Conservative management in the form of strict stall confinement for 6 to 12 weeks has been recommended for certain olecranon fractures. Complications associated with conservative therapy include angular deviation of the opposite limb and flexural deformity of the fractured limb. Thus unless finances dictate otherwise, surgical therapy should be applied.

The prognosis is good to excellent for nondisplaced fractures not involving the elbow joint. Fractures in young horses that involve the growth plate have a good to excellent prognosis for future soundness. Fractures involving the elbow joint have a guarded prognosis until elbow function can be evaluated 2 to 3 months after surgery.

OLECRANON BURSITIS (SHOE BOIL OR CAPPED ELBOW)

Olecranon bursitis occurs most frequently in draft horses and is caused by repeated trauma

to the point of the elbow (**olecranon**). This results in swelling and the formation of a **false bursa** (a fluid-filled, saclike cavity at an area of friction) at the site. Inflammation is induced by the horse hitting itself with the shoe of the affected limb, most often when the horse is lying down.

Diagnosis is made on the basis of the history, physical examination, and X-ray studies (to rule out any underlying bony abnormalities). Treatment of horses in the acute stages of the disease is similar to that described for carpal hygroma (*see* above). The injection of anti-inflammatory medication into the site may also be beneficial. More commonly horses are presented to the veterinarian with a chronic form of the disease, in which case treatment is much more challenging. Chronic cases can be managed by the injection of irritants such as iodine into the bursal swelling; by cutting into the bursa and **cauterizing** (applying a caustic substance to destroy tissue) its inner lining with an irritant; or surgically removing the false bursa.

The prognosis is good in acute cases if additional trauma can be prevented. The prognosis for chronic cases of olecranon bursitis is more guarded.

Disorders of the Humerus

HUMERAL FRACTURES

Fractures of the humerus are an uncommon occurrence because of the bone's short, thick configuration and its generous overlying musculature. Such fractures only rarely involve the shoulder or elbow joint. The **radial nerve,** which is necessary to support weight on the limb, courses directly over the body of the humerus and may be traumatized by a humeral fracture. Humeral fractures can result from direct trauma, such as an encounter with a motorized vehicle, or by running into a solid object. In racehorses, fractures of the humerus occur most frequently in association with a preexisting stress fracture and while galloping at a moderate pace. Clinically, the region over the humerus may be mildly swollen and the horse will often carry its limb with a "dropped elbow" appearance.

Diagnosis is based on the history, physical examination, and results of an X-ray examination. Treatment is dependent on the fracture's configuration, the age of the horse, and the degree of bone displacement. Some fractures with mild displacement may be managed conservatively without surgery. In such cases it is important to protect the opposite forelimb and, through the use of splints, prevent persistent flexion of the carpus on the affected limb.

Surgical management of humeral fractures involves either the application of one or two bone plates, or the insertion of one or more rods into the central marrow cavity of the bone. These rods may be combined with wires or bands around the surface of the bone to prevent further movement of the bone fragments. During the surgical procedure it is important that the radial nerve be evaluated to determine if it has sustained any damage.

The prognosis for horses with humeral fractures is guarded. Laminitis, flexural contracture of the affected limb, and angular deviation of the opposite limb unfortunately are common complications. The overall prognosis is poor, particularly if there is evidence of damage to the radial nerve.

Radial Nerve Paralysis

The radial nerve supplies the extensor muscles of the forelimb and allows the horse to bear weight on the leg. Paralysis of the radial nerve results in an inability to extend the forelimb or to bear weight on it. The underlying cause is usually traumatic. As mentioned above in the section on humeral fractures, the radial nerve courses over the surface of the humerus and can be traumatized by a humeral fracture. Radial nerve paralysis can also result from blunt trauma which does not result in a fracture but does damage the nerve. One of the most common causes of radial nerve paralysis is general anesthesia. A horse placed on its side on a hard surface for a lengthy surgical procedure may experience radial nerve damage with subsequent paralysis of the musculature the nerve supplies.

There are few good treatments for radial nerve paralysis. Horses that have suffered complete severance of the nerve are generally untreatable and should be humanely destroyed. Horses that develop radial nerve paralysis as a consequence of general anesthesia can occasionally be treated with success. Treatment consists of the intravenous administration of dimethylsulfoxide (DMSO) and an anti-inflammatory medication. The opposite limb should be protected with a support bandage and the horse given 1 to 2 weeks to recover its ability to bear weight. If the paralysis persists, it is unlikely that normal limb function will return in a reasonable period of time.

The prognosis for horses with radial nerve paralysis secondary to severe trauma (e.g., a humeral fracture) is grave. Horses with radial nerve paralysis secondary to general anesthesia have a guarded prognosis for a future soundness.

Diseases of the Shoulder

Bicipital Bursitis

The *bicipital bursa* lies underneath the biceps tendon, protecting it from the humerus. Inflammation of this bursa is rare in the horse, although it can occasionally occur as the result of direct trauma. Another potential cause is the horse's falling on a limb when the shoulder is flexed and the elbow extended.

The diagnosis of bicipital bursitis can be difficult to make. Clinical signs include an inability or reluctance to advance the limb, stumbling on the affected limb, and resenting flexion of the shoulder joint (i.e., pulling the limb back). Swelling of the bursa is often present, although due to its large size and muscle coverage, this swelling may be difficult to detect. Direct pressure over the bursa often elicits a painful response. Flexion of the shoulder, combined with simultaneous extension of the elbow, will usually cause pain in a horse with bicipital bursitis.

Bicipital bursitis is treated by the administration of anti-inflammatory medication directly into the bursa, normally once a week for a total of four or five injections. Such treatment must be combined with stall rest in order to minimize further trauma to the bursa. The prognosis is guarded. Acute cases that respond to therapy may return to their previous level of performance. In more chronic cases the prognosis tends to be less favorable.

OSSIFICATION OF THE BICEPS TENDON

Ossification (production of bone, in this case within a tendon) of the biceps tendon occurs in young horses and is thought to be either the result of direct trauma or a developmental disorder. The diagnosis is difficult to make and relies on the history, physical examination, and results of an X-ray examination. The physical examination usually reveals signs similar to those observed in bicipital bursitis (*see* above), i.e., horses resent flexion of the shoulder joint as the elbow is extended. There may also be atrophy of the shoulder muscles, particularly of the biceps muscle. Horses may be reluctant to advance the affected limb. X rays will reveal ossification of the biceps tendon.

There is no definitive treatment. The administration of anti-inflammatory medication may improve the horse's gait for a period of time. As the lameness becomes progressively more severe, the horse may have to be retired for breeding. The prognosis thus is poor to guarded for future athletic soundness, although the prognosis for breeding soundness is usually quite good.

SWEENY

The term "sweeny" is used to describe a condition wherein the **supraspinatus** and **infraspinatus muscles,** located over the **scapula** (shoulder blade), atrophy as the result of damage to their nerve supply (the **suprascapular nerve**). The suprascapular nerve is usually injured by a direct blow over the point of the shoulder, or by a horse's sudden fall with the limb behind the horse. In the acute stage there is a partial dislocation of the shoulder, causing both owner and veterinarian to suspect a fracture or luxation of the shoulder. As the condition becomes more chronic, however, the affected muscles atrophy, causing the outline of the spine of the scapula to become very prominent. A definitive diagnosis can be made using **electromyography (EMG;** examination of the electrical activity of muscles and associated nerves; *see* APPENDIX C, "DIAGNOSTIC TESTS"). X-ray studies should be performed to rule out any underlying bony abnormalities.

Treatment of this condition remains somewhat controversial. For acute cases some surgeons advocate conservative therapy in the form of anti-inflammatory medication, intravenous administration of DMSO, and stall rest. Others feel that surgical intervention should be performed immediately upon diagnosis. Surgical treatment involves release of pressure on the suprascapular nerve, a procedure in which the scapula underneath the nerve is notched to help relieve tension.

The prognosis is guarded for return of nerve function. Horses should be given a period of 6 to 9 months following either conservative or surgical treatment before a definitive prognosis for long-term soundness is rendered (it often requires this much time for the damaged nerve to resupply the muscles overlying the scapula).

SHOULDER LUXATION

Shoulder dislocations are rare in horses. When they do occur they are usually the result of a horse's falling on a forelimb when the limb is held in flexion. Injured horses exhibit shoulder swelling and severe lameness and are non–weight-bearing on the affected limb.

Diagnosis is made on the basis of the history, physical examination, and results of X-ray studies. Shoulder luxations are treated by surgically realigning the joint. After surgery horses should be stall-rested and possibly kept tied up for 4 to 6 weeks. The prognosis is good if the luxation is repaired shortly after the injury has occurred. Otherwise degenerative arthritis may develop and limit the future athletic abilities of the horse.

SCAPULAR FRACTURES

Scapular fractures are an uncommon occurrence in horses. The suprascapular nerve, which courses over the neck of the scapula, may be traumatized in some cases. The cause of scapular fractures is usually direct trauma to the scapula. Affected horses exhibit variable degrees of lameness and swelling over the scapula. Fractures that do not involve the shoulder joint may not cause significant lameness. In chronic cases the scapular muscles will atrophy, aiding in diagnosis. The diagnosis usually is confirmed with X-ray studies.

Treatment is dependent on the region of the scapula affected. Fractures of the neck or body of the scapula can be repaired with bone plates and screws. Fractures involving the shoulder joint are more difficult to repair, although screw fixation or screw and plate fixation may help speed healing.

The prognosis for fractures of the scapular spine, neck, or body that can be successfully stabilized is good for return to athletic soundness. For fractures involving the shoulder joint the prognosis is poor to guarded. Horses with these latter fractures, however, can usually be used for breeding.

Disorders of the Tarsus

BONE SPAVIN

Bone spavin is a term describing degenerative arthritis of the lower joints of the hocks. Bone spavin is the most common cause of hindlimb lameness in horses. The hock consists of several distinct joints, with the uppermost joint allowing the greatest degree of motion. The lower two joints, which are low-motion joints, are the ones most commonly affected by bone spavin.

Bone spavin is observed most frequently in older performance horses, including western performance horses, Standardbred racehorses, jumpers, and polo horses. Bone spavin is thought to result from cyclical forces that cause compression and rotation of the lower tarsal bones. Bone spavin has a much higher prevalence in horses with poor hock conformation, e.g., those that are cow-hocked or sickle-hocked. Bone spavin can develop also in foals with fractures of the central tarsal bone.

Horses with bone spavin exhibit a gradual onset of lameness, and tend to become more lame if worked hard. Reining horses and horses that must turn quickly often refuse to pivot on the affected limb. There is a tendency to gallop with a stiff gait because of pain on flexion of the hock. Generally, affected animals will be most lame when they are first put to work for the day, but will warm out of the lameness.

Diagnosis relies on the history, physical examination, and results of X-ray studies. Treatment is dependent on the severity of the disease and the age and intended use of the horse. For horses with mild bone spavin, corrective shoeing, administration of anti-inflammatory medication, and consistent, moderate exercise to maintain muscle tone will alleviate pain in many animals. For Standardbred racehorses it is common to inject the lower joints of the hock with a long-acting anti-inflammatory to alleviate swelling and pain. The initial injection usually works quite well in alleviating lameness, the effect lasting sometimes for as long as 3 or 4 months. Each successive injection works less well, however, and for a shorter duration, so that by the time a horse has received four or five injections very little effect is observed. Often horses require therapy only at the start of the season, the medication acting to alleviate the pain sufficiently to allow the horse to begin exercising and improving muscle tone. With increased muscle tone, the joints experience less stress, and the horse usually exhibits less pain.

Other treatments described for bone spavin include tendon cutting and surgical drilling of the lower hock joints. The goal of drilling the joints or of injecting an agent that destroys the articular cartilage, is to achieve actual fusion of the joints. With fusion the pain within the joints disappears. Since there is very little motion in these joints normally, a horse's gait is not adversely affected by the procedure. Unfortunately, unsuccessful fusion may exacerbate arthritis, causing an even greater degree of lameness.

The prognosis is always guarded. Some horses will exhibit evidence of mild bone spavin for years and need only be managed by corrective shoeing and the occasional administration of anti-inflammatory medication. Others will rapidly develop severe degenerative changes that ultimately limit the horse's athletic life. Horses that undergo fusion of the lower hock joints usually end up being sound, although there may be some alteration of gait and typically a bony protuberance is permanently evident on the inside of the hock.

CUNEAN BURSITIS

Cunean bursitis describes a condition wherein the bursa underneath the **cunean tendon,** which travels over the front and inside of the hock, becomes inflamed. It is an unusual condition that occurs mostly in young Standardbreds early in their racing careers. As described for bone spavin (*see* above), cunean bursitis is thought to result from the stresses placed on the hock as the horse trots or paces. Shoes that limit the motion between the shoe and ground, such as those that have been altered with heel calks, grabs, or trailers, often increase stress across the hock and predispose horses to cunean bursitis.

The diagnosis is sometimes difficult to make. A typical case would involve a young Standardbred early in race training, with the report that the horse is stiff in the back or suffers from a stifle lameness. Direct pressure on the cunean tendon often elicits a painful response. The diagnosis is usually confirmed by demonstrating temporary resolution of the lameness following injection of a local anesthetic agent into the cunean bursa. X-ray studies should also be performed to rule out bone spavin as the primary cause of lameness. (Bone spavin and cunean bursitis can exist simultaneously in the same horse and both cause hindlimb lameness.)

Treatment of horses with cunean bursitis centers on reduction of inflammation within the bursa by anti-inflammatory medication, and changes in the horse's work schedule. Fast work should be restricted and long, slower miles instituted in the horse's training regime. The administration of anti-inflammatory medication orally or by injection into the cunean bursa will help alleviate the inflammation. Although cunean **tenectomy** (severing of the tendon) has been described as a treatment for both bone spavin and cunean bursitis, current thinking questions the benefit of this procedure. The overall prognosis is good for return to athletic performance.

Bog Spavin

Bog spavin describes swelling of the upper joint of the hock. The most common cause is **osteochondritis dissecans (OCD)** (*see* "Osteochondrosis," page 203). Other causes of bog spavin include trauma and poor hindlimb conformation (horses with straight hocks tend to be predisposed to the condition).

Swelling of the hock joint, most prominent over the inside front of the joint, is a characteristic clinical sign of bog spavin. A significant but smaller swelling is usually present over the outside back portion of the joint as well. The degree of lameness is variable; horses with bog spavin may exhibit no lameness or be mildly or moderately lame, depending on the underlying cause. The diagnosis is relatively straightforward, based on the history and the presence of the typical swellings. The cause is often less clear. Horses with OCD can often be diagnosed by X-ray examination. Other causes of bog spavin are more difficult to diagnose.

Treatment of bog spavin is dependent on the reason for the swelling. For horses with OCD, the fragments should be removed by arthroscopy. Horses with bog spavin secondary to trauma may respond to two or three injections of an anti-inflammatory medication into the joint. The application of a compressive bandage helps minimize any return of the swelling.

Horses with OCD often resolve the swelling following surgery and suffer no limitations in athletic ability. By contrast, horses with bog spavin secondary to excessively straight hocks may never be lame but always have a swelling present in the upper tarsal joint. The prognosis for bog spavin secondary to trauma is dependent on the degree of trauma and whether or not the horse responds to initial therapy.

Thoroughpin

This is swelling of the tarsal sheath that encloses the deep digital flexor tendon of the hind limb in front of the Achilles tendon. The cause of thoroughpin is typically unknown, but may be related to conformational problems. Typically, there is no history of injury or inflammation of the site.

The diagnosis is made by digital palpation and visual examination of the tarsal sheath. Thoroughpin varies in size and typically does not cause lameness. Thoroughpin usually is not treated and is considered a blemish. If treatment is necessary due to increasing swelling of the tarsal sheath, injection of an anti-inflammatory agent such as a corticosteroid has been used successfully. Unfortunately, steroid injection into the tarsal sheath is often a temporary solution.

FRACTURES OF THE CALCANEUS

Fractures of the **calcaneus** (heel bone) are uncommon injuries that are almost always caused by trauma, such as a kick from another horse or a horse's kicking a solid wall. For these fractures a presumptive diagnosis is relatively straightforward, with heat, swelling, and pain over the affected site and reduced weight-bearing on the affected limb. For smaller "chip" fractures, however, the diagnosis can be more difficult. The definitive diagnosis is usually made by X-ray studies.

Treatment is dependent on the severity of the fracture. For small chip fractures that do not involve the joint, removal of the fragment may not be necessary. If the joint surface is involved, the fragment can be removed by arthroscopy. For larger fractures of the body of the calcaneus, surgical repair with one or more bone plates may be necessary to achieve adequate stabilization. This procedure is often followed by the application of a long-legged cast to stabilize the hock.

The prognosis for horses with chip fractures of the calcaneus is good to guarded, depending on whether the joint is involved. For fractures of the body of the calcaneus, the prognosis is guarded for the patient's return to athletic performance.

LUXATION OF THE TARSUS

Dislocation of one or more of the tarsal joints is a relatively common occurrence in horses. The luxation is usually caused by a kick from another horse or by catching the hindlimb in a fence. Clinical signs include non–weight-bearing lameness on the affected limb, swelling over the hock, and deviation of the lower limb, either to the inside or to the outside, depending on the luxation and its exact orientation. X-ray examination of the tarsus is necessary to determine whether the bony structures within the hock have also been traumatized.

For simple luxations without fracture, the horse is anesthetized and the luxation is reduced. Luxations of the upper tarsal joint are much more difficult to treat and are often associated with fractures. Following reduction of the luxation, the limb should be placed in a long-legged cast to stabilize the structures. For horses with larger fractures, the fracture should be reduced and stabilized with screws.

The prognosis for horses with luxation without fracture is fair to good if the luxation involves the lower joints of the hock. By contrast, luxations of the upper hock joint and luxations associated with fractures have a guarded to grave prognosis for soundness.

CAPPED HOCK

Capped hock describes a traumatic bursitis over the point of the hock, usually caused by the horse's kicking a solid structure. The point of the hock is usually swollen and in the acute stages is hot and painful to palpation. Treatment consists of the application of ice, cold hydrotherapy, and the administration of anti-inflammatory medication. It is also important that further trauma to the site be prevented. Drainage of the fluid distending the bursa and local injection of an anti-inflammatory medication may help resolve the swelling. This treatment should be combined with the application of a pressure bandage. In horses with chronic cases of capped hock, treatments similar to those described for carpal hygroma (*see* above) should be instituted. These include incision and drainage of the bursa and cauterization of the inner surface of the bursa with an irritant such as iodine.

The prognosis is fair to good if horses are treated in the acute stages of the disorder. Chronic cases may have a permanent swelling at the site, although rarely if ever is there any lameness.

PERONEUS TERTIUS RUPTURE

The *peroneus tertius* is a tendon that flexes the hock when the stifle is also flexed. When the peroneus tertius is ruptured, the stifle will flex but the hock does not. Rupture of the peroneus tertius occurs secondary to overextension of the hock, as may happen if the leg is caught behind the horse as the horse then struggles to free itself. Rupture may also occur while a horse is wearing a long-legged cast and catches the cast behind itself in attempting to rise.

The diagnosis is made during the physical examination by flexing the stifle with the hock in extension. Often a "dimpling" of the powerful *Achilles tendon* can be observed during this maneuver, just above the point of the hock.

Treatment involves strict box-stall confinement for 6 to 8 weeks, followed by limited exercise for an additional 2 months. The prognosis is good to guarded. Horses that respond to such conservative therapy usually can return to their previous level of performance. By contrast, horses that do not respond within 2 to 3 months may never heal and should be given a guarded prognosis.

STRINGHALT

Stringhalt describes a condition wherein a horse involuntarily hyperflexes the hock as it walks. The cause of this disorder is unknown, although it is suspected that the primary abnormality lies in the nervous system. In North America cases are usually seen as isolated occurrences. This is in contrast to New Zealand and Australia, where actual outbreaks of stringhalt occur in groups of horses during the late summer and autumn.

Individual horses are affected to variable degrees. Some have only a mild flexion of the hock, while others exhibit such marked jerking of the limb that they actually hit the belly wall with the fetlock. The signs are usually exaggerated if the horse is backed or turned. The diagnosis is easily made.

Treatment involves surgical **resection** (cutting, removal) of a portion of the lateral digital extensor tendon. This tendon is not necessary for normal limb use, and its removal often improves an affected horse's gait. The prognosis is guarded to good. Almost all horses improve following surgical resection, although some may retain a degree of abnormality in their gait. It is difficult to predict before surgery which horses will fully improve and which will not.

Disorders of the Tibia

TIBIAL FRACTURES

Fractures of the tibia are a relatively common occurrence in horses. They most commonly result from external trauma, such as a kick, or from a combination of compression and twisting such as might occur during a fall or by stepping in a hole. The diagnosis is relatively straightforward for complete fractures. Affected horses are typically non–weight-bearing on the affected limb. Swelling over the tibia is often present. Crepitus may be evident upon manipulation of the limb. Foals with growth-plate fractures of the tibia often have a severe angular deviation of the limb centered at the fracture. Partial or incomplete fractures of the tibia are often more difficult to diagnose. In such cases horses are usually lame but exhibit only minimal swelling over the tibia.

Diagnosis is based on the history, physical examination, and results of X-ray studies. Treatment is dependent on the nature of the fracture and the age of the horse. Usually two bone plates are needed to give hope of stabilizing the fracture (conservative management using splints and casts is largely unsuccessful since it is impossible to immobilize the stifle joint). For some growth-plate fractures in foals, stall rest or application of a single bone plate may be sufficient to provide healing of the fracture.

The prognosis for tibial fractures in mature horses is poor. Even in the best of circumstances, stabilization of tibial fractures in adult horses is difficult to achieve. By contrast, foals have a fair prognosis for long-term survival and soundness.

OSSIFYING MYOPATHY

Ossifying myopathy describes a condition that most commonly affects the hindlimbs of horses where scarring and/or bone formation occurs within injured muscles. Affected muscles can include the semitendinosus, semimembranosus, and biceps femoris, each of which courses along the back of the thigh. Injuries of this nature are most commonly suffered by horses that perform "stop-and-go" performance work, such as Quarter Horses.

Affected horses exhibit a short, "slapping" gait in the hindlimbs. Typically a horse advances each limb normally, then suddenly pulls it backwards and slaps it onto the ground. The gait is most noticeable at a walk. Palpation of the musculature over the back of the thigh will reveal a firm scar or ossified structure in the affected area. Horses that have had the condition for a long time may also exhibit a secondary lameness associated with pedal osteitis or bruised soles (*see* above). The secondary conditions occur because of the hard slapping of the hoof wall on the ground.

Treatment consists of surgical resection of the semitendinosus tendon at the level of the stifle, which frees the damaged muscle and allows for a freer gait. The prognosis is guarded. Most horses exhibit some improvement following surgery, although only about half of horses so treated ultimately return to complete soundness.

Disorders of the Stifle

UPWARD FIXATION OF THE PATELLA
Upward fixation or displacement of the **patella** (knee cap) may occur in any breed or size of horse, although ponies appear to be more frequently affected. Fixation of the patella over the end of the femur prevents flexion of the affected hindlimb, effectively locking the leg in extension. The cause is often related to conformation, in that horses with a straight hindlimb appear to be predisposed. Upward fixation of the patella can also occur as the result of trauma to the patella. Debilitated horses with severe muscle wasting may also be affected by the condition.

Diagnosis is fairly obvious when the limb remains locked in extension. An affected horse cannot flex the stifle or hock, although it can flex the fetlock. Horses with periodic upward fixation of the patella are more difficult to diagnose. In such horses the leg may "catch" each time the horse places weight on the limb, but the limb does not lock into extension. The catching of the patella is most noticeable when the horse is circled. Manipulation of the stifle will usually elicit a painful response. X-ray studies of the stifle should be performed to rule out any other bony abnormalities.

Treatment is dependent on the severity of the condition. In mild cases with periodic catching of the patella, trotting exercises may increase muscle tone sufficiently to eliminate the problem. In horses that are locked or that do not respond to exercise, surgically cutting the medial patellar ligament will resolve the condition. The administration of anti-inflammatory medication is beneficial for alleviating the inflammation and pain associated with the disorder. Following surgery the horse should be rested for approximately 6 weeks in a small paddock before being put back to work. The overall prognosis is good.

PATELLAR LUXATION
Patellar luxation is a **congenital** (present at birth) abnormality that occurs only rarely in horses. The patella can displace in any direction, but most often luxates to the outside of the limb (lateral luxation). The disorder usually results from inadequate development of the lower end of the femur. Without a normal groove to ride in, the patella can move in and out of its normal position.

Clinical signs of patella luxation are dependent on the severity of the displacement. In complete luxation the horse is unable to extend the affected limb and will stand in a "crouched" position. If the luxation occurs periodically or is only partial, the horse will often move fairly normally but then suddenly lose its ability to stand on the stifle.

Diagnosis is made on physical examination. In horses with complete luxation, the patella will be readily palpable outside of its normal position. In horses with partial luxation, the patella can be manually moved outside its normal position.

Treatment involves surgical realignment of the patella. In horses with a poorly developed lower femur, it may be difficult to maintain the patella's position. Following surgery horses are usually kept in box-stall confinement for a time. The prognosis is guarded. Horses with only partial luxation, however, have a better prognosis. Some investigators feel that this disorder has a hereditary component and that owners of affected horses should be advised of this possibility.

PATELLAR FRACTURES
Fractures of the patella are a rare occurrence and usually result from direct trauma. This can be in the form of a kick or a sudden fall where the horse lands directly on the patella. Horses often demonstrate acute pain on the affected limb, with swelling present over the site. They

resent palpation of the stifle and crepitus may be present. The diagnosis is usually confirmed by X-ray studies.

Treatment is dependent on the orientation and severity of the fracture. For fractures in which the fragments are not displaced, conservative therapy in the form of rest may be sufficient to allow healing. For complete fractures with displacement, surgical fixation using screws and/or wires is recommended. Following surgery, the horse should be stall-confined for 3 to 4 months until the fracture has healed.

The prognosis is guarded. Horses with joint involvement or severely fragmented fractures have a much poorer prognosis because they may develop degenerative joint disease following surgery.

Disorders of the Femur

FEMORAL FRACTURES
Fractures of the **femur** (thigh bone) are a relatively common occurrence in horses and foals. In young horses the growth plates may be involved. The underlying cause is usually traumatic; in young horses it may be associated with halter-breaking or initial handling.

Affected horses are usually severely lame. Examination will reveal a physically shortened limb, since the fracture ends often override each other. Swelling and crepitation at the site of the fracture are usually present. Fractures of the head of the femur (the portion that fits into the pelvis) through the growth plate are much more difficult to diagnose. In these horses, shortening of the limb may be evident but crepitus and swelling may not be observed. Femoral head fractures are very similar in appearance to hip luxations (*see* below).

The diagnosis of a femoral fracture is confirmed by X-ray examination. Unfortunately, in fractures involving the upper half of the femur, portable X-ray machines may not be able to penetrate the thigh sufficiently to provide a diagnosis. In fractures of the femoral head, general anesthesia may be required to X-ray the hip joint.

Treatment is dependent on the size of the horse. Femoral fractures are very difficult to repair, and in horses weighing more than 400 or 500 pounds, humane destruction is usually recommended. For young foals, surgical repair can be performed in the form of plate, rod, or screw fixation, depending on the type of fracture. For fractures of the femoral shaft, rods and plates are often used. For femoral head fractures involving the growth plate, screw fixation may be sufficient to achieve stabilization. Following surgical repair of the fracture, horses should be box-stall confined until the fracture has healed.

The prognosis is poor to guarded. Adult horses and horses over 500 pounds have a guarded to grave prognosis and are often euthanized without an attempt at repair. Young foals have a much more favorable prognosis.

FEMORAL NERVE PARALYSIS
The **femoral nerve** supplies the muscles that extend the stifle (knee) joint; paralysis of this nerve thus results in an inability to extend the stifle. Horses affected with this condition usually stand in a "crouched" position. The most common causes of femoral nerve paralysis include trauma secondary to general anesthesia and lying on the nerve; overextension of the limb during exercise; and injury caused by a kick or slipping.

The diagnosis is made upon physical examination, with the horse demonstrating the stance described above. The diagnosis can be confirmed by electromyography (EMG) 10 to 14 days after the injury. X-ray examination should also be performed to rule out any underlying bony abnormalities.

Treatment is similar to that described for radial nerve paralysis (*see* above). In horses with paralysis of only one hindlimb, conservative management (administration of anti-inflammatory medication and DMSO) and good nursing care may help minimize inflammation around the nerve and allow return of normal function. Such treatment should be attempted for at least 30 days, in order to determine if the limb will regain nerve function. Horses that are affected in both hindlimbs can often be managed for only a short period of time before humane destruction must be considered. Unfortunately, the overall prognosis for horses with femoral nerve paralysis is guarded to grave.

TROCHANTERIC BURSITIS (WHORL BONE)

Trochanteric bursitis describes inflammation of the bursa that lies beneath the tendon of the *middle gluteal muscle* as it passes over the point of the hip. The condition occurs most often in Standardbred racehorses. It can be caused by a horse's falling on the hip, by straining of the tendon during race training, or by a direct traumatic blow to the hip, such as a kick. Hock lameness such as cunean bursitis (*see* above) in Standardbreds may also predispose a horse to trochanteric bursitis.

Affected horses are painful upon palpation of the point of the hip. They tend to rest the affected leg in flexion, and when walking or trotting will land on the inside of the hoof walls. If the condition persists the muscles of the hip become atrophied.

Diagnosis is made by the history and physical examination. Although not commonly associated with lameness, trochanteric bursitis can be confused with hock lameness or hip-joint abnormalities. In lame horses injection of the bursa with an anesthetic agent will temporarily resolve the lameness, thus making the diagnosis.

Trochanteric bursitis is treated by injection of the bursa with anti-inflammatory medication. An oral pain reliever may also be given. In severe cases the cartilage beneath the bursa can become damaged, leading to chronic pain and inflammation.

The prognosis is guarded. Horses that respond to therapy within 4 to 6 weeks may return to athletic soundness. Horses that do not respond typically remain lame for indefinite periods of time.

HIP LUXATION

Dislocation of the hip joint is relatively uncommon in horses. When it does occur, it affects ponies and young horses most frequently. Trauma, usually the result of falling or slipping, is the most common cause. Hip luxation can also result from a horse's catching a hindlimb in a fence or rope. Luxations are often associated with fractures of the **acetabulum** (the "cup" or "socket" portion of the hip joint).

Clinical signs associated with hip joint luxation include severe lameness, apparent shortening of the limb (the femur usually luxates upward), external rotation of the limb so that the toe is facing outward, and a shortened stride.

Treatment is dependent on whether or not a fracture of the acetabulum has also occurred. In horses without fracture, the luxation can be reduced under general anesthesia (often, an incision down to the hip joint is necessary to return the head of the femur to its normal position). For horses with an associated fracture of the acetabulum, euthenasia must be considered because successful surgical repair is unlikely.

The prognosis is guarded to grave. If the acetabulum is not fractured, reduction of the luxation is successful, and the horse does not luxate the joint again within the first 3 months after surgery, there may be a return to complete soundness. Most horses, however, are only useful for breeding after such an injury. If there is an associated acetabular fracture, the prognosis is grave.

Disorders of the Pelvis

AORTIC OR ILIAC THROMBOSIS

Thrombosis (blockage by a clot) of the *aorta* or *iliac arteries*, the vessels that provide the blood supply to the hindlimbs, is a rare occurence in horses today. In the past, thrombosis of these vessels occurred secondary to the migration of **strongyle larvae** (internal worm parasites) around these vessels. With the widespread use of dewormers and advent of the drug ivermectin, this condition has become very uncommon. (*See* CHAPTER 33, "INTERNAL PARASITES.")

Clinical signs associated with thrombosis include lameness that worsens as the horse exercises. The limb becomes cold owing to the decrease in blood supply. As the lameness develops the horse begins sweating and appears anxious.

Diagnosis is made on the basis of the history and physical and laboratory examinations. Treatment includes aggressive deworming with preparations designed to kill strongyle larvae. The prognosis is guarded. Some horses may reestablish blood supply to the limb and resolve the lameness, while others will deteriorate and require humane destruction.

PELVIC FRACTURES

Pelvic fractures are relatively frequent in horses, fractures of the wing of the pelvis being the most common. Wing fractures occur in older horses and are usually the result of jumping accidents. Fractures of other portions of the pelvis typically occur in young horses. The clinical signs are variable and dependent on the severity of the fracture and whether or not the hip joint is involved. For fractures of the wing of the pelvis, horses may exhibit very little lameness. However, when observed from behind they appear to have a flatter than normal hip, i.e., a so-called "knocked-down hip." If the fracture extends through the hip joint or results in displacement of the hip joint, horses will exhibit severe lameness and/or an apparent shortening of the affected limb. There is often a history of severe trauma to the affected side, such as a fall or slip.

The diagnosis may be very simple to make, as in a fracture of the wing of the pelvis, or may be much more difficult, as in nondisplaced fractures of the body of the pelvis. Diagnosis is made by means of the history and physical examination. X-ray studies of the pelvis can be pursued if the diagnosis is questionable. Unfortunately, X-ray examination of the pelvis requires general anesthesia.

At present there are no successful surgical procedures for treatment of pelvic fractures in horses. Treatment is therefore conservative, consisting of box-stall confinement to limit motion of the fracture. Horses may have to be rested for as long as a year before fracture healing occurs.

Although the prognosis for horses with pelvic fractures is guarded, young horses with fractures not involving the hip joint appear to have a better prognosis than most. Horses with fractures of the hip joint often develop degenerative arthritis and debilitating lameness. Other complications of pelvic fractures include laceration of the major vessels that course along the pelvis and a reduction in size of the pelvic canal, which may limit the ability of brood mares to foal.

SACROILIAC SUBLUXATION

The *sacroiliac joint* is the joint where the pelvis connects with the spine. There is a strong bony ligament attaching the **sacrum** (bone formed by the fusion of the sacral vertebrae, at the lower end of the spinal column) which is a portion of the spine) to the pelvis. Horses that fall, slip, or suffer injuries that cause a large twisting force on the pelvis may traumatize or rupture this ligament, resulting in a partial dislocation of the sacroiliac joint.

The clinical signs associated with sacroiliac subluxation are variable and dependent on the magnitude of the injury. Often horses are stiff, resent manipulation of the pelvis, and may be lame on one or both hindlimbs. When viewed from behind, affected horses exhibit excessive motion of the pelvis on the affected side.

Treatment is designed to allow the injured joint sufficient rest for healing of the ligament. This rest should ideally be in the form of box-stall confinement for 4 to 6 weeks. If the horse improves, it should be placed slowly back into training. For cases that do not respond to such conservative therapy, some practitioners recommend the injection of irritants into the joint to induce scarring. The sacroiliac joint exhibits very little if any motion normally, so that scarring of the joint to prevent motion usually will not adversely affect a horse's gait.

The prognosis is guarded. Horses responding to conservative therapy within 4 to 6 weeks may become sound and experience no further difficulties. Horses that do not respond or that continually reinjure the joint have a much more guarded prognosis, since continued subluxation of the sacroiliac joint will in all likelihood result in progressive and continued lameness.

CHAPTER 23

Fluid and Electrolyte Disturbances

by Gary P. Carlson

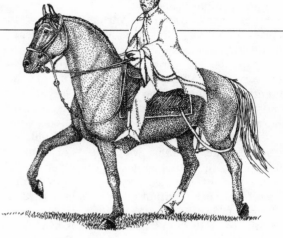

Water is an essential element for all forms of life. Approximately two-thirds of the body weight of an adult horse and nearly three-quarters of the body weight of a foal is water. The body fluids exist in two major fluid "compartments": the *extracellular* or *sodium-containing fluids*, which make up one-third of the body water, and the *intracellular fluid*, which accounts for the remaining two-thirds.

Electrolytes are simple, inorganic salts that act as charged particles in water solutions. In the **extracellular fluid** (the fluid outside cells) the two most important electrolytes are sodium and chloride, i.e., common salt. Potassium, magnesium, and calcium are largely **intracellular** (existing within cells), although their concentrations in the extracellular fluid serve important functions. It is the relative concentration of electrolytes in each of the two fluid compartments that creates an electrical charge across cell membranes—a charge that is responsible for the electrical events of the heartbeat, nerve conduction, and muscle contraction.

It is important to realize that water and electrolytes function *together* in the body fluids. As imbalances develop, changes in electrolyte content and concentration produce important physiological effects and may determine the outcome of a given disease situation.

Water Intake and Output

The normal water intake of a resting, adult horse in a temperate climate is between 20 and 30 liters per day. Since there are approximately 4 liters in a gallon, this amounts to nearly 8 gallons of water per day. Water intake is normally regulated to meet water output and is influenced by environmental factors (temperature, humidity), exercise, feed intake, and salt supplementation. Approximately 75–80 percent of water intake normally occurs within 1–2 hours of feeding time in resting horses fed hay rations twice daily. Horses fed heavy grain rations normally drink less water than those fed hay rations. Horses fed alfalfa hay as the sole feed tend to consume more water than horses fed oat or grass hay.

Horses should always have free access to fresh, clean water. Extremely fatigued, exhausted, or overheated horses should be allowed access to water in a carefully controlled manner. It is possible for these horses to rapidly consume enough cold water to produce digestive upsets that may result in abdominal pain (**colic**) or founder (**laminitis**). It is, however, a serious mistake to withhold all water from heavily worked horses in a hot or humid climate.

Fluid losses occur by a variety of routes. In horses on full feed, the principal loss of water is in the manure (normally formed fecal balls are approximately 75 percent water). The next most obvious source of fluid loss is in the urine. The quantity of urine formed depends in large measure on the amount of water consumed and on the nitrogen and electrolyte composition of the diet. Salt-supplemented horses on an all-alfalfa ration may have urinary water losses of 12 to 16 liters daily, i.e., 3 to 4 gallons of urine per day. If horses are not provided access to salt, or if they are off feed, urine output may be as little as 2 or 3 liters per day, i.e., less than a gallon. The third obvious route of fluid loss in horses is sweating. Like people, horses sweat profusely. Sweating is an essential means of regulating body temperature in the exercising horse. Substantial fluid and electrolyte losses occur with heavy sweating. Horses may lose 10 to 15 liters (3 to 4 gallons) of water *per hour* through heavy sweating.

We all know that sweat is salty, and when horses (or people) sweat they lose a large amount of salt as well as water. The chief electrolytes lost in sweat are sodium and chloride, along with some potassium. Heavy sweating can result in serious dehydration if fluid losses are not promptly replaced by voluntary consumption.

The final route of fluid loss is as "insensible" losses from the respiratory tract and skin. Fluid lost from these sources does not contain any electrolytes but is simply lost as water.

Consequences of Fluid and Electrolyte Imbalances

Dehydration refers to a loss of body water. It is said that dehydration first becomes evident when fluid loss exceeds 5 percent of body weight. In a 1,000-pound horse this would rep-resent a loss of approximately 50 pounds of water, or nearly 6 gallons. Clinical signs of dehydration become severe when the loss of fluid exceeds 10 percent of body weight. In the same horse this would be the loss of about 100 pounds of water, or just over 12 gallons.

With dehydration—particularly when there is a loss of sodium-containing fluid, as occurs in diarrhea, colic, or heavy sweat loss—there will be an abnormal decrease in the volume of blood in the circulation. This condition, known as **hypovolemia**, can have a profound effect on a horse's health and may ultimately result in the onset of **shock**. It is thus important to appreciate the clinical circumstances that might lead to severe fluid loss, and to learn to recognize some of the obvious clinical signs of dehydration.

One of the simplest and most useful procedures to evaluate the degree of dehydration is to observe the response of the horse's skin to a pinch on the neck, just in front of the shoulders, or on the upper eyelid—a procedure known as "tenting" the skin. In the normal well-hydrated horse, the pinched skin will snap back to normal very quickly, within a second or two. With slight dehydration (about 5 percent of body weight) the skin will remain raised or "tented" for 2 or 3 seconds following the pinch. With progressively more severe dehydration, up to 10 percent of body weight or more, the skin may remain tented for 5 to 10 seconds. The severely dehydrated horse will have a dry mouth and the eyes may be sunken deeper in their sockets. If these signs are evident, severe dehydration is present and veterinary assistance should be sought immediately.

There are significant differences among horses in their response to a skin pinch. Newborn foals and very thin horses have little fat under the skin. Their skin will tent up fairly markedly, certainly much more so than that of an overweight horse with a great deal of fat under the skin. *It is important for an owner to assess how a horse responds to tenting of the skin under normal circumstances, so that a dehydration abnormality, if and when it occurs, can be easily recognized.*

The heart of a horse normally beats between 30 and 40 times per minute. The heartbeat can be felt with the palm placed on the chest wall just behind the left elbow; the heart itself can be heard with a stethoscope or with the ear pressed against the chest. It is also possible to measure the pulse rate in the **digital arteries** of the feet or the **submandibular artery,** which runs along the inner aspect of the lower jaw. A persistent elevation of the heart rate above 60 beats per minute in a nonexcited, nonexercised horse may be an indication of dehydration.

Elevating the upper front lip of the horse will expose the gums, which normally are pink in color. With dehydration and the onset of shock, the gum color may change from pink to an injected red, and finally to a bluish, almost purple hue. The bluish color is a sign of serious dehydration or **systemic** (bodywide) illness. If thumb pressure is applied to the gums they normally will blanch. The time it takes for the blanched area to return to a normal pink color after thumb pressure is removed is called the **capillary refill time.** In a normal horse the capillary refill time ought to be less than 1 or 2 seconds. In a dehydrated horse it may be as long as 3 or 4 seconds—an indication of serious fluid and electrolyte deficits.

Clinical Conditions in Which Fluid and Electrolyte Disturbances Play a Major Role

FOOD AND WATER DEPRIVATION

Food and water deprivation may occur under a variety of circumstances, from the severely injured animal that is unable to reach the water trough to horses with **choke** (physical blockage of the esophagus) or neurologic dysfunction that are unable to eat or drink. Management deficiencies in which water pipes freeze or horses are inadvertently locked in an area without access to water can result in dehydration. In all but extremely hot or hot and humid conditions, horses can withstand 2 to 3 days of water deprivation without major adverse effects. If the environmental temperature and humidity are high or if the horse has been exercising, dehydration can occur quickly if water is not readily available.

Until profound dehydration develops most horses remain bright and responsive. There usually will be a marked decrease in the amount of manure and urine produced. The abdomen will often have a tucked-up appearance. Unless there are neurologic disturbances, a dehydrated horse usually is very thirsty when water first becomes available. Some care should be taken to provide water that is not extremely cold. It also should be provided in graded amounts so that the horse can begin to replace its fluid deficits without causing digestive disturbances. (*See* CHAPTER 26, "THE DIGESTIVE SYSTEM AND VARIOUS DISORDERS.") In circumstances in which horses are unable or unwilling to eat or drink, it may be necessary to provide water intravenously or through a stomach tube.

WEAK, ILL, OR INJURED NEWBORN FOALS

Newborn foals represent a special circumstance. Any injury or condition that makes them too weak to rise and nurse will quickly result in serious dehydration. Newborn foals are dependent on the mare's milk for water, electrolytes, and energy. They have very high energy requirements and very low energy stores. If they are not able to nurse frequently, newborns will not only become dehydrated owing to the lack of fluid intake but also will become energy deficient. Blood **glucose** (sugar) will drop to critically low levels and they may lapse into a coma. It is imperative that newborn foals be able to rise and nurse frequently (normally several times an hour). If they are unable to do so, they must be supplied with fluids. If they can be assisted to stand, it is best for them to nurse on their own. If they are unable to stand but can remain in a **sternal position** (resting on the breast bone) while lying down, it is possible to feed them from a bottle. If they are unable to assume a sternal position or lack a strong suck response, veterinary assistance should be obtained so that the life-saving fluids can be provided by stomach tube or by intravenous administration.

COLIC

Colic is a broad term indicating abdominal pain. It is often associated with a blockage of the intestine or displacement of the bowel. This can lead to an accumulation of fluid and gas within the intestine at a time when the horse is unable to take in fluids to meet continuing losses. Horses with milder forms of colic normally remain relatively well hydrated. Those with a more serious form of the disease—such as a twist or **torsion** of the intestine, causing a blockage and loss of local blood supply—become dehydrated very quickly and enter a stage of shock. It will be necessary to provide intravenous fluids to correct these deficits. (*See* CHAPTER 26, "THE DIGESTIVE SYSTEM AND VARIOUS DISORDERS.")

ACUTE DIARRHEA

Diarrhea can result from a variety of causes. So long as a horse eats normally and drinks readily, it will often be able to maintain a relatively normal state of hydration despite rather large fluid losses from diarrhea. But as the horse becomes more depressed, goes off feed, and fails to drink adequately, the continuing fluid losses can rapidly lead to serious, even life-threatening, dehydration. The fluids that are lost with diarrhea contain a substantial amount of salt and it is important that this be replaced along with the water; thus, supplemental salt should be made available. It may also be advisable to provide a dilute salt solution in addition to fresh, clean drinking water to encourage fluid intake during the course of the diarrhea. Horses with severe diarrhea should receive veterinary attention as soon as possible.

EXHAUSTIVE DISEASE SYNDROME

Endurance horses, three-day event horses, and horses on long trail rides may develop a significant level of dehydration, owing both to massive losses of fluid and electrolytes in sweat and to decreased fluid intake. One of the most reliable indicators of impending exhaustion in endurance horses is the recovery of the heart rate once the horse has arrived at a rest stop. Ordinarily the heart rate should decrease to below 60 beats per minute within 15 to 20 minutes of entering a rest stop. *A persistent elevation of the heart rate during this time period is an indication of significant fluid loss.* Clinical signs of this *exhaustive disease syndrome* include:

- Depression and dehydration
- Little interest in food or water despite apparent dehydration
- Decreased intestinal sounds, often with muscle cramps or spasms
- Rectal temperature significantly elevated (in some cases exceeding 41°C [106°F]) for a substantial period of time

Affected horses may exhibit evidence of prior sweating but may not be actively sweating at the time they are examined. Those with persistently elevated temperatures may require external cooling in the form of cool water that is sprayed over the body.

Problems can develop on long rides in poorly conditioned horses, or on long rides when it is particularly hot or hot and humid. Such factors can contribute to excessive sweat losses and the development of dehydration and electrolyte disturbances. As a horse owner it is important to recognize dangerous circumstances, to provide adequate numbers of rest stops with opportunities to drink, and to assess the response of the horse to the ride and environmental conditions. Exhaustion is a serious problem, and if it is suspected, veterinary attention should be sought as quickly as possible. It is always better to recognize a problem at an early stage, when simply getting off the horse and providing it with some external cooling, food, and water may be all that is required.

CHAPTER 24

The Nervous System and Various Disorders

by Sherril L. Green

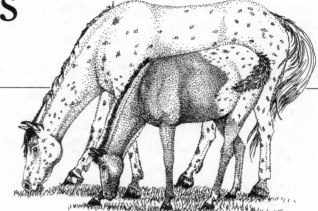

The Nervous System

The nervous system of the horse can be divided anatomically into two complex interconnected systems, the **central nervous system (CNS)** and the **peripheral nervous system (PNS)**. The CNS is composed of the *brain* and *spinal cord*, while the PNS consists of the *cranial*, *spinal*, and *peripheral nerves* supplying the muscles and body organs.

The brain is the ultimate control center of the body. It maintains consciousness, governs behavior, and coordinates voluntary movements and gait. It also regulates **autonomic** nervous processes, i.e., those that do not require conscious control, such as regulation of body temperature, food and water intake, heartbeat, breathing, sleep cycles, production of **hormones** (molecules produced by an organ or tissue, usually in extremely small quantities, that have specific regulatory effects on the activity of another organ or tissue), and passage of food through the digestive tract. Neurologic disorders can overtly affect a horse's mental status or gait or its ability to regulate autonomic nervous functions.

The brain and spinal cord are encased within the *skull* and the *spinal column,* respectively. The spinal column is composed of a lengthy series of blocklike bones called **vertebrae**, each with a central opening through which the spinal cord runs within the **vertebral canal.** Both the brain and spinal cord are covered by a tough outer layering of tissues called **meninges** and are bathed in a watery liquid called **cerebrospinal fluid (CSF).** These features help protect the CNS from invasion by infectious disease agents, exposure to toxins, and the concussive forces of direct trauma. The peripheral nerves are also covered by a tough outer sheath of tissues and are further shielded by the surrounding bones and muscles. Despite such protective features, the unique vulnerability of nerve cells (**neurons**) and their general inability to repair and regenerate limit the capacity of the nervous system to recover following an injury. Signs of a neurologic disorder thus warrant immediate veterinary attention, since the best hope for restoring optimal neurologic function is early diagnosis and treatment.

The diagnosis of neurologic disease is based on the history, physical examination, and a neurologic examination. A primary aim of the neurologic examination is to determine the location of the disease within the nervous system. The examination includes the evaluation of:

- Mental attitude and behavior, which assesses higher brain systems
- Cranial nerves, in which the visual and auditory systems, and other nervous system functions involving the head, are examined
- Spinal nerves, in which muscle tone, reflexes, and skin sensation are tested
- Gait analysis, which tests coordination and strength of the limbs

Once the general location of the disorder within the nervous system has been determined, further neurodiagnostic tests may be performed, including:

- Collection of a CSF sample
- Skull, neck, spine, or long bone **radiographs** (X rays)
- **Electromyography**, which tests the electrical function and nerve supply of muscles

Nervous System Disorders

Fortunately for horses and their owners, the incidence of neurologic disease in horses is relatively low when compared to the many respiratory, orthopedic, and gastrointestinal disorders. However, because horses with neurologic dysfunction may be unable to rise, eat, or drink, may lose athletic usefulness or become a danger to themselves or their handlers, they often must be humanely destroyed. For this reason equine neurologic disease is of special concern despite its low incidence. The diseases discussed in this chapter represent some of the most common neurologic disorders seen in horses, with the exception of rabies and eastern equine encephalomyelitis (EEE). These latter two diseases are uncommon in horses but are of public health concern.

FAMILIAL/INHERITED DISORDERS

Cerebellar Abiotrophy
This is an inherited disorder, seen in some Arabian family lines. It is caused by loss of neu-

rons in the **cerebellum** (the part of the brain responsible for the coordination of movement). The signs usually are recognizable in foals older than 1 month of age. Affected animals assume a wide-based stance at rest and exhibit jerky, rhythmic head movements and an uncoordinated gait. There is no effective treatment. Affected foals should be humanely destroyed.

Hyperkalemic Periodic Paralysis
This is a familial, inherited disease of heavily muscled, stock-type horses such as American Quarter Horses, Appaloosas, and Paints. It is characterized by intermittent episodes of muscular weakness and **fasciculations** (frequent small, localized muscle contractions), accompanied by transient elevation of the blood potassium concentration (**hyperkalemia**). Episodes may be precipitated by exercise or a period of rest after exercise. The disease does not appear to be fatal in most cases; however, it may limit a horse's athletic usefulness.

Cervical Vertebral Malformation
This disorder, also called **wobbles** or **wobbler syndrome**, is a common cause of incoordination in young horses, particularly Thoroughbreds. The neurologic signs result from spinal cord compression caused by narrowing of the vertebral canal, malalignment of **cervical** (neck) vertebrae, or **proliferation** (excessive growth) of surrounding soft tissue. The underlying cause is probably multifactorial in nature. Familial predisposition, high dietary energy intake, and injury to the cervical vertebrae and spinal cord probably all play a role. Young, large, fast-growing animals (often males) are most commonly affected. They may appear "clumsy" in the hind end. A recent accident or injury to the horse's neck is sometimes reported by the owner. Surgical techniques have been developed to treat wobbler syndrome, but the success rate is moderate at best. Surgically treated wobblers may improve neurologically, but residual neurologic deficits often persist. The prognosis in general is poor.

Equine Degenerative Myeloencephalopathy
This is a disease of young horses of any breed, although a familial tendency has been observed

in certain Appaloosa, Standardbred, and possibly Morgan lines. The cause is thought to be related to a vitamin E deficiency and is associated with lack of green forage or the feeding of heat-processed pelleted rations. Loss of neurons in the **brain stem** (basal portion of the brain) and spinal cord result in gait abnormalities. The disease is chronic and progressive, but clinical signs usually stabilize once the animal reaches about 1 year of age. Affected horses are otherwise in good health. Some signs may improve or stabilize with vitamin E supplementation. (*See* CHAPTER 8, "DISEASES OF DIETARY ORIGIN.")

INFECTIOUS DISORDERS

Equine Encephalomyelitis

Western equine encephalomyelitis (WEE), eastern equine encephalomyelitis (EEE), and *Venezuelan equine encephalomyelitis (VEE)* are virus-induced diseases of the brain and spinal cord. Both EEE and WEE occur in the United States. VEE occurs in Central and South America but has not been diagnosed in the United States for more than twenty years. The causative viruses are transmitted by mosquitoes and occasionally other blood-sucking insects to horses (or people) from wild birds and rodents, which serve as reservoir hosts. These diseases thus are of public health significance because human beings as well are susceptible to infection.

Outbreaks of equine encephalomyelitis tend to occur in late summer. EEE, WEE, and VEE overall are similar in their clinical manifestations, differing only in detail and degree of lethality (EEE being associated with a particularly high mortality rate, i.e., up to 90 percent). Infected horses develop fever, inappetence, depression, elevated heart rate, diarrhea (in VEE), and abnormalities in white blood cell counts. The animals become unresponsive or irritable. Head-pressing, leaning on walls or fences, compulsive circling, or blindness may occur. Death is usually preceded by coma and convulsions. Horses that survive often have residual neurologic deficits. There is no effective therapy. For prevention, **inactivated** ("killed") vaccines against both EEE and WEE viruses are available in the United States. (*See* CHAPTER 30,

"VIRAL DISEASES," and APPENDIX B, "VACCINATIONS AND INFECTIOUS DISEASE CONTROL.")

Rabies

Rabies is a viral disease primarily of bats and carnivores, the latter including the domestic dog and cat. In most of the developing nations, domestic dogs are the primary reservoir hosts for rabies and the principal source of human exposure. Rabid animals shed large amounts of rabies virus in saliva, which accounts for the primary means by which the virus is transmitted, i.e., by the bite of an infected animal. For both animals and people, rabies is an inevitably fatal illness once clinical signs are evident.

Fortunately, rabies occurs only rarely in horses. In most cases it is transmitted by the bite of an infected wildlife host. Less frequently a domestic dog or cat is the source. The range of signs seen in equine rabies can make it a difficult problem to diagnose (and thus an especially dangerous one for owners and veterinarians). Aggressiveness and indiscriminate attack are suggestive clinical signs, but rabies in horses is not always associated with aggressive behavior. Signs often include progressive gait abnormalities and incoordination, lameness, colic, hypersensitivity, or fever. Loss of tail and **anal sphincter** (circular band of muscle surrounding the anus) tone, and loss of sensory perception in the hind limbs also occur. Death is due to cardiac or respiratory arrest 4 days or so after the onset of clinical signs.

Rabies is a reportable disease. Horses exhibiting suspicious signs or with confirmed exposure to a suspected rabid animal should be isolated and the proper public health authorities notified. The diagnosis can only be made following **necropsy** (animal autopsy), using specific tests performed on brain tissue. Annual vaccination of horses against rabies is recommended in geographic areas where wildlife rabies is prevalent. (*See* CHAPTER 30, "VIRAL DISEASES," and APPENDIX A, "ZOONOTIC DISEASES: FROM HORSES TO PEOPLE.")

Equine Herpesvirus Myeloencephalitis

The cause of *equine herpesvirus myeloencephalitis,* an inflammatory disorder of the brain and spinal cord, is the abortion-inducing strain of equine herpesvirus type 1 (EHV–1). Respiratory disease or abortion outbreaks (abortion "storms") may or may not precede the onset of neurologic signs, which include fever, abnormal gait, "dog-sitting" (hind end on the ground), and recumbency. Decreased tail tone and loss of sensation around the **perineum** (region between the thighs encompassing the anus and genitalia) may be evident, along with constipation. Signs involving the head (cranial nerve dysfunction, depression, head tilt) are less often observed. Affected horses generally are alert and responsive and have a good appetite. Complete recovery is possible, although there may be residual neurologic deficits. (*See* Chapter 30, "Viral Diseases.")

Tetanus

Tetanus is an acute, often fatal disease caused by a **neurotoxin** (toxin targeting the nervous system) produced by the bacterium *Clostridium tetani*. This bacterium is a normal resident of the soil and is also found in small numbers amid the bacterial population of the lower gastrointestinal tract. In general, bacterial contamination of dead or dying tissue in a penetrating wound is the most common means by which tetanus is produced. **Spores** (survival forms) of *Clostridium tetani*, which are widely present in the soil, soon **germinate** (grow into mature bacterial forms) after entering a wound. Germination is accompanied by production of the neurotoxin, which affects neuromuscular responses in different areas of the body. The toxin blocks nerve impulses that normally inhibit muscular contractions. As a result the large muscle groups are trapped in a state of contraction, which is often accompanied by prolonged, painful spasms.

The clinical signs are characterized by gait stiffness, but generally progress to include elevation of the tail head, erection of the ears, **trismus** ("lockjaw"), flaring of the nostrils, and **prolapse** (protrusion) of the **third eyelid** (located in the inner angle of the eye, between the lower eyelid and the eyeball, and normally pulled back out of view). Difficulty eating and drinking, muscle tremors, and fever often develop, with recumbency and death rapidly ensuing.

The prognosis for survival is better if an affected horse receives early veterinary care, remains **ambulatory** (able to walk) and able to eat and drink, and has been vaccinated against tetanus within the previous year. Owing to the extreme susceptibility of horses to tetanus and the potential for wound contamination, yearly immunization is advised. Since the advent of commercially available tetanus vaccines, occurrence of this highly fatal disease in horses has become much less common. (*See* Chapter 31, "Bacterial Diseases.")

Parasitic Disorders

Equine Protozoal Myeloencephalitis

This inflammatory disorder is caused by infection of the brain and spinal cord with a poorly characterized protozoan parasite, tentatively designated *Sarcocystis neurona*. The life cycle and mode of transmission of the organism are unknown, so the source of infection remains unidentified. Affected horses develop incoordination, muscle weakness, and occasionally behavior changes. Therapy is based on the use of medications known to have an effect on other, possibly similar protozoan parasites, such as *Toxoplasma gondii*. Many horses relapse after therapy is discontinued, however. Humane destruction of the horse may be required owing to muscle **atrophy** (shrinkage or wasting) and loss of athletic capability. (*See* Chapter 33, "Internal Parasites.")

Toxic/Nutritional Disorders

Leukoencephalomalacia

Also known as *cornstalk disease*, *moldy corn poisoning*, *forage disease*, or *blind staggers*, this is a sporadic cause of mortality in horses. The underlying cause appears to be a toxin produced by the mold *Fusarium moniliforme*. This mold grows on the kernels of cereals (particularly corn) that have been damaged by drought and insects and that are subsequently harvested under conditions of high moisture or humidity. Clinical signs include inappetence, depression, incoordination, abnormal gait, cranial nerve dysfunction, blindness, and **mania** (frantic behavior). Seizures, recumbency, and coma precede death. There is no treatment for this disorder and the prognosis is grave. (*See* CHAPTER 8, "DISEASES OF DIETARY ORIGIN," and CHAPTER 32, "FUNGAL DISEASES.")

Yellow Star Thistle Poisoning
In horses, ingestion of yellow star thistle (*Centaurea solstitialis*) or Russian knapweed (*Centaurea repens*) causes destruction of specific areas of the brain. Affected horses usually have been eating the plants for several weeks and may be addicted. Characteristically, jaw tone becomes rigid and the animal cannot chew, open, or close its mouth completely. Horses may try to lap feed and water with the tongue, the lips retracting to produce a "smiling" appearance when attempting to eat. Aimless wandering or compulsive circling may also be seen. Death usually occurs due to starvation and dehydration. There is no specific therapy. Affected horses should be humanely destroyed. (*See* CHAPTER 41, "POISONOUS PLANTS.")

TRAUMATIC DISORDERS

Head Trauma
Of all the neurologic conditions affecting horses, trauma is probably the most frequently encountered. A horse that has fallen over backwards and landed on its **poll** (back of the head) may remain recumbent and semiconscious for varying lengths of time. If it is successful in its attempts to stand, it may exhibit profound depression and a wide-based stance, along with a head tilt, circling, leaning toward the affected side, or facial paralysis. Occasionally, seizures will occur after head trauma. The prognosis for horses with head trauma is guarded, particularly if stupor or coma persists beyond a few days, or the pupils of the eyes become fixed and **dilated** (enlarged or widened). A head tilt associated with a skull injury may persist indefinitely, although many horses seem to accommodate quite well.

Vertebral Fractures
Fractures of the cervical and **thoracolumbar** (upper trunk and back) vertebrae are quite common injuries in horses. Horses (or foals) with fractured vertebrae will exhibit a range of neurologic signs, broadly characterized by incoordination and paralysis. In general clinical signs are more likely to be present if concomitant spinal cord injury has occurred. **Radiography** (X-ray studies) often is helpful in determining the site of the fracture. However, it is not always practical for veterinarians to obtain X rays in field situations. Determining the site of the injury in such cases relies therefore on careful examination of the clinical signs exhibited.

The prognosis for spinal cord trauma associated with fractures or **luxations** (dislocations) of vertebrae is guarded. Patients remaining ambulatory and exhibiting only mild **ataxia** (incoordination) have the best chance for complete recovery (although residual gait abnormalities may persist). If a horse remains unsuccessful in its attempts to stand after 3 to 4 days of recumbency, the prognosis for recovery is grave.

Horner's Syndrome
The term "Horner's syndrome" refers to a set of clinical signs resulting from partial interruption of the nerve supply to the eyes and head. (Johann Horner was a nineteenth-century Swiss physician who first described the syndrome in human beings.) In horses, it is characterized by constriction of the pupils and protrusion of the third eyelid. Drooping of the upper eyelid may also develop. Sweating of the face and neck on the affected side is also characteristic. Horses are particularly susceptible to Horner's syndrome because the involved nerves become quite superficial in their course down the horse's neck.

Common causes of Horner's syndrome include trauma to the neck, localized infections, foreign bodies, perivascular injection (intravenous injection of a substance wherein some of the material accidentally leaks into the tissues surrounding the blood vessel and serves as an irritant), and infection of the **gutteral pouch** (internal sac that represents an outgrowth of the **eustachian tube,** the short canal connecting the middle ear with the back of the throat that acts to equalize pressure within the ear). Reversibility of the disorder is related to the severity of the injury. In general the prognosis is good to fair, but complete recovery may require several weeks to months.

Radial Nerve Paralysis

Injury to the *radial nerve* results in paralysis of the muscles of the elbow and forearm and loss of sensation in these areas of the forelimb. A common cause is direct trauma applied to the nerve as it crosses the **humerus** (the uppermost bone of the forearm) (*see* CHAPTER 16, "ANATOMY"). Such trauma often accompanies fractures of the humerus, kicks or falls on the lateral (outer) surface of the humerus, or prolonged *lateral recumbency* (lying down, as might occur when a horse is placed on its side on a hard surface for a lengthy surgical procedure). Radial nerve paralysis may also result from:

- Stretching of the nerve secondary to hyperextension of the forelimb
- Fractures of the first rib
- Compression of the nerve by enlargement of local lymph nodes, tumors, or **abscesses** (walled-off lesions filled with pus)

Clinical signs of radial nerve paralysis include a dropped elbow, inability to draw the affected limb forward, scuffing of the toe, and inability to extend the lower limb joints. Affected horses exhibit great difficulty in the simple task of getting up and down and stand with the shoulder partially extended. The foot usually is knuckled over at rest and the animal cannot bear weight on the limb. If the injury occurs at the point of the shoulder secondary to a fracture of the humerus, the *suprascapular nerve* may be paralyzed, causing wasting of the shoulder muscles (a condition known as **sweeny**).

Treatment is purely **palliative** (aimed simply at alleviating the clinical signs, in the absence of specific treatment for the underlying disorder) and involves stall rest. The prognosis for both radial nerve paralysis and sweeny is guarded to grave, depending largely on the location and extent of the injury. If significant nerve regrowth is required for recovery, the prognosis is grave. (*See* CHAPTER 22, "THE MUSCULOSKELETAL SYSTEM AND VARIOUS DISORDERS.")

Cauda Equina Neuritis

This is an inflammation of the nerve roots at the termination of the spinal cord, a region known as the **cauda equina.** The cause is unknown, but trauma, viral infection, or abnormal immune responses may play a role. Initially, affected horses may exhibit hypersensitivity around the tail head and rump. As the disease progresses, loss of sensation around the tail and perineum is observed. The urinary bladder, **urethral sphincter** (circular band of muscle that controls release of urine from the bladder), **rectum** (lowermost portion of the gastrointestinal tract, immediately adjacent to the *anus*), anal sphincter, and penis or vulva eventually become paralyzed, leading to retention of feces and **urinary incontinence** (loss of voluntary control over urination). Dribbling of urine causes scalding of the perineum and inner thighs. Atrophy of the muscles of the hindquarters can also develop. There is no effective therapy. Affected horses often must be humanely destroyed, owing to the severity of the clinical signs, progressive nature of the illness, and poor prognosis for recovery.

CHAPTER 25

The Respiratory System and Various Disorders

by W. David Wilson and
Jeffrey E. Barlough

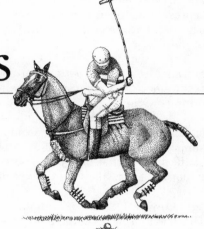

The Respiratory System

The equine respiratory system is composed of the **upper respiratory tract** (nasal passages, hard and soft palate, sinuses, pharynx, larynx, upper portion of the trachea) and the **lower respiratory tract** (lower portion of the trachea, bronchi, bronchioles, lungs, pleura). During inhalation the inspired air passes from the upper respiratory tract to the lungs, where the oxygen in the air is transported across the thin walls of the smallest airways (the *alveoli*) and into the blood. During exhalation carbon dioxide, a waste product of body metabolism, passes in the reverse direction, moving from the blood into the airways and so out of the body.

THE UPPER RESPIRATORY TRACT

The upper respiratory tract consists of the nasal passages, sinuses, hard and soft palate, **pharynx** (the back of the throat), and **larynx** ("voicebox"). The **palate** is divided into a rearward "soft" part near the larynx and a forward "hard" part (also known as the "roof" of the mouth). The soft palate separates the *pharynx* into an upper part (the **nasopharynx**) and a lower part (the **oropharynx**). The **guttural pouches** of horses are unique and represent extensions of the **eustachian tubes,** the structures that connect the nasopharynx with the middle ear and serve to equalize pressure in the middle ear with atmospheric air pressure (the opening of the eustachian tube is the "popping" sound heard in the ears when gaining altitude on a mountain road or in a small aircraft). There is one guttural pouch on each side of a horse's head, associated with each eustachian tube. The exact function of the guttural pouches remains obscure.

Within the nasal passages is a series of delicate, scroll-like bony structures known as the **nasal turbinates.** The membrane lining the turbinates is endowed with a generous nerve and blood supply and contains both fluid- and mucus-secreting glands, to moisten and warm the inhaled air and to filter out contaminating particles.

The interior of the nasal passages is divided by a vertical plane (the **nasal septum**) into two equal-size compartments called **nares**. The sense of smell originates within **olfactory nerves** found in the turbinates, the nasal septum, the sinuses, and parts of the bony nasal cavity. These nasal chambers all act to filter, warm, and humidify the incoming air. The seven **paranasal sinuses** of the horse (*rostral maxillary, caudal maxillary, frontal, sphenopalatine, dorsal conchal, middle conchal,* and *ventral conchal* sinuses) represent air-filled extensions of the nasal passages and are lined by a delicate mucous membrane.

The larynx or "voice-box" is located at the entrance to the trachea and protects the lower respiratory tract from contamination with food during swallowing, in addition to its major function in vocalization. It is composed of several cartilage-containing structures and muscles that support the vocal chords in a box-like structure at the back of the pharynx. The larynx is most important for swallowing and vocalization.

THE LOWER RESPIRATORY TRACT

The **trachea** or "windpipe" is the tubular connection between the upper and lower respiratory tracts. At its lower end it divides into two main air passageways (the *right* and *left mainstem* **bronchi**) leading to the right and left lungs. Within the lungs the mainstem bronchi branch into smaller bronchi and ultimately into small airways known as **bronchioles**. The mucous membranes lining the upper airways, trachea, and bronchi are important for trapping inhaled particles, which can potentially damage the gas-exchange areas of the lung. The airways from the trachea to the bronchioles are covered by specialized tissue containing many tiny, hair-like projections called **cilia**. An important function of this tissue is to generate the **mucociliary escalator** (a forceful, coordinated wave-like movement of the cilia) that, together with the cough reflex and the mucus coating, is essential for clearing debris, bacteria, and mucus from the airways.

Within the lungs the bronchioles terminate in tiny, thin-walled air sacs known as **alveoli** (singular = **alveolus**). Each alveolus is enmeshed in an intricate network of delicate blood vessels (**capillaries**) and is lined by a single layer of cells. When oxygen in inhaled air enters the alveoli it moves across this thin layer of cells

and into the capillaries, thereby entering the bloodstream. Conversely, carbon dioxide within the capillaries is transferred in the opposite direction into the alveoli, from where it passes up the airways and is exhaled.

The inner surface of the chest cavity and the surfaces of the organs within the chest are covered by a thin, continuous, transparent membrane called the **pleura**. Normally a small amount of lubricating fluid is present in the potential space (the **pleural cavity**) between the pleura covering the organs (the **visceral pleura**) and the pleura lining the chest cavity (the **parietal pleura**). The volume of fluid is maintained by a delicate equilibrium between production and reabsorption. A disturbance in any of several factors maintaining this equilibrium can result in excessive fluid accumulation in the pleural cavity, a disease condition known as **pleural effusion.**

Disorders of the Respiratory Tract

SINUS EMPYEMA (SEPTIC SINUSITIS)

Sinus empyema (pus in the sinus) is by far the most common disease of the paranasal sinuses. It occurs in horses of all ages but the peak incidence is in young adults. No breed or sex predilection has been recognized. The underlying cause in many cases is dental disease, e.g., tooth-root infection, periodontal disease, or extension of infection from other sites. Other causes include trauma, penetrating foreign bodies, and complications resulting from tumors or cysts. Clinical signs include a **unilateral** nasal discharge (i.e., a discharge from only one nostril), which is often malodorous; head-shaking; facial asymmetry and distortion, with swelling over the affected sinus; and weight loss. Diagnosis is based on the history, clinical findings, and the results of supportive tests, which may include sampling of the sinus contents and/or **radiography** (X-ray studies).

Cases without dental involvement A **catheter** (thin, flexible tube) is inserted through a hole drilled into the affected sinus so that the sinus can be flushed and drained daily for 1–2 weeks. An appropriate antibiotic should be given concurrently to help speed recovery. Feeding the horse on the ground and light exercise may promote drainage of the sinus. If the problem persists despite these efforts, surgical exploration of the sinus may be necessary.

Cases with dental involvement Extensive infection, inflammation, and **necrosis** (tissue death) within the sinus are often present in such cases, precluding treatment by sinus drainage and antibiotics alone. Removal of the diseased tooth is then necessary.

Most affected horses make a satisfactory recovery with treatment, but resolution of the clinical signs may require a lengthy period of time. Facial swelling and evidence of impingement on the upper airway (such as reduced airflow through one nostril or a snoring noise) usually indicate more long-standing disease, and this may adversely affect the prognosis. In general, the earlier treatment is initiated the better the overall prognosis for recovery.

CYSTS, TUMORS, AND GRANULOMAS OF THE NASAL PASSAGES AND PARANASAL SINUSES

Cysts are simple, sac-like, fluid-filled cavities that can develop in any of a number of different tissues of the body. Growth of cysts in the paranasal sinuses (usually the maxillary sinus) is an uncommon condition affecting young horses less than 2 years of age and is probably **congenital** (present at birth). Typically a thick or spongy membrane, sometimes incorporating a thin **osseous** (bony) shell, surrounds the yellowish cystic fluid. Clinical signs are similar to those seen in empyema, reflecting increased pressure within the sinus accompanied by secondary bacterial infection. The nasal discharge is often intermittent and not malodorous. Diagnosis relies on X-ray studies and identification of the characteristic amber fluid on aspiration of the affected sinus. Treatment consists of surgical exploration of the sinus and removal of the cystic membrane, followed by sinus **lavage** (irrigation, washing out).

Tumors and **granulomas** (walled-off lesions characterized by the accumulation of white blood cells and fibrous tissue around an offending agent) are rare and carry a grave prognosis. Most occur in old horses. Several different types of tumors have been reported, while granulomas are usually caused by fungi of the genera *Cryptococcus* or *Aspergillus*. Clinical signs vary depending on the degree of invasiveness of the lesion; most are similar to those reported for empyema. X rays, endoscopy, exploratory surgery, and biopsy are used in diagnosis.

GUTTURAL POUCH TYMPANY

Guttural pouch tympany is a relatively uncommon condition of young animals (foals, weanlings, yearlings), seen more often in fillies of all breeds and Arabians. It is characterized by an abnormal accumulation of air at greater than atmospheric pressure that causes distension (**tympany**) of the guttural pouches. It may be the result of a congenital defect that allows air to enter but not leave the pouches. Secondary infection and empyema are potential complications. Acquired tympany secondary to inflammatory conditions can also occur.

Clinically the condition is characterized by the development of a large, soft, nonpainful swelling just behind the lower jaw, on either one or both sides of the head. The swelling can be very large and sometimes is temporarily deflated by applying manual external pressure. Often there are no other signs except for a nasal discharge (in cases with secondary infection or pneumonia). The head and neck may be held in an extended position, and **dysphagia** (difficulty swallowing), respiratory distress, and **stridor** (loud, strained, high-pitched noise on inhalation) secondary to compression may be evident. In severe cases involving dysphagia, food or milk may be aspirated into the lungs or guttural pouches and then flow out from the nostrils as the foal nurses.

Diagnosis is made on the basis of the history, clinical findings, and X-ray studies. Placement of a semipermanent catheter to drain the pouches may provide a long-term solution. In other cases surgical intervention may be necessary.

GUTTURAL POUCH EMPYEMA/CHONDROIDS

Guttural-pouch empyema occurs frequently in association with or following upper respiratory tract infections, especially *strangles* (*see* below), as an extension of a generalized infection of the mucous membrane lining the upper airways. *Streptococcus* bacteria are the most common cause. Horses of any age and breed are susceptible, but the condition is said to be more common in ponies and miniature horses. Either one or both guttural pouches can be involved. In long-standing cases the pus in the pouch(es) becomes **inspissated** (thickened, congealed) into variously sized, "cheesy" concretions known as **chondroids**.

Clinical signs include a continuous or intermittent nasal discharge from one or both nostrils (the discharge is usually worse on the affected side). It often is more profuse when the head is lowered or following exercise. Swelling behind the lower jaw, coughing, weight loss, and enlargement of local lymph nodes may also be observed. Strangles should be suspected in cases with a high fever.

Diagnosis is based on the history, clinical signs, and identification of pus in the guttural pouch(es) by endoscopic or radiographic examination. Treatment primarily involves draining and flushing the affected pouch(es). This can be done using a temporary catheter or may require surgical intervention, particularly if chondroids are present. Antibiotics are usually administered in conjunction with local treatment.

GUTTURAL POUCH MYCOSIS

Fungal infection of the guttural pouch is infrequently encountered in the western United States but occurs regularly in the Midwest and on the eastern seaboard. Globally, fungal infections are the most common guttural pouch lesion of stabled horses in Britain and many other countries. This is probably a reflection of climate, i.e., rain during hay-making encourages fungal growth on hay. *Aspergillus nidulans* and *Aspergillus fumigatus* are the fungi most commonly involved, but other fungi as well may cause guttural pouch **mycosis** (fungal disease). These agents can be isolated from the guttural pouch of normal horses; the predisposing factors that allow the fungi to become invasive remain unclear, but may include prior inflammatory disease (e.g., bacterial infection) or **vascular** (blood-vessel) anomalies. The condition is usually unilateral and occurs most commonly in mature stabled horses.

Usually the disease process has been building for several months before clinical signs become evident. The signs are often variable in nature (largely reflecting invasion of associated structures), and can include:

- Recurrent **epistaxis** (nosebleed), mild to severe. This is the most common clinical sign. It may be preceded by a nasal discharge
- **Dysphagia** (difficulty swallowing, another very common sign), respiratory distress, and stridor. These are due either to compression or to paralysis secondary to nerve damage
- Pain in the area immediately behind the jaw
- Abnormal head carriage (head held extended or low), with head-shaking, head shyness, occasionally a head tilt
- Edema and swelling of the head, caused by impaired blood circulation
- Neurologic signs secondary to nerve involvement

Diagnosis is based on the history, clinical signs, and evidence of fungal growth in the affected pouch. Samples for biopsy can be obtained by **endoscopy** (procedure wherein a small viewing tube [an **endoscope**] is inserted into the guttural pouch).

Treatment is difficult and may not be successful. Horses without an underlying vascular problem can be treated conservatively by inserting a catheter into the pouch to promote ventilation. The horses should be maintained in an open, dust-free environment (preferably outdoors). If a vascular problem is present, anesthesia or major surgery to close the affected vessel may be indicated. A few horses may recover spontaneously, but this is rare. Topical treatments may be used to supplement either conservative or surgical therapy, e.g., daily flushing of the pouch with dilute disinfectants and antifungal medications. The prognosis for survival is about 50%; for complete recovery it is less. Damaged nerves will not regenerate, although horses may be able to overcome mild degrees of neurologic dysfunction.

CHRONIC PHARYNGEAL LYMPHOID HYPERPLASIA (CPLH)

Also called *chronic pharyngitis* or *follicular pharyngitis*, this is the most commonly diagnosed cause of partial upper-airway obstruction in young athletic horses. It occurs primarily in horses under 5 years of age, with the highest incidence in 2- and 3-year-old Thoroughbred and Standardbred racehorses. The condition is characterized by an abnormal increase in size of the lymphocyte-rich tissues lining the pharynx, and as such shares a number of similarities with *tonsillitis* of children. The cause is unknown. Some authorities suggest that all horses develop the condition in their early years, and that at least the milder cases may reflect the normal physiological maturation of the immune-system cells in the pharynx.

Clinical signs of CPLH can include one or more of the following:

- A history of reduced performance or failure to achieve expected performance
- Exercise intolerance
- Upper-airway noise, usually most apparent on inspiration during or after exercise
- Coughing or "choking" precipitated by exercise
- Nasal discharge
- Difficulty swallowing

Diagnosis is based on the history, physical findings, and results of an endoscopic examination of the pharynx. Many treatments have been tried, with mixed results. The major prerequisite for recovery is prolonged rest (1–2 months). Work and training should be suspended during this time and the horse turned out in a clean, dust- and pollutant-free environment such as a grassy pasture. Antibacterial and anti-inflammatory medications may be of benefit for some patients. In some cases the medications can be delivered by spraying them into the nose (this is most often beneficial in mild cases and may permit continued training and racing). A number of other treatments have been reported, including radiation therapy and laser treatment by means of an endoscope. The diversity of reported treatments probably is an indication that none is totally satisfactory and thus raises doubts as to the clinical significance of this disease as a cause of exercise intolerance. Horses with significant exercise intolerance and/or coughing should be examined very carefully for evidence of lower-airway disease, since the presence of severe CPLH is often an indicator of disease elsewhere in the respiratory tract.

STRANGLES

Strangles is an extremely important, highly contagious bacterial disease caused by *Streptococcus equi*. It is most often a problem on breeding farms, affecting mainly young animals (weanlings, yearlings, young adults). Also known as *distemper*, strangles is characterized by inflammation of the nasal and pharyngeal mucous membranes, with swelling, inflammation, and abscess formation in the associated lymph nodes. The name "strangles" refers to the **stenosis** (narrowing) of the upper airway produced by the swollen, enlarged lymph nodes in the head, jaw, and throat regions.

Outbreaks of strangles have a tendency to cycle every few years, reflecting the proportion of immune individuals in the population at risk. Overcrowding, movement and mixing of horses from different sources, and other stressful events seem to be important predisposing factors. Outbreaks occur when young horses are densely concentrated at breeding farms, boarding stables, training centers and, less often, racetracks and shows. Strangles is highly contagious but tends to spread less rapidly than equine influenza (*see* below). The **morbidity rate** (percentage of susceptible horses that become ill) may reach 100%, but this figure depends on the proportion of immune horses in the farm population. The **mortality rate** (percentage of susceptible horses that die from the disease) is generally low (1–5%) but can be higher in severe outbreaks. On farms where new horses are constantly being introduced new cases of strangles can appear all year long, with infection carried over to each succeeding foal crop.

The strangles bacterium is most often introduced into a group by an animal that is incubating the disease, is clinically ill, or is recovering from it. Spread can occur by direct contact, by inhalation of the bacterium, and by objects (feeders, water buckets, tack, bedding, pitchforks), insects, animals, or people contaminated with infective discharges. Affected horses remain contagious for at least 3 weeks, but rarely more than 6 weeks, after they have clinically recovered. A small percentage of recovered horses become **asymptomatic carriers,** i.e., they are clinically healthy but shed bacteria in nasal secretions. This carrier state can last for nearly a year. Strangles bacteria are sensitive to drying and sunlight but can remain infective for several months (perhaps up to a year) in discharges deposited in a moist, protected environment.

Infection usually occurs by inhalation or ingestion of *Streptococcus equi*, which attaches to cells in the tonsils and associated lymphoid tissues in the upper respiratory tract and pharynx. The release of enzymes and toxins from the organism induces inflammation at these sites, causing **rhinitis** (inflammation of the nasal passages), **pharyngitis** (inflammation of the pharynx; "sore throat"), and fever. The organism then spreads to the draining lymph nodes in the area, where its multiplication produces **lymphadenitis** (lymph-node inflammation) and abscess formation. During the early stages the bacteria can also gain access to the bloodstream and by this means be transported to lymphoid tissue in other areas of the body.

Approximately 75% of affected horses develop a solid, enduring immunity following recovery from the disease. The remaining 25% apparently fail to develop appropriate, protective immune responses, rendering them susceptible to reinfection with *Streptococcus equi* within 6–12 months. Protection against the organism is mediated by a combination of locally produced antibodies in the upper airways and other antibodies circulating in the blood. The locally produced antibodies are directed against the *M-protein* of the organism, a protein that renders the bacterium resistant to engulfment by white blood cells. M-protein antibodies are present in the **colostrum** (first milk) and milk of immune mares and generally provide protection to nursing foals up to the time of weaning.

The **incubation period** (period between infection and when clinical signs of illness become apparent) is usually 4–14 days, but can be as short as 2 days. The fever (39.5–41°C, 103–106°F) develops early and often subsides, only to return as lymph-node swelling develops and abscesses

mature. Associated clinical signs include depression, malaise, inappetence, painful swallowing, and a profuse, cloudy nasal discharge (usually from both nostrils). The accumulation of pus in the nasal passages may cause "snuffling" or "rattling" noise in the upper airway. The pharyngitis can become so severe that the horse stands with its neck extended. Attempts to swallow food or water may be followed by retching and expulsion of the material through the nostrils.

The lymph nodes of the head and neck become hot, swollen, and painful about 1 week after infection. Fluid may ooze from the overlying skin as the abscesses in the lymph nodes mature, then rupture to release a creamy pus. The lymph-node swellings can put pressure on the upper airways and cause respiratory distress and difficulty swallowing. Abscesses around the eyes may cause swelling of the eyelids, and swelling of the lymph nodes at the entrance to the chest can compress the trachea, potentially resulting in **asphyxia** (suffocation) and death. Extension of infection to the guttural pouch is not uncommon. Infection of young foals may result in a massive **septicemia** (presence of bacteria in the bloodstream, with accompanying clinical signs of illness) and abscessation of lymph nodes in many areas of the body. The clinical signs of fever, depression, and inappetence are often most severe just before rupture of an abscess. Thereafter recovery is rapid and usually complete within 1–2 weeks if further abscesses do not develop.

The herd history and findings of fever, nasal discharge, and lymph-node enlargement with abscessation are usually sufficient to provide a tentative diagnosis of strangles in an individual horse. The following points, however, warrant additional consideration:

- Early clinical cases with fever, depression, nasal discharge, and cough are difficult to differentiate from viral infections such as equine influenza or rhinopneumonitis (*see* below)
- Swelling and abscessation of lymph nodes of the head and neck can also be caused by other bacteria, including other streptococci, *Actinobacillus*, and *Corynebacterium pseudotuberculosis*

To confirm the diagnosis of strangles, laboratory culture and identification of the causative bacterium must be performed.

Treatment relies on several important principles:

- Suspected cases, and horses in contact with suspected cases, should be immediately isolated to prevent further disease spread. The handler must not pass any infective nasal discharges on to other animals on his/her clothes, shoes, hands, feeding equipment, or tack. Completely strip the horses' stalls of bedding and other materials. Thoroughly disinfect the stalls, tack, grooming equipment, and feeding utensils. The most effective disinfectants are the phenolics, povidone iodine, chlorhexidine, and glutaraldehyde. *Bleach is not effective.* Allow the stalls to dry and leave them empty for 4 weeks.

- Rest, good nutrition, and nursing care must be provided in a warm, dry, draft-free stall. Soft, moist, palatable feeds such as bran mashes are easier to swallow and are recommended. **Analgesics** ("pain-killers") often improve appetite by reducing pain and fever. Severe cases with marked respiratory distress and/or dysphagia may require a **tracheostomy** (surgically created opening through the skin into the trachea, for insertion of a breathing tube), feeding by stomach tube, and fluid therapy. The suspect cases and in-contact horses should be kept isolated for at least 1 month after complete resolution of clinical signs.

- Abscessed lymph nodes should be lanced, drained, and flushed with a dilute povidone-iodine solution for several days until the discharge ceases. The area around the draining abscess should be protected from **scalding** (burn from a liquid) with Vaseline or a similar ointment.

If the affected lymph nodes have not abscessed, two alternatives are possible—conservative therapy and antimicrobial therapy:

- With conservative therapy, hot-packs, poultices, or linaments are used to speed abscessation. This is a reasonable course to follow in mild cases that are not markedly ill and have no evidence of airway blockage.

- With antimicrobial therapy, an antibiotic (penicillin) is administered for at least 10–14 days (i.e., for at least 5 days past resolution of clinical signs).

Caution: Inadequate doses of penicillin for too short a time only serve to suppress the disease, delaying (but not aborting) abscess formation, and possibly also increasing the risk of developing internal abscesses ("bastard" strangles, *see* below). Such a prolonged course of antimicrobial therapy is expensive, stressful, and time-consuming, and may be difficult to implement when large numbers of horses are affected

Many authorities believe that the potential for complications in strangles warrants vigorous antimicrobial therapy *combined with* the surgical drainage of abscesses. Penicillin therapy is definitely indicated in nursing foals and in severe, acute cases exhibiting fever, inappetence, depression, and partial upper-airway obstruction and/or dysphagia, without overt evidence of lymph-node abscessation. High-dose intravenous penicillin therapy is indicated in cases with severe airway narrowing caused by abscessation, where conservative therapy would be associated with an increased risk of fatal airway obstruction. All horses receiving a tracheostomy should be given antibiotics. Penicillin treatment after drainage of abscesses appears to speed resolution of the disease and reduce complications. Record the rectal temperatures of all exposed horses at least once a day. Horses exhibiting a temperature rise or other early clinical signs of strangles should be isolated and treated with penicillin for 10–14 days.

Complications occur in approximately 20% of strangles cases and are responsible for most of the deaths associated with the disease. Pneumonia is reportedly the complication most commonly resulting in death. Complications may nevertheless have a *systemic* (bodywide) impact and severe consequences. Among the latter are "bastard" strangles and purpura hemorrhagica:

"Bastard" Strangles

Abscesses can occur in areas other than the head and neck, including the **mesenteric lymph nodes** (lymph nodes associated with the intestinal tract), **mediastinal lymph nodes** (lymph nodes located in the chest), lung, brain, spleen, kidney, liver, or in the skin of the **perianal** (around the anus) region and extremities. Rupture of infected lymph nodes in the chest or abdomen can cause life-threatening **pleuritis** (inflammation of the *pleura*, the thin transparent membrane covering the lungs and lining the chest cavity) or **peritonitis** (inflammation of the **peritoneum**, the thin transparent membrane lining the abdomen and the abdominal organs). Abscesses in the mesenteric lymph nodes are the most common. The treatment of choice for internal abscesses is a prolonged (weeks to months) course of penicillin.

Purpura Hemorrhagica

This is an immunologically mediated condition that can be associated with a number of different inciting factors, most often streptococcal infections. In strangles there is good evidence that the M-protein of *Streptococcus equi* is the molecule that the disease-causing immunologic reaction is directed against. This particular complication of strangles occurs more often in mature horses than in young horses. It is characterized by **edema** (swelling), primarily of the limbs, and widespread hemorrhages, varying in severity from a mild transient reaction to a severe fatal condition. Effective treatment is often difficult in advanced or severe cases, and relapses may occur if therapy is stopped prematurely. Antibiotics and anti-inflammatory steroid medications are indicated. Supportive therapy includes leg wraps, walking exercise, nursing care, **diuretics** (medications that promote urination), and hydrotherapy.

Routine management recommendations to control strangles (as well as other equine infectious diseases) include the following:

- Maintain well-defined herd subgroups
- Limit the movement of horses to different locations
- Quarantine new arrivals for at least 3 weeks

- Keep resident mares and foals separated from visiting mares and foals
- Keep breeding stock separated from show or racing stock
- Double-fence pastures
- Provide appropriate nutrition and preventive medicine

Several inactivated strangles vaccines are currently available, but none is completely effective in preventing strangles (although they do reduce the overall incidence and severity of illness in a herd). All strangles vaccines have a tendency to cause reactions at the inoculation site, particularly if given in the neck muscles. As a result vaccination against strangles is not routinely recommended except on certain premises, particularly breeding farms where the disease has become a continuing problem, or in individual horses that are being transported to a high-risk facility. (For immunization recommendations *see* APPENDIX B, "VACCINATIONS AND INFECTIOUS DISEASE CONTROL").

VIRAL RESPIRATORY DISEASES

Viral infections of the equine respiratory tract occur frequently and are among the major causes of economic loss to the equine industry. The clinical signs caused by the different viruses are similar, so that it is not possible to distinguish between the different infections on the basis of the signs alone. Antibody testing and appropriate virus isolation procedures are required for making a definitive diagnosis. Currently available vaccines are not completely effective in controlling equine viral infections, in part because the immunity conferred by vaccination is short-lived. Management practices at breeding farms, racetracks, boarding stables, and shows virtually ensure a high contact rate and dissemination of infections. The increased number and concentration of light horses and rapid national and international transportation also have contributed to the apparent increase in occurrence of viral infections of the equine respiratory tract during the last decade. Equine influenza virus and equine herpesviruses (**EHV**) types 1 and 4 are the most common and important causes of viral respiratory disease in horses. Of lesser importance are equine arteritis virus (**EAV**), equine rhinoviruses, and equine adenoviruses. (*See* CHAPTER 30, "VIRAL DISEASES.")

The clinical picture of the different viral respiratory diseases can vary considerably, depending on the **virulence** (ability to cause disease) and dose of the infecting virus, age of the horse and its level of acquired immunity, and environmental and management factors. What is typically observed is a rapidly spreading respiratory illness involving many horses, frequently following the introduction of one or more new horses onto a farm. (When a high degree of immunity is already present in a herd, only a small proportion of the horses will be affected.) Signs are of sudden onset and include cough, nasal discharge, increased respiratory rate, fever, inappetence, depression, and malaise. In general younger horses are more severely affected. Other, less common signs include mild **lymphadenopathy** (enlargement of lymph nodes), muscle soreness and stiffness, limb swelling, diarrhea (in some EHV–1 and adenovirus infections), and severe pneumonia in foals (particularly with severe influenza virus infections). In some outbreaks the clinical signs are quite mild or are only precipitated by exercise, e.g., coughing and exercise intolerance. It is now well recognized that low-level infections are common with many of these viral agents and may be completely inapparent or manifested simply as poor performance.

The different viral infections cannot be distinguished on the basis of clinical signs alone. However, the following points may serve as valuable clues:

- In equine influenza, the cough tends to be more frequent and explosive than in the other viral infections. Influenza spreads with lightning-like speed among a group of horses. There may be muscle stiffness caused by **myositis** (muscle inflammation), transient limb swelling, or *anemia* (low red blood cell count). Infection with highly virulent A_2 influenza virus strains can cause severe pneumonia in horses with no previous exposure.
- In EHV–1 infections, nonrespiratory signs may be evident in members of the herd,

e.g., abortion in pregnant mares or neurologic disease.
- EAV is also associated with abortions or embryonic death, a skin rash, and swelling of the eyelids, limbs, and male genitalia.

A tentative diagnosis of a viral infection of the respiratory tract can be made when an outbreak of respiratory disease with similar clinical signs occurs in a group of horses. Confirmation of the diagnosis requires isolation of the virus in the laboratory and/or demonstration of specific antiviral antibodies in the blood (**serologic diagnosis**). Serologic diagnosis relies on the finding of a significant (generally fourfold or greater) increase in antibody in acute and convalescent samples collected 10 to 28 days apart.

Treatment is largely **symptomatic**, i.e., the specific clinical signs rather than the underlying infection are addressed. Good nursing care, clean water, and palatable feed should be provided. Affected horses should be rested in a well-ventilated environment free of dust, drafts, and odors for at least 3 weeks after the onset of clinical signs (this is the minimum length of time needed for the damaged respiratory tract to repair itself). Owners should wait at least 2 weeks after abatement of clinical signs before resuming training, which should be re-introduced slowly and only if coughing is not aggravated by the exercise. *A good rule of thumb is to allow 1 week of rest for each day the horse had a fever.* Other stresses such as transportation should be avoided during convalescence.

Antibacterial therapy may reduce secondary bacterial infections but is not routinely recommended unless severe clinical signs are observed. Persistent fever (longer than 4 days), a nasal discharge containing pus, and evidence of pneumonia or pleuritis are all indications for the use of antibiotics. Nonsteroidal anti-inflammatory medications do not have the immunosuppressive properties of corticosteroids and are often used in horses with high fever, depression, and inappetence.

Most horses recover without complications within 2–3 weeks, although their athletic performance may be less than normal for a prolonged period. Severely affected horses and those developing complications may require several months to recover completely. Complications can be greatly reduced by enforcing rest and minimizing stress. Bacterial pneumonia, pleuritis, chronic pharyngitis with persistent cough and/or nasal discharge, and guttural pouch infections are the most common complications encountered. Influenza virus infections also predispose some horses to the later development of *chronic obstructive pulmonary disease (COPD)*, also known as "heaves" or "broken wind" (*see* below).

Control and Prevention During an outbreak, affected horses should be isolated for at least 3 weeks from other, susceptible horses, preferably in a different airspace (respiratory viruses can spread 30–40 yards in aerosols produced by coughing horses). If isolation is not possible, contact between affected and healthy horses should be minimized. Separate feeding and grooming equipment and tack should be maintained. Each day the healthy horses should be fed and handled before the sick horses are attended to. No horses should be taken off the premises for a minimum of 3 weeks. Any new arrivals should be adequately vaccinated and should be isolated for at least 2–3 weeks before they are allowed to mingle with the herd.

Vaccination during an outbreak remains a controversial procedure but many favor this approach, especially if the initial cases are quickly identified and isolated. There is usually insufficient time to wait for confirmation of a diagnosis, so vaccines containing several viral agents (equine influenza virus, EHV–1, EHV–4) are often used unless there is strong evidence implicating one particular agent. Efficacy of vaccination in the face of an outbreak is based on the assumption that many horses have had previous contact with the virus involved, either naturally or through prior vaccination, and have developed a primary immune response that can now be boosted by vaccination. If the proportion of immune animals can be made sufficiently high by vaccination of unaffected horses, enough transmission "blocks" will be established to prevent efficient transmission of the virus through the herd. (Such an approach is unlikely to work when the majority of animals in the herd are young and unvaccinated, however.) Vaccination of clinically ill horses is *not* recommended.

Routine prevention is based on vaccination and enforcement of health and vaccination requirements for incoming horses. New arrivals should be isolated away from the herd for at least 2–3 weeks. Show or racing bands of horses should be kept away from broodmares and foals. Herd groups defined by function should be maintained and kept as small as possible. Overcrowding should be avoided whenever possible. The quality of barn air can be maximized by ventilation to reduce humidity and the concentration of infectious disease agents, dust, and gases. Noxious barn gases and odors can be reduced by proper drainage and sanitation. Dust can be kept to a minimum by choice of bedding and flooring and the positioning of stalls in relation to hay storage and corrals.

Vaccines are available for immunizing horses against equine influenza virus, EHV–1, and EHV–4 (*see* APPENDIX B, "VACCINATIONS AND INFECTIOUS DISEASE CONTROL"). Frequent revaccination is necessary for optimal protection. An EAV vaccine is also available for use under special circumstances when the risk of exposure is high.

Equine Influenza

Influenza viruses are **RNA** (ribonucleic acid) viruses belonging to the Orthomyxoviridae family and are classified as either type A, B, or C. (*See* CHAPTER 30, "VIRAL DISEASES.") Equine type A influenza viruses are a major cause of respiratory disease among horses worldwide. Infections occur in a cyclic manner every few years and are characterized by rapidly spreading, explosive outbreaks involving 90–100% of susceptible horses on a farm. Two subtypes of equine influenza virus, A_1 and A_2, are currently recognized. All outbreaks of equine influenza in recent years have been caused by the A_2 subtype.

The degree of existing immunity from previous exposure or vaccination determines the pattern of infection. Horses not previously exposed develop the most severe clinical signs, shed the most virus, and are the easiest animals from which virus can be isolated. Pre-existing immunity either blocks infection completely or results in development of a mild illness with restricted virus shedding. Virus shedding by clinically healthy, partially immune, infected horses is important for disease spread and persistence of infection in the general population between outbreaks. Outbreaks can occur at any time of the year but are most common during mixing, confinement, and concentration of young susceptible horses for weaning, training, transportation, showing, or sale. Such activities stress the animals and provide ideal conditions for virus transmission. Subsequent relocation of the animals to other farms, shows, or training areas then results in dissemination of infection to other groups of horses.

Immunity following natural infection lasts for only about a year, i.e., horses can be infected with the same virus more than once. There is no cross-protection between subtypes A_1 and A_2. Preventive measures are based on management to reduce the risk of introducing and transmitting infectious disease and on vaccination. All currently available commercial vaccines are **inactivated** ("killed"), contain both subtypes, and are administered by intramuscular (**IM**) injection. (*See* APPENDIX B, "VACCINATIONS AND INFECTIOUS DISEASE CONTROL.")

Equine Herpesvirus Types 1 and 4

The herpesviruses are a large and diverse group of **DNA** (deoxyribonucleic acid) viruses causing very important diseases in many species, including human beings. (See CHAPTER 30, "VIRAL DISEASES.") In horses the disease commonly called **rhinopneumonitis** is now known to represent two separate conditions caused by two different herpesviruses, EHV–1 and EHV–4. EHV–1 causes respiratory disease, abortion in pregnant mares, early neonatal death, and neurologic disease, while EHV–4 rarely causes disease outside the respiratory tract. At least three other equine herpesviruses have been recognized (EHV–2, EHV–3, and EHV–5). Of these, only EHV–2 has been associated with respiratory illness.

Both EHV–1 and EHV–4 are widespread in the horse population and most horses have been exposed to them. Infection usually occurs by either inhalation or ingestion. Young horses usually become infected during the first year of life. After an incubation period lasting 2–10 days, clinical signs of respiratory disease of variable severity develop and then resolve within a few weeks. Resistance to reinfection persists for only 3–4 months. (Reinfections typically are milder, however.) Nursing foals often have sufficient *maternal immunity* derived from the mare's colostrum and milk (*see* CHAPTER 29, "THE IMMUNE SYSTEM AND VARIOUS DISORDERS") to reduce the severity of infection and thus may exhibit few if any signs of illness.

The immune response is frequently unsuccessful at clearing herpesviruses from the body; the majority of clinically recovered horses thus remain infected, probably for life. Such *latent infections* in chronic carrier horses are very important to the spread of herpesviruses in nature and explain why disease due to EHV–1 or EHV–4 can occur in closed populations without the introduction of new horses. Chronic carriers do not exhibit clinical signs but excrete virus under stressful circumstances, e.g., weaning, overcrowding, transportation, or concurrent illness.

EHV–4 EHV–4 is probably the most common cause of respiratory disease in young horses and is **enzootic** (widespread and always present, but producing disease at only low levels) in most horse populations. Outbreaks of respiratory disease occur annually, particularly in the fall and winter, and usually involve sucklings, weanlings, yearlings, and young adults on breeding farms, at racetracks, and at other assembly points. Older horses often are unaffected owing to the immunizing effect of multiple prior exposures.

Management practices largely explain the seasonal incidence of EHV–4-induced respiratory disease. Generally foals are reared outdoors in well-dispersed groups during the summer, and then are stressed when brought together in the fall for weaning, showing, training, or sales—precisely when maternal immunity is waning, making them maximally susceptible to infection. Stress-induced reshedding of EHV–4 from latent carriers or introduction of infection with new horses provides an ample source of virus. Concentration and confinement of the young horses are ideal conditions for subsequent virus transmission. Infected young stock moved to training areas, shows, and sales serve to disseminate the infection to other farms.

EHV–1 EHV–1 is enzootic on most equine breeding farms. Stress-induced reshedding from latent carriers or introduction of infected, virus-shedding horses creates a primary focus of infection. Infection of pregnant mares may lead to abortion, which creates a further focus of infection for propagation of an abortion "storm" or outbreaks of neurologic and/or respiratory disease.

Infection of the pregnant mare with EHV–1 or reactivation of a latent infection can lead to viral invasion of the placenta and fetus. The result is spontaneous abortion of an infected, "fresh" fetus 14–120 days later (usually the last trimester). Commonly the mare exhibits no signs of illness and the placenta is usually not retained. Such abortions may occur as isolated, sporadic incidents or in the form of an abortion storm affecting several mares. Infection late in pregnancy may result in the birth of a weak, nonviable full-term foal.

A neurologic syndrome caused by EHV–1 has been recognized in horses of all ages, either in sporadic individual cases or in the form of an outbreak. Neurologic disease may or may not occur in association with concurrent outbreaks of EHV–1-induced abortion or respiratory disease. The syndrome most likely reflects re-infection rather than a primary infection with EHV–1. The signs are usually of acute onset, varying in severity from mild incoordination in the hindquarters to *quadriparesis* (partial paralysis in all four limbs) and **recumbency** (lying down, unable to rise), loss of bladder function, **urinary incontinence** (loss of voluntary control over urination), and reduced muscle tone in the tail and anus. Treatment involves supportive care and short-term corticosteroid therapy. The prognosis for horses that remain standing is favorable, but poor for horses that become recumbent. The underlying lesion is a prominent **vasculitis** (blood-vessel inflammation) involving small vessels in the brain and spinal cord, leading to **ischemic injury** (injury caused by loss of blood

supply to a tissue). It is thought that certain EHV–1 strains are more likely to cause neurologic disease than are others.

Control and prevention Control and prevention of EHV–4 and EHV–1 outbreaks follow the general principles set down for all viral diseases, with the additional consideration that the products of EHV–1 abortions are important sources of infection. However, control measures for herpesviruses are less effective than they are for an agent such as equine influenza virus because EHV–4 and EHV–1 are enzootic in most horse populations and commonly establish lifelong, latent infections in healthy carriers.

Vaccination is important for disease control, but limitations still exist owing to the short duration of protection achieved. There are two major indications for vaccination of horses against EHV–4 and EHV–1:

- To prevent abortion in pregnant mares
- To prevent respiratory disease (rhinopneumonitis) in foals, weanlings, yearlings, and young performance and show horses at risk of exposure (owing to high levels of stress and contact with outside horses)

Although the current vaccines do not provide absolute protection, they do apparently modify the incidence and severity of illness and limit the occurrence of abortion storms. It should be noted that none of the available vaccines is effective in preventing EHV–1-induced neurologic disease. (*See* APPENDIX B, "VACCINATIONS AND INFECTIOUS DISEASE CONTROL.")

Equine Herpesvirus Type 2
Also known as *equine cytomegalovirus*, EHV–2 is ubiquitous in the equine population. It has been recovered from nasal scrapings and circulating white blood cells of both healthy and diseased horses. As with the other herpesviruses, a latent carrier state is common. Although the true disease significance of this virus is not yet known, it has been associated with respiratory disease in foals and with ocular and pharyngeal disorders in mature horses. It has been suggested that EHV–2 may cause immunosuppres-

sion and increased susceptibility to bacterial infections of the respiratory tract. There is also good evidence to indicate that EHV–2 may be important in enhancing latent EHV–1 (and perhaps EHV–4) infections.

Equine Arteritis Virus

Equine arteritis virus (EAV) is an RNA virus in the *arterivirus* genus (formerly a member of the Togaviridae family). The virus was first isolated from an outbreak of respiratory disease and abortion on a Standardbred breeding farm in Ohio in 1953. Infections have now been diagnosed in many parts of the world. Surveys in the United States indicate that 70–90% of Standardbred mares and stallions have antibodies to the virus, compared to only 2–3% of Thoroughbreds. The virus is highly contagious and is shed in respiratory secretions and aerosols, vaginal secretions, urine, and feces of acutely infected horses. In cases of abortion it is also present in the fetus, placenta, and placental fluids.

The two most important routes of transmission are venereal (chiefly from an infected stallion to a mare) and respiratory (in aerosolized respiratory secretions of an acutely infected horse). Venereal transmission by chronic carrier stallions represents the major means by which the virus is maintained in equine populations. Stallions become infected by the respiratory route or venereally by breeding with an acutely infected mare. A relatively high percentage of infected stallions become persistently infected and shed the virus in semen more or less continuously for months or years. Such stallions appear to shed virus solely by the venereal route and can transmit it during natural breeding or by artificial insemination. Establishment of clinical or inapparent infection in the mare is associated with a period of profuse virus shedding from the respiratory tract, resulting in transmission to herdmates. The virus is also shed from the reproductive tract, i.e., acutely infected mares can transmit it venereally to stallions. There is no evidence that a persistent carrier state similar to that in stallions can be established in either mares or foals.

In horses exhibiting illness the clinical signs can include fever, depression, inappetence, limb **edema** (swelling), stiff gait, **conjunctivitis** (inflammation of the **conjunctiva**, the mucous membrane lining the inner surface of the eyelids), **rhinitis** (inflammation of the nasal passages), nasal discharge, a skin rash (**urticaria** or "hives"), swelling of the male genitalia, swelling of the mammary glands, and abortion. Less frequently noted are coughing, respiratory distress, incoordination, and diarrhea. Affected horses usually recover within 2 weeks; deaths are rare. EAV-related abortions have been reported between 3 and 10 months of gestation. Abortion rates can be as high as 60% in some outbreaks. Lifelong immunity follows natural infection.

A modified-live vaccine is available for use as an adjunct to testing and management practices to reduce the occurrence of EAV infection and disease. Vaccination provides protection against illness for at least 1–3 years (but does *not* prevent infection) and restricts virus shedding. The primary indications for use of the vaccine are:

- To prevent clinical infection in susceptible mares being bred to carrier stallions
- To prevent establishment of the carrier state in susceptible, mature stallions
- To prevent infection by the respiratory route during outbreaks of respiratory disease

The decision to use the EAV vaccine should be carefully considered since vaccinated horses test positive in blood tests for the disease and are thus ineligible for exportation to many countries.

Equine Adenoviruses

Adenoviruses are DNA-containing viruses and are found in a wide variety of animal species. Adenovirus infections are widespread in the equine population but are only rarely associated with clinical illness. Disease is seen primarily in foals with compromised immune systems, e.g., Arabian foals with severe combined immune deficiency (*see* CHAPTER 29, "THE IMMUNE SYSTEM AND VARIOUS DISORDERS.")

Most normal foals probably acquire adenovirus infections from the mare shortly after they are born. Most of these infections are mild or inapparent, but some may be associated with cough, nasal discharge, conjunctivitis, fever, increased respiratory rate, diarrhea, and ulceration around the lips. In immunodeficient foals the signs are much more severe; secondary bacterial, fungal, or protozoal infections can lead to pneumonia, intestinal inflammation, and death.

Immunity following infection is not permanent and reinfection is common. Adenoviruses can persist for lengthy periods in equine populations isolated from outside contact, indicating that prolonged shedding by carrier horses is an important factor in transmission. There is no available vaccine.

Equine Rhinoviruses

Three distinct RNA-containing rhinoviruses, designated equine rhinovirus (ERV) types 1, 2, and 3, have been recovered from horses in recent years. They are very similar to the more than 90 different "common cold" rhinoviruses known to exist in human beings. Ample evidence indicates that infections with all three ERVs are widespread in equine populations throughout the world.

Sources of infection include clinically ill horses, healthy carrier horses, and recovered horses that are still shedding virus. ERV–1 has been isolated from the throat, feces, and urine of horses for up to a month following infection. There is evidence that a chronic infection of the urinary tract with persistent shedding of ERV–1 occurs in approximately 20% of infected horses. Inapparent infections with ERV–1 are common. Other ERV–1 infections are characterized by a fever (usually below 40°C, 104°F) lasting for 1–2 days and a copious nasal discharge. Depression, inappetence, coughing, and painful swallowing may be evident in some animals. Recovery is usually rapid and uneventful. There is no available vaccine.

LARYNGEAL HEMIPLEGIA ("ROARING")

Laryngeal hemiplegia is a paralysis affecting one side of the larynx and is caused by damage to either of the two recurrent laryngeal nerves. Although it may develop as a complication of another condition such as strangles, more often it is **idiopathic**, i.e., the original inciting cause is undetermined. Idiopathic laryngeal hemiplegia occurs mainly in males of the taller, long-necked breeds and almost always affects the left side of the larynx. Signs often become evident at 2 or 3 years of age. Why only the left recurrent laryngeal nerve is predisposed to degenerative changes in these cases is still unclear. There is some evidence, however, that inherited factors may be involved, perhaps related to conformation and the fact that the left recurrent laryngeal nerve is longer than its companion on the right.

The prominent clinical sign is a loud, strained, high-pitched sound ("roaring," "sawing," or "whistling") on inhalation that becomes evident while a horse is being exercised at a gallop (it is usually not evident at a trot). This is often accompanied by exercise intolerance and poor performance. The obvious source of the sound is the protrusion of the paralyzed laryngeal tissue into the airway, creating excessive turbulence to airflow through the upper respiratory tract and trachea.

Diagnosis is based on the history, physical findings, and endoscopic examination of the larynx to observe the protruding tissue. Over the years various surgical techniques have been developed for correcting this problem, with varying degrees of success. The technique of choice today is the **combined laryngoplasty/ventriculectomy,** in which one portion of the protruding laryngeal tissue is surgically removed while the remainder is pulled back out of the way and tied down, in order to widen the airway and reduce turbulence. Some horses may develop complications from surgery, however, including aspiration of food into the airway and/or chronic coughing; thus the prognosis for return to optimal performance is guarded.

FOAL PNEUMONIA

Pneumonia is an inflammatory condition of the lung characterized by filling of the air spaces with fluid, impeding gas exchange. It is a common problem in foals of all breeds and causes significant economic losses to the equine industry worldwide. Foals between 4 weeks and 6 months of age are most susceptible. The morbidity rate on a national basis in the United States has been estimated at about 9%, although 50% or more of the annual foal crop on an individual farm may develop pneumonia. Mortality rates of 5–15% are not uncommon. In extreme cases an outbreak may claim up to 80% of affected foals, especially when *Rhodococcus equi* is the disease agent involved (*see* below). The disease prevalence varies from year to year and from location to location, emphasizing the important roles of climate and management factors.

The causes of foal pneumonia are complex and involve interactions between a number of predisposing factors and a variety of microorganisms. Viruses such as EHV–1, EHV–4, EHV–2, equine influenza virus, equine rhinoviruses, equine adenoviruses, and possibly others, are thought to be initiating factors in many cases. By the time the foal develops signs of pneumonia, however, secondary bacterial complications have usually set in. In general viruses act by directly damaging tissue and compromising the lung's normal defense mechanisms. The bacteria then take advantage of this pre-existing damage to engineer a pneumonia. Parasites, such as *ascarid* worms (*Parascaris equorum*, or large roundworm; *see* CHAPTER 33, "INTERNAL PARASITES"), can injure lung tissue and produce a mild pneumonia during their migration through the lungs. Fungi such as *Pneumocystis carinii* may serve as opportunists in immunodeficient foals or in horses receiving prolonged antibiotic therapy.

Bacterial pneumonia in newborn foals is usually associated with generalized **sepsis** (widespread presence of the bacteria in blood and tissues) and the mortality rate is correspondingly high. Bacteria causing such severe disease include *Escherichia coli*, *Actinobacillus*, *Klebsiella pneumoniae*, and certain streptococci. Bacterial pneumonia in older foals is usually caused by opportunistic microorganisms that are either normal inhabitants of the upper respiratory tract or gastrointestinal tract, or are present in the environment. It is not unusual to find several different species of bacteria involved. *Streptococcus zooepidemicus* and *Actinobacillus suis spp.* (multiple species) represent the most important opportunistic disease agents in pneumonia affecting foals from 4 weeks to 6 months of age. *Streptococcus equi*, the cause of strangles (*see*

above), is often found in foals and young horses but is not commonly recovered from the lungs of foals with pneumonia. *Rhodococcus equi* usually causes disease only sporadically but on certain breeding farms may represent a devastating cause of foal pneumonia.

Of all the interactive environmental and management factors predisposing a foal to develop pneumonia, the most important appears to be a high ambient temperature (with or without associated humidity), in particular when dry, dusty conditions prevail. The respiratory tract in many animals is important for the regulation of body temperature and it may be that foals are less able than mature horses to tolerate extremes of climate. Harsh fluctuations in ambient temperature, such as the hot day/cold night conditions prevalent in arid regions, may exacerbate the problem. In colder climates, chilling and overprotection from the cold, e.g., blankets or reduced ventilation in a barn, also appear to be detrimental. Overcrowding may produce stress and increase the concentration of potentially dangerous microorganisms, thereby facilitating their transmission. Dust acts as an irritant to the respiratory tract and can compromise the lung's normal defense mechanisms as well as transmit infectious disease agents.

Indoors, warmth and humidity promote the survival and transmission of microorganisms. Bedding, as well as being a potential source of dust and **allergens** (substances inducing allergy), may act as a growth medium for certain bacteria and fungi. Poor stall drainage, poor sanitation, high temperatures, and faulty ventilation can contribute to the buildup of noxious gases such as ammonia, which can compromise lung defenses. Transportation, showing, and weaning produce stresses on young foals. Weaning also results in the concentration of young, susceptible animals and thus promotes disease spread. The common practice of transporting mares and foals to other farms for breeding and the mixing of visiting mares and foals or show horses with the resident foal crop also increase the likelihood of acquiring new infections. Nutrition, including overfeeding of young foals for halter shows or sales, may also play a role.

One of the most important bacteria causing

foal pneumonia is *Rhodococcus equi*. It is normally an inhabitant of the soil and can be recovered from horse feces. It is resistant to many disinfectants and tolerates a wide range of soil dryness and pH, especially when the feces of herbivores such as horses or cattle are present. *R. equi* can survive in soil containing equine feces for at least a year, if not longer. It has been recovered from the gastrointestinal tract of most grazing herbivores and appears to multiply in the digestive tract of foals. (Although it can survive passage through the intestinal tract of mature horses, its multiplication in these animals normally is inhibited). After it is passed out in the feces the organism proliferates rapidly in the fecal pat. Under ideal conditions of temperature and humidity a 10,000-fold increase in the number of organisms can occur over a period of a few weeks. On farms where *R. equi* infection is widespread, the organism has been found in highest numbers in dust from stables, holding pens, exercise areas, and aisleways where infected foals have been kept. These areas thus pose the greatest risk of infection for young, susceptible foals.

Mare feces and contaminated soil or dirt appear to be important sources of *R. equi* for colonization of the newborn foal's intestinal tract during the first few weeks of life. The **coprophagic** (feces-eating) behavior of foals may be important in this regard. This initial colonization probably does not result in infection of the foal but instead amplifies shedding of the organism in the feces of both foals and mares. This, along with reduced moisture and increased environmental temperature, promotes multiplication of the organism in fecal pats. Dry, windy conditions present during the summer months facilitate dispersal of the bacteria into the air at a time when large numbers of susceptible foals are present.

The clinical signs associated with foal pneumonia vary considerably from horse to horse and from farm to farm. The spectrum ranges from an otherwise normal-appearing foal with intermittent coughing and a mild nasal discharge, to a foal with high fever, marked depression, abnormally rapid breathing, increased respiratory effort, inappetence, profuse nasal discharge, severe respiratory distress, and **cyanosis** (bluish discoloration of the mucous membranes caused by decreased levels of oxygen in the blood).

Diagnosis is based on the history, physical examination, and the results of supportive laboratory tests. **Tracheobronchial aspiration** (retrieval of secretions from the lower respiratory tract; also called a **transtracheal wash**) with microscopic examination and culture of bacteria from the aspirated material is the most definitive diagnostic procedure available. Currently there are no diagnostic blood tests available for any of the bacterial species commonly associated with foal pneumonia, with the possible exception of *R. equi*.

Treatment requires an integrated approach in order to destroy the causative microorganisms, improve respiratory function, minimize stress, and maximize patient comfort and environmental quality. Restricting exercise is important initially in severe cases in order to reduce stress on the respiratory system. In milder cases and those improving with therapy, limited exercise may be helpful to promote **expectoration** (coughing up mucus). Confinement in a cool, clean, dust-free, odor-free, well-ventilated enclosure is indicated in order to minimize activity and exposure to the elements. Screened doors and wall panels are useful for promoting ventilation. Sprinklers can be used to control dust in paddocks and pastures. If possible, feeders should be removed to grassy areas. Dusty aisles and stalls should be cleaned and watered down regularly during hot periods. Barns with poorly insulated roofs can be cooled by water sprinklers on the roof. Confinement in an air-conditioned stall may be necessary for foals experiencing severe respiratory distress.

Antibiotics should be chosen based on herd history and the result of culture and sensitivity testing to determine succeptibility of the bacteria to an antibiotic. Antibiotic therapy should be continued for at least 1 week after clinical signs of pneumonia have resolved, i.e., it is important not to discontinue treatment too early. If an affected foal does not exhibit clinical improvement within 3–5 days after initiation of treatment, the choice of antibiotic should be reevaluated. Chronic cases of foal pneumonia in general will respond more slowly than acute cases. Nonsteroidal anti-inflammatory medications such as phenylbutazone or flunixin meglumine may be of value in limiting the inflammatory reaction within the lungs, reducing fever, and improving attitude and appetite. Maintenance of adequate hydration is important to promote normal clearance mechanisms within the respiratory tract. Medications that aid in clearing respiratory secretions are also of benefit. As a general rule, most foals with bacterial pneumonia will survive if given appropriate treatment.

The cornerstone of prevention is good herd management. This involves:

- Providing optimal hygiene and sanitation
- Avoiding overcrowding
- Reducing dust
- Strict parasite control
- Vaccinating to prevent viral respiratory infections
- Enforcing rest if viral respiratory infections do occur
- Maintaining fixed herd groups
- Separating resident horses from visiting horses
- Isolating new arrivals and clinically ill horses
- Booster-vaccinating mares against respiratory disease agents before foaling
- Ensuring adequate and early intake of colostrum by foals
- Attending to the foal's umbilical cord at foaling
- Avoiding transportation and mixing of young foals from different sources
- Providing adequate shade for horses pastured in hot, sunny climates

Early diagnosis of pneumonia is important if treatment is to be cost-effective and successful. Foals should be observed closely for signs of nasal discharge, coughing, elevated respiratory rate (more than 30 per minute), abnormal respiratory effort, depression, and inappetence. The best time to evaluate respiratory rate and character is during the cool early morning hours. Appropriate diagnostic and therapeutic mea-

sures should be taken immediately if abnormalities are noted.

BRONCHOINTERSTITIAL PNEUMONIA AND RESPIRATORY DISTRESS IN FOALS

A sporadic, rapidly progressive, highly fatal, acute respiratory-distress syndrome has been described in foals between 1 week and 8 months of age. The cause is unknown. Clinical signs include a markedly elevated respiratory rate, flaring of the nostrils, extended head and neck position, increased respiratory effort, and reluctance to move or eat. Most affected foals have a fever and are **cyanotic** (having blue mucous membranes, indicative of oxygen deprivation) at rest, or become so following minimal exertion.

This syndrome constitutes a respiratory emergency necessitating aggressive and intensive therapy. The high mortality rate in spite of different treatments that have been applied indicates that no one treatment is highly effective. Of the foals with this syndrome seen at the University of California, Davis, those that survived (about 50%) received prompt treatment with corticosteroid medications.

Particular care should be taken to control ambient temperature and to protect foals from direct exposure to the sun on hot days. Transporting foals during hot weather should be avoided. Any necessary transportation should be scheduled for the early morning while it is still cool. Appropriate ventilation of the trailer should be provided. Available evidence suggests that some foals surviving the syndrome have permanent lung damage that could potentially impair their future athletic performance.

CHRONIC OBSTRUCTIVE PULMONARY DISEASE ("HEAVES," "BROKEN WIND")

Chronic obstructive pulmonary disease (**COPD**) refers to a number of conditions leading to chronic or recurrent obstruction of airflow within the lung. In people, the common conditions responsible for COPD are asthma, chronic bronchitis, bronchiolitis, and emphysema. The terms *heaves* and *broken wind* are often used to describe severe cases of equine COPD.

This syndrome occurs worldwide but is more common in temperate climates, where it is the most common cause of chronic coughing in horses. Stabled horses are affected more often, so the syndrome is more prevalent in winter and early spring. Dusty atmospheres, particularly those generated by moldy hay or bedding, represent a predisposing factor in most instances. A variant of COPD occurs in the summer and represents an allergy to certain pollens. Outbreaks of viral respiratory disease (e.g., influenza) may also contribute to susceptibility.

The clinical signs usually develop insidiously but may occur suddenly in some horses. They can vary markedly from horse to horse and may wax and wane in any individual animal. The signs may be exacerbated following indoor housing or work. Mildly affected animals may exhibit reduced performance or work capacity, while others may suffer periodic "asthmatic" attacks with coughing, wheezing, nasal discharge, depression, and exercise intolerance. Severely affected horses exhibit marked respiratory distress with flaring nostrils, rapid breathing, increased (forced) expiratory effort, inability to exercise, inappetence, and weight loss. Cyanosis may be present when the animals are forced to move. Long-standing cases may assume a "heave line" along each side of their lower abdomen and a "barrel-chested" appearance caused by an inability to force enough air out of their lungs.

Diagnosis is based on the history, clinical signs, inspection of the horse's environment, and the horse's response to treatment, environmental changes, and allergy testing. Many cases of COPD are reversible if the syndrome is diagnosed early and if control measures are rigorously followed. Environmental management to minimize exposure to dust is the cornerstone of therapy. *Therapeutic efforts will fail unless the horse's environment is altered.*

Exposure to potential allergy-causing substances (**allergens**) and irritants can be reduced by:

- Maintaining the horse at pasture (provided the horse is not sensitive to pollen)
- Feeding complete cubed or pelleted feed. If hay must be fed it should be of the highest quality (*see* CHAPTER 7, "FEEDING HORSES") and should be soaked thoroughly at a distant site before feeding. Vacuum-packed hay or grass silage represent acceptable alternatives
- Substituting for straw any of the following forms of stable bedding: shredded paper, hardwood shavings, or peat
- Ensuring good ventilation
- Subjecting all horses sharing the same airspace to these same environmental controls
- Not storing hay or straw in or near the horse's stable (preferably not within 50 yards)
- Resting the horse until clinical signs subside

Clinical signs in most COPD-affected horses will subside within 1–2 weeks if the above measures are instituted and the animal is rested. More severely affected cases respond more slowly and may not resolve completely.

Specific drug therapy—anti-inflammatory medications, **bronchodilators** (medications causing expansion of vital airways in the lungs), and **expectorants** (medications that promote the coughing up of mucus from the lungs)—is indicated in patients with severe respiratory distress as an adjunct to environmental management, or in those situations where environmental alterations are not feasible.

LUNGWORMS
See "RESPIRATORY PARASITES: NEMATODES" in CHAPTER 33, "INTERNAL PARASITES."

PLEURAL EFFUSION, PLEURITIS, AND PLEUROPNEUMONIA
As indicated earlier, the term **pleural effusion** refers to an accumulation of fluid within the pleural cavity, the potential space between the visceral pleura, covering the surface of the lungs, and the parietal pleura, which lines the inner surface of the chest cavity. There are many different causes of pleural effusion in the horse, by far the most common being inflammatory in nature. The causes of pleural effusion can include:

- Bacterial infection secondary to pneumonia or lung abscesses, a condition known as **pleuropneumonia** (the most common cause of **pleuritis** [inflammation of the pleura] in the horse)

- Primary pleuritis, i.e., pleuritis unassociated with any other disease process
- Chest trauma involving a puncture wound of the chest wall
- Ruptured esophagus
- Internal abscesses
- Coccidioidomycosis (a fungal infection) or nocardiosis (a bacterial infection)
- Tumors, such as lymphosarcoma
- Trauma
- Heart failure
- Diaphragmatic hernia

Although pleuropneumonia can occur spontaneously, it is often associated with a stressful event, prolonged transportation, a recent acute viral illness (such as influenza), or prolonged recumbency during general anesthesia. A typical history often includes an inadequately short period of treatment and rest from a virus infection, followed by prolonged transportation, anesthesia, surgery, or premature resumption of training and vigorous exercise. There is also a marked "occupational" predisposition to the disease: The vast majority of affected horses are Thoroughbred and Standardbred racehorses. Aspiration of dirt or blood into the lungs during exercise may play a significant role in disease development. In some animals, surgery involving the upper respiratory tract may result in complications affecting the larynx, allowing inhalation of foreign material during feeding or at other times.

The clinical signs associated with pleural disease vary somewhat depending on the cause, other underlying diseases, and duration and severity of the condition. Pain is evident early on but tends to diminish as the disease progresses. Other early signs include an abnormally rapid heartbeat, fever, depression, a stiff gait, and reluctance to move or lie down. An affected horse usually stands quietly and often has an anxious facial expression, reflective of discom-

fort. Breathing is shallow and rapid, with restricted movement of the chest wall. Chest expansion often is markedly reduced during inspiration. Nostril-flaring and other signs of respiratory distress may be evident. Pain when the chest wall is touched may be exhibited by flinching, muscle spasm, grunting, biting, or kicking. A painful grunt may be heard when the horse coughs or strains to defecate. The problem is common in racehorses and can esily be confused with other conditions such as influenza, **laminitis** (founder), and **myositis** (muscle inflammation), the latter two conditions being characterized as well by stiffness and pain.

As the disease progresses and more fluid accumulates in the pleural cavity, the predominant clinical signs can include recurrent or constant fever (especially when pneumonia or lung abscesses are present), respiratory distress, inappetence, depression, edema, and moderate to severe weight loss.

Diagnosis is based on the history, clinical signs, and results of supportive tests (e.g., diagnostic ultrasound, X-ray studies, transtracheal wash, examination of fluid obtained from the chest cavity). Specific treatment must be based on the underlying cause of the fluid accumulation. For horses with bacterial pleuropneumonia, a prolonged course of antibiotic treatment is essential. The prognosis is always guarded. In general, the more chronic the condition the poorer the prognosis.

Note: It is important to evaluate medically any horse that develops fever, depression, inappetence, and respiratory difficulties within a few days of racing or other strenuous exercise, transportation, or surgery. The response to treatment and the prognosis for complete recovery are greatly improved if appropriate therapy is administered early in the disease course. Any delay will greatly increase the chances that a horse will develop life-threatening or incapacitating complications, such as lung scarring, pleural **adhesions** (abnormal tissue attachments), systemic infection, laminitis, and so forth.

CHAPTER 26

The Digestive System and Various Disorders

by Steven Zicker

The digestive tract is essentially an elongated, continuous tube that begins at the mouth and ends at the anus, the diameter of the tube varying at different points along its length. Its most important function is the digestion of raw food materials for use by the body. **Digestion** can be defined as the breakdown of larger substances into smaller subunits, which can be more readily carried into the body for use in energy production and the construction of body tissues. Disturbances in the transport or digestion of food may result in alterations of normal function that are detrimental to the animal. Indeed, digestive-system disorders are among the most common problems observed in domesticated horses.

Equine Digestive Physiology

Each section of the **digestive tract** (mouth, stomach, small intestine, large intestine) has a specific function in the processing of foodstuffs. The horse differs from other species—such as the cow or the dog—in how the order of food processing is arranged along the digestive tract.

Because of this unique ordering of digestive processes, horses are classified as **nonruminant herbivores.**

Nonruminant herbivores can subsist entirely on fiber-rich vegetative matter, such as hay or pasture, just as a cow or goat may. Cows and goats (both of which are **ruminant herbivores**) process their high-fiber diets by ingesting the food and passing it immediately to the **rumen**, the first part of a compartmentalized stomach. The rumen is essentially a large vat containing microorganisms that **ferment** (break down) the fiber into smaller, more usable subunits.

Horses, being nonruminant herbivores, have no rumen. Instead, the food a horse ingests is passed down into a simple, noncompartmentalized stomach, then on to the small intestine, and finally to the large intestine (*see* CHAPTER 16, "ANATOMY"). The large intestine of the horse is able to ferment fiber-rich plant material, much like a rumen does, to produce usable fuel for the horse's body.

Adequate functioning of the digestive system as a whole is needed for maintaining good health, growth, reproduction, and performance.

Each segment of the equine digestive tract has a special function in the digestion and processing of food. These functions will be reviewed and compared to those of other species, to illustrate their uniqueness to the horse and their importance with regard to the digestive processes.

THE MOUTH

The mouth of the horse is responsible for the initial processing of food. Horses are unable to regurgitate food; i.e., food cannot move from the stomach back to the mouth, as it does when cows chew their "cud," or when a sick animal or a person vomits. The horse's mouth thus assumes a very important role in the primary processing of food. It is the responsibility of the mouth, through **mastication** (the action of chewing), to prepare food for passage into the **esophagus** (the muscular tube connecting the back of the mouth to the stomach) and for further digestion farther down the digestive tract.

The horse has both **deciduous** (temporary) and *permanent* teeth. Adult horses normally have 40–42 permanent teeth. The positions of the teeth are defined by a *dental formula*, which describes the configuration of the teeth from the midline back toward the rear (*see* CHAPTER 16, "ANATOMY"). Thus, the dental formula delineates the order of the teeth for one-half (i.e., one side) of the upper and lower arcade. For the top row of teeth the formula from front to rear is: 3 incisors, 1 canine, 3 or 4 premolars (the first premolar is called the **wolf tooth,** and its presence is variable in some horses), and 3 molars. The formula for the bottom teeth is exactly the same except that there are only three premolars, never four.

The upper teeth are positioned in the jaw so that they are slightly wider and forward of the lower set of molars and premolars. Because of this, and because horses' teeth continue to grow throughout life, the potential for uneven wear is substantial. It is, in fact, quite normal for sharp edges (**enamel points**) to develop on the outside of the upper teeth and inside of the lower teeth, owing to the offset. The development of enamel points on the front of the upper second premolar and rear lower molar is also common (*see* "DENTAL DISORDERS OF THE ORAL CAVITY," below).

The horse has only 24 deciduous teeth, all of which are lost when the permanent teeth erupt. The horse has no deciduous molar teeth, only permanent molars. The approximate timing of the eruption of the permanent and deciduous teeth is shown in Table 1.

Horses chew about 60,000 bites per day when they are subsisting on a diet of hay. The purpose of this extensive chewing is twofold:

- To process the feed into smaller particles that can pass through the digestive tract
- By breaking the feed into smaller particles, the surface area of the feedstuff is increased, thus providing more space for the action of digestive **enzymes** (the molecules that break down food) farther down the digestive tract

The chewing process not only produces small 1¼- to 2-centimeter (½- to ¾-inch) particles, but also mixes these particles with saliva. Horses produce about 5 to 10 liters (5¼ to 10½ quarts) of saliva per day. This saliva is very viscous and

Table 1
Timing of the eruption of equine deciduous and permanent teeth

Tooth	Eruption Time
Deciduous	
1st Incisor	Birth to 1 week
2nd Incisor	4–6 weeks
3rd Incisor	6–9 months
Canine	Variable
1st Premolar	Birth to 2 weeks
2nd Premolar	Birth to 2 weeks
3rd Premolar	Birth to 2 weeks
Permanent	
1st Incisor	2.5 years
2nd Incisor	3.5 years
3rd Incisor	4.5 years
Canine	4–5 years
1st Premolar	5–6 months
2nd Premolar	2.5 years
3rd Premolar	3 years
4th premolar	4 years
1st Molar	9–12 months
2nd Molar	2 years
3rd Molar	3.5–4 years

has large amounts of bicarbonate but few digestive enzymes. The main function of saliva is to lubricate and buffer the food for passage down the esophagus to the stomach. (The esophagus has no recognized digestive function other than to transport food from the mouth to the stomach).

The Stomach

The stomach holds 8 to 10 liters (about 8½ to 10½ quarts), about 8–10 percent of the total capacity of the equine digestive tract, and has two parts: a *nonglandular* area closer to the esophagus, and a *glandular* area closer to the small intestine. The nonglandular area appears to have a storage function, while the glandular area secretes substances that aid in the digestion of food.

The secretions from the glandular area of the stomach include digestive enzymes and acid. Because of this the acidity of the stomach increases as food moves from the entrance of the stomach to the exit. Acidity is required so that the digestive enzymes can begin breaking the food down into smaller pieces, for subsequent processing by the small intestine. The time ingested food is retained in the stomach is short (usually under 2 hours), allowing for little digestion to be performed there.

The Small Intestine

Once partially digested food enters the small intestine it passes very rapidly (usually in less than an hour) into the large intestine. However, because of the large surface area of the food particles and of the small intestine itself, a sizable amount of digestion occurs. Food in the small intestine is bathed in digestive juices secreted from the pancreas which are high in digestive enzymes and bicarbonate. The bicarbonate is necessary to counteract the acid from the stomach and allows the digestive enzymes to work more efficiently. Horses also have other digestive enzymes that originate within the walls of the small intestine.

Together these enzymes allow fats, proteins, and simple carbohydrates to be digested in the small intestine.

The small intestine is also responsible for mineral absorption and some water absorption,

but it is unable to digest much (if any) fiber. In horses the small intestine also loses the ability to digest milk sugar (**lactose**) at about 3 years of age. Any food or water that is not digested or absorbed in the small intestine is passed on to the large intestine for further processing.

The Large Intestine

The large intestine, which includes the **cecum** (the first segment of the large intestine, consisting of a large dilated pouch), performs several very important physiological functions. In some ways the equine large intestine is similar to the rumen of the cow, but in others it is quite different. Its primary function is to ferment the fiber that has not been digested in the small intestine. The fermentation is carried out by the bacteria that reside in the large intestine. The resulting fermentation products supply about 30–50 percent of a horse's daily energy requirements. The bacteria also synthesize some important B vitamins that the horse needs.

The large intestine is also responsible for most of the water absorption in the horse. About 80 liters (over 21 gallons) of water (representing ⅙ to ⅐ of a horse's body weight) are absorbed from the large intestine *each day* in an average, nonworking horse.

Signs of Digestive-System Disorders

Close observation is critically important in pinpointing the cause of any digestive-system disorders that may arise in a horse. Disorders of the digestive tract can manifest themselves in a variety of ways, and may have a sudden or insidious onset. Careful observation of regular eating patterns, body weight, and fecal consistency are important for the early recognition of digestive-system disorders. Common clinical signs can include weight loss, colic, or diarrhea.

Weight loss may occur rapidly or gradually over an extended period (weeks to months). When normal horses are deprived of food for 2 days or more they can lose as much as 10 percent of their body weight, just from evacuation of feed from the large intestine. Thus it is important not only to recognize weight loss but also to determine whether it is a true loss of muscle and fat or whether it simply represents emptying of the digestive tract.

Colic is defined as abdominal pain or discomfort. Horses may exhibit signs of colic in several different ways. With severe discomfort they may sweat, paw at the ground, or lie down and roll. With less severe discomfort they may make attempts to stretch out the abdomen by placing the rear legs farther back, may refuse to eat when feed is presented to them, may grind their teeth, or may look back at their side. Other signs may include excess **flatulence** (gas), increased gurgling sounds over the rear part of the abdomen, dry hard feces, mucus-covered feces, or lethargy.

Diarrhea is usually manifested by an increase in the water content of the feces. Fecal consistency may range from "cow pie" to very watery, the latter being indicative of a more severe problem. The number and frequency of bowel movements may increase or decrease. The odor of the feces may also become more foul or **putrefied** (smelling of decomposition) as the diarrhea worsens. A lack of appetite (***inappetence*** or **anorexia**) may accompany the diarrhea. Inappetence that continues for a long period of time is usually a poor prognostic sign, i.e., the outcome is usually unfavorable.

Disorders of the Digestive System

Health problems can arise that mimic digestive-system disorders. For instance, the most common causes of weight loss in the horse are inadequate nutrition, dental problems, and intestinal parasites. Some of these problems can easily be prevented with proper management.

DENTAL DISORDERS OF THE ORAL CAVITY

Most problems arising in the mouth are related to the teeth. They may involve a single tooth or a group of teeth, such as the cheek teeth. The most common signs include weight loss, dropping of feed, abnormal chewing patterns, intolerance of the bit, and head-shaking. With severe dental disease the poorly chewed food may increase the possibility of a blockage of the digestive system, either in the esophagus (resulting in **choke**) or the large intestine (leading to **impaction colic**).

Dental Malformations

A variety of malformations can occur in tooth eruption and jaw position in the horse. Some of the more common abnormalities include extra teeth, overextended upper jaw (**parrot mouth**), and underextended upper jaw (**sow mouth**). If a dental malformation is suspected, the owner of the horse should consult with a veterinarian to confirm the observation and to discuss treatment options.

Caps

Caps are remnants of deciduous premolars that are left behind when the permanent premolars erupt. In younger horses caps may develop at 2 to 4 years of age. They can be removed by a veterinarian with a relatively simple procedure.

Wolf Teeth

Wolf teeth (the **first premolars**) usually cause no medical problems unless they are large, impacted, or infected. They may, however, interfere with the lay of the bit in the mouth and it is common practice to have the wolf teeth removed. A veterinarian can perform this procedure with the horse lightly sedated.

Enamel Points

One of the most common dental problems is the development of sharp enamel points, owing to the normal positioning and growth of the teeth in the horse's mouth. Horses may drop feed because of the sharp points' impingement on the cheek and tongue during chewing. The condition can be corrected by having a veterinarian grind down the sharp points with a special instrument called a **dental float.**

Wave or Step Mouth

This abnormality of older horses is characterized by a wavelike or stair-step configuration of the premolars and molars from front to back. The cause is unknown. The condition may be ameliorated by having a veterinarian grind the teeth down. The more severe the condition, the more work will be required to improve the teeth. Even with the best of veterinary assistance, however, the abnormality may not be amenable to complete correction.

Smooth Mouth

In extremely old horses the teeth may lose their rough edges and become smooth or be lost entirely. Smoothing of the teeth results in improper grinding of the food. Clinical signs may include weight loss or dropping of feed. There is no treatment. Affected horses should be managed by providing highly digestible feeds that are not too coarse.

Patent Infundibulum

In the center of each premolar and molar tooth is a soft core of **cementum** (specialized type of connective tissue that covers the tooth roots) contained within the **infundibulum** of the tooth. The funnel-shaped infundibulum runs from the surface to the root of the tooth. If the infundibulum becomes infected, is lost, or is incompletely formed, an opening extending essentially from the oral cavity to the root of the tooth is created, allowing infection to develop at the base. Depending on the exact location of the tooth root, the following signs may be observed:

- Swelling with or without a draining tract (pus actively draining out) in the jaw
- Nasal discharge (white pus) if the sinus is infected
- Bad breath (**halitosis**) arising from the infected tooth
- Weight loss
- Dropping of feed

Infected teeth may be identified by **radiographs** (X-ray studies) of the jaw. Treatment usually requires extraction of the tooth. However, some root-canal surgeries are now being performed to correct this problem.

NONDENTAL DISORDERS OF THE ORAL CAVITY

Cleft Palate

Cleft palate is a birth defect that is most often observed in newborn foals. Occasionally, if the abnormality is not too severe, it may not be detected until the foal is a few months of age. The defect is characterized by an abnormal connection between the oral cavity and the nasal cavity. As a result, small amounts of milk may be seen dripping from the nostrils when the foal suckles. More seriously, milk may run down into the lungs and produce a pneumonia. Aside from attempts at surgical correction there is no treatment for cleft palate in the horse; affected foals are usually euthanized.

Foreign Bodies

Horses eating coarse hay or hay contaminated with barbed grass awns (e.g., yellow bristle grass, foxtails) or chewing wood, may get sharp fragments of feed, awns, or wood splinters lodged in the soft tissues of the mouth. In some cases these items may produce wounds in the tissues without actually becoming embedded. Clinical signs can include bad breath, weight loss, dropping of feed, or even draining tracts if infection arises in a wound. When foreign bodies become lodged in the mouth they should be removed by a veterinarian, who will also see to it that the affected tissues are thoroughly cleansed so that proper healing will occur.

Trauma

Trauma can result in fractures of the bones surrounding the oral cavity. The upper jaw, lower jaw, and bones of the **throatlatch area** (area of the throat under which the strap of a bridle or halter passes) potentially can be involved. The clinical result is usually an unwillingness to eat and swelling at the site of the trauma. Horses may eat but be unwilling to swallow if the throat bones are fractured. Most of these fractures can be surgically repaired by a veterinarian.

Salivary Gland Disorders

Salivary glands can be found under the jaw, between the two halves of the **mandible** (lower jaw), and just behind the jaw, below the ear and throatlatch area. These glands drain into the mouth through a series of tiny tubes or ducts. If the tubes become blocked with small stony concretions (**sialoliths**), swelling of the salivary glands may occur.

Occasionally, inflammation of the salivary glands may be seen. This condition has been associated with the spring season and may be related to the bloom of new plants in pasture. Clinical signs include an unwillingness to chew and pain in the salivary-gland area. This problem can be treated by a veterinarian and in most cases should resolve without complications.

DISORDERS OF THE ESOPHAGUS

Choke

The most common disorder of the esophagus is an obstructive disorder commonly referred to as **choke**. The clinical signs include stretching of the head and neck, restlessness, drooling (or excessive salivation) attempts to swallow that may result in coughing, a feed-tinged discharge from the nostrils, bad breath, and possibly a lump at the site of obstruction. Choke may have many different causes, e.g., feed, wood, or foreign bodies.

A common predisposing factor for choke is improper **mastication** (chewing). Causes of poor mastication include poor teeth in older horses, erupting teeth in younger horses, greedy eating, exhaustion, and depressed swallowing reflexes from general anesthesia (as would occur following a surgical procedure). Other possible causes include a narrowing (**stricture**) of the esophagus, and tears or outpouchings (**diverticula**) of the esophagus that become impacted and occluded with feed.

Most cases of simple choke resolve spontaneously; however, the more quickly they are relieved, the less injury will be sustained by the esophagus. Feed and water should be removed from a horse if choke is suspected. An examination by a veterinarian is recommended to ascertain the cause and to provide a course of treatment. If the choke cannot be attributed to a simple cause—such as bad teeth or greedy eating—the prognosis may be less optimistic, as is the case with strictures and diverticula of the esophagus.

DISORDERS OF THE STOMACH

Disorders of the equine stomach are difficult to diagnose and require special equipment. The clinical signs include (but are not limited to) weight loss, poor body condition, colic, diarrhea, excessive salivation, and poor appetite. Problems may occur at any age, but the underlying causes may differ.

GASTRIC ULCERS

Gastric ulcers may occur in horses of any age. In foals the clinical signs include grinding of the teeth, salivation, and colic with rolling onto the back; in older horses the signs are often more obscure. As many as 50 percent of some horse populations may be affected by gastric ulcers. Ulcers may be found in apparently healthy horses, making the exact significance of the lesions confusing. In some horses ulcers may perforate the stomach and result in leakage of stomach contents into the abdomen, causing a **peritonitis** (inflammation of the inner lining of the abdomen) that can lead to death.

The only way to definitively diagnose ulcers that have not perforated the stomach is to pass a long, fiberoptic viewing instrument (an **endoscope**) into the stomach and visually identify the lesion. Treatment relies on the administration of anti-ulcer and anti-acid medications that protect the stomach wall against gastric acidity. This allows the ulcer to heal, and should produce a resolution of the clinical signs. Ulcers associated with stress require a change in the horse's environment or use for resolution.

Gastric Impaction

Occasionally, the stomach of a horse may become impacted with feed. Clinical signs include an unwillingness to eat and colic. Impactions may be treated medically, or may require surgery if they are particularly severe and resistant to medical therapy.

Gastric Dilation and Rupture

Retrograde (backward) motion of the intestinal contents, owing to disease of the small or large intestine, may result in the reverse flow of fluid back into the stomach. Because horses cannot vomit the fluid can build up in this organ, causing distension. Occasionally gastric distension may occur as a primary disease in and of itself, rather than as a secondary effect of another digestive disorder.

Distension of the stomach is very painful to the horse and the resulting signs of colic may be severe. If left untreated too long, rupture of the stomach may occur. Rupture is usually accompanied by a lessening of the signs of colic, followed by death of the horse.

Note: Signs of colic do not necessarily mean that gastric dilation has occurred. Many other digestive disorders can result in colic.

Gastric dilation may be relieved by a veterinarian passing a tube into the stomach. Usually, however, there is an underlying problem that has caused the distension, so that relief will only be temporary. It is imperative that a veterinarian be called immediately to assess the cause of the colic. All feed and water should be removed and the horse should be kept up and walking until the veterinarian arrives.

Stomach Cancer

Cancer of the stomach is very rare in horses. When it does occur, it is usually in older horses and more often than not is of the *squamous cell carcinoma* type. Clinical signs include weight loss, poor appetite, and colic. Diagnosis is very difficult, and usually relies on visual identification of the tumor through an endoscope, or identification of cancer cells in fluid drawn from the abdominal cavity. There is no treatment. (*See* Chapter 34, "Cancer.")

DISORDERS OF THE SMALL INTESTINE

Anterior Enteritis
(Proximal Duodeno-Jejunitis)

This syndrome is more common along the Gulf Coast of the United States, although it may be seen anywhere. The cause is unknown. It is characterized by severe inflammation of the upper portion of the small intestine. When the intestine becomes severely inflamed its **motility** (ability to move) is lost and fluid begins to accumulate in its upper reaches. This results in distension of both the small intestine and the stomach, causing colic. Treatment is aimed at relieving the distension and inflammation. Once the distension and inflammation have been neutralized, the intestine will begin healing on its own. The outcome of treatment is variable; some horses will recover while others will succumb.

Obstructive Lesions

A variety of disorders can result in a blockage of the small intestine; they include:

- Twisting of the bowel on itself
- **Lipomas** (benign fat tumors) that hang in the abdomen by a fat string, and can wrap themselves around the bowel like a bola
- Squeezing of the bowel through tears (**hernias**) in the abdominal wall
- Intraluminal (within the intestine) strictures
- In weanling horses, **ascarids** (roundworms) can produce a very painful lesion that usually results in violent colic

Almost all of these causes must be corrected surgically. The outcome will depend on the severity of damage to the bowel.

Malabsorption Syndrome

This syndrome usually occurs in adult horses and is characterized by weight loss in the face of a ravenous appetite. The cause is unknown, but the result is a "leaky" intestine that does not absorb nutrients properly. Diarrhea accompanying the condition indicates concurrent involvement of the large intestine in the disease process.

Blister Beetle Poisoning

Ingestion of alfalfa hay infested with blister beetles (*Epicauta* **spp**. [multiple species]) can result in signs of colic in horses. Blister beetle poisoning usually occurs during the late summer and is caused by a toxic compound, **cantharidin**, that is present in the beetles. Additional clinical signs include fever, increased heart and respiratory rates, depression, sweating, and diarrhea. There is no antidote for the toxin, and treatment is purely supportive, the outcome depending upon the amount of toxin ingested. (*See* Chapter 8, "Diseases of Dietary Origin.")

Disorders of the Large Intestine

Disorders of the large intestine can be divided into two very general categories: those characterized primarily by colic, and primarily by diarrhea. Some overlap of these clinical signs is possible, however, depending on the nature of the underlying disease process.

Obstructive Disorders

Several disorders can produce a mechanical or functional obstruction of the large intestine. Bowel distension from the accumulation of gas and intestinal fluid occurs secondary to these types of conditions. The distension causes pain and signs of colic. The outcome is dependent on the nature and duration of the lesion.

Feed impaction of the large intestine occurs most commonly at the **pelvic flexure**, where the large intestine narrows and folds back on itself. Impaction colic may be secondary to dental problems that result in poorly chewed food. Impaction colic also occurs when there is a sudden change in feed, a horse's access to water is limited, or when environmental conditions promote dehydration.

Torsion of the large intestine is a serious but infrequent problem. A **torsion** is simply a twisting of the bowel upon itself in a clockwise or counterclockwise direction, like the twisting of a wet towel that is wrung out to dry. The result is an interruption of the blood supply to the bowel and an obstructive lesion. The cause is unknown, but there appears to be a higher than expected incidence in mares 1–2 months after foaling. Surgical intervention is necessary to correct a torsion. The outcome is dependent on how quickly the problem is discovered and corrected.

Enteroliths are stony concretions that can develop in the large intestine of the horse. They may grow to the size of a bowling ball, but seem to occur only in horses from certain regions of the United States. The cause of these concretions is unknown but may be related to diet or water content of the feed. Horses may pass smaller enteroliths in the feces on their own accord, but larger enteroliths require surgery to be removed. Some have advocated a cup of vinegar once a day as a preventive measure but the efficacy of this method has not been determined.

Ingestion and deposition of sand in the large intestine may lead to irritation and impaction of the large colon resulting in signs of colic. Other signs associated with this problem include weight loss and intermittent diarrhea. Attempts should be made in sandy, soiled areas to feed horses off the ground. In addition, the feeding of psyllium fiber may help to decrease and clean out sand buildup in susceptible horses in high-risk areas. If sand buildup is severe, surgery may be necessary to alleviate the problem.

Poor or ineffective motility of the large intestine is reflected in an inability of the bowel to push feed contents through to the anus at a normal pace. The resulting functional obstruction will produce signs of colic similar to those caused by a physical obstruction of the bowel, with the only differences that functional obstructions are much more difficult to diagnose and the outcome is very poor.

Nonobstructive Disorders

The major disorder in this category is what is commonly called **gas colic** or **spasmodic colic.** *The majority of colics in horses are of this form and have a very favorable outcome.* The cause is unknown but may be related to the ingestion of highly digestible feeds, overeating, or temporary spasms of bowel motility. The result is the overproduction of gas and subsequent distension of the large intestine. Unlike other colics there is no obstructive lesion present; thus, the gas may be passed on to the rectum and the pressure released. The majority of such colics may be managed medically and will resolve within a few hours.

Diarrhea

The underlying causes of diarrhea in the horse remain largely unknown, although most cases are associated with disorders of the large intestine. Diarrhea may occur in animals of any age, from foals to adult horses. The onset may be either gradual or sudden, and the diarrhea may be brief or, rarely, may last for the horse's lifetime. The clinical outcome depends on the cause and severity of the diarrhea. The appearance of diarrhea, especially if watery and accompanied by inappetence, colic, or lethargy, should necessitate immediate concern and a call to your veterinarian. Severe cases of diarrhea, if left untreated, may result in the death of the horse.

Diarrhea in foals Diarrhea in foals may have an infectious (bacteria, viruses, parasites) or noninfectious (nutrition) cause. A normal physiological diarrhea known as **foal heat scours** is often observed during the first heat cycle of a mare after foaling, usually between days 7 and 14 after the foal's birth.

Diarrhea in foals less than 7 days of age may be an indicator of disease that is more widespread in the body. Foals of this age with diarrhea in conjunction with lethargy or a poor suckle reflex should be examined thoroughly. Foals with diarrhea may also exhibit signs of colic, making diagnosis of the primary problem very difficult.

The best preventive measures are proper foal husbandry and maintenance of a clean environment. Adequate transfer of antibodies from the mare to the foal in the **colostrum** (first milk) is vital for ensuring the health of the foal. (*See* CHAPTER 29, "THE IMMUNE SYSTEM AND VARIOUS DISORDERS.")

Proper sanitation is also of vital importance; even foals with adequate immunity from the mare may be overwhelmed by filthy living conditions.

A variety of bacterial and viral agents may cause foal diarrhea, although some are more common than others. The most common bacteria are *Clostridium* and *Salmonella*, while the most common virus is rotavirus. Bacterial invasion of the digestive tract is more dangerous in foals than in adult horses; the chances that bacteria will move from the digestive system into the blood, thus spreading throughout the body, are much higher in foals under 2 months of age than in adults. Rotavirus primarily affects foals in this same age group but is less likely to cause widespread disease. (*See* CHAPTER 30, "VIRAL DISEASES," and CHAPTER 31, "BACTERIAL DISEASES.")

Diarrhea in foals can result in dehydration. *Severe diarrhea must be treated aggressively with intravenous fluids to replace the lost water.* If bacteria have crossed into the blood, antibiotics must also be administered. Most foals with diarrhea will recover uneventfully if involvement of other body systems is not extensive.

The best way to avoid bacterial or viral diarrhea is by appropriate preventive measures. Ensure an adequate colostral transfer of antibodies, maintain a hygienic environment, and, if diarrhea does occur, wear gloves or wash hands immediately after handling the affected foal to prevent further spread of the disease agent.

Parasitic infestation with the intestinal threadworm *Stongyloides westeri* is common in foals. The parasite can be transmitted to nursing foals in the postcolostral milk (days 4–47 after birth), with eggs appearing in the feces in as little as 1 week. Infections are readily diagnosed by fecal examination, and several effective antiparasitic drugs are available for therapy. (*See* CHAPTER 33, "INTERNAL PARASITES.")

Foal diarrhea of nutritional origin has been attributed to the overingestion of milk, improper feeding of milk replacers, and transient **lactase** (intestinal enzyme that breaks down milk sugar) deficiency. The diagnosis of nutritional diarrhea is complicated and usually anecdotal. Most nutritional problems seem to result in a mild diarrhea, are self-correcting, and without long-term complications.

Diarrhea in adult horses Diarrhea in adult horses may be of infectious or noninfectious origin, and may have a rapid (**acute**) onset or a lengthier (**chronic**) duration. The most commonly diagnosed cause of acute diarrhea in adult horses is *Salmonella*. Another bacterium that has been identified as a cause of *toxemic colitis* (or *colitis X*) and diarrhea is *Clostridium*. Several other bacteria have been isolated from adult horses with diarrhea, but no consistent associative pattern has been recognized. (*See* CHAPTER 31, "BACTERIAL DISEASES.")

Another important bacterium that causes acute diarrhea in adult horses is the rickettsial bacterium *Ehrlichia risticii*, the cause of *Potomac horse fever*. This is a disease primarily of horses in the eastern half of the United States, but isolated cases have been documented in some western states. A vaccine is now available. (*See* CHAPTER 31, "BACTERIAL DISEASES," and APPENDIX B, "VACCINATIONS AND INFECTIOUS DISEASE CONTROL.")

Treatment for any of the acute causes of diarrhea in horses may include oral or intravenous fluids, anti-inflammatory or anti-ulcer medications, and oral coating agents. The outcome of the diarrhea depends on the severity of the underlying disease. The more severe the disease, the more severe the dehydration and **systemic** (bodywide) complications. A serious complication of toxic diarrhea in horses is **laminitis** (founder). If laminitis occurs it usually necessitates euthanasia of the horse. (*See* CHAPTER 22, "THE MUSCULOSKELETAL SYSTEM AND VARIOUS DISORDERS.") Even after resolution of acute diarrhea, a chronic diarrhea may persist.

Chronic diarrhea may be caused by a number of problems that are very difficult to identify. It may result from a bout of acute diarrhea, or may be secondary to a systemic illness, toxicity, nutritional intolerance, or physiological problems of the large intestine. It is one of the most frustrating problems for veterinarians to diagnose and is rarely resolved.

A variety of diagnostic tests, treatments, feed changes, and management alterations may be performed; more often than not these endeavors will meet with little or no success. As long as the horse is able to maintain its normal weight and activity level and is otherwise healthy, chronic diarrhea is often best left alone. Occasionally a spontaneous resolution may occur, but is the exception rather than the rule.

CHAPTER 27

The Liver and Various Disorders

by Gary P. Carlson

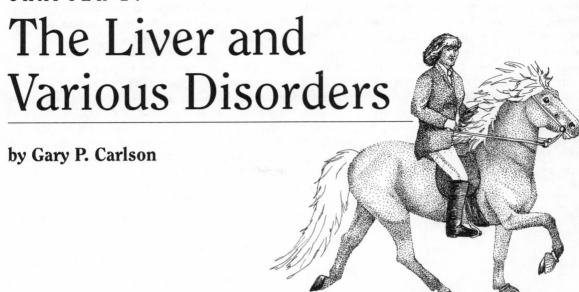

The Liver

The liver is the largest internal organ in the body, occupying the upper or forward part of the abdominal cavity. All the blood draining from the gastrointestinal tract passes through the liver, which plays a central role in the metabolism of carbohydrates, fats, and proteins. The liver is also responsible for the breakdown and excretion of many potentially toxic compounds. In this important and vulnerable position, the liver is easily damaged; yet this remarkable organ has an amazing capacity for regeneration and repair. Mild injuries to the liver often are sustained without any recognizable clinical signs. Signs of liver disease appear only when there has been massive damage in which most of the liver tissue has been destroyed or replaced by scar tissue. Clinical signs of liver disease largely represent a failure of the damaged organ to fulfill its various vital functions, thus allowing toxic compounds to accumulate in the body. The signs are often nonspecific and may include depression, loss of appetite, weight loss, neurologic dysfunction,

and **photosensitivity** (sensitivity to light) reactions in the white areas of the skin. (*See* CHAPTER 17, "THE SKIN AND VARIOUS DISORDERS.")

Icterus or **jaundice**, a yellow discoloration of the gums and **sclera** (the white of the eye), is caused by an abnormal accumulation of the pigment **bilirubin**. Icterus is an important clinical sign of liver disease, but is more variable in the horse than in any other domestic animal species. Acute liver failure usually results in profound icterus, while other forms of liver disease may produce variable degrees of icterus. In horses, many **systemic** (bodywide) disorders that cause a horse to go off feed will produce a slight yellowing of the gums and sclera. It thus may be difficult to differentiate icterus caused by liver disease from icterus associated with lack of feed intake. To complicate matters further, some forms of **anemia** (low red blood cell count) can also produce icterus in horses. Laboratory evaluation of blood samples is generally necessary to make an accurate differentiation, which is very important when considering prognosis. Most horses with clinical signs of liver disease and evidence of liver failure have a poor prognosis for recovery. It is, therefore, very important that a veterinarian be consulted to determine whether a horse has anemia, nonspecific icterus associated with being off feed, or liver failure.

Disorders of the Liver

IRON OVERLOAD IN NEWBORN FOALS
This condition occurred some time ago, when a specific microbial culture product containing supplemental iron was administered orally to a number of valuable newborn foals for the prevention of **scours** (diarrhea). The youngsters absorbed excessive amounts of the iron, producing massive damage to the liver, liver failure, and death in many of the foals during the first week of life. The product in question has been off the market now for years, but owners should be cognizant that iron supplementation—particularly during the first 2 or 3 days of a foal's life—can have potentially fatal consequences.

TYZZER'S DISEASE
Tyzzer's disease is an extremely rare and highly fatal **hepatitis** (inflammation of the liver) of young foals, usually 1 to 8 weeks of age. It is caused by a spore-forming bacterium, *Bacillus piliformis*. The organism is a normal inhabitant of the intestinal tract of mice, and foals are thought to acquire infection by ingesting fecal matter contaminated with the bacterial spores. The onset of the disease is extremely rapid. A fever, depression, loss of appetite, and mild jaundice may be followed by collapse, respiratory distress, and death. In many cases, foals are simply found dead. The clinical course is usually very brief, ranging from a few hours to a few days. There is no effective treatment or vaccine. (*See* CHAPTER 31, "BACTERIAL DISEASES.")

SERUM HEPATITIS (THEILER'S DISEASE)
Serum hepatitis is an acute form of liver failure in adult horses that has been recognized for many years. In most (but not all) cases it has been associated with the injection of some biological product of equine origin, 4 to 8 weeks prior to the onset of illness. While a variety of biological products have been associated with this disorder, the problem in the United States

has been most often associated with the administration of tetanus antitoxin in adult horses. This is one of the reasons why veterinarians strongly recommend that all horses be vaccinated with tetanus toxoid (*see* APPENDIX B, "VACCINATIONS AND INFECTIOUS DISEASE CONTROL.") All adult horses should be immunized with tetanus toxoid as a part of their routine vaccination program, under the supervision of a veterinarian.

Serum hepatitis does not appear to be a problem in foals. To the author's knowledge, there have been no instances of serum hepatitis following the routine administration of tetanus antitoxin to newborns.

Clinical signs of serum hepatitis include an abrupt onset of severe depression and loss of appetite. Affected horses often develop a variety of neurological abnormalities, including excessive yawning, wobbly gait, and in some cases circling, head pressing, convulsions, coma, and death. The one consistent feature is a profound and severe jaundice of the white of the eye and the visible mucous membranes. The urine is often darkly colored, owing to the presence of breakdown products of red blood cells. The prognosis is poor for most horses with massive liver damage and functional failure. Treatment largely consists of supportive care.

PYRROLIZIDINE ALKALOID INTOXICATION
The ingestion of plants containing *pyrrolizidine alkaloids* may result in severe liver damage and liver failure in horses. **Pyrrolizidine alkaloids** are toxins that produce a very specific type of liver damage and are the most common cause of chronic liver failure in horses in the western United States (although this toxicity has been recognized worldwide as well). A list of the most common pyrrolizidine alkaloid-containing plants is presented in Table 1.

Most toxic plants containing pyrrolizidine alkaloids are unpalatable and tend to be avoided by livestock and horses. Intoxication ordinarily does not occur at pasture unless poor pasture conditions or overgrazing has led to a marked reduction in the more palatable forage. *The immature stages of some of these plants may contain higher concentrations of the toxic alka-*

Table 1
Toxic Plants
Containing Pyrrolizidine Alkaloids

Common Plants	Scientific Names
Fiddleneck, fireweed	*Amsinckia intermedia*
Common groundsel	*Senecio vulgaris*
Threadleaf groundsel	*Senecio longilobus*
Tansy ragwort	*Senecio jacobaea*
Woolly groundsel	*Senecio ridelli*
Rattlebox	*Crotalaria* **spp.** (multiple species)
Viper's bugloss	*Echium plantagineum*
Common heliotrope	*Heliotropium europaeum*
Hound's tongue	*Cynoglossum officinale*

loids than do the mature plants. Poisoning is more likely to occur when feeding hay contaminated with one or more toxic plants. Pelleted or cubed hay poses a special risk since it is not possible to detect the presence of these poisonous plants by simple inspection.

Massive liver damage will occur if very large amounts of these toxic plants are consumed. Liver failure has occurred in as little as 4 to 6 weeks after the feeding of heavily contaminated hay. More commonly, limited exposure to toxic plants results in gradual, progressive destruction of the liver. This eventually leads to liver failure, which may appear to have an acute onset despite the fact that the damage has been steadily progressing over a long period of time (months to years). All horses on a given property that have had access to a contaminated feed source are likely to have suffered some degree of liver damage. Clinical signs and death are known to have occurred as long as 6 months to a year after ingestion of a contaminated feedstuff has ceased.

Pyrrolizidine alkaloid poisoning is usually associated with gradually developing depression, loss of appetite, and weight loss, together with a variable degree of jaundice. Body temperature, pulse, and respiratory rates are usually within normal limits unless the horse has become agitated or has been convulsing. Neurological signs often range from a change in attitude to aimless wandering to compulsive walking (in the past pyrrolizidine alkaloid poisoning was often referred to as "walking disease"). Affected horses tend to yawn, have a wobbly gait, may appear blind, and begin to head-press against solid objects. This can then progress to convulsions, coma and death. Self-inflicted trauma is often the presenting complaint in horses that have become oblivious to their surroundings and have injured themselves.

A tentative diagnosis can be made on the history and clinical signs but confirming it requires microscopic examination of liver tissue for the typical lesions of pyrrolizidine alkaloid poisoning.

Treatment consists largely of supportive care. Affected horses should be kept indoors out of the sunlight, particularly if their skin shows white areas and evidence of photosensitive reactions. (*See* CHAPTER 17, "THE SKIN AND VARIOUS DISORDERS.") Horses that continue to eat stand a reasonable chance of recovery. They should be fed grain, and good-quality grass, timothy, or oat hay. Older reference sources suggest that alfalfa hay should be avoided owing to its higher nitrogen content, which can potentially contribute to a buildup of toxic ammonia in a horse with impaired liver function. Practical experience suggests, however, that it is much better for a horse to eat alfalfa hay than to refuse to eat hay it doesn't like. *The key feature is to keep the horse eating*. Horses that are off feed will require intense supportive care under the supervision of a veterinarian.

The prognosis for recovery is guarded. If the condition is recognized promptly and the toxic plants are removed from the feed, regeneration and repair of liver tissue can occur in many affected horses. Pyrrolizidine alkaloid poisoning is also eminently preventable, by assuring that horses are not fed contaminated hay or exposed to potentially poisonous plants at pasture.

CHAPTER 28

The Endocrine System and Various Metabolic Disorders

by Noël O. Dybdal

There are two main categories of glands in the body, exocrine and endocrine. **Exocrine glands** secrete their contents through **ducts** (tiny tubes), and include the salivary glands and the exocrine portion of the pancreas. **Endocrine glands** secrete their contents directly into the bloodstream and, in some cases, into the **interstitial fluid** (the fluid surrounding cells). Secretions from endocrine glands are of two basic types: **steroid hormones**, manufactured by the body from cholesterol and protein, and **peptide hormones**, manufactured from amino acids, sometimes with the addition of **carbohydrates** (sugars). Many endocrine glands are present as paired structures, one member of each pair on either side of the body. Paired endocrine glands include the parathyroids, adrenals, and **gonads** (ovaries and testes). **Solitary** (unpaired) endocrine glands include the pituitary, thyroid (with right and left lateral lobes), and pancreas (actually small "islets" of cells scattered throughout the exocrine portion of the pancreas).

The **pituitary gland**, sometimes called the "master gland" of the body, is located at the base of the brain and secretes a variety of pro-

tein hormones that control or modulate the growth and secretory behavior of other endocrine glands. The pituitary in turn is under the control of the portion of the brain overlying it (the **hypothalamus**) and consists of three main parts, the *anterior*, *intermediate*, and *neural lobes*.

The cells of the anterior lobe produce hormones that directly control the production and secretion of hormones from the thyroid gland (**thyroid-stimulating hormone**, or **TSH**), adrenals (**adrenocorticotropic hormone**, or **ACTH**), and gonads (**follicle-stimulating hormone**, or **FSH**, and **luteinizing hormone**, or **LH**). The anterior lobe of the pituitary also produces **growth hormone (GH)**, which has generalized effects on growth, and **prolactin**, which is involved in milk production (**lactation**).

The function of the intermediate lobe of the pituitary is poorly understood but is believed to involve modulation of the body's response to stress. The intermediate lobe is the site of the most common endocrine disorder of horses, *Cushing's disease* or *hyperpituitarism*, in which excessive amounts of ACTH and certain related hormones are produced. The neural lobe of the pituitary produces **antidiuretic hormone,** which acts on the kidneys to conserve water, and **oxytocin**, which affects the reproductive organs.

The *thyroid gland* is located just below the angle of the jaw. It is divided into right and left lobes, situated on either side of the **trachea** ("windpipe"). In response to TSH from the pituitary, the thyroid gland produces and secretes the hormones **thyroxine (T_4)** and **triiodothyronine (T_3)**. These hormones are important in maintaining the metabolic rate of the body. Loosely associated with the thyroid gland and extending down either side of the neck are the four **parathyroid glands**. These glands are not under pituitary control but instead respond to the concentrations of calcium and phosphorus in the blood by secreting the hormones **parathyroid hormone (PTH)** and **calcitonin**.

The **endocrine pancreas** is composed of small clusters of cells, called **islets of Langerhans**, which are scattered throughout the exocrine portion of the pancreas. A variety of peptide hormones are produced by the islet cells. The most important are **insulin** and **glucagon**, which are primarily responsible for maintaining blood sugar levels within a normal range. As with the parathyroids, the islet cells are not under the direct control of pituitary hormones but respond directly to changes in blood-sugar concentration.

The **adrenal glands**, located just in front and to the central side of each kidney, are composed of an outer portion (the **cortex**) and an inner portion (the **medulla**). The cortex in turn is composed of three layers. The cells of the outer layer, the **zona glomerulosa**, produce and secrete the steroid hormone **aldosterone**. The function of the zona glomerulosa is independent of the pituitary. The cells of the middle layer, the **zona fasciculata,** produce and secrete the steroid hormone **cortisol** in response to ACTH from the pituitary. This pituitary–adrenal interaction is critical in the body's adaptation to stress. The cells of the inner layer, the **zona reticularis**, produce and secrete the steroid sex hormones *estrogen*, *progesterone*, and *testosterone* (the ovaries and testes, however, represent the primary sources of these hormones). The adrenal medulla produces **epinephrine (adrenaline)** and

norepinephrine (noradrenaline). The cells of the medulla are under the control of the nervous system and so can respond very rapidly to perceived stress. They are not controlled by the pituitary hormones or by concentrations of various compounds in the blood.

The *gonads* are the primary source of the sex steroid hormones. Cells in the *interstitium* of the testes produce and secrete testosterone, while cells in the insterstitium of the ovaries produce and secrete estrogen and progesterone.

Endocrine and Metabolic Disorders

Disorders of the endocrine system result when there is too little or too much of a given hormone secreted. An under- or overproduction of a hormone leads to imbalances that can in turn lead to the under- or overproduction of other hormones as the body tries to compensate and rebalance its metabolism.

Hypothyroidism

Although a diagnosis of **hypothyroidism** (abnormally decreased thyroid function) is often considered in individual cases, the condition has not been reported in adult horses except following surgical removal of the thyroid. Hypothyroidism in foals, however, is a well-documented but uncommon disorder.

Hypothyroidism in the foal is most often the result of the dam's ingesting excess iodine (usually in the form of kelp-containing feed supplements) or plant **goitrogens** (compounds causing goiter) during pregnancy. (A few cases of unexplained foal hypothyroidism, all from western Canada, have also been reported.) Although the mare's **placenta** (the tissue connecting the dam to the fetus) is permeable to iodine and plant goitrogens, it is impermeable to T_4 and T_3. The excess iodine or goitrogen reaching the foal blocks the production of T_4 and T_3 in the foal's thyroid. In response to low blood T_4 and T_3 the foal's pituitary secretes TSH, which stimulates the thyroid to enlarge, although it still cannot produce either T_4 or T_3.

The thyroid may appear greatly enlarged ("**goiter**") or normal in hypothyroid foals. Microscopic changes can persist for some time following an episode of goiter; if confirmation of the condition is necessary a **biopsy** (tissue sample) is the best diagnostic test. Foals normally have very high blood T_4 and T_3 concentrations shortly after birth—10 to 20 times higher than in the adult—so in some cases a blood test can also aid in diagnosis. Treatment of hypothyroidism usually relies on the administration of synthetic thyroid hormone (**L-thyroxine**) or iodinated casein.

The condition often diagnosed in the adult horse as "hypothyroidism" is actually not caused by underproduction of T_4 and T_3, but instead is the result of the overproduction of hormones from the intermediate lobe of the pituitary gland. This results in a clinical syndrome suggestive of low T_4 and T_3 production; the functional levels of T_4 and T_3 are actually normal. Confusion over the diagnosis of hypothyroidism has resulted from the lack of a good diagnostic test for the condition in the adult horse. Measurement of baseline T_4 and T_3 concentrations in the blood can be misleading; the concentrations measured can vary greatly depending on the time of year, time of day, whether the horse is sick (particularly with liver disease), if the horse is receiving medication (particularly phenybutazone), or if the horse has a poor appetite.

HYPERTHYROIDISM

Hyperthyroidism (abnormally increased thyroid function) has not been reported to occur spontaneously in the horse. Hyperthyroidism can result, however, if horses receive oversupplementation with thyroid hormone replacement therapy. Clinical signs include weight loss, nervousness, hyperactivity, elevated heart rate, and excessive or inappropriate sweating. In some cases weight loss is the only recognizable sign. Treatment involves reducing the level of thyroid hormone administered.

THYROID TUMORS

Nonfunctional, benign thyroid tumors (thyroid *adenomas*) are relatively common in older horses in some parts of the country. They occasionally are large enough to **palpate** (feel with the hands), but usually are too small to notice.

They are very slow growing, requiring years to change noticeably in size.

The possibility of a malignant tumor, a thyroid *carcinoma*, should be considered if a rapidly enlarging mass (i.e., a mass that enlarges noticeably over a period of one or two months) is seen in the region of the thyroid. The veterinarian will probably obtain a biopsy of the mass to confirm the diagnosis. The recommended treatment is surgical removal.

CUSHING'S DISEASE (HYPERPITUITARISM)

This is the most common endocrine disorder of horses. It occurs in a high percentage of horses over 15 years of age (the average age at diagnosis being 20 years), and is seen with equal frequency in mares and geldings. No specific breed of horse has been shown to have an increased susceptibility to the disease, although it does appear to occur more commonly in ponies than in horses.

Cushing's disease is associated with enlargement of the intermediate lobe of the pituitary and overproduction of the intermediate-lobe hormones **b-endorphin** and **melanocyte-stimulating hormone** (**MSH**), as well as ACTH. This in turn leads to enlargement of the zona fasciculata of the adrenal cortex and overproduction of cortisol. In this complicated disorder, clinical signs develop for a variety of reasons: the excessive levels of circulating cortisol, physical destruction of the pituitary neural lobe, and possibly the increased circulating concentrations of ACTH, b-endorphin, and MSH.

Because this syndrome in many ways resembles human Cushing's disease (which has a different cause, i.e., excessive secretion of ACTH from a tumor in the anterior lobe of the pituitary) it has been called equine Cushing's disease, although the two diseases are not strictly identical. Nevertheless equine Cushing's disease may *progress* to a tumorous state in the pituitary. In horses the intermediate lobe is controlled primarily by inhibition from a chemical in the brain called **dopamine**. Dopamine reaches the pituitary intermediate lobe directly via nerves extending from the hypothalamus. If dopamine is removed, the cells of the intermediate lobe produce and secrete hormone; if dopamine is present, the cells are blocked from producing and secreting hormone. In horses with Cushing's disease there is a complete loss of the dopamine-containing nerves in the intermediate lobe. With dopamine removed the cells produce and secrete hormone in an uncontrolled fashion, leading to serious and widespread metabolic imbalances. The reason for the loss of the dopamine-containing nerves has not yet been discovered. It appears to occur over an extended length of time, however, since the disease is usually very slow to develop. The underlying mechanism may differ, however, in certain rare cases in which the disease appears to develop more rapidly.

Common clinical signs of Cushing's disease in the horse include:

- Growth of a heavy, long and/or curly hair-coat at inappropriate times of the year
- Excessive water consumption and urination
- Increased appetite
- Bulging eyes, bulging fat pads above the eyes
- Enlarged abdomen
- Obesity

Affected horses have a depressed immune system and so may also develop infectious disease conditions, including dental disease, pneumonia, and sole abscesses. They are also very susceptible to gastrointestinal parasitism. A thin horse with Cushing's disease thus should be examined for other conditions, such as pneumonia, liver disease, or parasitism, which should be treated aggressively if found. Affected horses often can be built back up by regular deworming, dental care, and the feeding of softened, pelleted rations.

Diagnosis is based on the history, physical examination, and results of supportive laboratory tests. The veterinarian may perform several blood tests including a dexamethasone suppression test, which requires two days to complete, and a blood chemistry panel, to help establish the diagnosis and to determine how advanced the condition is.

Medical treatment of equine Cushing's disease is only in the experimental stages at this time, so if an affected horse appears to be stable the veterinarian may not recommend any medical therapy. Often horses with Cushing's disease will live many years with careful management, which includes regular dental and deworming programs, routine hoof care, body clipping as necessary, and attention to diet. If the horse is in very poor condition (i.e., no longer able to fight off secondary infections despite antibiotic support), the veterinarian may recommend trying one of several experimental treatments currently being investigated. The most promising medication under investigation is a long-acting dopamine replacement called pergolide. Cyproheptidine is another medication that is being investigated, with approximately 35 percent of horses treated reportedly showing improvement.

ADRENAL INSUFFICIENCY
(HYPOADRENOCORTICISM, ADDISON'S DISEASE)

Adrenal insufficiency (*hypoadrenocorticism* or *Addison's disease*) is not a common problem in horses. When it does occur it is most often a complication of long-term corticosteroid therapy. Use of **corticosteroids** (steroid hormones produced by the adrenal cortex) over a long period of time inhibits the pituitary gland's production of ACTH, which in turn leads to understimulation of the adrenal gland and adrenal suppression. Some of the more common corticosteroids used in horses are dexamethasone, prednisolone, prednisone, and triamcinolone. Each of these medications produces different degrees of adrenal suppression for varying lengths of time. Treatment times of less than one month with dexamethasone or prednisolone generally do not lead to significant adrenal suppression. If a horse must be treated for a longer period (as might be necessary for a severe allergic or hypersensitivity reaction), careful attention must be paid to the corticosteroid used and its dosage in order to avoid adverse adrenal effects.

Conditions referred to variously as "turn-out" or "let-down" syndrome are poorly documented conditions thought to be related to adrenal insufficiency. However, electrolyte abnormalities, low corticosteroid values, and poor responses to ACTH have not been reported in racehorses or endurance horses that have been evaluated for this condition. The adrenal glands are a "shock organ" in the horse, and can be damaged as a result of very low blood pressure. This sometimes occurs during severe bouts of colic, intestinal inflammation, severe hemorrhage, or **anaphylaxis** (a rapidly developing, exaggerated, and potentially life-threatening allergic reaction). If the damage is severe enough it is possible that adrenal insufficiency could develop; this has actually never been shown to occur, however.

Clinical signs of adrenal insufficiency include depression, loss of appetite, weight loss, and (sometimes) a dull haircoat. Diagnosis is based on the history, physical examination, and the results of supportive laboratory tests. The history may indicate that the horse has recently come off the track or completed some other form of intensive training, has had corticosteroids administered, or has recently experienced an episode of severe colic or dehydration. The veterinarian usually will first perform a screening blood test (basic chemistry panel and complete blood count). If a diagnosis of adrenal insufficiency is suspected a second blood test (ACTH challenge test) will be performed to determine the degree of adrenal suppression.

Therapy is dependent on the cause and severity of the condition. It may only be necessary to provide supportive care and shield the horse from stressful conditions for a few months. If the condition is very severe, medical therapy (electrolyte administration, hormone replacement) may be required.

ADRENAL TUMORS

Functional tumors of the adrenal medulla, called **pheochromocytomas**, are only rarely diagnosed. Clinical signs are intermittent and include excessive sweating, increased water consumption and urination, anxious behavior, recurrent colic, increased heart rate, and dilated pupils. To aid in a diagnosis the veterinarian may collect blood for evaluation of epinephrine and norepinephrine levels in addition to a standard chemistry panel. Unfortunately this condition is difficult to diagnose because the abnormal release of hormones is usually intermittent.

At present surgical removal is the only therapeutic option. Surgery on the adrenal glands is extremely difficult and risky because of the glands' close association with a major blood vessel, the *vena cava*. It is further complicated by the tumor's disruption of the adrenal gland and by the unstable condition of the patient caused by epinephrine release.

DIABETES MELLITUS

Primary *diabetes mellitus* is caused by an inability of the islet cells of the pancreas to produce insulin; fortunately, it is rare in the horse. When diagnosed it is usually the result of physical damage to the pancreas. In most cases there has been concomitant destruction of the exocrine pancreas, with a resulting loss of digestive enzymes; thus insulin replacement alone cannot return an affected horse to normal. In these rare cases destruction of the pancreas has most commonly been the result of the unfortunate localization in the pancreas of an internal abscess (as caused by *Rhodococcus* or *Streptococcus* bacteria), or has been secondary to a severe migration of parasitic worms (**strongyles**). (*See* CHAPTER 31, "BACTERIAL DISEASES," and CHAPTER 33, "INTERNAL PARASITES.")

Secondary, or insulin-resistant, diabetes mellitus is more common in the horse than primary diabetes mellitus because it eventually develops in most cases of equine Cushing's disease. Owing to the overproduction of the hormones ACTH and cortisol, blood sugar levels are elevated and the action of insulin to promote the uptake of sugar into cells is blocked. Early on, circulating insulin levels will be high as the islet cells try to produce enough insulin to reduce blood sugar levels; with time, however, insulin levels drop as the islet cells effectually "burn out." Insulin therapy cannot reverse this condition.

NUTRITIONAL SECONDARY HYPERPARATHYROIDISM

This condition is very rare today, but in the past—in the days of the great work horses—it was much more common. The synonyms for the disorder, which include "bran disease," "bighead," and "rubberjaw," reflect either the clinical signs shown by affected horses or the nutritional management causing the condition. **Hyperparathyroidism** (hyperactivity of one or more parathyroid glands) results when a horse is fed a diet high in phosphorus but low in calcium. In response the parathyroids produce large amounts of PTH, which causes calcium to be pulled out of the bones in order to balance the blood concentrations of calcium and phosporus. Over time the loss of calcium from the bones results in a weakening of their structure. The body reacts by laying down excessive amounts of connective tissue to help support the weakened bony framework. Clinical signs are most obvious in the jaw because the action of chewing causes more connective tissue to be deposited around the teeth and muscle connections; hence the terms "bighead" and "rubberjaw." The term "bran disease" refers to development of the disease in work horses that were fed a diet composed primarily of bran.

PSEUDOHYPERPARATHYROIDISM

In this disorder blood calcium levels are high but are not a result of the excessive production of PTH by the parathyroids. Instead, they are caused by production of a PTH-like substance by a tumor. Malignant tumors that have been associated with elevated calcium levels include lymphosarcoma, squamous cell carcinoma of the stomach, and mesothelioma. (*See* CHAPTER 34, "CANCER.")

CHAPTER 29

The Immune System and Various Disorders

by Jeffrey E. Barlough

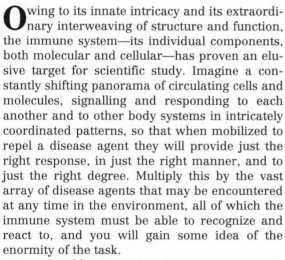

Owing to its innate intricacy and its extraordinary interweaving of structure and function, the immune system—its individual components, both molecular and cellular—has proven an elusive target for scientific study. Imagine a constantly shifting panorama of circulating cells and molecules, signalling and responding to each another and to other body systems in intricately coordinated patterns, so that when mobilized to repel a disease agent they will provide just the right response, in just the right manner, and to just the right degree. Multiply this by the vast array of disease agents that may be encountered at any time in the environment, all of which the immune system must be able to recognize and react to, and you will gain some idea of the enormity of the task.

A smoothly operating immune system is essential to the health and well-being of all higher living organisms. Without the complex circuitry of the immune system, higher organisms would be virtually defenseless, cast adrift in a perilous environment populated by opportunists—viruses, bacteria, fungi, and parasites—ready and able to colonize a host and produce

disease. Furthermore disease conditions intrinsic to the body itself, such as cancer, would more often than not gain the upper hand were it not for the complex interplay of cells and molecules comprising the immune response.

It has been said that the immune system oversees an armory containing some of the most powerful molecular and biological "explosives" ever devised by nature. When unleashed against an aggressor, the firepower of the immune response would surely be the envy of any microbiological field commander; thus the importance of maintaining firm and uncompromising control over such an arsenal, for if turned against the host itself—as in the **autoimmune diseases**—the consequences can be devastating. It is a tribute to the marvelous efficiency and balance of this control system that most infections pass unnoticed by the host.

What will be discussed in this chapter, in relation to horses, are among the more well-accepted aspects of the anatomy and physiology of the immune response, with descriptions of some equine disorders whose origins lie within the immune system itself. These include diseases resulting from an overactive immune response as well as those resulting from immunodeficiency. Readers with a deeper interest in these topics are referred to any of several excellent texts available in veterinary or human immunology. It should be noted that, in general, the introductory discussion of anatomy and physiology may be readily applied to the human immune system as well.

Anatomy and Physiology of the Immune System

The immune system is composed of a complicated network of molecules and cells, all precisely balanced in both their individual and overlapping functions. Immune responses are closely allied to the activities of two other body systems, the *blood circulatory system* and the *lymphatic system*. The blood circulatory system is responsible for transporting oxygen and other vital nutrients to the tissues and for removing metabolic waste products. Among the materials transported are some of the most important constituents of the immune system: **antibodies**, specialized proteins able to recognize molecules and cells foreign to the host; **lymphocytes** and **monocytes**, white blood cells capable of responding to the presence of such foreign material; and **cytokines**, "messenger" molecules by which cells of the immune system signal and instruct one another and, in some cases, direct other activities occurring in body tissues. Among the more important cytokines are **gamma-interferon** and the (at least) 12 known **interleukins**. In addition, the spleen acts as an important immunological filter to trap and destroy foreign material and host **cellular debris** (dead or dying red blood cells, for example) that pass through the spleen by way of the blood circulation.

The lymphatic system is composed of a highly specialized, interconnected lacework of delicate vessels or channels that transport a viscous fluid called **lymph** from body tissues back to the blood circulatory system. Lymph consists of a clear admixture of tissue fluids, various proteins, **solutes** (dissolved substances), and other minor constituents. Many lymphocytes circulating within the lymph fluid itself traffic regularly between the system's *lymph nodes* and the blood circulatory system and back again. Lymph nodes are the small specialized structures within the lymphatic system that act as barrier filters for the removal of foreign material, which is then subjected to destruction by the immune response. The lymph nodes' immunological filtering of lymph can be considered analogous to the spleen's immunological filtering of the blood.

The end result of this filtering and circulating is a highly desirable network of *immune surveillance*, wherein the molecules and cells of the immune system constantly "scan" the blood and lymphatic channels for signs of foreign intruders, abnormal cellular components (tumor cells or virus-infected cells, for example), and host cellular debris, all of which are appropriate targets for immunological attack.

The tissues or organs comprising the immune defenses of the body can be classified into either of two convenient categories: the *primary lymphoid organs* and the *secondary lymphoid organs*. **Primary lymphoid organs** are those in which the production and maturation of lymphocytes take place. In mammals, primary lymphoid organs consist of the **bone marrow**, the **mucosal-associated lymphoid tissue** (MALT—lymphoid tissue found lining the digestive, respiratory, and urogenital tracts), and the **thymus**, an organ in the chest that regulates the maturation of specialized lymphocytes known as **T lymphocytes** or simply **T cells**. Secondary lymphoid organs are those in which **antigens**, i.e., substances capable of being recognized by the immune response, are trapped and destroyed. Secondary lymphoid organs consist of the lymph nodes, spleen, and portions of the bone marrow and MALT.

Antigens (which occur as component parts of bacteria, fungi, viruses, parasites, toxins, or altered host body cells) are normally taken up by specialized white blood cells called **macrophages**, which can be found in large quantities in secondary lymphoid organs. Following ingestion of an antigen the macrophage, by means of cytokines and other molecules, begins signaling local lymphocytes—those that have already detected the antigen's presence—to mount a highly specific immune response against the antigen.

A subset of T cells, known as **helper T cells** or **T$_H$ cells**, assists other lymphocytes called **B cells** to produce antibody against the antigen. (The cells that actually secrete the antibody are end-stage B cells known as **plasma cells**.) The mounting of an antibody response to an antigen is referred to as a **humoral immune response**. Helper T cells also assist in the maturation of another subset of T cells known as **cytotoxic T cells** or **T$_C$ cells**. Cytotoxic T cells are responsible for tracking down and eliminating altered or infected body cells (for example, a cell infected with a virus, or a tumor cell carrying altered surface molecules that the body interprets as foreign or "non-self"). Also important in destroying such cells are the macrophages themselves, which not only aid in directing the immune defenses of the body but also inactivate many ingested antigens. (Other white blood cells known as **neutrophils** can ingest and destroy foreign substances, particularly bacteria, but they do not "direct" the activities of lymphocytes the way macrophages do.) A population of specialized lymphocytes known as **natural killer cells** or **NK cells** also is important in detecting and eliminating tumor cells and virus-infected cells. The mounting of a T$_C$ cell/macrophage/NK cell response to an antigen is referred to as a **cellular** or **cell-mediated immune response.**

The net effect of the activities of these two interrelated arms of the immune system is to attack the inciting antigen simultaneously from several different angles, in order to enhance the probability of its successful destruction. Such a multipronged, "fail-safe" strategy is particularly desirable because of the varied nature of the different antigens with which the immune defenses are confronted. Not all immune mechanisms perform as efficiently against all antigens (e.g., an enveloped virus versus a roundworm parasite); hence, the greater the number and variety of immune defenses alerted and activated, the greater the chance for a favorable outcome. In some cases, antigens even stimulate preferentially the precise immune mechanisms that are the most effective against them—a tribute to the marvelously wily and adaptive capabilities of the immune system.

Antibodies, also called **immunoglobulins** (abbreviated **Igs**), are vital players in a number of different immune mechanisms. Several types or *classes* of immunoglobulins exist. The most common class, **immunoglobulin G (IgG)**, circulates in the blood and tissue fluids and in human beings is able to cross the mother's placenta into the circulation of the developing fetus (transmission to the fetus does not occur to any extent in the horse, however). In horses a subset of IgG known as **IgG (T)** is involved in the immune response to parasites and tetanus toxoid.

A second class of immunoglobulin, **IgM**, is a much larger molecule than IgG and is found almost exclusively in the bloodstream. IgM is the first immunoglobulin type to be produced in the blood following initial exposure to an antigen. A third type, **IgA**, is the major immunoglobulin found in the mucous secretions that constantly bathe the surfaces of the body's mucous membranes—primarily the linings of the digestive, respiratory, and urogenital tracts. These surfaces are frequent first sites of contact between antigens and the immune system; IgA plays a crucial role in patrolling these surfaces and preventing potential disease agents from gaining deeper access to the body. This IgA-mediated surface-monitoring system is often referred to as the **secretory immune system**.

A fourth type of immunoglobulin, **IgE**, exists in vanishingly small quantities in the blood but is also found adhered to the surface of cells called **mast cells** and **basophils**. These cells and IgE (along with another cell known as the **eosinophil**) are important in protecting the body against invasion by certain parasites. Unfortunately mast cells, basophils, and IgE are also largely responsible for the annoying signs and symptoms of *allergy*. The final immunoglobulin type, **IgD**, is found on the surface of certain lymphocytes where it functions chiefly as a **receptor** or "sensor" for the detection of antigens.

Functionally, antibodies are "detector" molecules and do nothing more than attach to antigens; they have no capacity in and of themselves to destroy them. (Antibodies thus are just another group of complex messenger molecules with which the immune system is replete.) Attachment of antibody to an antigen sets into motion a chain of events that results ultimately in the antigen's removal by other, so-called "effector" mechanisms. In the case of IgG and IgM, the presence of these antibodies adherent to the surface of an antigen is a signal to certain cell types—macrophages, neutrophils, eosinophils, some lymphocytes—that a foreign antigen is present and requires elimination. In addition antigen–antibody complexes, known as **immune complexes**, act as attractants for components of a specialized series of blood proteins known as the **complement system**, whose major role is to disrupt the surface structure of microbes and altered body cells.

The immune system possesses two vital characteristics: *specificity* and *memory*. "**Specificity**" refers to the ability of antibodies and lymphocytes to recognize specific, individual antigens. Each individual antibody molecule recognizes *one and only one* antigen; the same is true for each individual lymphocyte. In other words, the receptors present on each antibody or on each lymphocyte are each specific for only a single antigen. When a particular antigen appears in the body, only those lymphocytes carrying the proper receptors for that antigen are stimulated, and only those antibody molecules capable of binding to it are bound, so that humoral and cell-mediated immune responses to the antigen are produced. In this way the energies of the immune system are focused very specifically on the inciting antigen.

"**Memory**" refers to the fact that exposure of lymphocytes to an antigen results in the production of a population of *memory lymphocytes* that continue to circulate once the antigen has been eliminated. Should that particular antigen again be introduced into the body, memory lymphocytes in conjunction with macrophages will very quickly trigger a vigorous immune response. It is for this reason that with many infectious disease agents a single, symptomless exposure to the agent or a single bout with the disease will be sufficient to produce a solid, long-lasting immunity.

Maternal immunity is a form of temporary immunity that is passed from mother to offspring. Maternal immunity, primarily in the form of antibody, serves to protect the neonate until its own immune system becomes fully operational. In horses, maternal immunity is transferred in the **colostrum** (first milk) delivered to the suckling foal during the first 24 hours after birth. This initial "transfusion" of antibody is taken up from the digestive tract and passed directly into the blood circulation, where it serves to protect the foal temporarily against serious infection. Soon after this the digestive tract becomes impermeable to the absorption of maternal antibody. Instead, antibody passed in the milk during subsequent suckling serves to coat the tonsils, associated lymphoid tissue, and digestive tract to protect the foal against many different disease agents. In this way the foal is shielded against the disease agents prevalent in its environment until a few months of age, by which time its levels of maternal antibody will have decayed and its own fledgling immune system will be able to take over.

Anything that prevents adequate transfer of maternal antibody to the newborn will cause the foal to become prematurely susceptible to infection. The failure of a foal to receive sufficient colostrum from the mare can contribute to the development of a severe or even fatal infection during the neonatal period.

Veterinarians and horse owners are frequently confronted with infectious disease masquerading in a variety of disguises. Unfortunately, we are usually aware only of the most severe manifestations of a given infection. This severe form is often described in textbooks as the "classical" or "typical" form of that particular disease. In reality the severe form of the disease usually is *not* the most common form occurring in nature. Animals and human beings have evolved over time with their disease agents to the point that, following exposure, they often experience only a mild, self-limiting, or even clinically inapparent (**asymptomatic**) infection. As a general rule severe illness usually occurs only when a combination of host, disease agent, and environmental factors are particularly unfavorable. Not only is the primary illness apt to be more severe under such conditions, but the proportion of individuals developing a persistent infection will be increased, aberrant or chronic forms of the disease will be more prevalent, and overall mortality rates will be higher.

Disorders of the Immune System

Under certain circumstances the immune defenses of the body can malfunction, such that the harmful side-effects produced by the immune response are more serious than those produced by the inciting antigen itself. In such cases it is actually the inappropriate response of the immune system that leads to a so-called **immune-mediated** or **immunologically mediated** disease. In other situations the immune response is inadequate or even absent, resulting in a condition known as **immunodeficiency**. The remainder of this chapter will be concerned with some of the consequences of an improperly functioning immune response. It should be noted that some of the following topics are covered in greater detail in other chapters.

ALLERGY, ATOPY, AND ANAPHYLAXIS

True *allergies* result from an inappropriate response on the part of IgE, mast cells, and basophils to relatively innocuous antigens, e.g., house-dust mites, molds, pollen, dander, or other environmental substances. Contact with such *sensitizing* antigens (referred to as **allergens**) results in massive **degranulation** (release of granules) of IgE-coated mast cells and basophils lying beneath mucosal surfaces. The granules released from these cells contain an array of noxious compounds such as **histamine**, **serotonin**, and the **leukotrienes**. In any given individual, the degree of sensitivity to an allergen is directly proportional to the quantities of these compounds released by the cells. In some cases the tendency toward the development of allergies is inherited; this tendency is referred to as **atopy**, and an animal (or person) with such an inherited predisposition is said to be **atopic**. True atopic disease appears to be rare in the horse. Food allergies, also considered rare in horses, may be manifested by an allergic skin condition.

Treatment of allergic disease problems relies on accurate identification of the underlying cause of the allergy, followed by avoidance of the allergen, dietary modification, and possibly therapeutic intervention. Allergies in horses commonly are manifested by signs of irritant respiratory

disease (such as *chronic obstructive pulmonary disease*) or skin disease (such as *urticaria* and *Culicoides hypersensitivity*). For discussions of various allergy-related conditions in the horse, *see* CHAPTER 17, "THE SKIN AND VARIOUS DISORDERS," and CHAPTER 25, "THE RESPIRATORY SYSTEM AND VARIOUS DISORDERS."

Anaphylaxis or an **anaphylactic reaction** represents a rare but extreme example of an IgE-mediated response gone awry. Massive release of histamine and other unpleasant substances from mast cells and basophils produces a range of deleterious effects, such as constriction of airways and blood vessels within the lungs and contraction of smooth muscle in the walls of the digestive tract and bladder. The release of histamine also causes an intense itching about the face and head. The changes within the lungs (e.g., constriction of breathing passages and reduced outflow of blood) result in sudden respiratory distress. An anaphylactic reaction is a life-threatening emergency that arises abruptly following contact with the inciting allergen. The treatment of choice is **epinephrine (adrenaline)**, which must be administered immediately.

It should be kept in mind that anaphylaxis represents an inappropriate overreaction of an idiosyncratic nature; obviously, not all substances induce anaphylaxis in horses, nor are all horses sensitized to the extent that anaphylaxis will occur. Fortunately for both horses and horse owners, anaphylactic reactions are relatively uncommon occurrences.

IMMUNE-MEDIATED HEMOLYTIC ANEMIA

Immune-mediated hemolytic anemia (**IMHA**) is a disease condition in which broadly cross-reactive **autoantibodies** (antibodies directed against the "self," i.e., against the body) called **hemagglutinins** attach to red blood cells, resulting in their immunologic destruction and thereby producing **anemia** (a reduction in red blood cell numbers). The cause or causes are unknown, but the disease is usually found to be secondary to another underlying disorder or circumstance, e.g., cancer (particularly *lymphosarcoma*), bacterial abscesses, equine infectious anemia virus infection, respiratory infections, **purpura hem-**

orrhagica (disease syndrome of subcutaneous hemorrhages or bruises), or penicillin administration. It is thought that disease occurs when an antibody response directed against surface components of red blood cells is generated, indirectly causing the red cells' removal and destruction by the immune system. Although considered a common immune-mediated disorder in dogs, IMAH appears to be of infrequent occurrence in horses.

The onset of disease may be sudden or gradual, and in general the clinical signs exhibited by affected horses can be quite variable. Weakness, lethargy, pallor, **jaundice** (yellowish discoloration of the skin and mucous membranes), and increased heart and respiratory rates are some more common features.

Diagnosis is based on the history, clinical signs, and the results of supportive laboratory tests. The latter include a *Coombs test* to detect the presence of antibody directed against the patient's red blood cells, and a *Coggins test* for detecting antibody to equine infectious anemia virus (*see* CHAPTER 30, "VIRAL DISEASES"). Treatment relies upon the use of corticosteroids or other more potent immunosuppressive drugs to suppress the immune-mediated phenomena that are at the heart of the problem. All efforts must be made to identify and address the underlying cause. In some cases blood transfusions may be required, but compatible donors may be difficult to find. Gradual improvement usually will occur within a few days of initiating therapy. Full restoration of blood counts to normal may require months. The prognosis is usually poor, however.

HEMOLYTIC DISEASE OF THE NEWBORN

Hemolytic disease of the newborn, also known as **neonatal isoerythrolysis**, is an important condition that if left untreated can kill an otherwise healthy newborn foal. It is an unusual type of hemolytic anemia in that the antibodies directed against the foal's red blood cells are transmitted orally from the mare to the foal through the colostrum. The presence of such antibodies in the mare is the result of prior sensitization, usually from a traumatic birthing during which some of a previous foal's blood has leaked into the maternal circulation. The mare then forms antibodies against that foal's red blood cells, and in later pregnancies can transmit the antibodies to subsequent offspring. Should any of those offspring be sired by stallions having the same red blood cell antigens to which the mare has become sensitized, **hemolysis** (red blood cell destruction) of the foal's red cells may occur. Thus, affected foals are usually from the second or later pregnancies of a mare.

Clinical signs include weakness, lethargy, depression, jaundice, and elevated pulse and respiration rates within 1–4 days of birth. Diagnosis is based on the history, clinical signs, and results of supportive laboratory tests, i.e., a Coombs test to detect anti-red cell antibodies and/or a **cross-match** (procedure by which blood samples of the mare and foal are tested for compatibility).

Treatment is best aimed at prevention. When the diagnosis is made prior to birthing, the foal at birth can be immediately removed from the mare for 1–3 days and suckled on a "safe" foster mare or provided with a commercial milk replacer. The mare should be milked several times daily until the foal is returned. Appropriate supportive measures for treating acute hemolytic disease will be required if such precautions are not taken.

No data are available to suggest a familial susceptibility to sensitization. Thus horse owners need not assume that sires or dams of affected foals possess a transmissible liability that would ethically dictate their removal from the breeding pool.

IMMUNE-MEDIATED THROMBOCYTOPENIA

In immune-mediated *thrombocytopenia* (decreased blood platelet numbers) **(IMT)**, antibodies to platelet membranes cause circulating blood platelets to be removed and destroyed in the liver and spleen. Although equine IMT may occur secondary to another underlying disorder or circumstance, such as equine infectious anemia virus infection, cancer (especially lymphosarcoma), bacterial infections, immune-mediated hemolytic anemia, or drug administration, in most cases no predisposing cause can be identified. The blood platelets are indispensable for normal blood clotting and thus signs of deficiency are manifested as a bleeding syndrome. The most common clinical signs consist of small hemorrhages that appear as pigmented spots in the mucous membranes of the mouth, third eyelid, **sclera** (white portion) of the eye, or vagina. On occasion sporadic bleeding from the genital tract or nostrils may be noted.

Diagnosis is made on the basis of the history, clinical findings, and the results of supportive laboratory tests. The presence of low numbers of blood platelets with normal blood coagulation times are suggestive of IMT. Often the diagnosis may be tentatively confirmed on the basis of the animal's response to therapy.

Treatment relies on the use of one or more immunosuppressive medications (**corticosteroids**). A thorough attempt should be made to identify and address any underlying cause(s). The prognosis for recovery is good, provided that therapy is quickly and aggressively applied. Recovery usually occurs 2–3 weeks after treatment is initiated. Many horses will experience only a single episode of thrombocytopenia, but some will endure recurrent bouts. In horses with this more chronic form of the disease, long-term corticosteroid therapy may be required.

PURPURA HEMORRHAGICA

Purpura hemorrhagica (**immune-complex vasculitis**) is an immune-medicated condition that can be associated with various different inciting factors, most often streptococcal or viral infections. It is essentially a *hypersensitivity vasculitis*, i.e., an immunologic reaction targeted at blood-vessel walls, primarily those in the skin. In *strangles* (*see* CHAPTER 25, "THE RESPIRATORY SYSTEM AND VARIOUS DISORDERS") there is good evidence that the M-protein of *Streptococcus equi* is the molecule that the disease-causing immunologic reaction is directed against. The condition also occurs occasionally following respiratory disease caused by *Streptococcus zooepidemicus* or equine influenza virus.

As a complication of strangles, purpura hemorrhagica occurs more often in mature horses than in young horses. It is characterized by depression, reluctance to move, presence of hot, sensitive areas of swelling on the head, trunk, and/or extremities, and widespread hemorrhag-

ing in the skin. The condition varies in severity from a mild transient reaction to a severe fatal condition.

Diagnosis is based primarily on the history and clinical signs. Effective treatment is often difficult in advanced or severe cases, and relapses may occur if therapy is stopped prematurely. Antibiotics and anti-inflammatory medications are indicated. Supportive therapy includes leg wraps, walking exercise, nursing care, **diuretics** (medications that promote urination), and **hydrotherapy** (use of water externally as a therapeutic measure). Death may occur from any of several complications, including pneumonia, **laminitis** ("founder" or inflammation in the foot), and secondary bacterial infections.

SYSTEMIC LUPUS ERYTHEMATOSUS

Systemic lupus erythematosus (**SLE**, **lupus**) is a **multisystemic** (involving many body systems) disorder characterized by a general derangement of certain key immune defense mechanisms. It is considered to be the prototypic immune-mediated disease. In SLE a variety of immune mechanisms begin to attack basic structural components of the body, some as basic as the *deoxyribonucleic acid* (**DNA**)—the genetic material within the nuclei of cells. Autoantibodies directed against such host-cell components attach to cells in the blood, kidneys, skin, and elsewhere, resulting in a widespread immunologic assault upon the body.

Horses are only rarely diagnosed with SLE. Clinical signs that have been reported include fever, depression, weight loss, **edema** (swelling) of the limbs, **panniculitis** (inflammation of fat tissue in the skin), hair loss, and **polyarthritis** (inflammation occurring simultaneously in several joints).

The diagnosis is based on the history, clinical signs, and results of supportive laboratory tests, including the *antinuclear antibody* (**ANA**) *test*, which detects autoantibodies directed against the DNA in cell nuclei. The presence of such autoantibodies is one of the most important diagnostic criteria for SLE and is considered a hallmark of the disease.

Immunosuppressive medication (corticosteroids) represents the cornerstone of therapy. It is likely that affected horses will require long-term treatment, perhaps for life. The prognosis is guarded to poor.

IMMUNE-MEDIATED POLYSYNOVITIS

Polysynovitis (inflammation of the lining membranes of joints) of immunologic origin is a rare condition that has been observed in both foals and mature horses. It appears to be a manifestation of a general phenomenon known as **immune-complex disease**—a syndrome wherein antigens joined together with their specific antibodies into antigen–antibody complexes are filtered out of the circulation and deposited in certain vulnerable tissue sites such as the joints. The trapped complexes attract white blood cells and related components of the immune system, all of which interact to produce inflammation and tissue damage.

Clinical signs include swelling of the affected joints (often in all four limbs) and a stiffened gait. An underlying infection elsewhere in the body often is present and may be the ultimate source of the problem. The diagnosis is made by microscopic examination of joint fluids and by X-ray studies of the affected joint structures. Treatment must address the underlying cause, if it can be identified. Therapy of the immunologic complications requires anti-inflammatory medication (corticosteroids). The prognosis is guarded, and is dependent ultimately on the nature of the underlying infection.

AUTOIMMUNE SKIN DISEASES

Autoimmune skin diseases observed in horses include *pemphigus foliaceus* and *cutaneous lupus erythematosus*. For information on these disorders, *see* CHAPTER 17, "THE SKIN AND VARIOUS DISORDERS."

LYMPHOSARCOMA

Lymphosarcoma (**LSA**) is the most common malignancy of the blood-forming tissues of horses. Lymphosarcomas consist chiefly of solid masses of proliferating lymphocytes no longer responsive to the inhibitory signals that normally control cell division. The net result is runaway growth. This is compounded by the fact that many LSA tumor cells closely resemble the normal cells from which they were derived, and hence may evoke little response from the immune system. There are no recognized age, breed, or sex predilections. The cause of equine LSA is unknown. The feline leukemia virus is the causative agent of most such tumors in cats; to date no analogous equine tumor-inducing virus has been identified.

Several different forms of equine LSA have been described, based principally on variations in the anatomic distribution of the tumor masses. The four major forms are:

- *Multicentric LSA.* This form is characterized by primary involvement of many lymphoid tissues of the body, accompanied by invasion of other organ structures such as the liver, spleen, kidneys, intestine, central nervous system, eyes, or lungs. Clinical signs can include inappetence, depression, weight loss, wasting, **subcutaneous edema** (swellings in the skin), **lymphadenopathy** (enlargement of lymph nodes), jaundice, respiratory difficulty, and neurologic abnormalities.
- *Alimentary LSA.* The **alimentary** (digestive-tract) form of LSA is characterized by tumor-cell infiltration of the digestive tract and other organs, including the associated lymph nodes, liver, and spleen. Clinical signs can include inappetence, weight loss, wasting, subcutaneous edema, and mild colic.
- *Mediastinal LSA.* This form of LSA is centered on the chest cavity and is characterized by inappetence, weight loss, wasting, and respiratory difficulty.
- *Cutaneous LSA.* The **cutaneous** (skin) form is characterized by the presence of a few to many nodules and ulcerated masses infiltrating the skin. Cutaneous LSA usually assumes a chronic course of extensive duration, gradually progressing to involve more and more of the skin surface while at the same time slowly infiltrating internal organs.

The diagnosis usually is made on the basis of the history, presenting clinical signs, and results of appropriate laboratory tests, including serum chemistries and blood counts. Microscopic examination of the tumor cells themselves provides the most definitive diagnosis. Unfortunately there is no satisfactory treatment for equine LSA, although some horses may respond temporarily to the administration of corticosteroid medications.

MULTIPLE MYELOMA

Multiple myeloma is a very uncommon malignant tumor of **plasma cells** (the cells that make antibody) arising from the bone marrow. The cause is unknown. No age, breed, or sex predilections have been noted. The clinical signs are diverse and numerous, and can include inappetence, weight loss, intermittent fever, local swellings, generalized pain, bleeding disorders, lameness, kidney disease, anemia, paralysis of the hind legs, chronic infections, and bone fractures at the tumor site. Myelomas grow through and destroy the normal architecture of bone, and this is the underlying cause of many of the clinical features. In many species the cancerous plasma cells produce large quantities of antibodies or fragments of antibodies that can be detected in blood and sometimes urine, where they are known as *Bence-Jones proteins* (this occurs much less commonly in the horse).

The diagnosis is based on the history, clinical signs, blood counts, X rays (which may graphically reveal the extent of bone destruction caused by the tumor), and microscopic examination of the tumor cells themselves. Treatment with anti-cancer medication has been attempted. However, the prognosis for recovery is extremely poor.

Severe Combined Immunodeficiency (CID) of Arabian Foals This well-known and highly lethal disease of Arabian foals is inherited as an *autosomal recessive* disorder (*see* CHAPTER 13, "GENETICS"). Approximately 2 percent of Arabian foals are born with this condition; about 25 percent of all Arabian stallions and mares are carriers of the defective gene. The specific gene defect involved has not yet been identified, so no carrier test is available; however, the birth of an affected foal provides solid evidence of the carrier status of *both* its parents.

CID foals have no mature T or B lymphocytes and so cannot make antibody or generate any antigen-specific immune responses. (They *do,* however, possess neutrophils, macrophages, and complement, and so can mount certain nonspecific immune responses.) Once the temporary "infusion" of maternal immunity acquired in colostrum has been exhausted, these foals are essentially at the mercy of the microbial population of their environment. They usually succumb before 5 months of age to massive infections, chiefly by pathogens of the respiratory tract, e.g., equine adenovirus as well as bacterial and other opportunists. Antibiotics and infusions of blood plasma containing adenovirus antibodies may be given but will only postpone the inevitably fatal outcome.

Diagnosis is based on the history, physical findings, and supportive laboratory findings. The latter include:

- **Lymphopenia** (decreased number of circulating lymphocytes)
- Absence of circulating IgM
- **Hypoplasia** (underdevelopment) of the lymphoid tissues

All three of these abnormalities must be present for a definitive diagnosis of CID to be made. Because the parents of an affected foal are carriers of the defective gene, they should both be removed from the breeding pool.

SELECTIVE IGM DEFICIENCY

This immunodeficiency disorder affecting primarily Arabians and Quarter Horses was first reported in the late 1970s. As the name implies, the only immunologic abnormality is a subnormal level of circulating IgM. Three major clinical forms of the disease have been recognized:

- A highly fatal syndrome of pneumonia, arthritis, or **enteritis** (intestinal inflammation) in young foals (this is the most common clinical form)

- Chronic, recurrent infections in foals, usually responsive to antibiotic therapy but resulting in retarded growth and poor athletic performance
- Respiratory infections in mature horses, often associated with concomitant lymphosarcoma

Diagnosis is based on the history, clinical findings, and results of supportive laboratory tests, e.g., serum IgM levels. Treatment requires almost continuous antibiotic therapy because clinical signs usually recur when antibiotics are withdrawn. Even with treatment, affected horses will never be athletically "normal" even during periods of remission. The prognosis is guarded to poor.

PART VI

Infectious Diseases, Cancer, and Geriatrics

Here lies the body of my good horse,
The General. For years he bore me
around the circuit of my practice and all
that time he never made a blunder.
Would that his master could say the same.

—JOHN TYLER
TENTH PRESIDENT OF THE UNITED STATES
EPITAPH FOR HIS HORSE

CHAPTER 30

Viral Diseases

by Jeffrey E. Barlough and W. David Wilson

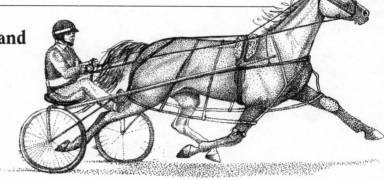

No virus is *known* to do good: it has been well said that a virus is "a piece of bad news wrapped up in protein."
> —P.B. Medawar and J.S. Medawar,
> *Aristotle to Zoos:*
> *A Philosophical Dictionary of Biology (1983)*

In the realm of the microbes, viruses and certain viruslike agents occupy a unique niche: they can infect and damage living hosts, yet they themselves are not alive. To human beings such a mode of existence may be somewhat difficult to imagine. Viruses for example do not ingest or process nutrients. They have no need for breathing or utilizing oxygen in any way. Because they have no independent metabolism they do not excrete waste products. They are incapable of movement and cannot sense their environment in any manner approaching our own powers of sensation. Their sole purpose for existing is to perpetuate and disseminate their own kind. From a broad evolutionary perspective, of course, such is the ultimate purpose of all nature's creatures; so in this a virus is really not that different from a housefly, or a

hadrosaur (duck-billed dinosaur), or a horse. But the way a virus goes about it provides a rare and fascinating glimpse of complex molecules hovering at the threshold of life.

In essence, a typical virus is composed of a segment or several segments of a **nucleic acid**—the virus's genetic material, essentially equivalent to the chromosomes of living cells—that is enclosed in a protective outer shell of protein known as a *capsid*. The nucleic acid is either *ribonucleic acid* (**RNA**) or *deoxyribonucleic acid* (**DNA**)—either one or the other, never both in the same virus. By contrast the nucleic acid of a living cell is made of DNA, while RNA shuttling through different compartments of the cell carries out important regulatory and protein-synthetic functions.

In some viruses the protein shell is itself encased in a soft outer **envelope** that confers certain special properties. Some viruses also carry with them a packet of **enzymes** (proteins that speed chemical reactions) to assist in the viral **replication** (reproduction) cycle. All viruses rely on the living cells they infect for their reproduction. Outside a cell a virus is nothing more than an inert bit of particulate matter; once taken inside, however, the virus commandeers the cell's biosynthetic machinery, converting the cell into a "biotechnology factory" for the assembly and release of countless new virus particles.

Many viruses through their activities kill their host cells, often producing disease as a result and usually initiating an attack by the host's immune defenses. In certain cases the immune response may be particularly aggressive and produce unwanted side-effects that can be more severe than the viral disease itself. Other viruses cause very little damage to host-cell machinery and provoke little if any immunological reaction; they may remain in a dormant or **latent** form for years. Fortunately, most virus infections are **asymptomatic**, i.e., they are so mild and the host response so stunningly effective that signs of disease never develop.

Because few viral diseases respond to specific medication, it is usually the secondary effects of a viral infection that are addressed medically. The immediate goal is to stabilize the patient and guard against secondary bacterial or fungal infections while an antiviral response is being generated by the immune system of the host. Antibiotics (which inhibit bacteria and certain fungi) and antifungal drugs in general have no appreciable effect on viral replication, while clinically useful medications having direct antiviral activity remain few in number and are restricted almost exclusively to some very specific viral infections. Examples of antiviral medications in use today include azidothymidine (AZT), acyclovir, amantadine, and ribavirin.

The *best* therapy for any viral disease, of course, is prevention, i.e., immunization through *vaccination*. (*See* APPENDIX B, "VACCINATIONS AND INFECTIOUS DISEASE CONTROL.")

Equine Viral Diseases

EQUINE VIRAL RESPIRATORY DISEASES

Viral infections of the equine respiratory tract are common and are among the major causes of economic loss to the equine industry. Equine influenza virus and equine herpesviruses types 1 and 4 are the most important causes of viral respiratory disease in horses. Of lesser importance are equine arteritis virus, equine her-

pesvirus type 2, equine rhinoviruses, and equine adenoviruses. The clinical signs caused by the different viruses are similar in nature and thus it is not possible to distinguish between the different infections on the basis of the signs alone. Antibody testing and appropriate virus identification procedures are required to make a definitive diagnosis. Treatment is largely symptomatic. (For complete information on the equine viral respiratory diseases, *see* CHAPTER 25, "THE RESPIRATORY SYSTEM AND VARIOUS DISORDERS.")

EQUINE INFECTIOUS ANEMIA

Equine infectious anemia (**EIA**) is one of the most important viral diseases of horses. It is characterized by a diversity of clinical signs and an exceedingly variable course. Equine infectious anemia occurs in a variety of clinical forms ranging from **acute** (rapid onset, severe) to **chronic** (long term), but in essence it is a chronic infection resulting in a **persistent** (lifelong) carrier state with periodic exacerbations of illness. It was first described in France in 1843 and since then has been reported in virtually all parts of the world where horses are raised. It has been recognized in the United States for more than 80 years.

The Cause

Equine infectious anemia virus (**EIAV**) is a member of the Lentivirinae subfamily of retroviruses (enveloped RNA viruses). Retroviruses carry with them a unique enzyme, **reverse transcriptase**, which allows them to transform their genetic material into DNA. This DNA copy can then be inserted into the chromosomal DNA of the host cell, where it remains for the life of the cell. The DNA copy of the viral RNA is replicated whenever the host cell divides and can serve as a template for the production of new virus particles. Because a version of their genetic material becomes a part of the total genetic blueprint of the cells they infect, retroviruses are among the most intimate parasites known in nature.

Occurrence and Transmission

Equine infectious anemia occurs frequently in rather restricted areas from which it exhibits little tendency to spread. The common name

swamp fever was derived from the observation that flat, swampy lands tended to favor perpetuation of the disease. The virus is shed in virtually all secretions and excretions of the body and is present in the blood. The regional distribution of the disease is due to virus transmission by insects, particularly blood-sucking flies. Horseflies are especially important in transmission because of the volume of infective blood they can carry on their mouthparts. Stable flies, deerflies, and mosquitoes can also spread the infection. The pattern of disease spread predictably is determined by the seasonal distribution of the insects and by their flight habits. Evidence indicates that EIAV can also be transmitted from an infected to a susceptible horse by the careless use of blood-contaminated hypodermic syringes, tattooing needles, or surgical instruments. Natural infection also occurs across the placenta from the mare to the developing fetus, and by the foal's ingestion of **colostrum** (first milk) containing infected white blood cells.

PATHOGENESIS

Once it has entered the body EIAV travels through the bloodstream and is readily taken up by certain white blood cells in which it is able to replicate to high levels. The presence of circulating virus results in fever and other clinical signs and stimulates the production of antibodies and immune cells by the horse's immune system (*see* CHAPTER 29, "THE IMMUNE SYSTEM AND VARIOUS DISORDERS").

Despite these highly charged responses, however, infected horses are unable to eliminate the virus from the body and remain infected for life. Such infected carriers are the only recognized reservoir of EIAV in nature.

The disease itself consists of a series of exacerbations of fever and anemia which coincide with the appearance of new EIAV variants in the bloodstream. Most likely these result from inborn errors of virus replication, which paradoxically are beneficial to the virus because they generate variant virus particles to which the immune system must respond anew. The anemia is due to a combination of impaired red blood cell production and immunologically mediated destruction of circulating red blood cells (an abnormality

seen in a number of different virus infections). Affected horses also develop a **thrombocytopenia** (an abnormally low number of circulating **platelets**, cell fragments that play an important role in blood clotting), which may be immunologically mediated as well.

Clinical Signs

Equine infectious anemia may assume an acute or chronic disease course. The acute form occurs most commonly when the virus is first introduced into a group of susceptible horses. The clinical signs during an acute attack include fever, inappetence, depression, rapid weight loss, **ventral edema** (tissue swelling affecting the underside of the body), anemia, and depressed blood platelet counts. Affected horses often sweat profusely during warm weather and may develop a nasal discharge. An acute attack usually lasts for 3–5 days, while the period between attacks may be months or years. During the first few months of infection, recurrent episodes may occur with surprising regularity; after this period attacks are much less frequent and severe. Any attack has the potential to kill a horse. Most infected horses recover, however, and become lifelong carriers of the virus. In the chronic form of EIA, attacks continue at periodic intervals until the horse becomes progressively more emaciated and anemic, and eventually dies.

Diagnosis

Diagnosis is based on the history, clinical findings, and results of supportive laboratory tests. Among these are low red blood cell and platelet counts, and a positive test for EIAV antibody by the *agar gel immunodiffusion (AGID) test* or *Coggins test*. (Because infection with EIAV is lifelong, the presence of antibody in a horse indicates that it is a virus carrier.) Recently a second antibody test, the *competitive ELISA (C-ELISA)*, has been approved for the diagnosis of EIAV infection. Horses suffering their first attack of EIA may be more difficult to diagnose because they may not yet have developed antibodies to EIAV at the time of examination.

Treatment

There is no specific therapy for EIA. Treatment is purely supportive in nature.

Prevention

Strict federal and state control measures are in place in the United States in order to identify carriers of EIAV. In most states it is required that all incoming horses test negative for EIAV antibody within a 6–12 month period prior to entering the state. Many states also require a negative EIAV antibody test at the time ownership of a horse is transferred. Many show and athletic events also require that participating horses test negative.

State regulations vary with regard to the disposition of horses testing positive for EIAV antibody. Options may include euthanasia, permanent identification and lifelong quarantine in a screened, fly-proof environment, or transfer to an EIAV research facility. Interstate transport of EIAV carriers is strictly prohibited, except when a horse is being shipped to its place of origin, to a slaughterhouse, or to a government-approved EIAV research facility.

In areas where EIA is prevalent the use of common equipment (bridles, combs, brushes, etc.) should be discouraged. Surgical instruments should be thoroughly sterilized before use on an animal. Syringes and needles should preferably be the disposable type and be used only once on each horse. Flies and other insects should be controlled through the use of insecticides and protective screening, wherever possible.

There is no available vaccine.

RABIES

The specter of rabies has haunted Europe and Asia since the dawn of recorded history. The first identifiable account of it may reside in this excerpt from the law tablets of ancient Mesopotamia: "If a dog is vicious and the authorities have brought the fact to the knowledge of its owner, (if nevertheless) he does not keep it in, it bites a man and causes (his) death, then the owner of the dog shall pay two-thirds of a mina of silver . . ." Rabies was also familiar to the ancient Greeks; Aristotle and Xenophon recorded instances of its occurrence.

Today rabies can be found on all continents of the world except Australia and Antarctica. Despite the availability of effective rabies vaccines for both animals and human beings, rabies remains a persistent cause of concern, particularly in the developing countries. In the western industrialized world, vaccination programs aimed at domestic dog populations have virtually eliminated human cases of rabies. In the United States rabies cases among domestic animals continue to be reported at a relatively low frequency, a reminder of the lingering presence of this ancient scourge.

The Cause

Rabies is caused by a bullet-shaped virus in the Rhabdoviridae family of RNA viruses. Rhabdoviruses have outer envelopes and thus are relatively easily destroyed by common household soaps, detergents, and disinfectants.

Occurrence and Transmission

Rabies virus cycles in nature through wild and domestic carnivores and through certain other wildlife species. Variation exists in the pattern of hosts in different areas of the world. In the United States, skunks have a major role in transmitting the disease, particularly in the midwest and west, where they are now the main reservoir of rabies virus infection. In the southeastern states raccoons are spreading the infection and moving it northward along the eastern seaboard. Wild foxes are very important reservoir hosts in Europe and to some extent in North America as well. In the Caribbean and much of the Americas, bats are important reservoirs of infection. In the Latin American countries, vampire bats are particularly notorious for spreading rabies to herds of cattle. The mongoose is another well-known reservoir host in certain regions, including South Africa and the Caribbean. The woodchuck appears to be the only rodent species of importance in rabies virus transmission, particularly in the mid-Atlantic and midwestern regions of the United States.

Of the domestic species only dogs and cats are important carriers of rabies virus. In most developing countries, domestic dogs remain the primary reservoir hosts for rabies and the principal source of human exposure. Rabid animals excrete large quantities of rabies virus in their saliva, which accounts for the primary mechanism by which the virus is transmitted, i.e., by the bite of an infected animal. Most rabid horses probably acquire the infection from wildlife. A number of cases of rabies have been documented in foals and young horses (1 year of age or younger). Such animals may be more likely to be bitten by rabid wildlife because they are more eager and inquisitive than older animals.

Pathogenesis

The **incubation period** (time between exposure and the onset of clinical signs of disease) for rabies in the horse is quite variable, generally ranging from 2 to 9 weeks. This variability apparently reflects the amount of time the rabies virus is retained within muscle cells at the site of inoculation (usually a bite wound). Following this early stage of infection, the virus crosses the **neuromuscular junctions** (connections between muscle cells and adjacent nerve cells) and advances into the nervous system, traveling directly up the nerve-cell bodies until it gains access to the spinal cord and eventually the brain. Invasion of the brain is followed by further virus spread—again within the nerves themselves—to additional sites important for subsequent transmission of the virus, e.g., the salivary glands, respiratory system, and digestive tract. Once clinical signs have developed the outcome is invariably fatal, although the precise cellular mechanism by which the virus causes death remains unidentified.

Clinical Signs

The clinical signs of rabies are similar overall in the different animal species, but those observed in individual cases can vary tremendously. In general, two major forms or manifestations of rabies are recognized: the excitatory or "furious" form (the better known and more graphic), and the paralytic or "dumb" form. In actuality, most cases of rabies exhibit one or more manifestations of both forms. The paralytic form always represents the terminal stage of the disease; however, some animals die during convulsive seizures while in the furious stage without progressing to the final, paralytic stage.

Rabies in the horse is often insidious in onset and clinically can resemble almost any other disease. Affected horses may be presented to the veterinarian for a variety of complaints, such as lameness or colic, that would not immediately bring rabies to mind as a possible diagnosis. Most rabid horses exhibit few if any signs of excitement or "madness," the clinical picture reflecting instead the effects of **paresis** (partial paralysis) or paralysis. **Hyperesthesia** (excessive sensitivity to touch or other external stimuli), fever, incoordination, and paresis beginning in the hindquarters and progressing forward, are among the clinical signs observed in most horses at some point in the disease course. Other signs that may develop as the disease progresses include **hypalgesia** (diminished sensitivity to pain) in the hind limbs and loss of tone in the musculature of the tail and *anal* **sphincter** (circular band of muscle that controls the expulsion of feces from the anus). Some horses develop swallowing difficulties owing to paralysis of muscles in the throat. Depression, **recumbency** (inability to stand), and coma precede death. Some recumbent horses may continue to eat and drink before suffering the final effects of the disease (usually respiratory or cardiac arrest). Convulsions may or may not occur.

For both horses and human beings, rabies is an inevitably fatal illness once the clinical signs have appeared. To date only a handful of human survivors are recorded in the medical literature. Survival time of horses after the onset of clinical signs is 4 or 5 days; rarely, horses may survive for 10 to 18 days.

Diagnosis

From the foregoing discussion it is evident that the clinical signs of rabies in the horse are not in and of themselves sufficient to arrive at a correct diagnosis; a definitive diagnosis can be made only by laboratory examination of brain tissue. In cases involving human exposure to a potentially rabid horse or other animal—taking into account the grave prognosis for recovery once clinical signs are apparent—the accuracy of the diagnosis in the suspect animal is of paramount importance.

Currently there are three available methods for the laboratory diagnosis of rabies:

- **Immunofluorescence microscopy,** the most rapid and accurate method and the one most recommended, in which brain tissue is directly examined for the presence of rabies virus using fluorescent-labeled antibodies and a fluorescent microscope

- **Histopathology**, in which brain-tissue smears are examined for the presence of *Negri bodies*, intracellular inclusion bodies that are formed in the brain in many (but not all) cases of rabies
- **Mouse inoculation,** which is often used to confirm positive results or to investigate further any strongly suspected rabies cases that have tested negative by other methods

Guidelines for the control of rabies virus infection in animals are available from the National Association of State Public Health Veterinarians, Inc. (**NASPHV**). Each year, usually in January, updated NASPHV guidelines are published in an issue of the *Journal of the American Veterinary Medical Association*, together with a compendium of currently licensed rabies vaccines for use in domestic animals. It is these guidelines in part that serve as the basis for the recommendations that follow.

Any wild or domestic mammal that has bitten a human being and is exhibiting clinical signs consistent with a diagnosis of rabies should be humanely destroyed. The head should be submitted to a qualified rabies diagnostic laboratory where the brain will be examined for the presence of rabies virus. *Regardless of clinical signs,* any bat or wild carnivorous mammal that has bitten a human being should be destroyed and the head submitted for diagnostic testing (this is because of the variable period of salivary shedding of rabies virus that can occur *before* clinical signs are manifested). Any bat that has bitten a human being should be presumed rabid until confirmed negative by laboratory examination.

An *unvaccinated* horse that has been bitten by or exposed to a known rabid animal should either be destroyed or quarantined for 6 months and vaccinated for rabies 1 month before release. *A properly rabies-vaccinated horse* that has been bitten by or exposed to a known rabid animal should be given a rabies booster immunization immediately and kept under observation for 90 days. If clinical signs of rabies should appear during the observation period, the ani-

mal should be humanely destroyed and the brain examined to confirm the diagnosis.

Treatment
Owing to the potential risk of exposing human beings to rabies virus, *attempted treatment of animals suspected of having rabies is not recommended*. Treatment of human beings exposed to a known or suspect rabid animal, however, must be aggressively applied. Any person bitten by a wild animal should immediately report the incident to his or her physician, who can evaluate the need for anti-rabies therapy. Treatment should consist of:

- Thorough flushing and cleansing of the bite wound with warm soap and water. *The importance of this simple measure cannot be overemphasized!*
- Administration of rabies virus antiserum to those exposed individuals with no previous history of rabies immunization
- Administration of human diploid-cell rabies vaccine in five doses, given on days 0, 3, 7, 14, and 28 postexposure

Further details regarding pre-exposure and postexposure rabies prevention and vaccine administration can be found in the current recommendations of the Immunization Practices Advisory Committee (**ACIP**) of the U.S. Public Health Service. These recommendations can be obtained at any state health department office.

Prevention
In the United States and most other countries, highly effective rabies vaccines are available for use in domestic animal species. Mass immunization programs for dogs have been employed for many years to control rabies virus spread by creating an "immunological barrier" between wildlife reservoirs of the disease and human beings (dogs frequently acquire the infection from wildlife hosts and then may transmit it to human contacts).

Some nations, notably Japan, England, Iceland, and the Scandinavian countries, have eradicated rabies through control programs and stringent quarantine regulations. Despite such successes, however, rabies is still a significant public health hazard in many developing countries of the world.

Immunization remains the best deterrent to the spread of rabies to human populations. Horses maintained in rural (particularly wooded) areas where rabies is known to occur in the local wildlife population are at risk and should be vaccinated. Several rabies vaccines, all containing **inactivated** ("killed") virus for intramuscular injection, are approved for use in horses and appear to be safe and effective. Manufacturers' recommendations specify primary vaccination of horses aged 3 months or older with a single dose of vaccine, followed by a second dose at 1 year of age with annual boosters thereafter. *However, the authors recommend that the primary series be initiated with two doses of vaccine given 1 month apart.* (*See* APPENDIX B, "VACCINATIONS AND INFECTIOUS DISEASE CONTROL.")

Rabies vaccination of pregnant mares is not currently recommended, pending further safety studies of vaccination during pregnancy. Mares should therefore receive their immunizations prior to breeding.

Public Health Significance

The clinical signs and course of rabies in human beings are similar to those of animal victims of the disease. Both excitatory and paralytic symptoms may be apparent. The incubation period, as in animals, may vary in length—from about 2 weeks to as long as a year — but usually averages between 3 and 6 weeks. Once symptoms appear the course of illness is brief—only a few days— *and the mortality rate is essentially 100 percent.*

The extent of human exposure to rabies virus during the examination, treatment, or postmortem examination of a rabid horse is dependent on the measures that have been taken to minimize exposure and the speed with which the suspect case was recognized. A horse suspected of being rabid should have a warning sign posted conspicuously on its stall, and all traffic should be diverted away from the immediate vicinity. Individuals who have handled the horse should be identified and the extent of their contact with the animal documented.

Although it has not been conclusively proven that infected horses are capable of transmitting rabies virus to people, it is prudent to minimize the number of personnel involved in the diagnosis and supportive care of a suspected case. Personnel providing supportive care should be vaccinated against rabies, wear rubber gloves and face shields and other protective clothing around the patient, and have as little contact as possible with the patient's mouth and saliva.

VESICULAR STOMATITIS

Vesicular stomatitis (**VS**) occurs primarily in horses, cattle, and pigs, and is characterized by fever and the development of **vesicles** (blisters) and **ulcerations** (severe sloughing of the surface tissue) of the mouth, tongue, **coronary band** (band of tissue from which the horn of the hoof grows), and teats. People and certain wildlife species are also susceptible to infection.

The Cause

Like rabies, VS is caused by a member of the bullet-shaped Rhabdoviridae family of RNA viruses. Three types of VS virus (**VSV**) are recognized: Indiana, New Jersey, and a variety of local strains. In general the New Jersey type produces a more severe illness and has been responsible for most of the outbreaks of VS recorded in the United States.

Occurrence and Transmission

The most recent equine outbreaks of VS in the United States occurred in New Mexico, Arizona, Colorado, Texas, and Utah in 1995. A previous outbreak occurred in the midwestern and western states (particularly Colorado) in the 1980s. In general outbreaks occur at more frequent intervals in the tropics and less often at more temperate latitudes, and there is a definite seasonal pattern. In the temperate zone the disease appears late in the warm season and disappears with the onset of killing frosts, while in the tropics it appears at the close of the rainy season and disappears as the countryside dries out. This feature, combined with VS's recognized rapidity of spread, predilection for well-watered areas, and at times idiosyncratic confinement to certain wooded pastures, suggests a possible role for insect or tick **vectors** (organisms that carry disease-causing microorganisms from an infected animal to a noninfected animal) in VSV transmission. One hypothesis holds that VSV is actually a plant virus that only becomes infective for mammals after passage through a vector. The disease can also be transmitted from one infected animal to another by means of oral secretions, which can contain immense quantities of virus.

Pathogenesis

The disease mechanism appears to be relatively straightforward. A fever and **viremia** (presence of virus in the bloodstream) of short duration develop soon after infection, with the virus eventually localizing in the oral tissues, mammary gland, and coronary band. Replication of the virus at these sites is followed by local cellular **necrosis** (cell death) and the formation of vesicles, which quickly rupture to leave raw, eroded areas. Like rabies virus, VSV apparently cannot penetrate intact skin but may enter through breaks or across mucous membranes.

Immunity to VSV is relatively short-lived (only 6 months or so). Animals thus can be reinfected with the same virus type and redevelop clinical illness. Unfortunately there is no cross-immunity between the different virus types.

Clinical Signs

Excessive salivation is often the first clinical sign of VS in the horse. The lesions are most evident on the lips, gums, and tongue. Because the vesicles develop early and are quite fragile they are rarely observed; instead, what one usually sees are the erosions and ulcers left in their wake. Affected horses often are depressed and reluctant to eat, but they may accept water. They champ their jaws and grind their teeth, drooling a clear, ropy saliva. They may rub their lips on the edges of mangers or other convenient surfaces. Lesions can also develop in the rear of the mouth and in parts of the nasal passages, resulting in **dysphagia** (difficulty swallowing), mild **epistaxis** (nosebleed), or respiratory distress. Oral ulcers usually begin healing within a week or two of onset.

Lesions developing on the feet include **coronitis** (inflammation of the coronary band) and subsequent ulceration of the coronary band, which can lead to cracking of the hoof wall and severe lameness. Secondary bacterial infection of the lesions can be a serious complication. Lesions of the teats, while common in dairy cattle with VS, are rarely observed in horses.

Diagnosis

A tentative diagnosis of VS can be made on the basis of the history and clinical signs. A definitive diagnosis can only be made in the laboratory, with isolation and identification of virus from lesion samples being the most trustworthy procedure.

Treatment

There is no specific treatment. Affected horses should be removed from woodlot pastures and isolated from healthy, susceptible animals. Water and a soft, readily palatable feed should be provided. Severely affected horses may require intravenous fluids and antibiotics. Foot lesions should be promptly and assiduously cared for to prevent hoof loss. Communal water troughs and feed bunks should be thoroughly cleansed and disinfected, and insect control measures instituted, if possible.

Prevention

At present no VSV vaccines are available for use in horses.

Public Health Significance

The vast majority of human VSV infections are clinically inapparent. When VS does occur in people it is characterized by mild, influenzalike signs. Occasionally vesicles are formed, particularly in the mouth and on the lips. Most cases have occurred in laboratory workers and researchers in contact with large quantities of virus derived from cell cultures. Nevertheless, owners and veterinarians should always use caution (and preferably wear rubber gloves and protective face- and eyewear) when handling infected horses.

Equine Viral Encephalomyelitis

In the United States equine viral **encephalomyelitis** (inflammation of the brain and spinal cord) is caused by either eastern equine encephalomyelitis (**EEE**) virus or western equine encephalomyelitis (**WEE**) virus. Venezuelan equine encephalomyelitis (**VEE**) caused by VEE virus, which occurs in the southern Americas, has not been diagnosed in the United States for over 20 years. All three viruses are transmitted from wild birds and/or rodents (which act as reservoir hosts) to horses by mosquitoes and occasionally by other blood-sucking insects. Human beings are also susceptible to infection and on occasion develop severe, sometimes fatal, neurologic disease.

The Cause

The equine encephalomyelitis viruses are alphaviruses in the Togaviridae family of enveloped RNA viruses. There are at least six known subtypes of VEE virus.

Occurrence and Transmission

In the United States EEE occurs during the late summer and early fall primarily in the eastern and southern parts of the country. The virus is transmitted chiefly by mosquitoes of the genus *Culiseta*, with waterfowl acting as reservoir hosts, i.e., they carry the virus but rarely develop disease. Outbreaks of EEE in horses and pheasants and occasional cases in people often occur in close proximity to freshwater swamp habitats where the virus is cycling through its reservoirs. People and horses are essentially "dead-end" hosts, i.e., they are susceptible to infection but cannot transmit the virus themselves to another host, becoming infected only incidentally when fed upon by infected mosquitoes.

Western equine encephalomyelitis occurs in the summer and early fall throughout much of the United States, particularly the western, midwestern, and southern states. It is transmitted chiefly by mosquitoes of the genus *Culex* and is harbored by wild-bird reservoirs and possibly rodents. As with EEE, horses and people are dead-end hosts for the virus.

Outbreaks of VEE occur periodically in Central and South America. The causative virus can be transmitted by many different blood-sucking insect species. Unlike EEE and WEE, horses serve as the principal reservoir hosts for outbreak strains of VEE virus. Human beings are only dead-end hosts.

Pathogenesis

After being introduced into the body by the bite of an infected insect, the viruses replicate in muscle and local lymph nodes. Most infections are quickly squelched by the immune system. If this does not occur, the virus can spread through the blood circulation to infect the liver, spleen, and nervous system, resulting in encephalomyelitis and severe neurologic dysfunction.

Clinical Signs

The disease syndrome is essentially similar for all three infections. Early clinical signs include fever, muscle stiffness, and inappetence, lasting for up to 5 days. If the disease progresses beyond this point, neurologic signs soon become apparent. These include depression, chewing movements, excessive salivation, compulsive walking or circling, and incoordination. (The common name "**sleeping sickness**" is used in reference to the depression and somnolence characteristic of the disease.) Further progression to severe encephalomyelitic illness may be manifested by head-pressing, drooping of the ears and eyelids, apparent blindness, inability to stand, and convulsions, leading to coma and death.

Many equine infections with EEE, WEE, and VEE viruses are clinically inapparent. The mortality rates for horses developing neurological disease are high, however, ranging from approximately 20–50% for WEE, the least pathogenic of the three, to 40–80% for VEE and as high as 75–98% for EEE.

Diagnosis

Diagnosis is based on the history, physical examination, evidence of seasonal insect vector activity in the vicinity, and the result of supportive laboratory tests (antibody assays, virus isolation, analysis of **cerebrospinal fluid** [fluid bathing the surface of the brain and spinal cord]).

Treatment

There is no specific therapy. Treatment is primarily supportive, and may include the administration of intravenous fluids and nonsteroidal anti-inflammatory agents. Affected horses should be protected from accidental self-trauma with leg wraps and head protection. Quality nursing care is essential. Animals that recover from neurological signs may exhibit permanent neurological abnormalities, including behavioral changes, incoordination, and depression.

Prevention

Preventive measures are based chiefly on insect control and vaccination of horses in areas where the viruses are active. Safe and effective vaccines for all three viruses are currently available. Vaccination should be timed to precede the mosquito season. (For current EEE and WEE immunization guidelines, *see* APPENDIX B, "VACCINATIONS AND INFECTIOUS DISEASE CONTROL.")

Public Health Significance

The presence of equine cases of viral encephalomyelitis are indicative of infected insect-vector activity in the area. Although the percentage of exposed human beings developing neurological disease is very low, such disease when it does develop can have devastating consequences. In affected areas, precautions should be taken to minimize exposure to mosquitoes during the warm months of the year. Useful preventive measures include avoiding outdoor activity at night (particularly at dusk and dawn), applying mosquito repellants, and wearing long-sleeved shirts and long pants.

OTHER EQUINE VIRUS INFECTIONS

Equine Rotaviral Enteritis

Rotaviruses are members of the Reoviridae family of viruses and contain several segments of double-stranded RNA as their genetic material. The name **rotavirus** is derived from the "spoked-wheel" appearance of the viral particles, which are nonenveloped but surrounded by a unique double-layered capsid that provides protection against environmental degradation. Rotaviruses are causative agents of diarrhea in the young of many species, including foals, calves, lambs, and human babies.

Rotaviral enteritis (intestinal inflammation) is most common and severe in young nursing foals. Equine rotavirus can produce profuse diarrhea, dehydration, inappetence, and depression in foals from 2 days to 6 months of age. Although many foals can become ill at one time, the mortality rate is usually low if appropriate supportive therapy is provided. Transmission occurs primarily by the fecal-oral route, i.e., the virus is ingested, replicates in the intestinal tract, and then is excreted in large quantities in the feces. Although infected animals shed rotavirus for short periods (days) while recovering, the general hardiness of the virus and its persistence in the environment are probably of equal, if not greater, importance in perpetuating infections. Foals that recover from rotavirus infection usually acquire a long-lived immunity.

A presumptive diagnosis of equine rotaviral enteritis can be made by the veterinarian on the basis of the history, clinical signs, and the results of supportive laboratory tests, the most valuable of which are the latex agglutination and ELISA tests for rotavirus in feces.

No specific antiviral therapy is available. Veterinary care is aimed chiefly at preventing and treating dehydration. The primary goal is to stabilize the foal until its normal immune defenses clear the infection and initiate recovery. Fluid and electrolyte solutions thus have become mainstays of therapy, and good nursing care is an absolute essential. *One cannot overemphasize the importance of fluid therapy, either oral or by injection, in the treatment regimen for rotaviral enteritis.* It is the massive loss of fluids and electrolytes that can occur in diarrheic feces, more than any other single factor, that is most contributory to an unfavorable outcome.

Once infection with rotavirus has occurred the virus may persist on the premises for many months. The resistance of rotavirus to environmental inactivation necessitates thorough cleansing (soap and water) of stall surfaces followed by disinfection with a phenolic disinfectant. All foaling stalls should be washed and disinfected, allowed to dry, and disinfected again prior to the foaling season and after each foaling. There is no available vaccine.

Equine Herpesvirus Type 3

Herpesviruses are enveloped DNA viruses that cause a wide variety of important diseases in a number of species. *Equine coital exanthema* is caused by equine herpesvirus (**EHV**) type 3. It is usually spread during breeding and is characterized by the development of small blisters and ulcers on the penis of the stallion and vulva of the mare. Lesions can also occur on the teats of the mare and the muzzle and lips of the nursing foal. No effects on fertility have been recognized, but affected stallions may be reluctant to breed until the penile lesions have healed. Infected horses are believed to carry the virus for life.

Diagnosis is based primarily on the history, clinical signs, and results of supportive laboratory procedures. Treatment involves temporary isolation and sexual rest (at least several weeks) and application of soothing ointments to promote healing of the lesions. There is no available vaccine.

Equine herpesvirus type 5 does not cause any recognized disease in horses.

Equine Viral Papillomatosis

Horses may develop infectious *papillomas* (warts) on the muzzle, around the lips, or on the extremities. Occasionally they are found on the genitalia or around the eyes. They can vary in number from a few lesions to several hundred warty masses. Papillomas essentially are benign tumors of the upper skin layers and are caused by *equine papillomavirus*, a member of the Papovaviridae family of double-stranded DNA viruses. The papillomas usually grow for 1–2 months and then spontaneously regress, with recovery complete in 4–6 months. Transmission occurs probably by direct contact and by contaminated implements (combs, brushes, tack, surgical instruments). Sometimes papillomas are found as **congenital** (present at birth) lesions in the skin of the head, neck, back, or croup of newborn foals, reflecting infection of the fetus before birth.

Diagnosis is based on the history and on the physical appearance of the warts themselves. Treatment is usually not necessary.

African Horse Sickness

African horse sickness (**AHS**) is an acute, severe to mild, insect-transmitted disease of horses, mules, and donkeys. It is restricted primarily to sub-Saharan Africa but outbreaks have been reported on the Asian continent and in southern Europe. As a former veterinary medical officer for the U.S. Department of Agriculture once wrote: "The disease has a history of following camel trains in the desert. Camels are not susceptible to this disease but there usually is a donkey leading the camel train. The donkey always knows where he is going, whereas that is not necessarily true for the camels."

The most recent outbreaks outside sub-Saharan Africa occurred in the late 1980s in Spain, Morocco, and Portugal. The causative virus, an orbivirus in the Reoviridae family of double-stranded RNA viruses, is not present in North America or any other part of the Western Hemisphere.

African horse sickness occurs in low-lying, warm, humid regions where the insects that spread the virus—primarily gnats of the genus *Culicoides*—can be found in abundance. There are four major clinical forms or syndromes:

- A fatal **peracute** or **pulmonary form**, in which the lungs rapidly fill with fluid and the horse virtually "drowns" in its own respiratory secretions
- A **subacute** or **cardiac form**, characterized by widespread swelling of various body tissues; approximately 50 percent of affected horses die
- An **acute** or **mixed form**, with clinical signs of both the pulmonary and cardiac form; the most common form of AHS, with a mortality rate of 50–95 percent
- A **horse sickness fever form**, a very mild illness characterized by fever and perhaps slight depression and inappetence, from which most animals recover

At least nine different AHS virus types have been identified. Animals that recover from AHS develop a solid immunity to the virus type with which they were infected, and do not carry or shed the virus for any appreciable length of time.

In countries where AHS is common, the history and clinical signs are frequently sufficient to provide a diagnosis. Otherwise, virus identification and serum antibody studies are required. There is no specific treatment. A number of experimental vaccines have been investigated for use in the field, and at least one commercial vaccine has recently become available. Control of the disease relies on a combination of vaccination and insect-control measures.

Getah Virus

Like AHS virus, *getah virus* is not known to occur in the United States. It is an alphavirus in the Togaviridae family of RNA viruses. It infects a wide variety of vertebrate hosts and is transmitted by mosquitoes. Although the virus is widespread throughout southeast Asia and Australia, disease has been reported thus far only in Japan.

In horses getah virus causes an acute illness characterized by fever, skin rashes, and swelling of the extremities. A nasal discharge and enlargement of lymph nodes in the head or neck may also be seen. Spontaneous recovery usually occurs within 1–2 weeks.

Diagnosis is based on the history, clinical signs, and the results of supportive laboratory tests (virus isolation, detection of specific antibodies). Treatment is purely supportive. Mosquito-control measures combined with vaccination are reportedly effective in controlling infections.

Japanese Encephalitis Virus

Japanese encephalitis virus (**JEV**) is a member of the Flaviviridae family of RNA viruses. It infects a variety of vertebrate hosts (including people) and is transmitted by mosquitoes. The virus is widespread throughout Asia and the Pacific islands. Outbreaks are most often reported in China, Japan, and Korea. The virus is not known to occur in the United States.

In horses and donkeys JEV causes an acute illness characterized by fever, lethargy, inappetence, and severe neurologic dysfunction (disorientation, staggering, excitation, blindness, seizures, coma) reflecting **encephalitis** (inflammation of the brain). The disease is seasonal in occurrence, coinciding with the activity of the mosquito vectors. Several species of waterfowl and probably pigs serve as reservoir and/or amplifying hosts. Horses and people are essentially dead-end hosts, becoming infected only incidentally when fed upon by mosquitoes that have acquired the virus from reservoir hosts.

Diagnosis is based on the history, clinical signs, and the results of supportive laboratory tests (virus isolation, detection of specific antibodies). Treatment is purely supportive. Mosquito-control measures combined with vaccination are reportedly effective in controlling infections in China and Japan.

Borna Disease

This is a rare, highly fatal disease of horses and sheep that has been recognized in Germany and Switzerland for over 150 years. It is apparently caused by an RNA virus that thus far has proved extremely difficult to characterize or classify. Spread of infection probably results from contamination of food or water with virus shed in nasal and salivary secretions of affected horses. The virus is also excreted in milk and urine. Borna disease is not known to occur in the United States or in any other country of the Western Hemisphere.

In horses the disease is characterized initially by fever, inappetence, excessive salivation, chewing movements, frequent yawning, and lethargy. As the disease progresses severe neurologic signs become evident, including incoordination, rapid eye movements, head-pressing, a "saw-horse" stance, partial paralysis, and loss of equilibrium. General restlessness and irritability, biting, and kicking are often seen. Eventually the horse is no longer able to stand, lapses into a coma, and dies.

Diagnosis is based on the history, clinical signs, and results of supportive laboratory tests. There is no specific therapy. The prognosis is extremely poor; more than 90 percent of animals developing neurologic signs die. A vaccine is available.

CHAPTER 31

Bacterial Diseases

by Jeffrey E. Barlough and
John E. Madigan

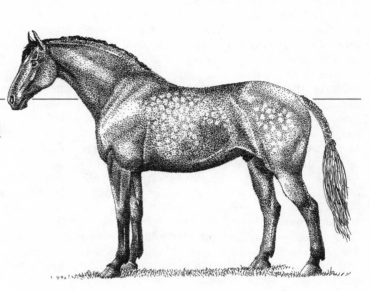

The bacteria represent a varied group of **unicellular** (single-celled) microbes whose family tree can be traced back to the very roots of life on earth. These minute, versatile organisms surround us in our everyday lives, existing not only in the environment but also on and within us, yet they remain essentially invisible to the naked eye. Bacteria (singular = *bacterium*) are complex, sophisticated, metabolizing, self-reproducing, living organisms—quite unlike the inanimate, particulate, **subcellular** (smaller than cells) biochemical entities known as viruses that were discussed in the previous chapter. Moreover, bacteria contain both types of nucleic acid, *deoxyribonucleic acid* (**DNA**) and *ribonucleic acid* (**RNA**), while viruses contain only one or the other. Bacterial cells are surrounded by a cell wall and have a central **nucleus** that contains the DNA but lacks a delimiting membrane. Most bacteria multiply by **binary fission**, in which the parental cell divides into two approximately equal offspring.

Many bacteria are free-living inhabitants of the biosphere and through their metabolic activities are instrumental in supporting local and global ecosystems. Other bacteria can be found on the skin and in the digestive and reproductive tracts of higher organisms where they exist in harmonious balance with the host, from whom they derive nourishment and for whom they often provide benefits in return. On occasion, if given the proper conditions, some of these otherwise beneficial bacteria may gain access to the deeper, normally sterile tissues of the host and produce disease.

Another extensive and somewhat specialized group of bacteria can be classified as true **pathogens**—agents of disease. These are bacteria that for the most part have a heightened potential for injuring the host. They are able to colonize tissue and for some period of time can evade the host's immune responses. In some cases they are not considered part of the normal bacterial flora and if present are almost always associated with a disease process. These organisms are the primary bacterial disease agents of importance to veterinarians and their equine patients.

Taxonomic classifications for bacteria are identified primarily by the genus, whose first letter is capitalized, followed by the species which is entirely in lower case. Both are always in italics. After the bacterium is named formally, it is thereafter identified by the initial of the genus and the species name. The genuses are divided into 19 groups with lower-case, italicized names such as *spirochetes* or *mycoplasmas*.

The **rickettsiae** are a group of specialized bacteria that differ from the more "conventional" bacteria in a number of important ways. Most rickettsiae multiply only within host cells (being somewhat viruslike in this requirement) and usually are transmitted to animals or people by lice, ticks, fleas, or mites. Two examples of rickettsial pathogens important in equine medicine are *Ehrlichia risticii*, the cause of Potomac horse fever, and *Ehrlichia equi*, the cause of equine granulocytic ehrlichiosis.

Included among the many equine bacterial diseases are a broad spectrum of infections that may develop at any time in a horse's life. During the neonatal period the foal receives its initial exposure to the bacterial population of its immediate environment. Should the maternal immunity the foal received in the mare's **colostrum** (first milk) prove insufficient, or should the foal be exposed to a pathogen during the time that maternal immunity is declining but before its own immune defenses are fully operational, serious infections may occur. In later years some bacterial infections may be promoted, at least in part, by **immunosuppression**, i.e., by a compromised immune system. Certain drugs, inherited tendencies, or viruses can to one degree or another interfere with the normal functional mechanisms of the immune response and predispose the host to bacterial infection. Arabian foals with severe combined immune deficiency (**SCID**, **CID**) are at an equal disadvantage, not because their immune system has been suppressed, however, but because it has failed to develop properly in the first place. (*See* Chapter 29, "The Immune System and Various Disorders.")

Fortunately many bacteria are sensitive to the action of compounds known as **antibiotics**. As a guiding definition, antibiotics are chemical substances that are produced by microorganisms and that are capable of inhibiting or killing other microorganisms. Antibiotics thus represent a first line of defense that some microbes use for protection and to provide themselves with a competitive edge. Although microbial cultures represent important sources of antibiotics, many of today's front-line products are either synthesized in the laboratory or are chemically modified from antibiotics obtained from laboratory cultures.

Antibiotics act in a number of ways, either by killing bacteria outright or by inhibiting their multiplication or some other vital cellular function. Some act by zeroing in on essential metabolic reactions of the bacteria while others interfere with the manufacture of important constituents of the bacterial cell wall. Antibiotics in common use in equine medicine today include penicillin, amoxicillin, streptomycin, gentamicin, erythromycin, and oxacillin.

Unfortunately, resistance to the action of antibiotics has grown among many bacterial species. The survival of antibiotic-resistant bacteria has actually been enhanced by the use of antibiotics, i.e., the antibiotics "select" for those bacteria able to survive in their presence, suppressing or killing their antibiotic-sensitive rivals and allowing the resistant strains to flourish. Control of antibiotic resistance is indissolubly linked to two important factors: the identification of new and unique antimicrobial substances and greater restraint in the clinical use of available antibiotics to preclude selection for new resistant strains.

Salmonellosis

Salmonellosis is the most commonly diagnosed infectious diarrhea of mature horses. It is caused by members of the genus *Salmonella*. These bacteria, representing more than 2,000 different member types known as **serovars**, are ubiquitous in the environment and infect a wide variety of wild and domestic host species. Horses acquire infection by ingesting feed or water contaminated with *Salmonella*-laden fecal matter. Rodents, reptiles, birds, other horses, and other domestic animal species can serve as sources of contamination. There is evidence that horses recovering from infection shed *Salmonella* in the feces for a period of a few weeks to a few months; longer periods of shedding are probably rare.

The vast majority of *Salmonella* infections in horses are inapparent. Clinical signs usually are observed only when the immune defenses of the host have been weakened, as by stress or disease, or following the prolonged administration of antibiotics, which may suppress much of the normal intestinal flora and allow *Salmonella* to thrive. In one recent outbreak over 90 percent of the horses developing salmonellosis had been receiving antibiotic therapy. Horses undergoing colic surgery or treatment for another gastrointestinal illness were the ones most often affected.

Signs of salmonellosis in the horse can include inappetence, lethargy, fever, weight loss, and a severe watery to bloody diarrhea. The most serious lesions are usually found in the cecum and ascending colon. Outbreaks of salmonellosis occur most often during the hot months of the summer and fall. Conditions of high humidity in lush pastures or within doors following frequent hosing and stall-cleaning may encourage transmission of the bacteria. Large numbers of horses may be affected and the mortality rate can be substantial.

Under certain conditions *Salmonella* may escape from the gastrointestinal tract and invade deeper tissues, producing **septicemia** (presence of bacteria in the blood, with accompanying disease signs) and serious **systemic** (bodywide) illness. This occurs most commonly in foals. The clinical signs often are related to the sudden onset of shock and/or respiratory or central nervous system dysfunction.

Diagnosis of salmonellosis is made on the basis of the history, clinical signs, and identification of the causative bacterium in feces, blood, or tissues. Early diagnosis combined with aggressive therapy offers the best chance for a successful outcome.

Affected horses should be isolated from all susceptible animals for up to 6 weeks. Treatment of uncomplicated cases should be directed primarily at replenishing the fluids and electrolytes lost in the diarrhea. Good nursing and supportive care are essential for recovery. To avoid selecting for a more aggressive, antibiotic-resistant *Salmonella* and to preserve the normal intestinal bacteria which act as a shield against more harmful microorganisms, antibiotics should be withheld unless systemic disease is either imminent or already present, i.e., unless the white blood cell count is dangerously low or the clinical signs indicate that the *Salmonella* has already spread beyond the intestinal tract.

Salmonellosis today is a disease of great public health significance. Owners of clinically affected horses should be aware that salmonellosis is a **zoonotic disease** (i.e., it is transmissible from animals to people) and that the organisms excreted in the feces of an infected horse represent a potential health hazard for human beings. Human infections with *Salmonella* can be particularly severe and in some cases can persist for months. Thus, owners must be especially cautious and observe strict hygienic measures while caring for horses suffering from salmonellosis. Hands should be washed often, particularly after attending to the ill animal, and protective boots and overalls should be worn. Contaminated stalls and breezeways should be thoroughly cleaned, preferably with hot pressurized water, to remove all traces of feces and animal tissue, and then disinfected with any of several approved products (which can be obtained from, or recommended by, the consulting veterinarian).

Young children, older adults, and individuals taking antibiotics or an immunosuppressive medication (such as a corticosteroid) should be kept away from an affected horse, especially for the first few weeks after infection, until the numbers of bacteria excreted in the feces have declined. Should any individual on the farm develop diarrhea, severe abdominal pain, and fever, the family physician should be consulted immediately and the possibility of salmonellosis presented. It is recommended that the physician contact the attending veterinarian for specific details about the case and the particular *Salmonella* serotype involved. (*See* APPENDIX A, "ZOONOTIC DISEASES: FROM HORSES TO PEOPLE.")

Neonatal Septicemia

Septicemia, a severe illness associated with the presence of disease-causing bacteria in the bloodstream, is not uncommon in foals less than a week of age. A number of factors have been recognized that can predispose a foal to this condition. These include:

- Failure of the foal to receive sufficient protective immunity from the mare in colostrum
- Poor sanitation
- Overcrowding
- Insufficient cleansing of the foal's umbilical stump
- Intrauterine infection during pregnancy

In most cases the septicemia results from a mixed bacterial infection, i.e., more than a single bacterial species is involved. Bacteria often implicated in neonatal septicemia include *Escherichia coli*, *Klebsiella pneumoniae*, *Actinobacillus*, *Streptococcus zooepidemicus*, and *Salmonella*. They may be ingested or inhaled by the foal or gain direct access to the bloodstream through an improperly disinfected umbilical stump.

Affected animals essentially are overwhelmed by a massive infection, with clinical signs developing a few days after birth. Early signs include weakness, inappetence, depression, and reluctance to move. As the septicemia progresses, fever, an increase in respiratory rate and effort, and small hemorrhages on the mucous membranes and ears become apparent. Diarrhea, swollen joints, or neurologic abnormalities may be seen. Coma followed by death can occur within 24–48 hours of onset. **Septic shock**, a massive systemic reaction to toxins associated with the causative bacteria, is a common cause of death. The mortality rate in neonatal septicemia is high: between 50 percent and 75 percent of affected foals will not survive.

Diagnosis is based on the history, clinical signs, and results of supportive laboratory tests. One important test that can be performed literally at the foal's side is the zinc sulfate turbidity test for determining the level of antibody in the foal's serum. The results of this test will tell the veterinarian whether the foal has received sufficient maternal immunity and so will provide an important clue for both diagnosis and therapy.

Early diagnosis and treatment are essential if the foal is to be saved. Moreover, therapy must be aggressively applied. Treatment measures include fluid and electrolyte replacement, infusions of antibody-rich blood plasma, administration of antibiotics, nutritional support, and good nursing care. The prognosis, even with the best of treatment, is guarded. In foals with a highly disseminated infection—particularly if the central nervous system has been invaded—the prognosis is grim.

Streptococcal Infections

Streptococcal bacteria often are involved in local or generalized **pyogenic** (pus-forming) infections in horses. They may act alone or in concert with other bacteria as part of a mixed bacterial infection. The two most important disease-causing streptococci in the horse are *Streptococcus zooepidemicus* and *Streptococcus equi*.

Streptococcus zooepidemicus is found in a wide variety of animal species and is a normal inhabitant of the skin and upper respiratory tract. It is the most common cause of equine wound infections and is a frequent opportunistic invader in viral upper respiratory infections of young horses. In foals *S. zooepidemicus* can colonize the stump of the umbilical cord, spread through the bloodstream and localize in joints, causing a *polyarthritis* (inflammation of the joints). It is an important cause of genital tract infections in mares.

Streptococcus equi is the cause of *strangles*, an extremely important respiratory disease of young horses. (For information on strangles, *see* Chapter 25, "The Respiratory System and Various Disorders.")

Diagnosis of streptococcal infections is made on the basis of the history, clinical signs, and identification of the causative bacteria. Fortunately, most streptococci remain susceptible to penicillin or penicillin-group antibiotics.

Staphylococcal Infections

Staphylococci are a widely distributed group of bacteria that cause disease in human beings and many animal species, including horses. Staphylococci are ubiquitous in nature and are more resistant than many other bacteria to drying and the action of disinfectants. Staphylococcal bacteria are often found on the skin and mucous membranes; many of them represent members of the normal bacterial flora of the host. Staphylococci are opportunistic agents of disease, usually causing illness only if presented with suitable conditions. Strains of staphylococci carrying the enzyme **coagulase** (*coagulase-positive staphylococci*) are the more virulent members of the genus and are more frequently implicated in disease processes. The major species involved in equine disease is *Staphylococcus aureus*.

Botryomycosis is a type of wound infection caused by *S. aureus* and occurs following trauma. Common sites include the lower extremities and **scrotum** (the dependent pouch of skin enveloping the testicles). Scrotal botryomycosis often is a complication of surgical castration. The lesions consist of small nodules and pockets of pus, which may ulcerate and begin discharging to the skin surface. Treatment usually consists of surgical drainage and/or excision. Staphylococci may also be involved in more superficial infections of the skin and in **mastitis** (inflammation of the mammary gland).

Diagnosis is made on the basis of the history, the presenting clinical signs, and identification of the causative bacteria. Treatment of uncomplicated local infections such as a superficial abscess usually involves hot-packing followed by incising the abscess, drainage of the pus, and instillation of a disinfectant or antibiotic solution. Unlike streptococci, many strains of staphylococci have developed resistance to the action of penicillin and penicillin-group antibiotics. Cephalosporins and trimethoprim-sulfa drugs are frequently used in their place to treat staphylococcal infections in a number of species.

Rhodococcus Equi Infections

Rhodococcus equi is an important cause of bacterial pneumonia in foals. (For information on this organism, *see* CHAPTER 25, "THE RESPIRATORY SYSTEM AND VARIOUS DISORDERS.")

Nocardiosis

Bacteria of the genus *Nocardia* are normal inhabitants of the soil. As agents of disease they cause pus-forming infections of human beings and a number of animal species, including the horse. Trauma and puncture wounds, and occasionally inhalation or ingestion, allow these organisms to gain access to normally sterile tissues of the body. Severe systemic disease is favored when the immune defenses of the host are compromised in some manner, either by concurrent illness or by long-term administration of an immunosuppressive medication. In horses *Nocardia* is a cause of local wound infections, which usually resolve without complication if they are surgically opened and allowed to drain. *Nocardia* is also a cause of systemic and pulmonary disease in immunodeficient Arabian foals.

Corynebacterium Abscesses and Ulcerative Lymphangitis

Large, painful abscesses caused by *Corynebacterium pseudotuberculosis* occur sporadically in horses in the western states, most often during the late summer and early fall. The condition is known by a variety of colorful names, including "pigeon breast," "pigeon fever," "dry-land distemper," and "Colorado strangles." It is suspected that the organism is carried by ticks or flies, which inoculate it into the skin of the horse while they feed. The abscesses develop most often in the chest muscles of mature horses, but some may be found in the area of the groin, lower abdomen, or **axilla** (armpit). Complications can include limb **edema** (swelling) and the development of secondary abscesses inside the abdomen. Occasional widespread, generalized infections can be fatal.

Diagnosis is based on the history, clinical findings, and isolation of *C. pseudotuberculosis* from the abscesses. Draining and flushing of the abscesses is the treatment of choice. Immature abscesses may need to be hot-packed before they are lanced. Antibiotics may also be administered, depending on the severity of the condition. Clinical relapses with reformation of abscesses are not uncommon; such cases may require long-term antibiotic therapy.

Ulcerative lymphangitis is an uncommon condition that can be caused by *C. pseudotuberculosis*, usually as the result of wound contamination. (A similar condition is caused by the fungus *Sporothrix schenckii*; *see* CHAPTER 32, "FUNGAL DISEASES.")

The lesions appear as nodules that develop most often on the hind legs below the hocks. The nodules eventually break down and ulcerate, releasing a thick greenish pus mixed with blood. Subsequent swelling of the affected limb is a common complication. If the condition is left untreated new succeeding nodules form, often along connecting lymphatic channels, transforming the area into a large mass of infected, decaying tissue.

Diagnosis is based on the history, clinical appearance, and isolation of the causative organism. Treatment requires thorough, repeated draining, cleansing, and disinfecting of the lesions, combined with the administration of an appropriate antibiotic. Good supportive and nursing care are essential. Advanced cases with extensive tissue destruction may not respond to therapy.

Tetanus

Tetanus is an acute, often fatal disease caused by a **neurotoxin** (toxin targeting the nervous system) of the bacterium *Clostridium tetani*, and is characterized by violent muscle spasms and contractions, hyper-reflexive responses, and "lockjaw." *Horses are highly sensitive to the action of tetanus neurotoxin,* and this combined with their propensity for acquiring puncture wounds and lacerations makes tetanus an exceedingly important disease in the equine species.

The causative bacteria are normal residents of the soil but can also be found among the bacterial population of the large colon of the horse. Special conditions must be present for the organism to produce disease, however. In general, bacterial contamination of dead or dying tissue in a penetrating wound is the most common means by which tetanus is produced. Spores of *Cl. tetani*, which are widely present in the soil, **germinate** (grow into mature bacterial forms) soon after entering the wound. Germination is followed by production of the neurotoxin. The toxin affects neuromuscular responses in different areas of the body, blocking nerve impulses that normally inhibit muscular contractions. As a result the large muscle groups are trapped in a state of contraction, which is often accompanied by prolonged, painful spasms.

The clinical signs of tetanus in horses include: stiffness of the limbs, resulting in a so-called "saw-horse" stance; erected ears, retracted eyelids, and flared nostrils; protrusion of the third eyelid; excessive salivation; swallowing difficulties, together with rigidity of the chewing muscles ("lockjaw"); and usually fever (secondary to prolonged tensing of the muscles). Painful spasms resembling convulsions (except that the horse remains fully conscious), **dyspnea** (respiratory difficulty), colic, and urine retention can occur. Spasms are often precipitated by external stimuli, e.g., loud noises. Serious, potential complications of tetanus include **laminitis** ("founder") and **aspiration pneumonia** (pneumonia caused by inhalation of food material, owing to paralysis of the laryngeal musculature). The clinical signs of tetanus may persist for as long as a month or more. Death is usually the result of respiratory insufficiency caused by paralysis of the breathing muscles.

The diagnosis in most cases is fairly straightforward, based on the history and the rather characteristic physical appearance of the patient. Therapy must be applied quickly and aggressively. *Thorough cleansing and disinfection of the wound, if it can be identified, to remove dead and dying tissue as well as the clostridial bacteria is an absolute necessity.* Penicillin is injected directly into the wound area to kill any remaining bacteria and is also given systemically. Tetanus **antitoxin** (an antiserum against the neurotoxin) to "soak up" unbound toxin is also administered. Following these initial critical measures, recovery will hinge on good nursing and supportive care. The horse should be maintained in a dark, quiet stall to minimize the impact of external stimuli. To prevent the horse from injuring itself, the walls should be padded and a generous supply of soft bedding provided. Several days may pass before any improvement in the animal's condition is noted; complete recovery usually requires weeks of therapy, and complications may arise. The prognosis is guarded and is directly related to the speed of onset of disease, i.e., the more quickly clinical signs develop after the injury, the poorer the prognosis for recovery.

All horses should be routinely immunized against tetanus using **tetanus toxoid** (a weakened form of the toxin). Available tetanus toxoid products are relatively inexpensive, safe, and induce a solid, durable immunity. (For immunization guidelines *see* APPENDIX B, "VACCINATIONS AND INFECTIOUS DISEASE CONTROL.")

Botulism

Botulism is a rare disease caused by a neurotoxin (*botulinal toxin*) produced by the bacterium *Clostridium botulinum*. It is contracted either by ingestion of preformed toxin in improperly canned food, raw meat, or decomposing carcasses, or by contamination of a wound with the bacteria, which subsequently produce the toxin in the damaged tissue ("wound botulism"). Botulinal toxin is one of the most potent biological toxins known in nature. It acts by blocking the transmission of nerve impulses, resulting in weakness progressing to paralysis, inability to swallow, and often death.

Three clinical forms of botulism are seen in horses:

- *Shaker foal syndrome* occurs following ingestion of *Cl. botulinum* spores and their transformation into mature, toxin-producing bacterial forms in the intestinal tract of 2- to 8-week-old, susceptible foals (foals without sufficient immunity). The disease is highly fatal. Clinical signs include an acute onset of weakness, tremors, **dysphagia** (swallowing difficulties), constipation, and **recumbency** (inability to stand), followed by death resulting from paralysis of the breathing muscles.

- *Forage poisoning* involves the ingestion of toxin produced by the bacteria in decaying plant material. The onset may be acute or gradual. Clinical signs can include weakness, muscle tremors, dysphagia, loss of tongue and tail tone, drooping of the eyelids, stumbling, and a stilted, "choppy" gait. Aspiration pneumonia represents a severe complication. Death when it occurs is usually the result of paralysis of the breathing muscles. Most horses with a gradual onset of signs recover, while those whose signs develop acutely often die.

- *Wound botulism.* Affected horses exhibit clinical signs similar to those indicated for forage poisoning.

The diagnosis is not always as clear as it is with tetanus. The history and clinical signs may or may not provide a high index of suspicion for botulism. A definitive diagnosis is based on detection of botulinum toxin in gut contents, vomitus, feces, or in a suspect food source (if available).

Treatment is almost entirely supportive, although in some cases antitoxin may be of help to neutralize any unbound toxin remaining in the circulation. The goal of therapy is to keep the patient alive and free of secondary infections or other complications until the bound toxin is naturally cleared from the body. As much as a week may pass before any evidence of improvement is seen. The prognosis is guarded and is directly related to the speed of onset of disease, i.e., the more quickly clinical signs develop following exposure the poorer the prognosis for recovery.

A vaccine is available for immunization against shaker foal syndrome (*see* APPENDIX B, "VACCINATIONS AND INFECTIOUS DISEASE CONTROL").

Leptospirosis

Leptospirosis is a zoonotic disease of worldwide occurrence. The causative bacteria, known generically as **leptospires**, are maintained in nature in a number of wild and domestic animal reservoir hosts. Leptospires are classified as **spirochetes** (filamentous, spiral-shaped bacteria) and are carried and shed in the urine of healthy reservoir hosts. Animals that have recovered from leptospirosis often continue to excrete organisms in the urine for periods of months to years.

Leptospires are not long-lived outside the body except under circumstances of ideal temperature and humidity. They frequently contaminate water supplies where livestock and wild rodents tend to congregate. Susceptible animals acquire the infection most often by direct contact with infected carriers or by ingesting organisms suspended in water contaminated with urine.

One manifestation of leptospirosis in horses is a recurrent inflammation of the eye known as **periodic ophthalmia.** The inflammation involves the *uvea*, the cell layer that contains blood vessels, the iris, ciliary body, and choroid (*see* Chapter 19, "The Eye and Various Disorders"). Clinical signs include **chemosis** (excessive swelling of the **conjunctiva**, the membrane covering the inner surface of the eyelids), tearing, **photophobia** (visual hypersensitivity to light), **miosis** (excessive contraction of the pupil), and **iritis** (inflammation of the iris). Blindness will result if the affected eye is left untreated.

Evidence indicates that periodic ophthalmia is caused primarily by an immunologically mediated reaction rather than by direct bacterial injury. Moreover, leptospires appear to be responsible for only a portion of the cases. The others apparently result either from infection with the threadworm *Onchocerca cervicalis* or are of unknown origin.

Leptospires have been associated with abortion and stillbirth in mares and an often fatal illness in foals characterized by variable signs of fever, respiratory distress, **jaundice** (yellow discoloration of the skin and mucous membranes), and kidney disease. There have been only sporadic reports of leptospire-associated kidney and/or liver disease in mature horses similar to the more familiar form of leptospirosis seen in dogs.

Diagnosis is based on the history, physical examination, and results of supportive laboratory tests. Serum from suspect cases may be submitted to a diagnostic laboratory for the *microscopic agglutination test (MAT)*, a standard **serologic assay** (test on serum, clear blood plasma without clotting factor) for the detection of antibodies to leptospires. A serologic diagnosis of leptospirosis in a horse exhibiting suspicious clinical signs can be made by demonstrating a fourfold or greater increase in antibody titers in paired serum samples, one taken at the time of active disease and the second approximately 2 to 4 weeks later. Isolation of the causative leptospires from blood, urine, or tissue may be attempted in cases where the diagnosis is difficult to achieve by other means. Treatment involves supportive care and the administration of appropriate ocular medications and antibiotics. There are no leptospiral vaccines approved for use in horses.

Dermatophilosis

Dermatophilosis is a superficial skin infection caused by an unusual bacterium, *Dermatophilus congolensis.* (For information on this disease, *see* Chapter 17, "The Skin and Various Disorders.")

Contagious Equine Metritis

This is a highly contagious disease of horses that was first described in Britain and Ireland in the late 1970s. Since that time it has been reported in a host of other countries. At the present time it is not known to exist in the United States. The causative agent is *Taylorella equigenitalis*, an **obligate parasite** (i.e., one that cannot live free on its own for a great length of time but requires a living host) of the genital tract of mares and stallions. Colts and fillies may also carry the organism. The primary means of transmission is venereal, most importantly from an infected stallion to a susceptible mare.

Clinical signs are limited to mares and are the result of inflammation of the genital tract, from the vagina to the uterus (**metritis** = inflammation of the uterus). Typically a thin, profuse, grayish-white discharge pours from the vulva, soiling the hindquarters and tail. The discharge usually becomes evident within 2 weeks of breeding with a carrier stallion and will persist for 1–2 weeks if left untreated. No constitutional signs are produced. Infection is inapparent in many mares, except for perhaps a brief period of infertility during the initial infection. A varying number of mares recovered from the infection will continue to harbor the organism in the genital tract, primarily in the area of the **clitoris** (the female analog of the penis), for months to years. Carrier mares can transmit the infection to their offspring, which in turn may become carriers themselves. Infected stallions are often long-term, healthy carriers and so constitute an important "silent" reservoir of infection.

Diagnosis is based on the history, clinical signs, and isolation of the causative bacterium from the genital tract. Choice of an antibiotic for treatment, when deemed appropriate, is based on antibiotic susceptibility testing in the laboratory. Most horses recover on their own without treatment.

Thorough washing and disinfecting of the genitalia of stallions and colts can aid in eliminating the carrier state in these animals. Similar procedures are much less effective in mares, however. Long-term reproductive performance of infected horses is usually not affected. There is no available vaccine.

Glanders and Melioidosis

Glanders is caused by *Pseudomonas mallei*. An ancient and once worldwide disease of equids, glanders is now a rare condition and is restricted to certain areas of the Middle East and Asia. In donkeys and mules glanders is an acute, systemic illness, while in horses it occurs chiefly in a milder chronic form. Following its inhalation or ingestion, the organism localizes in the lungs and mucous membranes of the upper respiratory tract and trachea. Characteristic lesions include ulcerations of the mucous membranes and the development of nodules in the lungs, resulting in pneumonia and related problems. Nodules can also occur in the liver and spleen. A skin form of glanders known as *farcy* is characterized by nodules, ulcers, and swollen lymph nodes and lymphatic channels, most often involving the legs or abdomen. *Pseudomonas mallei* also infects human beings, who can contract the disease by direct contact with affected equids. Because of the zoonotic aspects and the poor prognosis, treatment of affected animals is not recommended.

Melioidosis is a glanderslike disease caused by *Pseudomonas pseudomallei*, a **saprophytic** (living on dead and decaying matter) bacterium found in certain soils and waters in southeast Asia and a few other areas of the world. It is not known to occur in the United States. The disease can be found in a wide variety of animal species and is characterized by the development of small nodules in internal organs. The clinical spectrum is very wide, ranging from inapparent infection (which is the most common) to a rapidly fatal illness. Animals become infected either by inhalation or wound contamination. Clinical cases in horses (as well as in a few human beings) were reported in the late 1970s and early 1980s in France. Direct transmission from horses to people has not been reported; however, infected horses shed the organism and thus contribute to environmental contamination. Antibiotic therapy is available, although the prognosis is poor.

Lyme Borreliosis (Lyme Disease)

Lyme borreliosis is named for the town of Old Lyme, Connecticut, located a short distance inland from Long Island Sound. In the 1970s physicians in the area noticed an unusual pattern of transient, recurrent **arthropathies** (joint diseases) that occurred mainly in children during the summer and early autumn months. After a period of intense investigation a new **spirochete** (filamentous, spiral-shaped bacterium) called *Borrelia burgdorferi* was implicated in the causation of the disease. Lyme borreliosis (or more simply **Lyme disease**) has now been recognized in people throughout the world, and there is some evidence that it is increasing in incidence. This may be due to the increased urbanization of rural woodlands in endemic areas, i.e., by the growing encroachment of human civilization upon the woodland reservoirs of infection.

The majority of human cases of Lyme borreliosis reported each year in the United States are from the northeastern and mid-Atlantic regions of the country. The causative bacterium is carried and transmitted by **ixodid** (hard) ticks, different tick species serving as carriers in different geographical regions. In the Northeast and Midwest the deer tick *Ixodes dammini* (*Ixodes scapularis*), a tiny tick that infests wooded areas, is the primary *vector* (transmitter of infection). Typically 25–50 percent of *I. dammini* ticks in the Northeast are infected with the spirochete. The chief reservoir of *B. burgdorferi* infection in the wildlife population of the Northeast is the white-footed mouse. Deer ticks feeding on the mice inject spirochete-laden saliva into the bite wound and thereby perpetuate a cycle of infection that assures transmission of the organism to successive generations of mice. This tick also bites human beings and animals and is considered a major vector for transmission. In California the primary vectors are *Ixodes pacificus*, the western black-legged tick, and a second ixodid tick, *Ixodes neotomae*, both of which feed on a wildlife reservoir, the dusky-footed woodrat (also called the packrat). The California cycle is unique in that both ticks are required to perpetuate the disease in the human population.

Lyme Borreliosis in People

The spirochete multiplies at the site of infection for a period of several weeks. This local multiplication is followed by the appearance of a typical skin reaction called **erythema chronicum migrans (ECF)** at the site of the bite. It begins as a small red spot that then expands in a circular fashion with an area of central clearing. The appearance of ECM in humans is usually associated with varying degrees of fever, chills, malaise, fatigue, vomiting, headache, enlargement of lymph nodes, and neck stiffness. The ECM usually undergoes expansion for several weeks, clears in the center, and then fades.

Weeks to months after the primary ECM lesion has disappeared, a small proportion of infected individuals develop signs of chronic Lyme borreliosis. Neurologic complications are observed in about 15 percent of affected people, while heart problems are seen in about 8 percent. The most common complication, present in over 60 percent of affected individuals, is a **polyarthritis** (inflammation occurring simultaneously in several joints) that occurs as a series of attacks lasting for weeks to months, with subsequent recurrences developing over a period of years. This association of a specific infectious disease agent with chronic arthritis has spurred much promising new research into the causes (and possible cures) of arthritic ailments in people.

Lyme Borreliosis in Horses

In contrast to the picture in the human medical field, the significance of Lyme borreliosis for equine medicine is much less clear. Rates of infection in horses range from 6 percent to 35 percent or higher in the western and eastern United States, respectively. In all studies reported to date there has been no correlation between an antibody response and the presence of clinical signs suggestive of Lyme borreliosis. Thus a positive antibody test in a horse is indicative only of exposure to *B. burgdorferi* or a related organism and cannot be considered diagnostic for any disease. In our experience in California the majority of horses presented with clinical signs suggestive of Lyme borreliosis have been determined to be suffering from other conditions. Whether *B. burgdorferi* is the cause of any significant disorder in horses remains controversial at this time.

There is some public health concern regarding horses or other animals that have come into contact with the Lyme spirochete. Animals may physically transport infected ticks adhered to their bodies into barns, backyards, gardens, or homes, although the importance of this passive carriage in spreading the infection to people is not known at present. Currently public health authorities do not view animals in and of themselves as major factors in Lyme borreliosis transmission.

Tuberculosis

Tuberculosis is an ancient scourge. Its varied symptoms and disease course have been familiar to medical practitioners since the advent of recorded history. The cause remained a mystery until just over a century ago, however, when the German microbiologist Robert Koch presented his now famous paper on the subject before the members of the Physiological Society of Berlin. In the relatively brief period since then, much additional information has been gathered concerning the cause, cure, transmission, and prevention of this important disease of both human beings and animals.

The term "tuberculosis" derives from the many small nodules of inflammatory tissue ("**tubercles**") that are characteristic of the disease in some species. Tuberculosis is caused by several members of the genus **Mycobacterium**, including *Mycobacterium tuberculosis*, *Mycobacterium bovis*, and *Mycobacterium avium* (known collectively as "**tubercle bacilli**"). Today it is estimated that at least one-third of the world's human population is or has been infected with *M. tuberculosis*, the primary cause of tuberculosis in people. In the United States, between 22,000 and 25,000 new human cases of tuberculosis are being diagnosed annually, and this number is on the increase owing to the prevalence of human immunodeficiency virus (**HIV**) infection. Global morbidity and mortality figures now reflect *8 million new human cases* and approximately *3 million human deaths* each year. Any notion of human tuberculosis as a "disease of the past" must be seriously questioned in light of such statistics.

Most infections in horses are caused by *M. bovis* and are probably acquired by close contact with infected cattle or their secretions (e.g., raw milk, which can contain large numbers of mycobacteria). Affected horses may exhibit clinical signs referable to the respiratory tract, such as coughing, retching, and respiratory difficulty. Fever, inappetence, weight loss, and lymph node enlargement may be accompanying features. The infection can disseminate to other body sites such as the liver, spleen or vertebrae. Fortunately tuberculosis in horses is quite rare in the United States, owing to highly successful programs to eradicate tuberculosis from cattle populations.

Local public health authorities should be notified immediately if a diagnosis of tuberculosis is suspected. Owing to the danger of transmission of *M. bovis* to human contacts, attempted treatment of tuberculosis in horses is *not recommended*. A search for the source of infection, if unidentified, should be instituted as soon as a definitive diagnosis has been made. Vaccination of horses against tuberculosis is not currently feasible.

Anthrax

Anthrax is a rapidly fatal illness caused by multiplication and spread of *Bacillus anthracis* following ingestion of the bacterial spores. It is most often a problem of cattle but on occasion affects other species, including horses and human beings. The disease is encountered only in certain geographic regions where conditions favor the bacterium's survival in the soil. Exposure to spores in contaminated soil (e.g., by grazing on pastureland) is the major route of infection. Once inside the body, the spores germinate and release the bacteria, which then spread throughout the lymphatic and blood vessels. Massive multiplication of the organism takes place in the blood until the animal succumbs. Death is attributed to the release of powerful toxins that damage the nervous system and blood-clotting mechanism. The onset and course of disease are both very rapid. Clinical signs in affected horses can include depression, inappetence, colic, swellings in the throat region, neck, and shoulders, and bleeding from body openings. The mortality rate is very high.

Vaccines against anthrax have been available for over 100 years. In fact, one of the first vaccines ever made against any disease was the anthrax vaccine devised by Louis Pasteur in the 1870s. Because anthrax occurs only rarely in horses, and currently approved vaccines may be associated with some undesirable side-effects, vaccination is practiced only in rare circumstances when horses are pastured in a known contaminated area. A primary series of two doses given 2–3 weeks apart followed by annual boosters appears to provide adequate protection.

Tyzzer's Disease

Tyzzer's disease is an extremely rare and highly fatal disease caused by a spore-forming bacterium, *Bacillus piliformis*, and is characterized by acute liver dysfunction in foals. The organism is a normal inhabitant of the intestinal tract of mice, and foals are thought to acquire infection by ingesting fecal matter contaminated with the bacterial spores. Alternatively, it is possible that mares harbor the organism, which for some reason causes fatal illness in only a small percentage of infected foals. The incidence of *B. piliformis* infection in healthy foals is not known.

The onset of disease is exceedingly rapid; some foals are simply found dead without having appeared ill. Clinical signs in others may include inappetence, malaise, abdominal pain, jaundice, and diarrhea. The disease course is brief, typically lasting only 1 or 2 days. As a consequence the diagnosis is often made only after death, when the characteristic bacteria are identified in samples of liver tissue. Death is usually attributable to massive liver failure. There is no effective treatment or vaccine.

Potomac Horse Fever (Equine Monocytic Ehrlichiosis)

Potomac horse fever (**PHF**) was first reported in the late 1970s in horses in the eastern United States. Since then it has been diagnosed in other regions and also in Europe. Most cases occur during the summer months. The causative organism, *Ehrlichia risticii*, is classified as a *rickettsia*, a member of a specialized group of bacteria most of which multiply only within host cells. Many rickettsiae are transmitted to animals and people by **arthropods** (invertebrate organisms with a hard outer skeleton and a segmented body; examples include ticks, fleas, and lice). The mode of transmission of *E. risticii* is still unknown, however, although several lines of evidence point to the activity of an as-yet-unidentified arthropod or other intermediary. Because the rickettsiae are shed in large numbers in the feces, some have speculated that either an internal parasite or a **coprophagous** (feeding on feces) arthropod may be involved in the transmission cycle.

The clinical signs vary considerably from horse to horse and from farm to farm. In some horses little more than inappetence and depres-

sion may be observed. Others develop a high fever and diarrhea that may be watery and severe and result in severe dehydration. The underlying cause for most of the clinical signs is *colitis* (inflammation of the large colon). The mortality rate in untreated cases can be as high as 30 percent. Life-threatening colic may develop as a complication in some horses. Another potential complication of PHF is **laminitis** ("founder"), which may occur in up to 40 percent of affected horses in some areas. Recently it has been shown that some pregnant mares may abort after recovery from PHF.

Diagnosis of PHF is based on the history, clinical findings, and knowledge of *E. risticii* activity in the immediate area. Unfortunately there is no definitive diagnostic test available; many diagnoses of PHF thus are only presumptive in nature. The indirect fluorescent antibody (IFA) test currently available for detecting exposure to *E. risticii* is fraught with difficulties. Development of a rapid, accurate diagnostic test represents one of the great needs in PHF research today. Researchers at UC Davis have recently developed a nested polymerase chain reaction (**PCR**) test that has the potential to provide routine and accurate diagnosis of PHF in affected horses. Further evaluation of this new test is currently in progress.

Ehrlichia risticii is exquisitely sensitive to tetracycline antibiotics. Oxytetracycline given for 3–5 days, together with appropriate supportive care, is the current treatment of choice. A prompt decrease in fever often occurs within 12 hours of initiation of therapy (often this dramatic response is used to make a presumptive diagnosis). Other clinical signs such as diarrhea and laminitis, however, require additional time for resolution. The prognosis for recovery in most cases receiving adequate treatment is fair to good.

Once cases of PHF have been verified on a farm or in a particular geographic locale, it is likely that cases will continue to occur in subsequent seasons. Immunization with one of several **inactivated** ("killed") vaccines is recommended for horses residing in or traveling to such areas. (For immunization guidelines *see* APPENDIX B, "VACCINATIONS AND INFECTIOUS DISEASE CONTROL..")

Equine Granulocytic Ehrlichiosis

An equine rickettsial disease characterized by fever, depression, **leukopenia** (low white blood cell count) **thrombocytopenia** (decreased number of circulating blood **platelets** [blood-clotting cells]), and limb *edema* (swelling) was first recognized in northern California in the early 1960s. Since then cases of **equine granulocytic ehrlichiosis (EGE)** have been diagnosed in several other states as well as in South America and Europe. The causative agent is *Ehrlichia equi*. Horses of any age are susceptible, but clinical signs are more severe in older animals (greater than 2 or 3 years of age). In northern California most cases are seen in late fall, winter, and spring.

Ehrlichia equi appears to be transmitted to horses by ticks; the tick involved in California is most likely the western black-legged tick, *Ixodes pacificus*. Infected horses do not become chronic carriers of *E. equi* and so do not serve as an efficient reservoir of infection. Rather, horses are "dead-end" hosts, the organism being maintained in some as yet unidentified wildlife reservoir, e.g., deer or rodents.

The clinical signs tend to evolve over several days. Initial signs of fever and mild depression are soon followed by inappetence, incoordination, limb edema, reluctance to move, lethargy, jaundice, leukopenia, and thrombocytopenia. **Cardiac arrhythmias** (heartbeat irregularities) may be identified in some cases. Many of the clinical signs appear to result from **vasculitis** (blood-vessel inflammation) and/or bone-marrow suppression. The signs usually persist for 1–2 weeks before gradual improvement occurs. Younger horses may have a shorter duration of fever without accompanying signs. The mortality rate is low, but some deaths have occurred as a result of secondary bacterial infection or traumatic injury resulting from incoordination. Recovered horses appear to possess substantial immunity.

The diagnosis of EGE is made on the basis of the history, clinical signs, and identification of *Ehrlichia equi* in **neutrophils** or **eosinophils** (types of white blood cells) in blood smears. Detection of antibodies to the organism in paired blood samples will also confirm the presence of infection. Researchers at UC Davis have developed a nested polymerase chain reaction (**PCR**) test that is highly sensitive and specific for detecting *E. equi* in blood samples from affected horses.

Oxytetracycline given for up to 7 days is the antimicrobial therapy of choice. A prompt decrease in fever occurs in all cases within 12–24 hours of initiation of treatment. The prognosis for recovery in most cases is excellent. There is no available vaccine.

Equine granulocytic ehrlichiosis clinically resembles a newly recognized human disease, *human granulocytic ehrlichiosis* (**HGE**), which is transmitted by ticks and is caused by a rickettsia that is remarkably similar to *E. equi*. Indeed, researchers at UC Davis have shown that when the human rickettsia is inoculated into horses it produces a disease indistinguishable from EGE. Whether the two organisms are indeed the same or variant strains of each other has not yet been determined. It should be emphasized that there is no evidence that people can catch HGE from their horses; instead, humans and equines may be infected by ticks that are carrying the causative rickettsiae.

CHAPTER 32

Fungal Diseases

by Jeffrey E. Barlough and John E. Madigan

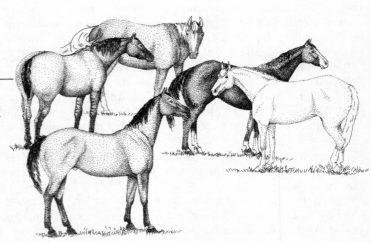

The term **"fungus"** encompasses the yeasts and molds, mushrooms, smuts, and rusts, all of which exist normally in the environment. Fungal cells are characterized by the presence of a rigid cell wall and the absence of **chlorophyll**, the green pigment used by plants, algae, and some bacteria to convert sunlight into energy. The primary life function of fungi is decomposition, i.e., the breakdown of inert organic material. Fungi are of great ecological importance because their digestive processes release nutrients trapped in organic debris and recycle them back to the biosphere.

A yeast is a **unicellular** (composed of single cells), budding fungus that forms bud-shaped spores, while a mold is a **filamentous** (thread-like) fungus. Some fungi, such as those causing sporotrichosis or the systemic mycoses (diseases caused by fungi), are **dimorphic**, i.e., they are able to exist in either of these two different physical forms: in the environment they occur as free-living molds, but once inside the body of the host they are transformed into a parasitic yeast.

Many fungi, if allowed the proper opportunities and conditions, are able to cause illness in animals and human beings. Often, fungal diseases occur because of some underlying defect in the immune defenses of the host, e.g., a **congenital** (present at birth) absence or deficiency of one or more immune-system components, or **acquired** defects produced by infection with an immunosuppressive virus or by long-term treatment with an immunosuppressive medication. In other cases, such as ringworm, infection occurs in the normal host but is usually of transient duration; once the immune system has been alerted, the fungus is gradually eliminated. Fungal diseases in the latter category can be managed fairly easily, while those in the former may be resistant to therapy and threaten the life of the host. Many horses have antibodies to different fungi in their blood as the result of environmental exposure.

Ringworm (Dermatophytosis)

Ringworm is one of the most common fungal diseases of animals. The highly contagious ringworm fungi, known as **dermatophytes**, invade the most superficial outer layers of the skin, hair, and nails (horn), subsisting on **keratin**, an insoluble, sulfur-rich protein derived from dead skin cells. Although ringworm is most commonly self-limiting, with spontaneous remission occurring within a few months of onset, treatment of some resistant cases may be long and costly. (*See* CHAPTER 17, "THE SKIN AND VARIOUS DISORDERS.")

Guttural-Pouch Mycosis

This fungal infection is infrequently encountered in the western United States but occurs regularly in the midwestern and eastern states. It is the most common lesion of the guttural pouch in stabled horses in Britain and many other countries. This may be a reflection of climate, i.e., rain during hay-making encourages the growth of fungi on hay. Fungi of the genus *Aspergillus* are the agents most often implicated, although other fungi can produce the condition as well. (*See* CHAPTER 25, "THE RESPIRATORY SYSTEM AND VARIOUS DISORDERS.")

The Systemic Mycoses

The systemic mycoses are a group of rare fungal diseases of animals and people, in which inhalation (usually) of the causative fungus is followed by widespread dissemination of fungal cells to internal organs or other tissues. The fungi reponsible for most of these disorders exploit specialized ecological niches, and so their distribution in the environment is often geographically restricted. In the majority of cases, exposure to these organisms results in the production of a strong immunity in the host rather than disease. In a small percentage of infections, however, the fungi are not checked by the immune response, but instead proceed to engineer a serious (often fatal) illness. It appears that certain inherited or acquired defects in the immune defenses of the host may underlie this susceptibility. The only systemic mycosis currently of importance to horses in the United States is *coccidioidomycosis*.

An important feature of the fungi causing the systemic mycoses is their dimorphic nature. In the environment they exist as filamentous fungi (i.e., molds). However upon inhalation or inoculation the filamentous form converts into a parasitic yeast that, unlike the mold form, is capable of growing in tissues of the host. One significant consequence is that, in general, infected animals or human beings are not directly contagious to others because the yeast form in their tissues is not infective. (*One caveat:* Under certain circumstances, there may be reversion to growth of the filamentous form on or within bandages placed over a draining tract or other fungal lesion, or in contaminated stalls containing an abundance of straw or other bedding. The potential for reversion from noninfective yeast to infective mold can be greatly decreased by frequent bandage changes and removal of litter.)

The change from the filamentous mold form to the parasitic yeast form is apparently an adaptation to survival in an unfavorable environment (in this case, the body of the host) and confers little additional advantage on the fungi. Diseased animals or people in essence are "dead-end" hosts who have accidentally become involved in a minor side-track of the fungal life-cycle. Growth in dead-end hosts is wholly irrelevant to the maintenance and propagation of these fungal species in nature.

COCCIDIOIDOMYCOSIS

Coccidioidomycosis ("valley fever") is the most severe and life-threatening of the systemic mycoses. It is caused by *Coccidioides immitis*, which resides in soil of the dry cactus country of the southwestern states from California to central Texas, particularly in areas where the creosote bush is common (an ecological niche known as the Lower Sonoran life zone). It is also found in Central and South America. The organism flourishes several inches down in the soil, where it is aided in its spread by the activities of burrowing rodents. Following a period of wet weather, wind and dust storms whipping up the surface soil may spread the filamentous mold forms, called **arthrospores**, across great distances. The fungus is normally dormant in the summer and is killed by freezing temperatures. In some people, inhalation of the infective arthrospores is followed by a very mild influenzalike illness characterized by fever, lethargy, partial inappetence, coughing, and sometimes joint pain or stiffness ("desert rheumatism"). The majority of human beings become solidly immune following this initial infection.

Most cases of equine coccidioidomycosis occur in mature horses. There is some evidence that Arabians may be at increased risk. No sex predilection has been recognized. Clinical signs include chronic weight loss (the most common sign), persistent coughing, musculoskeletal and/or abdominal pain, intermittent fever, and superficial **abscesses** (walled-off lesions filled with pus).

Diagnosis is made by identification of the **large spherule form** (the parasitic, tissue stage) of the organism in lesion or biopsy material. Microscopic visualization of spherules is normally sufficient to provide a clinical diagnosis. Treatment is usually unrewarding, owing to the poor clinical response of affected horses and the high cost of currently available antifungal medications.

The Subcutaneous Mycoses

The subcutaneous mycoses are a group of relatively rare fungal diseases affecting primarily the skin and underlying (subcutaneous) tissues. Occasionally they may spread to involve other areas of the body, including one or more organ systems. By and large, however, they are diseases of the more superficial body surfaces.

SPOROTRICHOSIS

Sporotrichosis is an uncommon chronic, pus-forming infection caused by *Sporothrix schenckii*. This fungus is widely distributed worldwide and can be found in soil, decaying vegetation, sphagnum moss, on rosebushes, tree bark, and other natural sources. In the environment *Sporothrix* exists as a mold, but transforms to a parasitic yeast at the higher temperatures of body tissues, i.e., it is dimorphic. Infection usually occurs by implantation following a penetrating wound, as by a thorn or wood splinter. Inhalation and ingestion are alternative (and probably less common) means by which the fungus gains access to the body.

Sporotrichosis occurs in two forms in horses:

- **Ulcerative lymphangitis,** characterized by the development of nodules along lymphatic channels, creating a "beaded cord" appearance. The nodules may abscess and ulcerate, releasing a pale yellow pus.
- A subcutaneous form characterized by the development of skin nodules, some of which may ulcerate

The lesions most often occur on the extremities and may involve one or more joints. There may be an associated swelling and thickening of the affected limb(s), owing to obstruction of normal lymph flow. The infection usually remains localized to the skin and underlying tissues.

Diagnosis is based on the history, physical examination, and biopsy and culture of lesion material. *Sporothrix* often is difficult to identify microscopically in tissues, pus, or fluid; it may require a number of attempts to locate the characteristic cigar-shaped yeast forms in the lesions. Thus the most reliable (but also the most time-consuming and expensive) diagnosis is made by culturing the organism in the laboratory.

Systemic antifungal medication combined with hot-packing or warm to hot hydrotherapy is the recommended treatment. The prognosis in most cases is guarded.

EQUINE PHYCOMYCOSIS

Equine phycomycosis is a general term describing several tropical and subtropical diseases caused by different organisms, one of which (*Pythium*) is actually not a fungus. The diseases have recently been classified into three main types: *basidiobolomycosis*, *conidiobolomycosis*, and *pythiosis*.

Basidiobolomycosis, which occurs only rarely in the United States, is caused by *Basidiobolus haptosporus*. Conidiobolomycosis is caused by *Conidiobolus coronatus*, while pythiosis is caused by *Pythium insidiosum*, a plant parasite found in water and on moist, decaying vegetation. In the United States both conidiobolomycosis and pythiosis occur most often in the southern states. Pythiosis is the more commonly encountered.

Lesions of pythiosis are frequently located on the lower parts of the extremities but may sometimes be found on the head and trunk. Swellings, skin ulcerations, lymph node enlargement, and draining tracts characterize many of the lesions, which are intensely **pruritic** (itchy). Occasionally, the disease process may spread to bone or other body sites. Lesions of basidiobolomycosis are similar to those of pythiosis but are found on the upper areas of the body (trunk, head, neck) rather than on the limbs.

Lesions of conidiobolomycosis develop primarily in the nasal passages and *nasopharynx* (the back of the throat), and occasionally in the mouth. Clinical signs include a thick nasal discharge, **halitosis** (bad breath), coughing, and **dyspnea** (difficult respiration).

Diagnosis is based on the history, clinical findings, and microscopic examination and culture of appropriate tissues or draining fluids. Treatment consists of surgical excision of the lesion(s), if possible, and topical or systemic antifungal chemotherapy. The prognosis is guarded.

PHAEOHYPHOMYCOSIS

Phaeohyphomycosis is an uncommon infection of the subcutaneous tissues caused by dark, pigmented fungi known as *dematiaceous* fungi. These organisms normally live in soil and on vegetation but on occasion can act as opportunistic pathogens, gaining access to tissues usually by means of a penetrating wound. Dematiaceous fungi can often be found in the home contaminating grout, toilet bowls, shower curtains, and other bathroom surfaces. Fungi of the genus *Drechslera* have been reported to cause lesions in the horse. The lesions consist of dark **plaques** (flattened areas) 1–3 centimeters in diameter that are covered with **pustules** (pimples) and **papules** (minute, firm, well-demarcated elevations of the skin). Topical antifungal therapy has reportedly been used with success.

RHINOSPORIDIOSIS

Rhinosporidiosis is an uncommon disease caused by an as yet poorly characterized fungus, *Rhinosporidium seeberi*. Rhinosporidiosis in animals and human beings is endemic in parts of Asia and South America, but occurs only sporadically elsewhere. It is a chronic, localized infection characterized by the formation of **polyps** (small fleshy masses protruding from the surface of a mucous membrane) in the nasal passages. Infection probably occurs when horses nose about in pools of stagnant water containing the infective stage of the fungus (the complete life history of this fungus is still relatively obscure). The fungus actively proliferates in the mucous membranes of the nasal cavity, inducing development of the tumorlike polyps.

Clinical signs include a nasal discharge and sneezing. Because of the chronic nature of the infection, signs may be evident for weeks to months before a diagnosis is reached. The diagnosis is made by microscopic identification of the causative organism in a smear of the nasal discharge or in a biopsy sample of an excised polyp. Treatment consists of surgical removal of the polyps (which may recur, necessitating more than a single surgical procedure).

CHAPTER 33

Internal Parasites

by David G. Baker

A parasite is an organism that lives in or on another organism, from which it draws nourishment but for which it provides no benefits in return. Parasites come in all shapes and sizes, ranging from microscopic protozoa a fraction of a millimeter across to giant tapeworms 3/4 meters long. Parasites differ from other organisms residing in or on a host in that parasites, for the most part, are ultimately detrimental to the health of the host.

Parasites can be classified into either of two broad general groups: **endoparasites** (internal parasites) and **ectoparasites** (external parasites). Endoparasites are found inside the host, chiefly in the gastrointestinal tract, while ectoparasites live in or on the skin. Horses can be host to many different kinds of parasites. Common internal parasites of horses include protozoa, nematodes, cestodes, and even some insects. Some of the consequences of host colonization by such parasites include:

- Inappetence
- Annoyance
- Allergic reactions

- **Anemia** (low red blood cell count)
- Increased susceptibility to other diseases
- Obstruction of blood vessels, lymphatic channels, or the gastrointestinal tract
- Tissue invasion, including destruction and occupation of tissues
- Depletion of nutrients needed by the host
- Toxic reactions
- Transmission to the host of disease agents carried by a parasite

This chapter will emphasize parasite biology and the clinical signs of the major parasitic diseases of horses. The parasites discussed are those that most commonly cause ill health in horses in the United States. Parasites can be classified into four major groups:

- *Protozoa.* Protozoa are the simplest **unicellular** (single-celled) members of the animal world. They move by gliding or by use of specialized structures such as **pseudopodia** ("false feet," temporary extrusions of the body wall), **flagella** (whiplike external structures), or **cilia** (minute, hairlike cellular processes). Protozoa feed by capturing food with their pseudopodia, by directing food into an opening called a **cytostome**, or by absorbing nutrients directly through the body wall. Many protozoa are capable only of **asexual** reproduction, i.e., self-division. Others are capable of either asexual or sexual reproduction, depending upon the host.

- *Nematodes.* Nematodes (**"roundworms"**) are unsegmented, cylindrical, cream-colored worms that exist in a wide diversity of species. Most adult nematodes infecting horses are large enough to be seen with the unaided eye. Roundworms possess a mouth, digestive tract, simple nervous system, excretory structures, muscles, and reproductive organs, including testes or ovaries.

- *Cestodes.* Cestodes (**"tapeworms"**) are highly adaptive internal parasites found in many aquatic and terrestrial species. They are long, flattened, ribbonlike worms lacking a body cavity or intestinal tract. Tapeworms possess rudimentary excretory and nervous systems and have muscles running through the body, which consists of numerous segments called **proglottids**. Tapeworms are **hermaphroditic**, i.e., each proglottid contains both male and female reproductive organs.

- *Arthropods.* Arthropod parasites include ticks, mites, and insects, most of which live outside the body. This chapter discusses those insects that spend a portion of their existence within the horse.

Gastrointestinal Parasites

The equine gastrointestinal tract is home to a large number of parasites, but five types stand out because of their high prevalence and/or potential impact on the host. These "big five" include the large roundworms, large strongyles, small strongyles, pinworms, and bots.

PROTOZOA

Cryptosporidium

Cryptosporidium parvum is an extremely minute protozoan, approximately 0.006 millimeter ($^1/_{4000}$ of an inch) in diameter, that infects many species of mammals. Asexual multiplication, followed by sexual reproduction, occurs in the cells lining the stomach and small intestine, resulting in the excretion of **oocysts** (encapsulated eggs) in the feces 3 days after infection.

Horses infected with *C. parvum* usually exhibit no signs of illness. Clinical disease (**cryptosporidiosis**) may occur, however, in debilitated or immunodeficient foals. Signs include severe diarrhea, dehydration, weakness, and occasionally death. Foals with normal immune function control the infection within a few weeks. Diagnosis of infection is sometimes difficult because the oocysts are very small and easily overlooked in a microscopic examination of the feces. No treatment is available.

Giardia

Giardia occurs in many vertebrate hosts. Although many species of *Giardia* have been named based on the host in which they are found, there may actually be far fewer species. There is no evidence that *Giardia* can be transmitted between horses and any other host species, including human beings.

Giardia infections are usually acquired by ingestion. Two forms of the parasite are recognized. The **trophozoite** is the feeding form and lives in the intestinal tract, where it attaches to the intestinal wall by means of a cup-shaped "sucker." For reasons that are not known, a trophozoite may round up, produce a protective coat, and pass out in the feces as a **cyst**, a resistant form that is infective to other animals. Cysts can survive for several months in cold water. Upon ingestion by a suitable host the cyst wall is broken down and the asexually dividing trophozoites are liberated to initiate another infection cycle.

Most infections with *Giardia* are **asymptomatic** (without clinical signs). In horses, *Giardia* can be an occasional cause of chronic diarrhea. Diagnosis is complicated by the fact that cyst formation and release are intermittent. It is possible that additional clinical cases might be detected if the condition could be diagnosed more consistently. Antiprotozoal medication is available.

Nematodes (Roundworms)

Stomach Worms

The stomach worms of the horse include *Habronema muscae*, *Habronema microstoma* (*Habronema majus*), and *Draschia megastoma*. Larval worms passed in the feces are ingested by the maggots of manure-breeding flies, where they remain during **pupation** (the second stage in the development of an insect). In the adult flies the larvae pass to the mouthparts and are deposited onto the horse as the fly ingests fluids on the lips, nostrils, eyes, penile sheath, skin wounds, etc. The horse becomes infected by ingesting the worm larvae or by swallowing infected flies in feed or water.

The worms either live free in the stomach or penetrate the stomach lining. When present in large numbers they may irritate the stomach, produce ulcers, and cause **nodules** (small lumps) to form in the stomach lining. Large nodules may interfere with normal stomach function. Diagnosis is difficult because few larvae are passed and they are not readily detected using routine fecal-examination procedures. Several **anthelmintics** (deworming medications) are useful for clearing the infection. An effective control program will also include fly control.

Far more serious are the lesions resulting from deposition of larvae at sites where flies sometimes feed, e.g., mucous membranes or skin wounds. The ensuing inflammatory response is characterized by fleshy masses that bleed easily, a condition known as **cutaneous habronemiasis** or **summer sores**. This highlights the importance of fly control, especially during the spring and summer months.

The small stomach worm *Trichostrongylus axei* inhabits the equine stomach and small intestine. Eggs are shed in the feces and the infective larvae are subsequently ingested with herbage. Light infections are asymptomatic. Heavy infections are more common in foals, particularly those sharing pasture with cattle. Signs can include **gastric** (pertaining to the stomach) disturbances, diarrhea, and constipation. A specific diagnosis can be difficult because the eggs of *T. axei* closely resemble those of the strongyles. Anthelmintics used to treat strongyle infections (*see* below) are also effective against *T. axei*.

Intestinal Threadworm

The intestinal threadworm, *Strongyloides westeri*, has two life cycles, a parasitic cycle and a free-living cycle. Parasitic female worms live in the small intestine and are **parthenogenetic**, i.e., they produce offspring from unfertilized eggs. The eggs are excreted into the environment and hatch, giving rise to larvae that become either parasitic females or free-living male and female worms. In the environment the free-living worms mate and produce infective, parasitic larvae that are then ingested by a horse or penetrate its skin. *Strongyloides westeri* can also be transmitted to nursing foals in the postcolostral milk (days 4–47 after birth), with eggs appearing in the feces in as little as 1 week.

Larvae of *S. westeri* thrive in moist, warm, soiled bedding. Foals housed under such conditions may develop skin lesions caused by direct penetration by the larvae. Migrating larvae may also damage internal organs such as the lungs. Heavy burdens of adult worms may cause severe, mucus- or blood-laden diarrhea in foals 3 weeks to 3 months of age. Infections in older horses are rarely significant clinically (except that infected adults can serve as a source of infection for foals). Infections are readily diagnosed by fecal examination. Several effective anthelmintics are available for therapy.

Large Roundworm

Parascaris equorum is a large, stout worm of the family Ascarididae (**Ascarid**). Females may reach over 45 centimeters (18 inches) in length, while males are smaller. Adult roundworms inhabit the small intestine of the horse, where up to 1 million eggs may be laid *per day*. In the environment the eggs develop to infectivity in as little as a week under ideal conditions of warmth and moisture—a fact that emphasizes the importance of prompt manure removal. Ingested eggs hatch in the small intestine. The released larvae soon penetrate the intestinal wall and migrate through the bloodstream to the liver and lungs. In the lungs they ascend through the airways to the **pharynx** (throat region) and are swallowed. Egg production begins approximately 10 weeks after infection.

Large numbers (1,000+) of worms can be found in foals aged 2–9 months and occasionally in geriatric horses. Heavily infected foals exhibit signs of coughing and nasal discharge (caused by larval migration to the lungs), foul-smelling diarrhea, **flatulence** (expulsion of air or gas from the anus), weight loss, stunted growth, and malaise. The hair coat is rough and some foals may have a "pot-bellied" appearance. Several of these signs are related to interference with nutrient absorption in the gastrointestinal tract. Occasionally, complications occur when worms migrate to an aberrant site, such as the bile duct. Also, if several adult worms "ball up" in a portion of the intestine, an obstruction can develop that can result in intestinal rupture. Fortunately, an age-related immunity to *P. equorum* develops by the time horses are 1–2 years of age.

Eggs of the large roundworm are remarkably long-lived and can survive for several years in a cool, damp environment. The eggs are also very sticky and can remain attached to a broodmare's teats and udder (thus serving as a source of infection for the nursing foal). The eggs can be readily transported to uninfected areas on clothing and farm implements. Prompt manure removal and anthelmintic therapy are essential for controlling the spread of this parasite.

Large Strongyles

Commonly called "blood worms" or "red worms," the large strongyles include some of the most important parasites of the horse. Fortunately the prevalence of these and many other equine worm parasites is steadily declining, owing to the introduction of improved anthelmintics and management practices.

Strongylus vulgaris is one of the most harmful parasites of horses. The male worm is approximately 1.7 centimeters (²/₃ inches) long and the female about 2.54 centimeters (1 inch). Adult females in the large intestine produce eggs that hatch and develop in the environment. If ingested, the larvae invade the walls of the intestinal **arterioles** (the smallest arteries) and

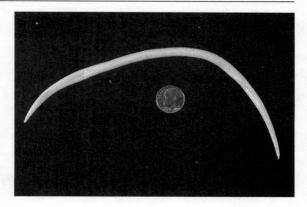

Figure 1. Adult roundworm. A dime is included for size comparison.

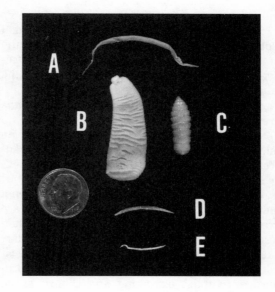

Figure 2. Selected adult parasites of the horse. A) Pinworm; B) Tapeworm (*Anoplocephala perfoliata*); C) Botfly larva; D) Large strongyle (*Strongylus vulgaris*); E) Small strongyle. A dime is included for size comparison.

migrate toward the large artery that supplies blood to much of the intestine. They may migrate as far forward as the heart. Eventually the larvae break out of the arterial walls and float freely in the bloodstream. Larvae entering the blood near the heart may be carried to virtually any site in the body. Many are transported to the large intestine, where they mature, mate, and produce eggs within 6–7 months after infection.

Larvae migrating through arterial walls are responsible for many of the health problems associated with this infection. As the larvae damage the vessel wall, weakened areas (**aneurisms**) containing blood clots (**thrombi**) form. The thrombi may detach and be carried downstream by the blood, eventually lodging and blocking blood flow, resulting in tissue death. Clinical signs associated with intestinal infection or arterial blockage include fever, inappetence, weight loss, constipation or diarrhea, colic, and occasionally death. Other signs are referable to the specific tissues affected, e.g., lameness may result after exercise when blood clots lodge in the large arteries supplying the hind limbs. Anthelmintic medications are effective against both the migrating larvae and the adult worms.

Strongylus edentatus and *Strongylus equinus* are less harmful species, since their larvae do not invade arterial walls. Instead, the larvae migrate through the liver (*S. edentatus*), pancreas (*S. equinus*), or abdominal cavity (both species).

For all three strongyle species there is often a marked seasonality in infection rates. Rates are greatest in the spring and summer when weather conditions favor the development of larvae on pasture. Older animals develop resistance to reinfection and may carry heavy worm burdens without exhibiting any clinical signs. Such animals represent a source of infection for foals because the infective larvae are quite long-lived on cool, moist pastureland.

Small Strongyles
Fifty-two species of small strongyles have thus far been identified. The adults live in the large intestine, where the female worms release eggs that pass out with the feces. The hatched larvae are ingested with the herbage and enter the lining of the large intestine, where they form nodules. Unlike other strongylid parasites, they do not migrate beyond the intestinal lining. Sexual maturity is reached 6–14 weeks after infection, depending on the species.

A marked seasonality to the parasites' life cycle is evident, with infection levels being greatest in the late winter and early spring. Small strongyles are less **pathogenic** (disease-inducing) than large strongyles, largely because of the limited migration of the larvae, although large numbers of worms can produce severe weight loss, intermittent diarrhea and constipation, colic, and occasionally death. Horses should be routinely treated for this infection.

The life cycle of the small strongyles is short, sometimes allowing two generations of worms to develop each year. As a consequence virtually all routine deworming schedules are directed toward controlling these parasites. Accordingly, many horses are given anthelmintics every 2 months, although eggs may reappear in the feces in as little as 4 weeks. Rapid worm turnover and frequent exposure to anthelmintics (sometimes at less than effective dosages), however, will facilitate the onset of drug resistance; this explains why certain drugs once effective against small strongyles are no longer useful. Because of this, manure should be promptly removed from paddocks.

All group-pastured horses should be given anthelmintics at specific intervals. Also, deworming and separating yearlings from mares and foals is particularly helpful for controlling small strongyle populations and can delay the onset of drug resistance. Yearlings tend to have the greatest parasite burdens and therefore contribute the most to pasture contamination.

Pinworms
The pinworm *Oxyuris equi* lives in the large intestine, where the males reach lengths of 1.27 centimeters (½ inch) and the females as much as 6 inches. Pinworms are so named because the tail of the female is narrow and long. After mating, the female moves to the rectum and crawls out through the anus, where she "glues" her eggs, in clusters of up to 60,000, to the skin of the **perianal** (around the anus) region. The eggs fall into the bedding and can survive for several weeks if kept moist (they die rapidly

when dried). Infection occurs following ingestion of infective eggs on feed, bedding, or fence posts. The eggs hatch in the intestine, the worms reaching maturity in about 5 months.

Infection with up to 20,000 worms is common in young horses. Clinical signs are associated with irritation caused by the egg-laying activities of the female worms. The perianal area itches intensely, causing restlessness and frequent tail-rubbing; the resulting hair loss at the base of the tail gives the horse a "rat-tailed" appearance. In addition, the annoyance causes appetite depression with loss of body and coat condition.

Pinworm infections can be diagnosed by applying a piece of clear Scotch tape to the perianal region, causing the eggs to adhere; the tape is then removed and the eggs attached to it are examined microscopically. Pinworm infections are easily treated with anthelmintics.

Probstmayria vivipara, the minute pinworm, also inhabits the equine large intestine. Infections with this worm are considered harmless.

CESTODES (TAPEWORMS)

Anoplocephala perfoliata, Anoplocephala magna, and *Paranoplocephala mamillana* inhabit the equine gastrointestinal tract. The most common species, *A. perfoliata*, attains a maximum length of 5 centimeters (2 inches). Frequently, adults congregate around the **ileocecal orifice,** the point at which the small intestine joins the large intestine. Adults of *A. magna* are nearly 76 centimeters (30 inches) in length and are found most commonly in the small intestine. *Paranoplocephala mamillana* also is found in the small intestine but like *A. perfoliata* is only about 5 centimeters (2 inches) long.

Free-living pasture mites are an essential component of these tapeworms' life cycle. The mites first become infected by ingesting tapeworm eggs. The mites are then eaten by grazing horses. Development of the larvae to mature tapeworm forms in the horse's gastrointestinal tract requires approximately 6 weeks.

Heavy infections may cause weight loss and diarrhea. Occasionally, heavy infections caused by *A. perfoliata* cause partial occlusion of the ileocecal orifice or even rupture of the wall of the **cecum** (a "blind pouch" protruding from the ileocecal orifice, representing an extension of the large intestine). Unlike many other parasitic infections, there is no apparent age resistance or acquired immunity to tapeworm infections. Infections are readily diagnosed but because most are considered harmless, treatment is seldom pursued.

ARTHROPODS

Bots

Bots are the larvae of hairy, beelike flies (*Gasterophilus* **spp**. [multiple species]) with nonfunctional, rudimentary mouthparts. In the spring and continuing until the first autumn frost, female botflies, each with an average lifespan of 7–10 days, attach their eggs (as many as 500) to the hairs of the horse. Three species of *Gasterophilus* are found in the United States. Each species deposits its eggs at specific body sites, such as the face, throat, legs, chest, or belly. The eggs may hatch spontaneously or may require warm, moist stimulation. The larvae develop within 1–2 weeks and are ingested by the horse during grooming. Invasion of the oral tissues follows, with the larvae ultimately passing to the stomach where they attach to the wall and grow. After a total of 8–10 months in the horse, the larvae leave the stomach to undergo further development in the soil. The mature flies emerge in the spring and summer.

Although botflies do not bite, horses may be disturbed by their presence and become irritable, sometimes injuring themselves or their handlers. Heavy infections (500+ larvae) may cause reactions in the oral cavity, including the development of pus pockets in the gums between the molar teeth. Attachment of the larvae to the stomach wall may cause ulcers, sometimes precipitating a fatal rupture of the stomach.

Treatment is usually recommended 1–2 months after the first hard frost in the fall. This may not be effective in removing "late arrivals" to the stomach, however. Regular removal of the eggs can reduce the level of infection. The eggs are readily visible and can be removed by plucking or trimming, although this can be quite laborious. Eggs found on the legs, chest, and belly may be stimulated to hatch and the larvae killed by washing with a sponge and warm, soapy water, or warm water containing an approved insecticide.

Respiratory Parasites

Parasitic infections of the respiratory tract are far less common than are infections of the gastrointestinal tract. The air-exchange surfaces within the lungs consist of thin, transparent layers of cells that permit oxygen and carbon dioxide to enter or leave the bloodstream (*see* CHAPTER 25, "THE RESPIRATORY SYSTEM AND VARIOUS DISORDERS"). Parasites invading the lungs may induce a thickening of these layers, impeding air exchange and thereby compromising the health of the horse.

NEMATODES

Lungworms
The equine lungworm, *Dictyocaulus arnfieldi,* is commonly found in donkeys, in which it causes little problem. Adult worms live in the larger airways, where the eggs are produced. As they hatch, the emerging larvae are coughed up, swallowed, and passed out with the feces. The larvae develop to infectivity in the environment. Following ingestion by another donkey they penetrate the intestinal wall and migrate to the lungs, where sexual maturity is reached in about 3 weeks. Adult worms may live for several years. Infective larvae do not survive drying on summer pasture, but may over winter and remain a source of infection in the spring.

Although clinical signs of infection are not seen in donkeys, infected horses may cough, breathe rapidly, and develop a nasal discharge. Because the horse is not the natural host for *D. arnfieldi*, worms frequently do not reach sexual maturity or produce eggs in this species. The diagnosis thus may be difficult to make, relying on suspicious clinical signs and evidence of coincident grazing with donkeys. Many anthelmintics are effective in treating this infection.

Musculoskeletal Parasites

NEMATODES

Onchocerca
Onchocerca cervicalis, a threadworm, lives in the **nuchal ligament**, a large, strong band of connective tissue that provides support for the neck. Another species, *Onchocerca reticulata,* lives in the nuchal ligament and in the flexor tendons and suspensory ligaments of the lower limbs. Adult females release minute prelarval forms called **microfilariae**, which travel through the bloodstream and localize in the skin of the **midline** (belly), head, neck, withers, and chest. Microfilariae must be ingested by biting **midges** (tiny flies) in order to develop further. Inside the midge the microfilariae transform into larvae, find their way to the mouthparts, and then they are transmitted to another horse when the midge feeds again.

The presence of worms in the suspensory ligaments of the fetlocks may result in swelling, lameness, and the formation of nodules. Affected horses may exhibit signs of intense itching at the sites of infection, due to allergic reactions to salivary secretions of the feeding midges. The *Onchocerca* larvae can be found in skin scrapings taken from these sites. Several anthelmintics are effective against the microfilariae but not against the adult worms. Confinement of horses in insect-proof stables from 4:00 P.M. to 7:00 A.M. during the warm months of the year can prevent attacks by midges, thereby interfering with the life cycle of the parasites.

Central Nervous System Parasites

PROTOZOA

Sarcocystis
Equine protozoal myeloencephalitis (**EPM**) occurs primarily in the United States and is caused by the protozoan parasite *Sarcocystis neurona.* Infections occur in the brain and spinal cord, where the parasite undergoes asexual reproduction. The life cycle of *S. neurona* has not been elucidated, so the source of infection is unknown.

Infected horses exhibit a variety of clinical

signs. If the infection is located primarily in the brain, signs such as head-tilt, facial paralysis, disorientation, and visual deficits may predominate. Spinal-cord infections are characterized by stumbling, incoordination, lameness, weakness, and inability to stand. Onset of signs may be sudden or gradual.

The diagnosis remains difficult to make at present, owing to the absence of a specific diagnostic assay. Infection with *S. neurona* cannot be differentiated on the basis of antibody tests from infection with other, harmless species of *Sarcocystis*. Moreover, clinical signs of EPM mimic many other neurologic diseases of horses.

NEMATODES

Micronema

Micronema deletrix is a free-living worm that lives in soil, manure, and decaying vegetation. Infections occur occasionally in horses. Clinical signs depend on the site of infection but are most severe following invasion of the nervous system, especially the brain and spinal cord. Affected horses may exhibit lethargy, incoordination, **recumbency** (lying down), and occasionally death. Lesions may form in other parts of the head, including the jaw and nasal passages, resulting in a nasal discharge and difficulty eating. The ease of diagnosis depends on the site of infection. Guidelines for treatment have not been established.

Miscellaneous Parasites

NEMATODES

Setaria

Setaria equina is a large worm that inhabits the abdominal cavity and occasionally the **scrotum** (dependent pouch of skin containing the testicles) of horses. The infection is transmitted by mosquitoes. Infected horses usually do not exhibit any clinical signs; infections for the most part are incidental findings during abdominal surgery or *postmortem examination* (autopsy). Clinical signs may develop, however, if the parasites lodge in an aberrant location, such as the eye. Aberrant infections are more common with other species of *Setaria*, such as *Setaria digitata*, which is normally a parasite of cattle. Diagnosis of an aberrant infection is nearly impossible. However, effective treatments of suspected infections are available.

Thelazia

The eyeworm *Thelazia lacrymalis* lives on the surface of the equine eye. Young larvae present in ocular secretions are ingested by certain flies, most notably the face fly. Later, infective larvae are redeposited on the horse's face and gain access to the eye. Infection may be associated with inflammation and an excessive production of tears. The worms can be identified visually on the surface of the eye. Effective treatments are available.

Prevention and Treatment of Internal Parasitisms

Horse owners can do a great deal to reduce the numbers of parasites in their horses. Efforts should be directed at preventing infection and treating existing infections. The following guidelines are useful for accomplishing these goals:

- Do not feed horses on the ground, where many of the infective forms (eggs, larvae) of equine parasites are found. Instead, provide a feed rack.
- Do not overstock pastures. Overstocking allows the parasite population to expand to dangerously high levels. A good rule of thumb is an acre of pasture per horse. If several pastures are available, horses should be moved (preferably 2–3 days after treatment) to fresh pasture.
- Prevent the accumulation of stagnant water on pastures. Water accumulating in potholes and poorly drained fields provides a breeding ground for many unwanted insects, such as mosquitoes and horseflies.
- Keep stalls clean. Remove manure and spilled feed daily during the summer and at least once a week in winter. In the summer keep bedding material to a minimum. Practice

weed control around stables and corrals. Keep areas as dry and airy as possible. Such practices will help reduce the number of parasites and remove breeding sites for many species of flies.

- Follow a regular program of deworming established in cooperation with the local veterinarian, who will be cognizant of the parasites prevalent in the area. The veterinarian also will know which medications to use to treat infections, what seasonal changes to expect in parasite populations in the area, and which parasites are more likely to be found in horses of different ages.

Opinions differ on the practice of alternating dewormers in an effort to delay the development of drug resistance. While some advocate this practice, others prefer using a single deworming medication until it is no longer effective. Those holding the latter opinion cite studies showing that alternating dewormers may actually accelerate the development of resistance to many compounds. Veterinarians can readily evaluate the efficacy of any deworming medication by comparing the number of parasite eggs in the feces before and after treatment. If the treatment results in less than a 90 percent reduction in the fecal egg count, the dewormer can be considered ineffective.

CHAPTER 34

Cancer

by Bruce R. Madewell

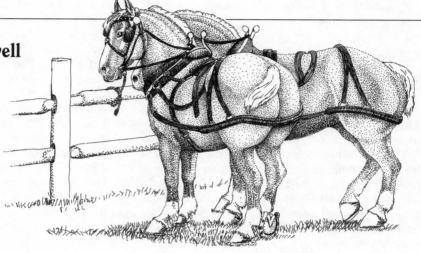

Most descriptions of tumors in horses are compiled from pathology collections of colleges of veterinary medicine; the actual frequency of occurrence of the different equine tumors among the total population of horses at risk is unknown. Surveys indicate, however, that the most frequently diagnosed tumors are derived from the skin, eye, and genital system, and that sarcoids and squamous cell carcinomas represent the most common tumor types in horses.

Causes of Cancer in the Horse

The causes of most equine tumors are unknown. Small DNA-containing viruses called **papillomaviruses** have been associated with the development of benign **papillomas** (warts) in horses, and these have been attributed to a species-specific equine papillomavirus (*see* CHAPTER 30, "VIRAL DISEASES"). There is no evidence that the horse is susceptible to human papillomaviruses. There is, however, good evidence to link the papillomavirus of cattle with connective-tissue tumors (**sarcoids**) in the

horse, and there is speculation that the equine papillomavirus may play a role in other malignant tumors of the skin and **mucous membranes** (lubricating membranes lining the internal surfaces of body cavities). RNA-containing **retroviruses** are associated with cancer in a variety of animal species and in people. *Equine infectious anemia virus* is a retrovirus infecting horses but is not known to be associated with the development of cancer.

Sunlight is an established risk factor for tumors affecting nonpigmented tissues around the eye (eyelids, third eyelid) in **skewbald** (having patches of white along with some other color except black) horses or in those with nonpigmented markings on the face. The areas around the eyes are the most frequent sites for the development of malignant tumors derived from skin surfaces (**squamous cell carcinomas**), a characteristic attributed to excessive exposure to sunlight.

Another important tumor in middle-aged to older horses is *malignant melanoma*. Although the cause of this pigmented tumor remains a mystery, an increased risk for melanoma in gray and white horses has been recognized for some time. The tumor also develops in those breeds of horses that undergo pigment changes as they age—breeds that include Arabians, Percherons, Lippizaners, and horses with foundation stock arising from these breeds.

Diagnosis of Cancer

The diagnosis of cancer in horses is based on the clinical history, physical examination, and results of supportive laboratory studies. Although there are no signs that are absolutely indicative of cancer, cancer must be considered in the differential diagnosis for any chronic **proliferative** (characterized by excessive tissue growth) or *ulcerative* (characterized by sloughing of the surface) lesion of the skin or mucous membranes, and for chronic maladies characterized by weight loss and failure to respond to routine therapies.

Because of the potential ramifications of a diagnosis of cancer, it is clear that the diagnostic process must be accomplished as expeditiously and accurately as possible. Laboratory examination of cells collected through fine needles (**cytologic diagnosis**) or of actual tissue specimens collected by **biopsy (histologic diagnosis)** is required to diagnose and categorize equine tumors. Because tumors may be confused with other infectious, developmental, or inflammatory lesions, it is imperative that representative specimens be collected properly for examination.

CYTOLOGIC DIAGNOSIS

The use of fine needles to secure cells for microscopic examination allows for the rapid evaluation of a lesion suspected of being cancerous. This procedure often requires local anesthesia. The collected cells are first stained and then examined under a light microscope. Cytology is generally used as a screening procedure to provide preliminary information on the nature of a growth or sore, although it has serious limitations in terms of accuracy. In general, decisions regarding the disposition of an animal with suspected cancer are not made on the basis of the cytological findings.

HISTOLOGIC DIAGNOSIS

For the majority of tumors, a formal *biopsy* procedure is required for an accurate diagnosis. Either a core or a wedge-shaped piece of tissue is usually collected for microscopic examination. For small lesions, the suspected tumor in its entirety may be removed, along with a border of normal tissue. This is referred to as an **excisional biopsy.** For larger or more deep-seated masses, a small tissue specimen is first collected, usually from the edge of the lesion (an **incisional biopsy**). Incisional biopsies are used to determine if the lesion is indeed a tumor, and if so, what type of tumor it represents. These findings can then be used to plan the most effective therapy possible.

The tissue specimen collected by incisional or excisional biopsy is fixed in a preservative such as **formalin** and stained for examination under the microscope. Examination of the specimen by a veterinary pathologist can provide information regarding the type of tumor present and, for excisional biopsies, an indication as well as to whether the tumor has been entirely removed (the pathologist looks for evidence of normal tissue completely surrounding the tumor biopsy). Finally, the pathologist provides information as to the degree of **malignancy** (ability to spread), which has significance with respect to treatment options and **prognosis** (outlook for recovery). Most veterinary diagnostic laboratories now provide rapid service for such biopsies, with a written report available to the clinical veterinarian within two days.

ENDOSCOPY

Endoscopy, the visualization of inner body structures by means of a specialized, tubelike viewing apparatus called an **endoscope**, is now a routine procedure in veterinary medicine. It provides direct visualization of anatomic sites previously accessible only by surgical or special **radiographic** (X-ray) methods. Equipment for fiber-optic and video endoscopy is available at many veterinary clinics. Endoscopy is applicable to the nasal passages and throat region, trachea, bronchi, esophagus, stomach, duodenum, urinary tract, female genital tract, and body cavities. Biopsy **forceps** (grasping instruments) are available to fit many types and styles of endo-scopes, to allow the collection of small biopsy specimens from internal areas under direct visual observation. Direct treatments such as **thermocautery** (destruction of tissue using a hot point or instrument) or laser therapy may also be performed using endoscopy.

RADIOGRAPHY

X-ray examination is an integral component of the diagnosis of some tumors in the horse. For tumors affecting skeletal structures, radi-ographic signs suggestive of cancer include changes in bone density, contour, or outline, and the appearance of newly formed bone. Radiography is especially helpful for evaluating lesions affecting the oral cavity, nasal cavity, and the surrounding sinuses. Because of the large size of adult horses, good-quality X-ray equipment is needed for a thorough examina-tion of body cavities. Tumors that **metastasize** (spread) to the lungs may appear as solid, round opacities on X rays, varying in size and distinct-ness of outline. **Thoracic** (pertaining to the chest) radiography is an insensitive method for the diagnosis of cancer, however, because tumors in the lungs must be 0.5 to 2 centimeters in diameter or greater before they can be seen on X rays.

ULTRASONOGRAPHY

Ultrasonography (also known as **diagnostic ultrasound**) is a noninvasive procedure for visu-alizing internal body structures by means of sound (echo) reflections. Ultrasonography is a valuable diagnostic tool in veterinary medicine; the equipment is available in many veterinary clinics and the procedure is safe and cost effec-tive. Ultrasonography is very useful for the examination of soft-tissue swellings, particularly those overlying long bones. Ultrasonography is also valuable for evaluating the heart and dis-eases within the thoracic cavity, particularly those characterized by the presence of free fluid. Ultrasonography can provide images of **abscesses** (walled-off lesions filled with pus), **granulomas** (lesions indicative of chronic inflammation, characterized by the accumula-tion of white blood cells around an offending agent), areas of lung **consolidation** (solidifica-tion), and tumors. In the abdomen, ultrasonog-raphy can be used to study the urinary bladder and its contents or free fluid within the abdomi-nal cavity itself. Ultrasonography using a special probe can also provide an image of the uterus, ovaries, and some suspect abdominal masses.

Treatment of Cancer

SURGERY

Surgical removal of a tumor is the most widely used treatment method. Surgery has the advan-tages of being quick, relatively inexpensive, and potentially curative. There are many considera-tions, however, in the use of surgery (or any other treatment method) for the management of cancer. These considerations include the size and location of the tumor and whether or not the tumor has already spread to underlying structures, regional lymph nodes, or distant sites. Large tumors, deeply invasive tumors, tumors located over complex anatomic struc-tures such as the head and neck, and tumors that have spread away from the primary site are more difficult to manage effectively. Another important consideration is the overall health of the horse—whether it is a suitable candidate for anesthesia. The utility of the animal following surgery may seriously limit the type or extent of surgical treatment used, and thus represents a serious consideration when a performance horse is involved.

The ideal candidate for surgical treatment of cancer would be an otherwise healthy animal with a small tumor affecting a readily accessible site away from joints, tendons, nerves, and other vital structures. In such a patient the tumor is **resected** (cut out) entirely, along with a wide margin of the surrounding normal tissue. The biopsy report will confirm that surgical excision is complete and that the tumor was either benign or of only low-grade malignancy upon microsopic examination. In this ideal patient, the surgical treatment would be consid-ered curative.

At the opposite extreme is the debilitated ani-mal with a deeply invasive tumor situated over a complex site, such as a joint. In such a patient, complete excision of the mass along with surrounding margins of normal tissue might not be possible; the surgical procedure might leave the horse either deformed or with loss of normal function. If the tumor is malignant and residual tumor tissue remains after surgery, it can be anticipated that the tumor will return unless additional therapy is provided.

RADIATION THERAPY

Radiation therapy (also called **radiotherapy**) is another established and time-honored method of cancer treatment. Although many horses with cancer have been treated with radiation therapy, this treatment modality is not readily available in veterinary practice except at university veterinary facilities. Because of certain limitations it is not always possible even at the universities to accomodate an animal as large as a horse for radiation treatment.

Implantation of radioactive devices has generally been used for radiation therapy in the horse, a technique referred to as **brachytherapy**. Brachytherapy may be preferable to surgical removal of some tumors if the tumor affects a structure such as the eyelid, where surgery might lead to a functional or cosmetic defect. Sources for irradiation include radioactive gold, cesium, cobalt, and iridium. For small and very superficial tumors, **b-irradiation** (consisting of electrons emitted from a radioactive substance) might be used. b-irradiation is most often employed as adjunctive therapy for tumors affecting the surface of the eye, once the main body of the tumor has been surgically extirpated.

CHEMOTHERAPY

Chemotherapy—treatment with medication—is a continually evolving method for dealing with cancer in small animals, but has had little application in the horse. Most anticancer drugs have not been tested for safety or toxicity in horses, and the costs for most drugs would be prohibitively expensive for such large animals. For horses with malignant lymphoma, particularly those with tumors affecting the skin, regression of disfiguring lesions might be accomplished with **corticosteroids** (hormones produced by

the cortex of the adrenal gland; or their synthetic equivalents). There have been occasional reports of the use of other anticancer drugs in horses with malignant lymphoma, e.g., when prolongation of survival was desirable to allow an affected mare to carry a foal to term.

Direct injection of anticancer drugs into tumors such as sarcoids and squamous cell carcinomas has been described. This method requires a series of once-weekly injections of a drug such as **cisplatin** (a platinum-containing compound). This treatment appears at present to be very effective for the control of superficial tumors of the skin, with minimal associated toxicity.

CRYOSURGERY

Cryosurgery involves the application of intense cold (below freezing) to destroy tumor tissue. The **cryogen** (substance producing cold) usually used is liquid nitrogen. Liquid nitrogen's extremely low temperature, $-198°C$ ($324.4°F$) is ideal for efficient and uniform freezing of tumors to the required temperature of $-25°C$ ($13°F$). Two freeze–thaw cycles are usually used to optimize results. Cryosurgery is most effective when the tumor can be directly visualized, so that the veterinarian can be certain that the entire mass has been frozen. Good results can be obtained for selected equine tumor types, including squamous cell carcinoma, malignant melanoma, sarcoid, and some others.

IMMUNOTHERAPY

A variety of innovative treatment methods has been developed over the years in an effort to enhance the patient's own immune or biological responses to cancer (**immunotherapy**). Most such methods in animals are still considered investigational, although it seems likely that true cancer cures will ultimately emerge from these strategies. Although most tumors have so far failed to respond to immunotherapy, the equine sarcoid is one lesion that often will regress following injection of a biological response modifier (substance that modifies immune responses) such as **BCG** (*Bacillus Calmette-Guerin*, containing cell-wall extracts of the bovine tuberculosis bacterium). Using a small-gauge needle, the tumor is directly injected with the BCG preparation, usually at 3-week intervals, for three to four treatments or until the tumor regresses. Such injections are most useful for sarcoid affecting the eyelids.

LASER THERAPY

A relatively new method for cancer treatment in veterinary medicine involves the use of a **laser** (*l*ight *a*pplication by *s*timulated *e*mission of *r*adiation). The far-infrared wavelength of the carbon dioxide (**CO_2**) **laser** provides precise tissue-cutting for surgical removal of a tumor or vaporization of a lesion. The CO_2 laser is particularly applicable to the management of superficial tumors of the eyelids, mucous membranes lining the eyelids, or the surface of the eye proper. Like hyperthermia (*see* below) and cryosurgery, laser treatment results in an open wound at the treatment site. These wounds heal slowly but completely within 6–8 weeks if no residual tumor remains.

The *neodymium:yttrium-aluminum-garnet (Nd:YAG) laser* emits energy in the near-infrared region of the spectrum. This wavelength can be delivered through a flexible fiber-optic system, thus allowing application to any site of the body accessible with an endoscope. Nd:YAG laser therapy is used most often for lesions of the upper gastrointestinal and respiratory tracts.

HYPERTHERMIA

Hyperthermia is a method of heating tumors to lethal temperatures. At the proper temperature, selective destruction of tumor cells occurs with preservation of normal tissue. Hyperthermia is used most commonly in concert with other treatment methods, such as radiation therapy, in an effort to enhance the effect of the other treatment. At present, most hyperthermia instruments available to veterinarians are applicable only to relatively small and superficial tumors. Hyperthermia has been the focus of considerable investigation in human cancer patients, and research is underway to develop instrumentation to heat large-sized tumors effectively for extended periods of time.

Tumor Types in Horses

Several surveys of tumors in horses have been conducted. Most such surveys have been derived from pathology collections, usually from veterinary schools or colleges, and therefore do not actually provide incidence data, i.e., they do not provide information on the numbers of new tumor cases diagnosed in a defined population at risk in a specific geographic area over a specific period of time. As a result, true incidence and prevalence rates for tumors of horses are not known. The pathology collections do, however, provide information about the most important tumors of the horse, that can alert the owner and veterinarian to the signs associated with specific tumor types. Surveys have indicated that the most important tumors in the horse are sarcoids, squamous cell carcinomas, melanomas, papillomas, and neurofibromas.

Terminology

The suffix "**-oma**" is used to designate a tumor. For example, a *benign* tumor (i.e., one that does not spread) derived from fat is termed a **lipoma**, one from fibrous tissue a **fibroma**, a tumor from smooth muscle a **leiomyoma**, one from the blood vessels an **hemangioma**, etc. **Malignant** tumors (tumors capable of spreading beyond the primary site) derived from surface components of a tissue are categorized as **carcinomas**. Malignant tumors of glandular structures are termed **adenocarcinomas**, while malignant tumors derived from deeper or supportive structures are termed **sarcomas**. A prefix is then used to indicate the tissue of origin. Thus a malignant tumor derived from fibrous connective tissue is termed a **fibrosarcoma**, one derived from fat a **liposarcoma**, one derived from blood vessels an **hemangiosarcoma**, etc. Some tumors are derived from specialized cellular components of the body, such as the **melanin-producing cells** in the skin (cells producing dark pigment). Such tumors are by convention termed **benign** or **malignant melanomas**.

This chapter will discuss the most commonly occurring tumors of horses, together with information about treatment methods and overall prognosis. The tumors will be categorized by anatomic site or body system.

TUMORS OF THE SKIN

The skin represents a complex organ, virtually every component of which can give rise to benign or malignant tumors. There are also nontumorous skin conditions that can mimic cancer; a biopsy is required to distinguish such developmental or inflammatory lesions from true tumors.

Benign tumors of the skin grow slowly, are well demarcated from surrounding tissues, and are easily removed surgically. By contrast, malignant tumors of the skin or subcutaneous tissues often grow rapidly, infiltrate adjacent tissues, invade blood vessels of the skin, and spread to local lymph nodes or to distant organs such as the liver or lungs.

Most skin tumors are treated surgically. However, virtually all of the currently available treatment options have a place in the management of malignant tumors of the skin, the choice of the most appropriate therapy being made on the basis of the tumor type, size, and site(s) of involvement.

Squamous Cell Carcinoma

Squamous cell carcinomas are malignant tumors derived from body sites covered by a specialized layer of cells, the **stratified squamous epithelium**. Important sites for squamous cell carcinoma in the horse are the skin and mucous membranes, including the eyelids, base of the tail, **perineum** (region between the thighs, encompassing the anus and genitalia), sheath and penis of the male, and vulva and clitoris of the female. Squamous cell carcinomas originating from the wall of the hoof are infrequently encountered. **Keratomas** (horny tumors of the hoof wall), a cause of hoof lameness, develop beneath the hoof wall or sole and must be differentiated from squamous cell carcinomas and infectious conditions of the hoof. Keratomas cause moderate to severe lameness with deformity of the hoof wall.

Sarcoid

Sarcoids are connective-tissue tumors unique to the horse, mule, and donkey, and vary in their gross and microscopic appearance from warty-appearing growths to lesions resembling **proud flesh** (exuberant tissue growth occurring during the healing of large skin wounds). The lesions may appear as small growths on a stalk (**pedunculated**) or as large, broad-based (**sessile**) masses. They may be solitary or multiple. Although sarcoids can occur anywhere on the body, important sites include the head (especially the ears and eyelids), lower abdomen, and limbs. In general sarcoids are considered to be of low-grade malignancy.

Melanoma

Melanomas can arise from the skin or mucous membranes virtually anywhere in the body. In horses they most frequently affect the skin, especially the regions around the anus, tail, and external genitalia. Melanomas may also originate from melanin-producing cells of the eye.

Papilloma

Papillomas (warts) are benign proliferations of the surface of the skin and mucous membranes. In the horse, papillomas generally occur in young animals and can affect the lips, nose, or skin of the limbs. Papillomas in young horses are related to infection with a virus, the equine papillomavirus (*see* CHAPTER 30, "VIRAL DISEASES"). Viral-induced papillomas may persist for as long as 9 months before regressing. **Congenital** (present at birth) forms of **papillomatosis** (development of numerous papillomas) have occasionally been described, suggesting infection **in utero** (in the uterus). Papillomas and squamous cell carcinomas have similar sites of predilection in the horse, and there is speculation that the equine papillomavirus may be involved in the development or progression of squamous cell carcinoma.

Neurofibroma

Neurofibromas are benign tumors of the nervous system, arising from **Schwann cells** (cells that form the **myelin sheath** around certain nerves, facilitating the conduction of nerve impulses). In the horse, neurofibromas generally involve the peripheral nerves and often affect the eyelids. They are usually small lesions measuring from one to several millimeters in diameter. Neurofibromas may be associated with the overlying skin or be freely moveable in the tissues beneath the skin. Although surgical removal should be curative, several surgical procedures may be required in some animals, particularly when a complex anatomic site such as the eyelid is involved.

Basal Cell Tumor

Basal cell tumors are extremely common tumors of the skin in human beings, dogs, and cats, but are only infrequently found in the horse. They are benign tumors derived from the basal cell layer of the **epidermis**, the outermost layer of the skin (*see* CHAPTER 17, "THE SKIN AND VARIOUS DISORDERS"). In horses basal cell tumors occur on the chest, tail, legs, back, or eyelids. They tend to invade local tissues but do not spread throughout the body. Surgical removal is usually curative.

Vascular Tumors

Tumors of blood vessels have been infrequently described in the skin of the horse. Most equine vascular tumors are benign **hemangiomas**, while a few are malignant **hemangiosarcomas**. Hemangiomas occur in the skin of young horses under a year of age. Some foals are born with congenital vascular tumors. Hemangiomas may grow rapidly at first, but soon ulcerate or bleed following irritation or trauma. Virtually any area of the skin may be affected, the lesions ranging in size from small **nodules** (lumps) less than a centimeter in diameter to large masses. Hemangiomas occasionally regress spontaneously. For persistent tumors, surgical removal is curative. Very few hemangiosarcomas have been described in the horse; such tumors are likely to be invasive.

Mastocytosis

Mast cells are normal constituents of the skin and are distributed widely throughout the body, particularly in the lungs, intestines, and near blood vessels. Although **mastocytosis** (abnormal infiltration of mast cells into a body tissue) in the horse is not considered a true tumor, it visually appears as a nodule or mass in or under the skin, especially on the head, neck, and extremities. Male horses over 7 years of age are most

frequently affected. Surgical removal is usually curative.

An unusual form of mastocytosis has been observed in foals. At birth or soon thereafter, multiple skin lesions develop that may either progress or regress. This form of mastocytosis resembles a disease in human patients termed *urticaria pigmentosa*.

TUMORS OF LYMPH- AND BLOOD-FORMING ORGANS

Malignant Lymphoma (Lymphosarcoma)

Malignant tumors derived from **lymphocytes** (specialized white blood cells capable of responding to the presence of foreign material in the body) are termed *malignant lymphoma* or *lymphosarcoma*. Although malignant lymphoma is a very commonly diagnosed tumor in dogs, cats, and cattle, it appears to affect horses less frequently. Nevertheless it is a tumor diagnosed with some regularity in aged horses and occasionally in foals.

Lymphoid (lymphocyte-containing) tissue is normally present throughout the body, and virtually any site may be affected by lymphoma. In horses the tumor may be localized or confined to a solitary site such as the skin, whereas in other animals it may be more generally distributed throughout lymphoid tissues including peripheral and internal lymph nodes and the gastrointestinal and/or respiratory tract. Great variation exists in the clinical appearance of this disease from horse to horse, depending upon the site(s) of involvement and the magnitude of the cancer present (the **tumor burden**). It is imperative, therefore, that the diagnosis be confirmed by microscopic examination. Because malignant lymphoma can be characterized by a fever, it must be distinguished from fever-causing inflammatory diseases. If the fever is also associated with **anemia** (low red blood cell count), then certain other diagnoses such as *equine infectious anemia* (*see* CHAPTER 30, "VIRAL DISEASES") will need to be considered. Malignant lymphoma affecting lymph nodes within the abdominal cavity often results in loss of appetite, weight loss, signs of colic, and fever—all of which may also be caused by abscesses.

Treatment of malignant lymphoma in the horse is a difficult undertaking. In most cases the tumor is not confined to a site that will permit simple surgical removal. Therapy for malignant lymphoma in both animals and people depends on the use of chemotherapy, i.e., anti-cancer drugs. In general, the costs associated with such medications in the horse are prohibitive. Further, drug treatment for this disease is generally **palliative** (able temporarily to relieve the clinical signs) rather than curative, and the utility of a performance animal such as the horse may be compromised as a result of treatment. For malignant lymphoma affecting the skin, effective remission of clinical signs may be achieved using corticosteroid drugs. Occasional reports in the literature describe the use of anti-cancer drugs for more widespread or systemic lymphoid tumors in the horse. The drug *L-asparaginase* has been used to achieve relief from signs in an affected pregnant mare, allowing full-term pregnancy of a valuable foal.

Leukemia

Tumors originating in the blood-forming organs (**bone marrow**) and affecting the blood have also been described in horses. These are rather unusual malignancies affecting a variety of cell types, including neutrophils, monocytes, and others. The diagnosis of leukemia requires microscopic examination of cellular smears obtained from blood and bone marrow, and often special stains are needed to elucidate the exact cell type that has become cancerous. Unfortunately, the veterinary literature offers no description of any effective therapy for equine leukemia.

TUMORS OF THE PITUITARY GLAND

Benign tumors derived from the **pituitary gland** (gland located at the base of the brain that stores or secretes an array of essential body hormones) have been associated with signs of **Cushing's syndrome** (hyperactivity of the adrenal cortex) in aged horses. These signs include increased thirst and urine output, weight loss, and increased sweating. The growth of long, shaggy hair coats, even in summer months, may indicate the presence of a pituitary tumor. Laboratory measurements of blood hormones and their stimulation are required to diagnose pituitary tumors as a cause of Cushing's disease in the horse. (*See* CHAPTER 28, "THE ENDOCRINE SYSTEM AND VARIOUS METABOLIC DISORDERS.")

TUMORS OF THE THYROID GLAND

Benign tumors of the **thyroid gland** (gland that produces hormones important in regulating the body's metabolic rate) are commonly encountered in aged horses, while their malignant counterparts have been only rarely described. Benign tumors are generally small and are usually only an incidental finding at **postmortem examination** (autopsy). Larger tumors may cause a swelling on the side of the neck, near the **larynx** (voice-box), but are not associated with swallowing difficulty or pain. The prognosis for surgical removal, when considered necessary, is good.

Malignant tumors of the thyroid gland must be distinguished from other swellings of the neck, including benign tumors, abscesses, **goiter** (generalized enlargement of the thyroid gland), and others. Scanning of the thyroid gland with a radioactive compound (a procedure known as **thyroid scintigraphy**), generally sodium [^{99m}Tc]-pertechnetate, can determine whether a neck mass involves the thyroid and also can provide some information regarding the size and extent of local tissue involvement. Malignant thyroid tumors may spread to lymph nodes or distant sites, making treatment difficult.

NASAL TUMORS

In general, tumors of the nasal passages and associated sinuses are uncommon in the horse. Among malignant nasal tumors, carcinomas are more often found than sarcomas. Clinical signs associated with nasal tumors include nasal discharge, swelling of the head, difficulty breathing or noise associated with breathing (**stertor**), a protrusive eye, and persistent shaking or rubbing of the head. Nasal tumors occur primarily in older horses, although some unusual tumors have been described in young horses and foals.

Diagnosis is made by X-ray examination and biopsy. Biopsy specimens can be collected with the aid of an endoscope. Unfortunately, there are few descriptions of successful treatment of nasal tumors in the horse. Conceivably, small lesions could be treated with the Nd:YAG laser, with endoscopic guidance.

ORAL TUMORS

Tumors of the oral cavity are diagnosed only sporadically in horses. Oral tumors can affect the lips, tongue, gums, or other structures in the mouth. Squamous cell carcinoma and fibrosarcoma are the most frequently observed malignant oral tumors in the horse. Affected horses exhibit difficulty eating and a foul odor from the mouth may be detected. Weight loss usually accompanies growth of the tumor. The tumor can be visualized by inspection of the mouth; diagnosis is made by biopsy. X-ray examinations are performed to determine if the bone underlying the tumor is involved. For small and noninvasive tumors, treatment options include surgical removal, cryosurgery, radiation therapy, and laser therapy.

TUMORS OF THE STOMACH

In general, tumors of the stomach affect horses between 6 and 14 years of age. The clinical signs resulting from stomach cancer are vague and nonspecific; they include loss of weight and condition, reluctance to eat, fever, and anemia. If the tumor spreads throughout the abdominal cavity, fluid may accumulate and masses within the abdomen may be palpable. Microscopic examination of fluid collected from the abdominal cavity may reveal the presence of tumor cells. Endoscopic examination of the stomach may allow the veterinarian to visualize the stomach tumor directly.

Most tumors of the equine stomach are malignant and are classified as carcinomas. On occasion, malignant lymphoma may involve the stomach. Unfortunately there are no reports of successful therapies for malignant tumors of the equine stomach. Most such tumors will have spread widely through the body by the time a diagnosis has been established.

TUMORS OF THE INTESTINES

Tumors arising in the intestines are uncommon in the horse. The tumor most likely to involve the intestinal tract is malignant lymphoma. Malignant lymphoma of the small intestine will produce signs of diarrhea, abdominal pain, **malabsorption** (faulty absorption of nutrients), and weight loss. Effective therapies for intestinal tumors in the horse have not been described.

TUMORS OF BONE

Malignant tumors arising in bone are uncommon in the horse. Benign **osteomas**, protrusive masses of dense bone, may affect the flat bones of the equine skull. Benign tumors derived from the **cartilaginous** (containing *cartilage*, a specialized type of connective tissue important in bone growth and the formation of joints) components of bone, termed **chrondromas**, are also found primarily in flat bones such as the skull, ribs, or other sites containing cartilage (larynx, ear, nasal cavity). Another benign tumor of the skeleton of the horse is the **solitary osteochondroma**, which may affect long bones. **Multiple osteochondromas**, also termed *multiple cartilaginous exostoses*, are inherited in horses as an *autosomal dominant* trait (*see* CHAPTER 13, "GENETICS"). These tumorlike malformations affect the long bones or flat bones of young horses and may already be present at birth. They usually appear as irregularly shaped, dense protuberances. A malignant tumor that may involve equine bone is **multiple myeloma** (derived from *plasma cells*, whose function is to produce antibodies), which may affect the flat bones of the skeleton (especially the vertebrae), causing multiple bony defects visible on X-rays (*see* CHAPTER 29, "THE IMMUNE SYSTEM AND VARIOUS DISORDERS").

Benign tumors of the skeleton may be treated surgically, depending upon their size and location. Treatment of multiple osteochondromas is generally unnecessary because these tumors will stop growing once the adjacent **growth plates** in the bone have closed (*see* CHAPTER 22, "THE MUSCULOSKELETAL SYSTEM AND VARIOUS DISORDERS"). Multiple myeloma could conceivably be treated with chemotherapy, although the cost would in all likelihood be prohibitive.

TUMORS OF THE LIVER

Liver tumors occur only sporadically in horses. Young horses occasionally develop **hepatocellu-**

lar carcinomas (malignant tumors derived from liver cells), while tumors derived from the **bile duct** (duct that discharges digestive fluids [**bile**] from the liver into the intestine) occur more often in older horses. The liver may also be affected by malignant lymphoma.

TUMORS OF THE KIDNEYS
Benign and malignant tumors of the kidney occur only infrequently in most domestic animals, including horses. Benign kidney tumors usually are small and not associated with any clinical signs. Horses with malignant kidney tumors usually are 10 years of age or older. They may exhibit signs of weight loss, abdominal pain, poor appetite, fever, and blood in the urine. A mass may be detected in the region of the kidney. Ultrasonography will allow direct imaging of the mass and a tentative diagnosis of cancer. Most kidney tumors described in horses are malignant (carcinomas), with spread throughout the abdomen into adjacent organs by the time of diagnosis.

TUMORS OF THE URINARY BLADDER
Tumors of the urinary bladder are uncommon in horses. When present they are usually malignant (squamous cell carcinomas) and occur in older horses. Clinical signs include straining to urinate, blood in the urine, and weight loss. A tentative diagnosis of bladder cancer can be made by palpation during a rectal examination. Other diagnostic methods include endoscopy, ultrasonography, and cytologic examination of urine.

TUMORS OF THE OVARIES
A variety of ovarian tumors have been reported in the horse, the great majority being *granulosa cell tumors* (*see* CHAPTER 12, "REPRODUCTIVE DISORDERS"). **Granulosa cells** are the cells that surround the developing ovarian **follicle** (the egg and its associate protective layers). Equine granulosa cell tumors may secrete hormones, including male and female sex hormones; it is these products that are responsible for the behavioral changes observed in affected animals. Changes include either male- or femalelike reproductive behaviors, alterations in the estrous

cycle, and **infertility** (diminished ability to produce offspring). Equine granulosa cell tumors usually affect only one ovary and are usually benign, although there have been descriptions of malignant forms.

Diagnosis of granulosa cell tumor is made on the basis of the clinical signs, a palpably enlarged ovary upon rectal examination, and laboratory confirmation of high circulating levels of sex hormones. Ultrasonography will permit direct imaging of the architecture of the ovaries. Ovarian tumors distort the normal architecture of the ovary, appearing as large, fluid-filled, **multilocular** (having many compartments) masses. The opposite ovary is usually small and inactive. Treatment is based on surgical removal of the affected ovary. Fertility usually is restored after successful surgery.

The second most common ovarian tumor in horses is the **teratoma**. Teratomas are benign tumors that do not produce clinical signs. They are usually recognized only incidentally upon rectal palpation or postmortem examination. Teratomas may contain **cysts** (fluid-filled sacs) as well as a bizarre combination of different embryonic tissues, such as bone, cartilage, hair, and teeth.

TUMORS OF THE UTERUS
Uterine tumors are uncommon in most domestic animal species. In the horse, uterine tumors are usually benign and classified as either **leiomyomas** (derived from smooth muscle) or **fibromas** (derived from connective tissue). Diagnostic methods include rectal examination, ultrasonography, and fiber-optic examination and biopsy with forceps. Benign tumors can be removed surgically.

TUMORS OF THE TESTICLES
Testicular tumors are infrequent in the horse; this may simply be because of the common practice of castrating young male horses. *Seminomas* are the most commonly described testicular tumors. The tumors are usually **unilateral** (on one side, i.e., present in only one of the two testicles), and may reach substantial size before a diagnosis is made. Undescended testicles appear to be at increased risk for testic-

ular cancer, a characteristic shared by dogs and human beings. Most equine seminomas are benign, with castration being curative. A small number of seminomas are malignant, however, and may spread to the opposite testicle as well as to local lymph nodes and abdominal organs. Other testicular tumors in the horse include *interstitial cell tumors* and teratomas.

TUMORS OF THE ABDOMINAL CAVITY

Lipomas, benign tumors derived from fat cells, are recognized most frequently in the abdominal cavity in horses. Lipomas are usually found incidentally in old horses during postmortem examination. On occasion they may be palpated during a normal rectal examination. Intra-abdominal lipomas occasionally have been associated with colic, as a result of their causing a strangulating obstruction of the small intestine or small colon. Lipomas of the **subcutaneous** (beneath the skin) tissues of the skin, although very commonly encountered in small animal practice, are only infrequently seen in horses.

Tumors most often encountered in the horse are derived from the skin, mucous membranes, and tissues around the eye. Malignant lymphoma and ovarian tumors are also described in most compilations and surveys. For tumors affecting the external surfaces of the body, early recognition, biopsy confirmation, and prompt treatment are the best measures for control.

Newer diagnostic methods, including fiberoptic and video endoscopy, ultrasonography, and special radiographic studies are now in routine use in many veterinary clinics. These methods have increased diagnostic precision and offer the possibility of an earlier diagnosis of tumors that previously had been inaccessible to noninvasive diagnostic procedures. Improvements in surgical techniques and the application of alternative treatment methods such as laser or radiation therapy have also favorably improved the outlook for many horses with cancer.

Great strides are now being made in human medicine in understanding the many causes of cancer. Accomplishments have been most noteworthy in the fields of molecular biology and genetics. Already the veterinary literature reports the application of these modern techniques to the horse. It is anticipated that such studies will eventually shed additional light on the causes and risk factors for equine tumors, improve their prognostic assessment, and aid in the design of optimal treatment and prevention strategies.

CHAPTER 35

The Aged Horse

by Mary A. Scott

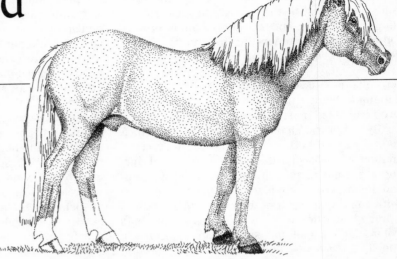

The natural life expectancy of the horse is difficult to define. According to the Guinness Book of World Records, the oldest horse on record was Old Billy, an English draft horse who lived to the grand old age of 62 years. Perhaps more remarkable is that Old Billy was retired from his job of towing barges *at age 59!* This example of equine longevity is astounding but illustrates the fact that, given the proper circumstances and care, horses can live for a long, long time. Although it is not unusual to hear of horses living into their mid-thirties, a more reliable approximation of the potential lifespan of the average horse is 25 to 30 years. One "horse-year," then, is roughly equivalent to three human years.

Horses evolved as grazing animals, living in herds on the grasslands of North America, and were subjected to the selection pressures of their natural environment. As herbivores, their teeth and digestive tract developed to provide for the most efficient processing of the vegetation that was available. These developments included:

- Incisor teeth for cropping grass
- Well-developed cheek teeth with surfaces best suited for grinding
- A small stomach with minimal storage capacity
- A large **cecum** (pouch-like extension of the large bowel) for fermentation of ingested nutrients

The pastoral existence of horses kept them on the move. This in turn kept their constantly growing hooves neatly shaped, prevented heavy parasitic infestations, and minimized disease transmission. Even today it is not uncommon to find wild horses that have survived to an advanced age without the benefits of vaccination, regular deworming, dental care, or the farrier's rasp.

In the managed environment of the domestic horse, however, the environmental pressures are quite different. High population densities and confinement in barns or corrals increase the potential for disease transmission, parasite infestation, hoof disease, and behavioral abnor-

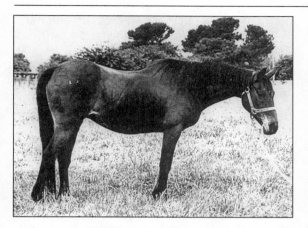

Figure 1. Grecian Lace, a 28-year-old brood-mare, exhibiting mild, age-related conformation changes, including a swayed back, protruding withers, and hollows above the eyes.

malities. These factors are of particular concern for the aged horse. As horses approach their late teens and early twenties, they become less resilient to the negative effects of stress, injury, and disease. Older horses often need individualized care, and those with chronic disease conditions may require specialized management that may be time-consuming and/or costly for the owner.

Strict attention to dietary needs, stable management, and routine health care can maximize the chances for an extended high quality of life for the older horse. This chapter will discuss some of the more common disorders associated with aging in the horse, and provide management suggestions that may aid in long-term maintenance.

Dental Disease

Certainly one of the most significant problems afflicting older horses is dental disease. In general, this includes not only conditions affecting the teeth but diseases affecting the gums as well, i.e., *periodontal disease*. Because it is not easy to examine a horse's full set of teeth, dental disease may progress unnoticed until it is quite advanced. Some conditions are painful, while others simply interfere with the mechanical efficiency of the chewing process. Any condition that prevents a horse from chewing properly can lead to poor digestion, compromised nutrition, and even digestive-tract disorders, such as choke or colic (*see* below).

ABNORMALITIES OF THE DENTAL ARCADES
A horse's permanent teeth continue to grow as it ages. At the same time the grinding action of chewing wears down the surfaces of the opposing teeth. Many aged horses have worn the grinding surfaces of their teeth completely smooth (a condition known as **smooth mouth**). Because the first molar (the fourth cheek tooth) is the first permanent tooth to erupt, it is typically the first to wear smooth, often by 18 or 20 years of age. Missing or broken teeth and poor alignment of opposing teeth (a condition known as **malocclusion**) will cause abnormal tooth wear. Many years of abnormal wear can result in conditions such as **wave mouth,** or **step mouth** (FIGURE 3). Either of these dental conditions can prevent a horse from chewing effectively. Moreover, because teeth become more

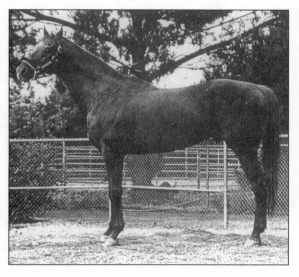

Figure 2. Grenfall, a 26-year-old fertile stallion in good body condition. The mother of this stallion died at the age of 35.

fragile and the tooth roots shallower with age, attempts to correct dental abnormalities can be risky in older horses, potentially resulting in tooth fracture and loss.

Gingivitis (inflammation of the gums) is not only painful but can cause "pockets" to form between the gum and teeth. Feed material lodged in these pockets can be a source of infection that may reach to the tooth roots. For upper cheek teeth whose roots extend into the **maxillary sinus** (one of the sinuses or airspaces in the skull), this can lead to a sinus infection.

Clinical signs of dental disease can be behavioral or physical. An affected horse may chew slowly, dribble grain, pack wads of feed material in its cheeks, or **quidd** (drop partially chewed feed material). The horse may seem to play with its tongue or exhibit an abnormal head posture while eating. Head-tossing may be seen and bridling the horse may become a problem. Often there is poorly-digested hay or grain in the manure. Pain associated with chewing can lead to a decreased appetite, with the reduced feed intake resulting in weight loss. The owner may notice a foul odor coming from the mouth. A nasal discharge or facial swelling may accompany a sinus infection caused by an infected tooth root. A lump on the border of the lower jaw

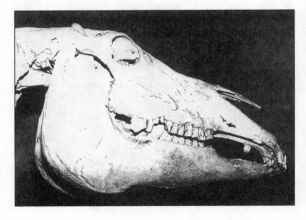

Figure 3. The cheek teeth in this horse skull exhibit the condition known as *step mouth*, which prevents proper chewing of hay. It is a common finding in aged horses.

may indicate an infected lower cheek-tooth root.

The ramifications of poor dental health are many. Consequently, dental care is a particularly important part of routine health management for aged horses. (*See* CHAPTER 3, "EQUINE HUSBANDRY.")

Digestion and Nutrition

To release stored nutrients from plant material, the horse must be able to grind the material sufficiently for proper digestion. Digestion begins in the mouth, where chewing reduces particle size and saliva initiates the breakdown of carbohydrates. A smooth-mouthed older horse may experience difficulty grinding hay fibers into pieces small enough for efficient digestion. In addition, the digestive processes in the large intestine are less efficient in the aged horse, causing decreased digestion of protein, phosphorus, and fiber. As a result, aged horses appear to have dietary needs similar to those of foals 6–18 months of age.

DIET

Many older horses can maintain good body condition on a diet of hay or pasture; alteration of the diet is necessary only if the horse begins to lose weight or condition. Feeding alfalfa hay plus a grain mixture of corn, oats, barley, and milo will provide high-quality protein and supplemental phosphorus. However, alfalfa hay is high in calcium and should be avoided in horses with reduced kidney function. In such cases, grass hay should be substituted and supplemented with linseed or soybean meal. In advanced age or if dental conditions necessitate, a diet of water-softened alfalfa pellets or alfalfa meal with molasses, supplemented with bran mashes and a pelleted concentrate, can be fed. Complete pelleted feeds that are specially formulated for aged horses have recently become available from commercial sources. The feeding of dry pellets should be avoided.

Requirements for vitamin C and the B-complex vitamins are increased in aged horses, and supplementation with zinc may be beneficial, particularly following injury. Suggested daily supplements include 50–200 ml of vegetable oil (for energy), 0.5–2 kg of dried brewer's grain (for protein, fat, and B-vitamins), 50 g of brewer's yeast (for B-vitamins), and 1–5 g of vitamin C (supplementing the diet with as much as 10–20 g per day has been suggested). Complete pelleted feeds may already contain adequate supplements except for vitamin C. (For complete information on the nutritional requirements of horses, *see* CHAPTER 6, "EQUINE NUTRITION," and CHAPTER 7, "FEEDING HORSES").

As a grazing animal the horse has evolved a digestive tract designed to handle small amounts of forage ingested in a continuous fashion. Unless they are on good pasture, horses should be fed at least twice daily. Horses with debilitating lameness may not be willing to move even short distances to eat or drink; in such cases the feed and fresh water should be easily accessible. Coarse, stemmy, or moldy hay should be avoided. Any changes in diet should be implemented gradually in order to avoid digestive disturbances.

SPECIFIC DISEASES OF THE DIGESTIVE TRACT

Older horses with poor dentition, a diet of stemmy hay, and decreased water intake may experience repeated bouts of *colic* or *choke*. Slightly-dry wads of poorly-chewed food do not move down the **esophagus** (muscular tube extending from the throat to the stomach) easily and may become lodged there, causing an obstruction (**choke**). Similarly, because poorly-chewed hay is not readily digested, such a diet may result in colic due to intestinal blockage (**impaction colic**). Surgery may be required to correct these conditions. (*See* CHAPTER 8, "DISEASES OF DIETARY ORIGIN"; CHAPTER 26, "THE DIGESTIVE SYSTEM AND VARIOUS DISORDERS"; and CHAPTER 37, "SURGERY AND POSTOPERATIVE CARE.") Older horses experiencing choke or impaction colic require a specialized diet and ready access to fresh water. These disorders are less likely to occur on a diet of water-softened alfalfa pellets, or alfalfa meal with molasses.

Another cause of colic in the aged horse is the **strangulating lipoma.** This is a fatty tumor on a long stalk that becomes wound around the intestine, causing a strangulating obstruction.

Strangulating lipoma occurs more frequently in geldings and horses over 17 years of age, particularly in overweight animals. Surgery is absolutely necessary to correct this condition. Horses that recover from the surgical procedure have reasonably good survival rates.

Squamous cell carcinoma is an uncommon tumor affecting the stomach lining, predominantly in older horses. Affected animals may exhibit intermittent colic, decreased appetite, weight loss, and **anemia** (low red blood cell count). There is no cure; horses diagnosed with this condition should be humanely destroyed.

Sand colic may occur whenever a horse is fed directly from the ground, or if a horse is "pastured" in a dry lot. Sand accumulation can be minimized by sound husbandry practices. Bran is an excellent bulk laxative, and bran mashes may be useful in eliminating some intestinal sand, although *psyllium* is the feed additive of choice for this purpose. Another type of impaction colic that may be encountered in older horses is that caused by intestinal stones, or **enteroliths**. This type of colic can only be corrected surgically. *Spasmodic colic* may result from a change in feed, ingestion of moldy hay, or simply stress. Pain is caused by spasms of the intestine. Colics of this type respond well to medical treatment. Regular deworming can prevent colics caused by a heavy parasite load. (*See* Chapter 8, "DISEASES OF DIETARY ORIGIN.")

Musculoskeletal Disorders

Horses can age gracefully when they are well cared for. Visible signs of advancing age, such as a swayed back, protruding withers, hollows above the eyes, and a drooping lower lip, may not appear until the age of 25 or even later, particularly if the horse is kept athletically fit (Figures 2 and 3). Indeed, one key to maintaining body condition and at least the appearance of youth in the older horse is routine exercise. The age at which a horse should discontinue strenuous athletic endeavors is highly individual, depending heavily on the horse's physical condition, athletic history, and current use. Horses in their late teens are often able to participate successfully in strenuous competition. In 1993, five of the 90 horses finishing the TEVIS Cup 100 Miles in a Day Endurance Ride were 18 years old, including the horse that placed fifth!

Aged horses tend to lose muscle tone and condition more quickly than younger horses. Thus, periods of inactivity should be followed by a gradual increase in the amount of work an older horse is asked to perform. Horses with minor lameness may benefit from routine exercise. Controlled exercise with strict attention to a schedule will usually provide the best results. For horses with **arthritis** (joint inflammation), it is best to avoid long periods of inactivity, which can result in decreased flexibility and range of motion in the affected joints.

Lameness resulting from *navicular disease* can often be managed with corrective shoeing and anti-inflammatory medications. Unrelenting cases may benefit from a permanent nerve block (**palmar digital neurectomy**) to the affected area, a procedure referred to as **nerving**. Horses that have been nerved require fastidious attention to hoof care. A hoof **abscess** (bacterial infection) in the desensitized region of the foot may go unnoticed until it is quite advanced. Horses older than 15 years of age are at low risk for developing navicular disease, however. (*See* CHAPTER 22, "THE MUSCULOSKELETAL SYSTEM AND VARIOUS DISORDERS.")

Chronic *founder* and recurrent *laminitis* are examples of debilitating lamenesses that may be encountered in the older horse. In addition to requiring specialized care, these conditions certainly prevent the use of the horse as a riding animal. Affected horses are often most comfortable if confined to a heavily bedded stall, with individual turnout in a small grass paddock. The decision to maintain a horse in this condition must include a thorough assessment of the animal's overall quality of life. (*See* CHAPTER 22, "THE MUSCULOSKELETAL SYSTEM AND VARIOUS DISORDERS.")

Cardiovascular Disorders

Heart murmurs, or unusual sounds caused by abnormalities of blood flow through the heart, are relatively common in aged horses. Typically they represent age-related changes in the functioning of the heart valves. Horses are capable of compensating for minor structural defects in the heart; often these murmurs do not affect the horse's level of performance and do not require medical treatment. The horse may limit its own performance to compensate for any deficiencies in heart function, however.

By contrast, abnormal heart rhythms (**cardiac arrhythmias**) can significantly affect performance, particularly if a horse is asked to do more than just light work. In severe cases, cardiac arrhythmias may even cause the horse to faint. The most common arrhythmia encountered in older horses is **atrial fibrillation**. In this condition the heart rate is uncontrolled, becoming very rapid during exercise; as a result it may go unnoticed unless the horse is asked to perform. The condition is treatable, although some horses may relapse. (*See* Chapter 20, "The CIRCULATORY SYSTEM AND VARIOUS DISORDERS.")

Rupture of the base of the **aorta**, the major blood vessel exiting the heart, has been the cause of sudden death in older stallions. This phenomenon occurs immediately after breeding; death results from cardiovascular failure. There are no warning signs. No treatment is possible.

Respiratory Disorders

Heaves, or **chronic obstructive pulmonary disease (COPD)**, may occur in older horses. Similar to reactive airway disease in people, heaves appears to be an allergic response of the respiratory tract. Horses with heaves breathe with an obvious effort on exhalation. Paroxysms of coughing often occur in response to certain feeds or a dusty environment. Depending on severity, clinical signs may develop in response to exercise or following exposure to dusts or molds, and may persist when the horse is at rest. Modifications in stabling management can help alleviate the problem, the aim being to minimize exposure to the offending substance. Stall bedding can be changed from straw or shavings to shredded paper. Stabled horses can be moved to grass pastures; conversely, pastured horses allergic to pollens or other plant material can be moved indoors. Medications may serve to lessen the severity of the clinical signs. (*See* CHAPTER 25, "THE RESPIRATORY SYSTEM AND VARIOUS DISORDERS.")

Tumors

Cushing's disease is caused by a tumor of the pituitary gland in the brain and is most commonly diagnosed in aged horses. The tumor stimulates the adrenal glands near the kidneys to secrete high levels of the corticosteroid hormone cortisol. Horses with Cushing's disease typically have a long, often curly haircoat that sheds late or in patches. They tend to drink and urinate large volumes and have a tendency to sweat heavily. Muscle wasting, delayed wound healing, and a "pot-bellied" appearance are also characteristic. Because of the abnormal levels of cortisol, affected horses are prone to a variety of infections of the skin, mouth, respiratory tract, and feet. With individualized attention and sound management practices, however, most horses can survive for many years with a high quality of life. Chronic or recurrent laminitis and sole abscesses are the most common reasons for euthanasia. (*See* CHAPTER 28, "THE ENDOCRINE SYSTEM AND VARIOUS METABOLIC DISORDERS.")

Melanoma is a tumor of pigment cells in the skin and is common in older horses. Unlike the situation in people, melanomas in horses do not appear to be caused by excessive exposure to sunlight; rather, the equine tumors are coat-color related. It may be accurate to call this the "old gray horse disease," since more than 80% of gray horses develop melanomas, typically after 15 years of age. The tumors are most commonly found on the underside of the tail or around the anus; however, they may arise anywhere on the body. Melanomas are firm in consistency and black or gray in color. Most often they grow slowly and are unlikely to spread; thus they are frequently left untreated. Melanomas can be surgically removed but complete excision often is difficult, depending on their location. In recent years *cimetidine*, a medication used for treating stomach ulcers, has been found useful for causing regression of melanomas in some horses.

Squamous cell carcinoma is another skin tumor that occurs predominantly in middle-aged and older horses. Unlike melanoma, this tumor tends to develop in non-pigmented skin and is correlated with exposure to sunlight. The breeds most likely to develop this cancer are Belgians, Clydesdales, Shires, Appaloosas, American Paints, and Pintos. The areas affected are typically the eyes, lips, nose, or genitals. The tumors are highly invasive and physically resemble a pink wart or cauliflower. They are often **ulcerated** (have a severely-sloughed surface) and grow rapidly. Surgical removal followed by radiation therapy is an effective treatment. In general the larger the tumor, the poorer the prognosis for recovery.

Squamous cell carcinoma of the genitals most commonly affects older geldings. An association between the accumulation of **smegma** (a grayish, oily material) on the penis and **sheath** (fold of skin enclosing the penis) and the development of this cancer has been suggested. Clinical signs include a swollen sheath and, if the **urethra** (membranous tube that transports urine from the bladder to the exterior of the body) is involved, intermittent bleeding and difficulty urinating. Amputation of the penis may be necessary if the tumor is highly invasive. Spread to local lymph nodes may also occur. In the mare, genital squamous cell carcinomas appear as ulcerative lesions on the vulva.

Disorders of the Eye

Moon blindness, also known as **recurrent uveitis,** is not a disease restricted to older horses, but owing to its recurrent nature may certainly occur in the aged animal. The clinical signs mimic acute trauma or injury to the eye; when examined closely, however, it becomes apparent that there is no damage to the **cornea** (transparent outer coat of the eye). One or both eyes may be affected. Recurrent uveitis is intensely painful and if left untreated can result in blindness. Cases that are refractory to treatment may require removal of the painful eye. (*See* CHAPTER 19, "THE EYE AND VARIOUS DISORDERS.")

Cataracts—opaque areas within the lens—most commonly result from injury or inflammation. Senile cataracts may develop after 20 years of age. Cataracts block the passage of light through the lens, resulting in impaired vision. Horses with cataracts may appear blind, particularly in bright daylight when the pupils are constricted. ((*See* Chapter 19, "The Eye and Various Disorders.")

A condition called **proliferative optic neuropathy** is an incidental finding in horses over 15 years of age. Typically only one eye is affected. When the eye is examined with an **ophthalmoscope** (instrument for viewing the inner reaches of the eye), a cauliflower-like mass can be seen attached to the **optic disk** (portion of the optic nerve visible at the back of the eye) and projecting into the inner eye chamber. Unless the mass becomes exceedingly large, the condition is not usually associated with loss of vision.

Any condition that results in a vision deficit may seriously limit the usefulness of a horse for riding or driving. A partially-blind horse is also likely to be a poor choice as a child's companion. Thus, prompt recognition of vision deficits and potential causes of vision problems is important.

Reproductive Disorders

Mares

Many mare owners ask if they should breed their older mares, and if so, what the chances of pregnancy might be. Many factors can affect reproductive performance. In the mare there is an age-related reduction in reproductive efficiency, e.g., pregnancy rates for 15- to 30-year-old mares average 32%, as compared to almost 100 percent for young mares. To decrease the chances of success even further, as many as 37% of mares over 24 years of age may not ovulate during the natural breeding season. Without ovulation, no egg is available for fertilization. (*See* Chapter 9, "Reproductive Physiology").

Old age in the broodmare is associated with damage to the uterus that ultimately decreases the chances of conception and maintenance of the embryo or fetus. Age-related changes in a mare's conformation can increase the susceptibility to uterine infections. The rates of pregnancy loss increase two-fold after 15 years of age, and there may also be an increased incidence of defective eggs. Even for older maiden mares there are natural age-related changes in the uterus that decrease the chances for a suc-

cessful pregnancy. To complicate matters further, older mares (especially those over 11 years of age) that have previously had several foals may have an increased risk of fatal uterine artery hemorrhage at delivery.

Artificial insemination (AI) rather than natural breeding is the method of choice for the aged mare because it limits the number of breedings per heat cycle and reduces the likelihood of uterine infection. (*See* Chapter 10, "Breeding Management.") It is important to check with the breed organization involved to be sure that this method of breeding is acceptable.

Because of these many factors, breeding an aged mare can be time-consuming and expensive. A thorough reproductive evaluation, including a uterine biopsy to assess the quality of the uterine lining tissue, is recommended prior to breeding. The information gleaned from this procedure can be used to determine the likelihood of the mare's carrying a foal to term.

Stallions

In contrast to mares, stallions can remain fertile until an advanced age. Conditions influencing a stallions' reproductive performance include semen quality, **libido** (sexual drive), and mating ability. Many stallions continue to produce high-quality semen throughout their lifetime.

A critical limiting factor to fertility can be the stallion's physical ability to cover a mare. Inability to cover can result from lameness or a lack of libido. With adequate libido, stallions having even severe forelimb lameness can be mated. By contrast, because the hindlimbs must support the weight of the stallion during the mating process, significant hindlimb lameness or pain may prevent successful breeding. Arthritis, particularly in the hindlimbs, may be managed with the use of anti-inflammatory medication prior to breeding. Alternatively, if AI is acceptable, stallions experiencing difficulty may be trained for semen collection using a "phantom" or "dummy" mare that can be adjusted to a comfortable position. (*See* Chapter 10, "Breeding Management.")

Infertility or subfertility may be encountered in the aged breeding stallion and may be due to a number of causes. Decreased production of sperm caused by testicular degeneration may be an age-related change, but more likely is the result of previous illness or injury. Stallions with low numbers of normal sperm in their semen can continue to produce foals if they are managed carefully. (*See* CHAPTER 12, "REPRODUCTIVE DISORDERS.")

General Management Tips

Being an observant owner is especially important as a horse ages. Because subtle behavioral changes may signal an early stage of disease, knowing your horse in health makes the rapid recognition of illness or injury more likely. Therefore, learn to recognize what is normal for your horse. Make a habit of observing your horse's attitude, how it moves, its eating and drinking habits. Inspect the horse daily in the light (natural or artificial). Be aware that a heavy winter haircoat can hide weight loss very effectively. Daily grooming provides an ideal opportunity for you to inspect the horse for signs of injury or illness. It is also a way to spend "quality time" with your older animal.

Another ideal opportunity to observe your horse is at feeding time. Is the usual interest in food there? Is the horse chewing normally? Is the manure of normal shape and consistency? Does the manure contain coarse hay stems or undigested grain? Such attention to detail can help maintain a high quality of care and maintenance for an older horse.

Housing and Stable Management

Proper husbandry is essential to assure a high quality of life for the aged horse. This includes stabling arrangements, nutrition, preventive health care, and exercise. Stress-free pasture and stable arrangements are essential because stress can alter nutritional requirements for an individual animal. Horses are highly social creatures and in general prefer the company of other horses. Indeed, horses deprived of companionship may refuse to eat or drink. In a herd situation horses establish a "pecking order," which can be hard on the older horse, who is often at the bottom of the list. Horses with debilitating lameness may do poorly if turned out with other horses, because they cannot defend their own

space or may be prevented from obtaining food.

Routine vaccinations, bi-monthly deworming, and regular hoof trimming or shoeing are standard maintenance for any horse, but are particularly important for aged animals. Strict attention to dental care and diet are essential for prevention of digestive disorders and loss of condition. Many factors influence the degree of specialized management required for older horses. The attending veterinarian can aid in determining the level and type of individualized care needed in a particular situation.

Older horses can be enjoyable and faithful companions. They are well adapted to their relationship with humankind, and tend to be more predictable and reliable than younger horses. Many aged horses are child-safe and are ideal as a "first horse." Maintaining an older horse in good health can be emotionally rewarding, and many owners feel a strong need to provide the best care possible for a retired old campaigner.

Saying Good-Bye

When an older horse's quality of life begins to deteriorate, the owner must eventually face the decision to have the horse **euthanized** (put down). Animals often seem oblivious to pain and many owners have difficulty judging their quality of life. A reasonable method is to assess the horse's overall appearance. A horse willing and able to eat and with good body condition has very likely a satisfactory quality of life. In times of illness or injury, however, the following questions may help the owner make a rational decision regarding euthanasia:

- How much is the horse suffering?
- What are the chances for recovery?
- What are the costs of recovery?
- What are the costs of maintaining a debilitated animal?

The knowledge and experience of the attending veterinarian can be of particular help in answering these questions.

The responsibilities of horse ownership undoubtedly weigh most heavily when the owner must decide to say good-bye to a long-time companion. Because of the expense involved in maintaining a horse, which may increase substantially owing to ill health, economic concerns are often a necessary part of the decision-making process. Decisions based on economics often carry with them a feeling of "not having done enough." The human-equine bond can be exceptionally strong, and elective euthanasia can stimulate feelings of grief and a deep sense of loss. These feelings are very real, and stem from the intangible bond that has existed between humankind and the horse for eons of time.

PART VII

Home Care

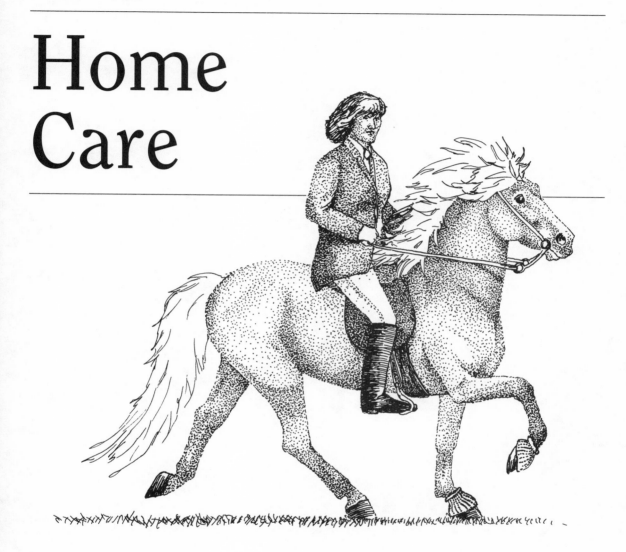

A canter is the cure for every evil.

—Benjamin Disraeli
The Young Duke

CHAPTER 36

Clinical Signs of Disease

by Johanna L. Watson

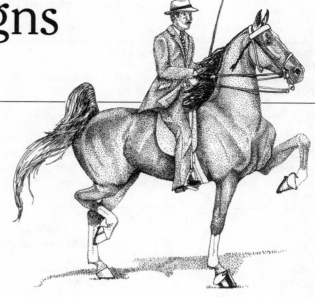

The Normal Horse

The clinical signs of disease in horses have been recorded over many centuries by many different observers. In the fourth century B.C., for example, the Greek philosopher Plato described the increased respiratory rate and difficulty breathing that he had observed in some horses. It is thought that he was describing a disease still seen in horses today known as "heaves" or chronic obstructive pulmonary disease (COPD).

All signs of disease have in common the fact that they are vital signs, behaviors, postures, patterns, appetites, or appearances that differ from what is considered "normal." The first important step in the recognition of disease, therefore, is the knowledge of what is or can be normal. Some measures of normality can be generalized to the entire species, such as a normal body temperature of 37.5-38°C (99.5–100.5°F), while others must be developed by the owner or caretaker for an individual horse, e.g., the knowledge that a particular horse lies down to sleep for a few hours each night. The first sort of measure, representing *vital signs* (TABLE 1), is something every horse owner should have avail-

able. The second sort, *individual animal patterns* (TABLE 2), is something an owner becomes familiar with during contact time with a horse. Both such measures of normality are valuable when one is attempting to determine if a horse is exhibiting normal behavior or signs of illness that may require veterinary attention.

Patterns of Clinical Signs

A clinical sign rarely occurs alone, and the types of signs that occur together often constitute a pattern that is characteristic of the malfunction of a given body system. There are clinical signs that are specific for a given body system, and others that are nonspecific and can occur with disease in any body system. An example of a specific clinical sign would be a cough, which is specific for the respiratory system. An example of a nonspecific sign would be a fever, which can occur with infection of any body system of the horse.

The causes of any particular clinical sign can range from the very common to the very rare. In Tables 3 and 4, specific and nonspecific signs of disease in the horse are listed with their com-

---

Table 1
Clinical Signs of Disease

Vital Signs

Vital sign	Adult horse	Foal
Temperature	37.5–38°C/99.5–100.5°F	38–38.6°C/100.5–101.5°F
Heart Rate	24–36 beats per minute	40–60 beats per minute
Respiratory Rate	12–24 breaths per minute	32–54 breaths per minute

---

mon (C), less common (LC), and rare (R) causes. If all the clinical signs exhibited by a horse are put together, they often form a pattern that denotes the nature of the underlying disease condition. For example, if a horse is exhibiting signs of cough, nasal discharge, fever, and inappetence, the pattern fits an infection of the respiratory system.

Table 2
Individual Animal Patterns

Behavior	Variations
Eating	How fast, how long, how much, preferred feeds, waste
Activity	Most active time of day, how much work will tire the horse
Defecation	Character of manure (wet, dry), amount of manure per day
Urination	Character of urine (color), posture while urinating
Sleeping	How often horse lies down, position chosen when down

---

Table 3
Specific Clinical Signs of Disease

Clinical sign	Body system	Causes
Cough	Respiratory	Dusty environment or feed (C)
		Upper respiratory tract infection (C)
		Influenza (C)
		Pneumonia (LC)
		Pleuritis (LC)
		"Heaves" (LC)
		Guttural pouch infection (R)
		Lung cancer (R)
Nasal discharge	Respiratory	Dusty environment (C)
		Upper respiratory tract infection (C)
		Influenza (C)
		Pneumonia (LC)
		Pleuritis (LC)
		Guttural pouch infection (LC)
		Sinusitis (LC)
		Abscessed tooth (LC)
		Mass or abscess in pharynx (R)

Table 3 (cont.)
Specific Clinical Signs of Disease

Clinical sign	Body system	Causes
Noisy breathing	Respiratory	During exercise: "roaring," abnormal function of the structures in the pharynx (C) At rest: Swelling of any structure in the pharynx (LC) Strangles (C) Foreign object caught in pharynx (LC) Mass or tumor in the pharynx (R)
Bad breath	Respiratory or dental	Not eating (C) Foreign object in mouth (C) Abcessed tooth (LC) Severe pneumonia (LC)
Diarrhea	Intestinal	Feed change (C) Moldy feed (C) Feed impaction (C) Sand impaction (LC) Incomplete bowel obstruction (LC) Intestinal infection with *Salmonella* (LC) Other intestinal infection (LC) Infiltrative bowel disease or malabsorption syndrome (protein-losing enteropathy) (R) Bowel cancer (R)
Hard dry manure	Intestinal	Feed change (C) Weather change (C) Lowered water intake (C) Feed impaction (C) Bowel obstruction (LC)
Straining to pass manure	Intestinal	Feed impaction (C) Bowel obstruction (LC) Mass or tumor of rectum or anus (R)
Colic pain	Intestinal	Spasmodic colic (C) Feed impaction (C) Meconium (first bowel movements of the newborn) impaction (foals) (C) Sand impaction (LC) Stone (enterolith) (LC) Displacement of large bowel (LC) Twisted large bowel (LC) Twisted small bowel (LC) Diaphragmatic hernia (R)
Frequent urination	Urinary	Females: in heat (C) Bladder infection (LC) Males: dirty sheath with partial obstruction of urethra (LC)

Table 3 (cont.)
Specific Clinical Signs of Disease

Clinical sign	Body system	Causes
		Overdrinking habit (LC)
		Cushing's syndrome (older horses) (LC)
		Bladder stones (LC)
		Kidney stones (R)
Discolored urine	Urinary or musculoskeletal	Dark yellow color: very concentrated urine (C)
		Coffee color: muscle breakdown ("tying up," exertional myopathies) (C)
		Red color: blood in urine (LC)
Straining to urinate	Urinary	Colic pain (C)
		Males: dirty sheath with partial obstruction of urethra (LC)
		Bladder stones (LC)
		Bladder infection (LC)
		Male foals: ruptured bladder (LC)
		Tumor in urethra or bladder (R)
Swollen sheath	Urinary	Decreased exercise regimen (C)
		Overweight horse (C)
		Dirty sheath (C)
		Infection in sheath (LC)
		Cancer on penis or sheath (LC)
Discharge from eye(s)	Ocular	Conjunctivitis (from dust, flies, wind, trailer ride) (C)
		Corneal injury or ulcer (C)
		Foreign body in eye (C)
		"Moon blindness" (recurrent uveitis) (LC)
		Ocular cancer (LC)
Squinting, blinking	Ocular	Corneal injury or ulcer (C)
		Foreign body in eye (C)
		"Moon blindness" (recurrent uveitis) (LC)
Cloudy eye(s)	Ocular	Corneal injury or ulcer (C)
		"Moon blindness" (recurrent uveitis) (LC)
Impaired vision	Ocular or neurologic	Corneal injury or ulcer (C)
		"Moon blindness" (recurrent uveitis) (LC)
		Cataract(s) (LC)
		Head trauma (LC)
		Retinal degeneration (R)
		Optic nerve damage (R)
		Ocular tumor (R)
Lameness	Musculoskeletal	Sole bruise (C)
		Sole abscess (C)
		Thin soles (C)

Table 3 (cont.)
Specific Clinical Signs of Disease

Clinical sign	Body system	Causes
		Infection from wound or puncture (C)
		Arthritis (C)
		Tendon injury (C)
		Ligament injury (LC)
		Fracture (R)
		Rabies (R)
Leg swelling	Musculoskeletal	Generalized:
		Change in exercise regimen (C)
		Infectious disease (influenza, equine viral arteritis, pleuritis, severe diarrhea) (LC)
		Localized (in one leg or one area):
		Trauma (C)
		Infection (C)
		Sprain or strain of a ligament or tendon (C)
Reluctance to move, lying down more frequently	Musculoskeletal	Founder (laminitis) (C)
		Any severe lameness (LC)
Hair loss	Skin	Abnormal shedding pattern (C)
		Rubbed off by tack or blanket (C)
		Ringworm (C)
		"Rain scald" (bacterial skin infection, dermatophilosis) (C)
		Fungal infection (LC)
		Hypersensitivity reaction to insect bites, topical sprays, or ointments (LC)
Bumps or masses in haired skin	Skin	Deep reaction to insect bite (C)
		Hives (allergic skin reaction) (C)
		Benign melanoma (C)
		Sarcoid (skin tumor) (LC)
		Malignant melanoma (R)
Growths or sores on non-haired skin	Skin	Fly bite reactions (C)
		"Proud flesh" (exuberant wound healing) (C)
		Sarcoid (generalized granulomatous disease) (LC)
		"Summer sores" (migrating parasite larvae) (LC)
		Skin cancer (white or light-colored areas) (LC)
		Immune-mediated skin disease (R)
Rubbing (itchy horse)	Skin	Fly sensitivity (C)
		Gnat sensitivity (C)

Table 3 (cont.)
Specific Clinical Signs of Disease

Clinical sign	Body system	Causes
		Sensitivity to topical sprays or ointments (C)
		Pinworms (tail rubbing) (C)
		Lice or mites (LC)
Incoordination	Neurologic	Head injury (C)
		Vertebral malformation in neck (C)
		Spinal cord infection (protozoal or bacterial) (LC)
		Rabies (R)
		Equine viral encephalomyelitis (R)
Personality change	Neurologic	Head trauma (C)
		Liver disease (LC)
		Rabies (R)
		Equine viral encephalomyelitis (R)

Table 4
Nonspecific Clinical Signs of Disease

Sign	Causes
Fever	Any infection
	Any cancer (R)
Inappetence (not eating)	Any respiratory (C), intestinal (C), or neurological (LC) disease
Depression	Any respiratory (C), intestinal (C), or neurological (LC) disease
Lethargy, exercise intolerance	Any respiratory (C), intestinal (C), musculoskeletal (C), or neurological (LC) disease

The keys to the recognition of disease in the horse are daily observation and good record-keeping. A safe rule of thumb for deciding whether or not to call in a veterinarian is: if any of the specific signs of disease occur in combination with one or more of the nonspecific signs of disease, then a veterinarian should examine the horse. For example, if the horse coughs in a dusty arena, but exercises normally, has no fever and a normal appetite, try wetting down the arena before exercise. However, if the horse has a fever and/or exercise intolerance, a veterinarian should examine the animal.

CHAPTER 37

Surgery and Postoperative Care

by John R. Pascoe

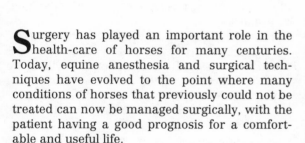

Surgery has played an important role in the health-care of horses for many centuries. Today, equine anesthesia and surgical techniques have evolved to the point where many conditions of horses that previously could not be treated can now be managed surgically, with the patient having a good prognosis for a comfortable and useful life.

Because many horses are used for athletic endeavors that are competitive in nature, owners often have an expectation that surgery will return a horse to complete, pain-free function. Such is not always the case, however. Despite the best surgical technique and rehabilitation efforts, a recovered horse may be comfortable at rest but nevertheless still exhibit soreness when exercised. It is important that the horse owner have a thorough and candid discussion with the veterinarian about the possible outcomes of surgical intervention. In this way, one is able to make an informed choice about the method of treatment. Should it become evident that a horse needs to be retired, the owner will at least know that he or she pursued the best medical options available. And as in human medicine, it is always prudent to obtain a second opinion before consenting to a major surgical procedure on a horse.

Surgery can be performed for a variety of different reasons. Chief among these are:

- Relief of pain and suffering
- Return of normal function
- Limiting the spread of a disease
- Repair of a wound
- Modifying a horse's behavior (e.g., castration)
- Correcting a developmental problem

Unfortunately, surgery is sometimes performed for unethical reasons, e.g., to satisfy certain breed-registry criteria or to accomplish certain appearances in the show ring. Such practices are not condoned by veterinary medical associations or equine veterinary associations. Surgery and anesthesia are not innocuous procedures; the decision to pursue surgical intervention must be made after the perceived benefit has been balanced against the potential risks. Moreover, the costs of anesthesia and surgery can be formidable. A clear understanding of such costs, and any additional obligations that may be incurred if complications arise, should be arrived at before any final decisions are made.

Emergency Surgery or Elective Surgery?

Surgical procedures can be either *elective* or *emergency* in nature. Elective surgical procedures are those in which an owner has a choice whether or not to proceed with surgery, i.e., the procedure is medically necessary but the timing is not critical. Examples of elective procedures include removal of a slow-growing mass, a **neurectomy** (surgical cutting of a nerve to relieve pain), and removal of an infected tooth. Emergency surgical procedures are not only medically necessary but must be performed immediately to save a horse's life or to prevent serious complications. Emergency surgical procedures may involve **colic** (abdominal pain), fractures of major bones, penetrating injuries of the foot, and wounds involving joints.

In the case of certain emergency surgical conditions—for example, severe blood loss or an acute intestinal obstruction, with loss of large amounts of fluid into the gastrointestinal tract—the patient must first be stabilized medically before proceeding with anesthesia and surgery. Intravenous administration of fluids or blood may be necessary before and during surgery to maintain circulating blood volume and blood pressure. Otherwise serious complications, such as kidney failure, **myopathy** (muscle disease), cardiac arrest, or even death, may ensue. In some circumstances it may not be possible to correct an abnormality completely until the underlying problem has been surgically repaired; sufficient fluids or medication will need to be administered during anesthesia and surgery in order to decrease the risk to the horse.

Responsibility and Costs Associated with Surgical Care

The costs of equine medical and surgical care can be substantial. Procedures requiring general anesthesia in a surgical theater often range from $500 to $1,500. Medications, **implants** (bone plates and screws), bandages, and hospitalization all incur additional costs, so that it is not unusual for total costs to range from $1,000 to $5,000. Should complications arise necessitating additional surgery or prolonged medication or hospitalization, the total cost may reach $15,000.

Equine medical and surgical insurance is available, but it is quite expensive and often is not practical for owners with more than a single horse. In addition, most policies have deductibles and limits on the amount of coverage. It is good practice for owners to have a frank discussion, before the need arises, of the financial limitations they may choose to place on medical or surgical care for a horse. Most owners are sufficiently upset and anxious, and often (unnecessarily) harbor feelings of guilt about their ability to meet financial obligations, such that a decision made in an emergency situation is later regretted. In difficult situations, **euthanasia** (putting a horse to sleep) is an acceptable choice. Owners should not feel uncomfortable about discussing this option with the attending veterinarian.

It is important to leave the veterinarian or care-givers explicit guidelines as to the extent of medical or surgical treatment one is willing to pursue, before leaving for vacations or extended trips. If an owner is unable to be contacted and a horse requires emergency care, the attending veterinarian is obligated to provide sufficient care to stabilize the horse's condition. *This may include surgery and as the owner, one is obligated to bear the costs associated with necessary treatment.* If a horse is insured for health care or mortality, it is the obligation of the owner to notify the insurance company when a horse requires veterinary attention, and also to notify the veterinarian that the horse is insured.

Insurance companies may require a second opinion before treatment or euthanasia. From a veterinary vantage point, mortality insurance usually covers only euthanasia associated with diseases causing intractable pain or suffering. If a horse develops a problem that may result in long-term treatment with little probability of a return to normal function, the insurance carrier may not authorize euthanasia and in fact may require the owner to proceed with necessary treatment to maintain a valid policy. This does not preclude an owner's decision to terminate treatment; it simply means that the carrier is unwilling to compensate the owner for a loss under the given conditions.

Costs of major medical or surgical care also become an issue when they involve horses that are leased or owned in partnership. It is always good practice to discuss these issues at the time of the original negotiations, and to include any important conditions or caveats in the lease or partnership contract. In general, it is the lessee's responsibility to cover all health care costs unless some other agreement has been reached. In a partnership it is useful to designate a spokesperson for the group, so that the veterinarian does not have to divert time away from patient care to speak to each individual owner of a horse. Often the trainer initially fulfills this role; however, the partners may wish to designate one person as the conduit for daily reports from the veterinarian to the group.

Hospital Visits

Most equine clinics will allow an owner to visit a horse after it has been admitted for a major medical or surgical problem. One should inquire whether the clinic has visiting hours or when it would be convenient to visit. It is important to respect these hours and not interfere with the functions of the nursing staff or veterinarians during a visit. Unfortunately, some common courtesies practiced in human hospitals are often forgotten in equine clinics.

One should restrict a visit to one's own horse. It is not appropriate for visitors to wander about the clinic or hospital wards looking at other patients, nor is it appropriate to question the staff about horses other than one's own. Questions concerning the progress and care of one's horse should be directed to the attending veterinarian unless one has been advised otherwise. Just as it would be improper to question custodial personnel about a family member's progress in a human hospital, so it would be inappropriate to expect barn personnel to provide accurate information concerning a horse's progress. Similarly, although nursing staff can provide information about a horse's general progress, one should rely on the attending veterinarian for detailed progress reports.

It is courteous to ask first if one can go into a patient's stall and if the horse can be taken outside for a walk. Sometimes these activities may not be in a horse's best interest; at other times they may be precluded by the risk of disease transmission. **Nosocomial** (hospital-acquired) infections can occur in horses just as they do in humans, so hospital staff may restrict an owner's access to his or her horse. This is another important reason why one should restrict one's visit to one's own horse alone. One should feel free to discuss one's concerns with the attending veterinarian, and to alert the staff of any special feeding requirements or behavioral traits of relevance. Sick and convalescing horses respond positively to visits from familiar persons just as hospitalized people do. Visits can be an important part of a horse's health care, but they should coincide with regular hospital activities. Common courtesies also should be observed.

Preparation for Anesthesia and Surgery

Once the decision to perform a surgical procedure has been made, an orderly sequence of events should be followed to prepare a horse for anesthesia and surgery.

PATIENT PREPARATION
Before surgery, the horse must be carefully evaluated for anesthetic risk. A thorough physical examination is usually performed first, with particular attention to **auscultation** of the chest, i.e., listening carefully to the heart and lung sounds for abnormalities that might increase the risk of complications associated with anesthesia. Blood is collected for analysis to ensure that the horse has an adequate red blood cell count (an index of the blood's oxygen-carrying capacity), white blood cell count (important for defense against infection), and blood platelet count (important for blood clotting). The fibrinogen concentration in the blood is also checked (the protein fibrinogen can be an important indicator of acute inflammation). It may also be important to evaluate the blood for a variety of other substances

that provide information about the status of the liver, kidney, muscles, or other organs. If a horse has a bleeding or blood-clotting problem, additional tests to evaluate the clotting system will be performed. When major blood loss during surgery is anticipated, or if a horse is severely **anemic** (has a very low red blood cell count), blood-typing tests may be necessary to identify a suitable blood donor. For some diseases it may be important to evaluate a urine sample prior to surgery. If abnormalities are detected on auscultation of the chest or in the various blood or urine tests, certain additional procedures such as chest X-rays or an **electrocardiogram (ECG)** (examination of the electrical activity of the heart) may need to be performed before anesthesia and surgery.

Most horses are held off feed for at least 12 hours prior to surgery, but are allowed access to water until immediately before the procedure. For some abdominal surgical procedures it is necessary to reduce feed intake for three to four days before surgery to decrease the volume of food in the large intestine. This may be to allow the surgeon better access to organs within the abdominal cavity, or to reduce the weight of the bowel lying over the abdominal incision after recovery from anesthesia. If a horse is being fed grass or rich alfalfa hay, it is often important to

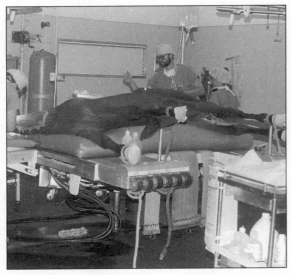

Photo by Mordecai Siegal.

restrict intake for 12 hours before surgery to prevent **bloat** (gas distension) of the large intestine. Bloat can make it difficult for the horse to breathe under anesthesia, and in extreme cases can lead to respiratory arrest and death.

PREPARATION FOR ANESTHESIA

After the preliminary examinations have been performed, the horse is assigned an anesthesia risk status based on the nature (elective or emergency) and type of surgical procedure to be performed and on the results of the various examinations. Decisions are made regarding:

- Drugs that will be used to induce and maintain anesthesia
- Type of intravenous fluids to be administered to support the circulation
- Other drugs that may be needed to support the patient during anesthesia and recovery from anesthesia
- Types of monitoring equipment needed during the procedure
- Special padding or positioning requirements

An intravenous **catheter** (flexible tubular instrument for insertion into a blood vessel) is usually inserted into one of the jugular veins in the neck. It is good practice to shave and prepare the skin over the vein, in a manner similar to that for the surgical site itself. The catheter provides continuous and ready access to the horse's circulation and is used for the administration of drugs and fluids, thus avoiding the need for multiple punctures of the vein.

The horse's mouth is washed to remove any feed material, so that when the **endotracheal tube** (flexible tube passed from the mouth into the **trachea** [windpipe] for the administration of anesthetic gas) is passed no foreign material will be carried into the lungs. A strong halter and tail rope are often used to control the horse from the standing to the **recumbent** (lying down) position during induction of anesthesia, in an effort to minimize physical injury to the horse and/or personnel.

Depending on the procedure and the likelihood of post-surgical pain, swelling, and infection, antibiotics and nonsteroidal anti-inflammatory medications may be given immediately before surgery. **Prophylactic** (preventive) antibiotic administration is commonly practiced in equine surgery, even for clean elective procedures, because it is difficult to get the horse and the operating-room environment completely clean, and because horses used for certain athletic activities seem to be at greater risk for chest infections after anesthesia and surgery.

Most horses, unless they are very sick, are given an intravenous sedative or tranquillizer to minimize apprehension during induction of anesthesia. These drugs can have a profound depressant effect on heart and lung function, and are usually given only in small quantities sufficient to make the horse more tractable. After sedation, a short-acting anesthetic agent is administered intravenously. Once the horse is recumbent a mouth gag is positioned and an endotracheal tube is passed through the mouth into the trachea. An anesthetic machine is connected to the endotracheal tube so that the anesthetic gas, typically halothane or isoflurane, can be delivered in oxygen to maintain anesthesia.

The horse is positioned most commonly on its side or back, depending on the surgical approach to be used. It is important that the horse be properly padded, in order to minimize muscle or nerve injury during the anesthetic period. In many clinics this is accomplished by the use of a foam pad or water bed. The water bed is particularly advantageous in that it distributes the horse's weight more evenly, and the use of warm water can help maintain the horse's body temperature during surgery.

Some surgical procedures are relatively short in duration and can be performed with intravenous anesthesia alone. Examples include castration, biopsy of suspicious lumps, repair of wounds, application or removal of casts, flushing of infected joints, and other procedures that can be accomplished in less than a half hour. Depending on the circumstances an endotracheal tube may be passed to provide access to the horse's airway and to administer supplemental oxygen. If necessary the period of recumbency can be lengthened by the administration of additional anesthetic drug or the use of gas anesthesia.

MONITORING ANESTHESIA

The anesthesiologist is a very important member of the surgical team. The surgeon relies on the anesthesiologist to prevent patient movement and to minimize pain perception. At the same time the horse cannot be too deeply anesthetized. In addition to monitoring the patient's physical signs, the anesthesiologist uses information from devices that monitor the heart rate and rhythm, respiratory rate, blood pressure, and, under certain circumstances, **blood gas** (oxygen and carbon dioxide) concentration, serum **electrolytes** (e.g., sodium, potassium), and anesthetic gas concentration. Blood pressure can be monitored by use of a cuff placed around the base of the tail (**indirect monitoring**) or by use of a monitor connected to a catheter placed in an artery (**direct monitoring**), either on the side of the face, under the jaw, or in a leg. This requires shaving and preparation of another site on the horse's body. Fluids are administered by the jugular catheter throughout the surgical procedure in order to replace any fluids lost during surgery and to help maintain the body's circulating blood volume.

SKIN PREPARATION

To minimize the likelihood of infection, careful preparation of the incision site and protection of the region from contamination are critical in preparing a horse for surgery. In addition to the obvious contaminants (dirt, feces), the hair and skin have a resident population of bacteria that must be substantially reduced in numbers to prevent infection of the tissues beneath the incision. This is accomplished by clipping the hair from a wide area around the incision site. For instance, when surgery is performed on a horse's knee, the hair is usually clipped from the coronet to the upper forearm. Often the immediate surgical area is then shaved to prevent short pieces of hair from contaminating the incision. After the hair has been clipped, the entire region is washed thoroughly with soap and water and rinsed clean. After shaving the surgical site and surrounding area are vigorously scrubbed with an antiseptic soap. This procedure is usually repeated at least twice. Then at least three washes with a surgical preparation solution, each followed by an alcohol rinse, are applied to the skin. After the final rinse the surgical preparation solution is again applied and allowed to remain in contact with the skin throughout the surgical procedure. The two most commonly used surgical preparation solutions are povidone-iodine (Betadine) and chlorhexidine (Hibiclens). To reduce the resident bacterial population of the skin, these solutions must be in contact with the surface of the skin for a period of at least five minutes.

Protection of the Surgical Site
After the skin has been prepared, the surgical field is protected from the rest of the horse's body by the use of sterile barriers (*drapes*). Often the initial barrier is a sterile plastic drape that is impregnated with povidone-iodine and has an adhesive that holds the drape against the skin. The surgical area is then isolated by the use of disposable paper drapes or cloth drapes. Towel clamps are used to anchor the drapes to the skin.

The surgical team will don gowns, masks, caps, and gloves to minimize contamination of the surgical site. Before gowning and gloving, the hands and forearms up to the elbows are prepared by washing, scrubbing, and rinsing with antiseptic solutions, in a manner similar to the preparation of the horse's skin at the surgical site.

Surgical Procedure
Surgery requires a principled approach combined with a thorough understanding of the regional anatomy, skill in tissue handling and operative technique, anticipation of potential complications and knowledge of how to deal with them, and an understanding of the complex interrelationships that occur in disease. Most surgical procedures require an incision through the skin, separation of tissue layers including muscle, correction of the underlying problem, and closure of the various tissue layers so that structures are realigned anatomically for cosmetic appearance and function.

Recovery from Anesthesia
Although distinct risks are associated with all stages of anesthesia and surgery, recovery from general anesthesia holds the greatest potential for complications. Unfortunately such complications are occasionally catastrophic, resulting ultimately in death of the horse. It is important for owners to understand the risks of anesthesia before consenting to a surgical procedure.

Why do such complications occur? Simply put, horses spend much of their life in a standing position. In fact, most horses spend less than an hour a day lying down. As a consequence, a horse's natural instinct when recovering from anesthesia is to stand as soon as possible. If one imagines a groggy, thousand-pound horse attempting to stand without the fine motor control required to coordinate such a maneuver and to maintain stance, it seems amazing that serious injuries do not occur more often. In the past two decades refinements in anesthetic management and surgical technique have substantially reduced the likelihood of serious complications' occurring during anesthetic induction and surgery; however, there have been relatively few major improvements in recovery of horses from anesthesia.

Most horses are recovered in a padded recovery stall, on a lawn, or occasionally in special devices such as recovery pools or slings. Horses should be observed during recovery so that they can be assisted, if necessary. Assisted or hand recoveries are practiced fairly routinely by some veterinarians, while others prefer to have the horse lie quietly in a dark or dimly lit stall until it can stand on its own. Arguments can be made in support of both methods of recovery. Some clinics use padded recovery stalls, some use large foam pillows, some protect the horse's head with a padded head stall, and others utilize a head and tail rope until the horse can stand unassisted.

Unfortunately some horses do not recover quietly, responding vigorously by fighting to stand while they are still incapable of doing so. Initially this is manifested by head-slapping, then leg-paddling or floundering. Some horses manage to stand early, only to fall when they attempt to move in their stuporous state. A steadying hand to prevent further movement until the horse is more aware of its surroundings and can stand without stumbling or falling can minimize injury, but is also of considerable risk to personnel. Common equine injuries that can occur during recovery include bruising or **lacerations** (tears in the skin) around the head or limbs, laceration of the tongue, sprains, and occasionally fractures. It is precisely because of such complictions that some long-bone fractures, especially in adult horses, may not be amenable to repair, and even if repair is possible the cost (which must be assumed by the owner) may preclude further treament.

Unfortunately there is no way to predict which horses, on the basis of temperament, will experience a good recovery and which will have problems. An innate desire to stand, the degree of pain experienced, responses to external stimuli, and the presence of casts or splints on limbs all contribute to the varied behaviors seen during recovery. Attempts to modify these behaviors can be achieved to a certain extent by the administration of sedatives and **analgesics** (pain-killing medications), or both, during the recovery period.

CARE AFTER SURGERY

Close monitoring of both the horse and the surgical site are important after recovery from anesthesia. The frequency of monitoring depends on the type of procedure performed and the general health status of the horse before surgery. Minimum monitoring can be performed twice daily, usually at feeding time or when treatments are administered. Minimum care should include general observation of the horse's demeanor, interest in eating and drinking, frequency and volume of urination and defecation, and monitoring of body temperature and, if possible, heart and respiratory rates.

Bandages or wound dressings should be changed on a regular basis and must be kept clean and dry. Medications should be given at the prescribed times, and every effort should be made to ensure that the entire dose is administered. This is especially critical for medications that are given orally or in the feed, i.e., it is important to see to it that the horse swallows all of the dose or that the feed in which the medication has been mixed is completely consumed. Some oral medications, like phenylbutazone

("bute") are very bitter, even when mixed with sweeteners like corn syrup or molasses, and will cause some horses to salivate, play with their mouths, quit eating, or pout. If this occurs, the veterinarian should be consulted about the best method of drug administration. Prevention of infection or control of an existing infection requires the appropriate administration of an antibiotic. In general, the specified amount of medication must be given at the specified times. Some drugs need to be given more than twice daily, and while this can be difficult to accomplish, adherence to the prescribed schedule is necessary if effective concentrations of these drugs are to be achieved in the blood and tissues.

Observation of eating behavior is important because stress associated with anesthesia and surgery can be further compounded by inappetence, leading to digestive upsets such as diarrhea. Certain types of stress-associated bacterial diarrhea can on occasion result in death. Care should be taken to avoid overfeeding horses that have had feed withheld before surgery. Overfeeding associated with decreased water consumption and internal fluid losses may lead to **impaction** (constipation) and colic.

It is usually best to continue feeding the same diet after surgery unless the veterinarian indicates otherwise. Most horses will eat normally after surgery, but some may be fussier than usual and not eat normally for several days. If a horse is not eating normally the attending veterinarian should be consulted.

After surgery, particular attention should be directed to a horse's feet for signs of soreness and **laminitis** (founder). This devastating complication can occur in association with surgical stress, digestive disturbances, toxemia, and inappropriate weight-bearing on one limb (*see* CHAPTER 22, "THE MUSCULOSKELETAL SYSTEM AND VARIOUS DISORDERS"). It is usually advisable to monitor the horse's feet for warmth, especially at the **coronary band** (ring of tissue, well supplied with blood vessels, along the upper edge of the hoof wall) and sensitivity to pressure around the coronary band, and to assess the character of the pulse in the digital arteries of the feet (**digital pulse**). The pulsation of the blood in these arteries can be detected at the back of the fetlock or pastern, and should be checked at least once a day. Unless instructed otherwise, it is advisable to walk the horse outside the stall when evaluating it for foot sensitivity or soreness. Increased hoof warmth, coronary band sensitivity, increased digital pulses, and soreness are all cause for immediate concern and veterinary attention.

Common Surgical Procedures

CASTRATION

Castration to remove objectionable male characteristics can be performed safely at any age but is most commonly done when a horse is one or two years old, when such behavior often becomes a management problem. Occasionally castration is indicated if the testicles are injured by trauma or during hernia repair, or when testicular abnormalities such as cancer (rare in horses) are present.

Castration can be performed as a standing procedure or with the horse under general anesthesia. Both methods are acceptable; the more tractable the horse, the more likely the veterinarian is to perform the procedure with the horse standing and sedated, using local anesthesia. Castration incisions usually are not **sutured** (stitched), to allow for adequate drainage after surgery.

Care of the horse after castration includes daily observation and exercise. The most common post-surgical complication is excessive swelling of the **scrotum** (dependent pouch of skin containing the testicles) resulting from inadequate drainage. This is best prevented and managed by vigorously exercising the horse twice a day for seven to ten days after castration. The day after surgery the horse is walked for five to ten minutes in the morning, and trotted on a line or in a pen for five to ten minutes in the afternoon. Twice-daily trotting is repeated for at least seven to ten days. If swelling increases or persists it is likely that the edges of the incision need to be reopened to allow drainage. This must be done cleanly to avoid introducing infection at the site. Occasionally cold-water hosing of the scrotum can help to reduce swelling. Phenylbutazone and antibiotics may be administered, depending on the preferences of the veterinarian. Tetanus toxoid administration is highly recommended, as horses are exquisitely sensitive to tetanus (*see* CHAPTER 31, "BACTERIAL DISEASES.").

Castration becomes a more complicated procedure as a horse gets older. In mature (more than 4 years old) horses or aged stallions, it may be necessary to separate out the **cremaster muscle,** which suspends the testicle, and crush and cut it separate from the **spermatic cord**, which contains the blood vessels that supply the testicle. The concept of "cutting a horse proud" is a myth that has been perpetuated for at least a century. With this technique, the **epididymis** (duct used for the storage, maturation, and movement of sperm) was separated from the testicle and left in the horse, in the hope that the stallionlike **phenotype** (visible, physical expression of a genetic trait) would be retained but the unwanted behavioral characteristics would be removed. *There is no scientific evidence to support this idea.* The epididymis acts as a reservoir for conditioning and storage of sperm and is not capable of producing the male hormone *testosterone*, which is responsible for stallion behavior (*see* CHAPTER 9, "REPRODUCTIVE PHYSIOLOGY"). Prepubescent (before one year) castration may result in reduced neck development, but otherwise has little effect on growth.

CRYPTORCHID CASTRATION

Normally colts are born with both testicles descended into the scrotum. In some, however, either one or both testicles does not descend completely, remaining either in the abdomen or in the **inguinal canal** (the passage between the abdomen and scrotum). Generally, if the testicles are not present by 12 months of age they will not descend into the scrotum. Castration of such a **cryptorchid** horse can be more complicated, especially if it is not possible to feel any part of the testicle in the inguinal canal or scrotum. General anesthesia is recommended for this procedure. Because of the potential for complications and the possibility that the abdomen may have to be entered, it is best that this type of surgery be performed in a clinic equipped with a surgical theater.

One serious and often fatal complication is **evisceration** (**herniation** or passage of intestines through the inguinal ring). The interior of the scrotum is in direct contact with the abdominal cavity. Because scrotal incisions are not routinely closed at the time of surgery, there is always some risk of herniation. Depending on the surgical technique used, this risk is usually considered to be less than 4%; with the technique of semiclosed castration commonly practiced in North America, the risk is considered to be less than 1%. Self-inflicted trauma to the herniated bowel and **peritonitis** (inflammation of the abdominal lining) are the most common causes of fatal complications.

ABDOMINAL SURGERY

The most common reason for abdominal surgery in horses is identification and correction of the cause of a colic that has not responded to medical treatment (*see* CHAPTER 26, "DIGESTIVE SYSTEM AND VARIOUS DISORDERS"). Once the diagnosis and the decision to operate have been made, the horse is prepared for general anesthesia. Exposure of the abdominal organs usually is accomplished through a midline incision in the bottom of the abdomen. Because many of the organs and some parts of the intestinal tract cannot be brought out through the incision, careful **palpation** (feeling with the hands) of the abdomen is necessary. Owing to the physical limitations on exposure of the entire intestinal tract, some colic problems cannot be surgically corrected.

The most common cause of colic requiring surgical correction involves an obstruction of the bowel. Internal obstructions of the bowel can be caused by intestinal stones (**enteroliths**), hardened manure (**fecoliths**), or foreign bodies swallowed by the horse (e.g., baling wire, sponges). There may also be external obstructions, as when another loop of intestine wraps around a segment of bowel, pinching off its interior and preventing the passage of food material. **Lipomas** (benign tumors of fat cells), more common in older horses, originate in the **mesentery** (the sheetlike membrane that suspends the intestine from the roof of the abdomen) and

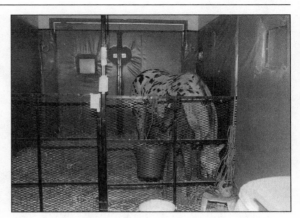

Photo by Mordecai Siegal.

often have a long stalk, which may wrap around a segment of bowel, blocking passage of its contents and cutting off its blood supply.

A variety of displacements, twists, and malpositions of the small and large intestines can occur, for reasons that remain poorly understood. Such changes in position often result in compromise of the blood supply to the intestine and partial to complete obstruction. Reduced blood flow to the intestine results in swelling, discoloration, and eventual death of that segment of bowel. Such devitalized segments of intestine need to be cut out during surgery, and the healthy ends of the intestinal tract joined back together. Sutures or staples can be used to accomplish this. For many problems, the surgeon will also evacuate as much of the feed material from the **large colon** (a part of the large intestine) as possible, so that there will be less weight on the abdominal incision and the horse will feel more comfortable after surgery.

After recovery from anesthesia, nursing care becomes critical to the survival of horses that have had major abdominal surgery. Such horses usually will remain in intensive care for two to seven days after surgery. Regular observation and monitoring and administration of intravenous fluids and medications are important for support of the horse during recovery. One complication associated with intestinal disease and surgery is **ileus**—a condition in which the bowel does not resume its normal **motility** (ability to move) after correction of an underlying problem.

Ileus results in a functional obstruction of the intestine, with **reflux** (backward flow) of fluid and intestinal contents back into the stomach, causing continued discomfort. Although medications are available to stimulate intestinal motility, they are not always effective and intensive care will be necessary for support until normal function resumes. Feed intake is also regulated during recovery; most horses are not back on full feed for four to seven days after surgery.

Other complications that can occur include peritonitis, formation of **adhesions** (pieces of bowel sticking together, causing another obstruction), diarrhea, founder, and an **incisional hernia** (a defect in the healing abdominal incision that results in a bulge in the belly wall). Each of these complications will result in increased risk for the horse and increased costs to resolve. Alone or in combination, they can be serious enough to result in death or necessitate euthanasia because the cost of treatment becomes prohibitive.

Horses that recover completely from colic

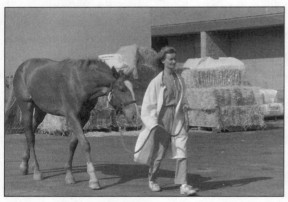

Photo by Mordecai Siegal.

surgery can usually be ridden again two to three months later and can return to their previous use. The survival rate following colic surgery has improved tremendously in the last two decades. For many intestinal diseases, survival rates of 80–95% are common, whereas for some conditions survival is still around 40%. Interestingly, the survival rate after surgery for related intestinal conditions is similar in both horses and humans.

ORTHOPEDIC SURGERY

Removal of bone chips from joints and repair of fractures are quite common procedures in athletic horses. Chip fractures are removed by **arthroscopic** techniques, wherein a small flexible tube for viewing is passed into the joint and instruments to remove the bone fragments and clean up the joint surface are inserted through a second small hole. This approach allows for improved observation and treatment of the joint without the need for a large incision. When bone chips occur there is often some degree of damage to the joint surface; the length of convalescence will be determined by the time it takes for the damaged surface to be restored. A typical layup time after surgery would include 30–60 days of stall rest with hand walking, 60–90 days of turnout in a small paddock, and another 60–90 days of turnout in a large paddock, before a return to training. There are several medications that may be recommended to aid healing and restoration of joint function during convalescence. The prognosis for return to athletic use is variable, depending on the type of injury and the severity of any associated degenerative joint disease. (*See* CHAPTER 22, "THE MUSCULOSKELETAL SYSTEM AND VARIOUS DISORDERS.")

CHAPTER 38

Convalescence and Home Care

**by Thomas B. Yarbrough and
John R. Pascoe**

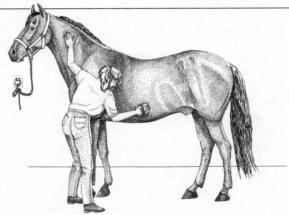

Home health care is an important part of equine practice. By carefully following the veterinarian's recommendations, the horse owner can provide quality nursing care and often substantially decrease the cost of medical care. For the process to work effectively, the veterinarian must describe for the owner the observations to be made, the treatments to be performed, and the potential complications that may arise. As an owner one needs to understand fully what needs to be done and be confident that one can comply with the veterinarian's instructions. One must also have the time to provide the necessary care and the insight to know when professional assistance is indicated. No one knows a horse better than its owner; careful observation of the animal during recovery from illness, injury, or surgery can facilitate the veterinarian's recommendations so that the horse can return to normal function as quickly as possible.

Many horses, especially those used to daily attention, will maintain a better attitude and recover more rapidly when they receive care from their owners in their usual environment. Some illnesses and injuries are sufficiently seri-

ous that hospitalization is required; in other instances the frequency of observation or administration of medication may be such that it is more practical for a horse to be lodged at an equine clinic or hospital where intensive care can be provided. When this level of care is no longer needed, and if one has the time, then appropriate nursing care can probably be provided at home.

Caring for a horse at home can be both a frustrating and a fulfilling experience. It is important to remember that careful observation and compliance with the veterinarian's instructions are both critical to a successful outcome. The economic advantages of home care will only be realized if the owner is willing to comply with instructions and work in partnership with the veterinarian as a caregiver.

Observation and Monitoring

Careful observation of a horse's behavior is a critical element in assessing the response to treatment. Evaluation of attitude, response to one's presence and other stimuli, and interest in eating are important behavioral indicators that can provide information about a horse's well-being. The rectal temperature, heart rate, and respiratory rate during recovery from illness are also useful measures of a horse's progress. Observation of the frequency, volume, and character of the urine and manure will provide additional insight into a horse's condition. Examination of the **mucous membranes** lining the mouth, eyelids, and vulva for color and moistness can provide an additional measure of health and hydration.

MUCOUS MEMBRANES

Normal mucous membranes should be pale pink to pink in color and slightly moist to the touch. If a finger is pressed against the surface of the **oral** (in the mouth) mucous membranes for 10–15 seconds, the color will blanch as the blood in the small vessels is squeezed away. As the finger is removed the color should return in less than two seconds if blood flow is normal. A return of normal color requiring more than two seconds is usually an indication of poor circulation and should be investigated further.

Hydration can be assessed by the degree of moistness of the mucous membranes and by the elasticity of the skin on the side of the neck. A small fold of skin can be "tented" up and in a well-hydrated horse will snap back into position immediately. With increasing dehydration, mucous membranes become dry and tacky and skin elasticity (**turgor**) diminishes such that the fold of skin will take progressively longer to return to its normal position. Abnormalities in these relatively simple tests usually indicate a loss of body fluids and in all likelihood the need for replacement fluids, which, depending on the circumstances, may be given by stomach tube or intravenously. Mucous membranes that are grossly red to purple-red in color usually indicate **toxemia** (toxins in the blood). Very pale mucous membranes may indicate blood loss, while yellowish membranes indicate that the horse either has not been eating or has liver disease. Identification of any of these variations in normal mucous membrane color warrants immediate veterinary examination.

RECTAL TEMPERATURE

A conventional thermometer or one with a digital read-out can be used. Standing in a safe position alongside the horse's left hind leg, the base of the tail is elevated and the thermometer is gently inserted through the **anal sphincter** (band or ring of muscle that controls the release of feces) into the rectum. The measurement should be made over a period of at least one minute. (It is a good idea to have a clip attached to the thermometer by means of a piece of string; the clip can be anchored to the tail hair while the temperature is being taken, in order to prevent loss of the thermometer within the rectum). Because body temperature changes in response to ambient temperature, it is good practice to take the temperature at the same time each day. Mornings are preferable, as there is less **diurnal** (having a daily cycle) variation in the early-morning body temperature. This is especially true in foals.

Normal rectal temperatures should be between about 37.5 and 38.6°C (99.5 and 100.5°F). Morning rectal temperatures higher than 102°F indicate that something is awry and should be investigated. Foals will have a slightly higher resting rectal temperature, and if they become excited during restraint may have temperatures between 38 and 38.6°C (100.5 and 101.5°F). Temperatures greater than 102.5–103°F should be investigated further.

RESPIRATORY (BREATHING) RATE

The respiratory rate can be measured by careful observation of flank, chest wall, or nostril movement. This is best done with a quiet approach, refraining from any disturbance of the horse or foal in its current activity. Awareness and interest in people often results in an irregular breathing pattern in the horse and will make the respiratory rate more difficult to assess. As with body temperature, it is important that measurements be made at the same time each day. If once-daily measurements are being taken they should be made early in the morning, because the respiratory rate increases as the ambient temperature rises. Normal respiratory rates are 8–12 breaths per minute for adult horses and 12–16 breaths per minute for foals.

HEART RATE

Less easily accomplished is an evaluation of the heart rate and character, which requires the use of a stethoscope positioned over the lower part of the chest wall just behind the horse's elbow. Normal equine heart sounds have two distinctly audible components, and it is important not to count both sounds when taking the heart rate. The heart rate should normally be measured over a period of a minute. Normal rates for resting adult horses are 28–40 beats per minute. Rates for foals are slightly higher at 36–60 beats per minute. As with the respiratory rate the foal's heart rate will vary considerably, depending on the degree of excitement and restraint during measurement.

It is good practice to listen to the character of both heart sounds, often for several minutes before counting. One should notice a decrease in the heart rate as the horse becomes accustomed to one's presence and realizes that it is not being threatened by use of the stethoscope.

Administration of Medication

Medications can be administered by mouth (**orally**), by injection (**intramuscular and intravenous routes** are the most common in horses), by topical or surface application, by stomach tube, and less commonly as an enema.

Medications should be used only as prescribed by a veterinarian or according to the manufacturer's instructions. Like other perishable items, drugs have a shelf life and should be safely disposed of when no longer needed. They should not be used if discolored or if the expiration date printed on the container has passed. Care should be taken to store medications as indicated by the manufacturer. Generally, drugs packaged in amber bottles should be considered light-sensitive; direct contact with light should be limited, especially if the drug is drawn into a syringe in advance. Most medications should not be exposed to extremes of temperature, particularly heat. Some drugs require refrigeration for normal storage or after the seal is broken. It is important to remember that some drugs may be poisonous to children or pets and should be kept in a secure location when not being used.

Before giving any medication it is critical that the route of administration be determined. Some drugs can be given only by the intramuscular route (e.g., procaine penicillin, most vaccines), while others, such as the injectable form of phenylbutazone ("**bute**"), are extremely irritating to the muscles and should only be given intravenously. The recommended routes of administration, as listed on the manufacturer's label or on the veterinarian's prescription label, should be checked before giving any medication. If one is at all uncertain, the veterinarian should be consulted.

Proper hygiene is essential when giving any injectable medication. Bacteria can grow in antibiotic preparations if they become contaminated. Contamination of the container by dirty needles, passing needles through a dirty top, or failing to disinfect adequately the top of the container can result in a serious infection in the horse. Likewise, inappropriate cleansing of the injection site can result in contamination of the underlying tissues, sometimes with devastating results.

INJECTIONS

Intramuscular Injections
Four regions of the body are recommended sites for the intramuscular injection of medications:

- The large muscles on the side of the neck
- The *gluteal* muscles over the rump
- The *pectoral* muscles at the front of the chest
- The *semimembranosus* and *semitendinosus* muscles at the back of the thigh

Intramuscular injections in the neck have the highest incidence of complications and are the most likely to involve vital structures. It is prudent to limit neck injections to volumes of 10 cc (or ml) or less, to avoid undue soreness at the site. The safest method for neck injection is to place the hand flat against the muscles of the neck, with the thumb lying over the bones of the neck and the smallest finger against the front of the horse's shoulder blade. The triangle formed between the outstretched thumb and forefinger outlines a safe region for deep injection. Injections in the chest generally result in more noticeable swelling; if a complication such as abscess should occur in this region, however, it can be easily drained. The muscles of the rump and thigh are the largest and therefore most appropriate for repeated intramuscular injections or injections of large volumes of medication.

Needle selection is important. The diameter (or *gauge*) of the needle should be large enough to allow ready flow of the medication through the needle, but small enough so that it causes the least discomfort to the horse. Clean, sterile needles should always be used; needles should *never* be reused. Care should be taken that the horse is adequately restrained to avoid injury to both horse and handlers. The handlers should be positioned so that they can avoid being hurt if the horse objects to the injection.

Perhaps the most common mistake when giving an intramuscular injection is advancing the needle too slowly into the muscle; such an approach usually causes more discomfort than a quick thrust into the muscle. If the needle is held between the thumb and forefinger and the injection site is tapped sharply two times with the heel of the palm before the needle is inserted on the third hit, the horse usually will not exhibit any obvious signs of discomfort or apprehension.

Before giving an injection, it is important to **aspirate** (draw back on the syringe) to make sure that the needle is not in a blood vessel. If no blood enters the syringe, one can proceed with the injection. If volumes larger than 15 cc are being injected, the needle should be redirected within the muscle once or twice during the injection, without pulling the needle back out through the skin. For repeated injections, sites should be alternated to minimize soreness.

Intravenous Injections
Intravenous injections should only be used when specified for a particular medication and should preferably be performed only by a veterinarian. Extreme care must be taken to prevent accidental injection into the **carotid artery** (which runs parallel to the jugular vein), which could result in death of the animal. Accidental injection of some drugs outside a vein can cause a severe tissue reaction, with tissue death and sloughing, leaving an ugly wound.

In the upper half of the neck a muscle separates the jugular vein from the carotid artery, making this a safer site for an intravenous injection. After appropriate skin preparation, the jugular vein is **occluded** (held off with the thumb or fingers) below the injection site, in order to distend the vein and facilitate needle insertion. The needle is then advanced into the interior of the vein and the syringe is attached. Correct positioning is indicated by the aspiration of blood into the syringe. If there is a pulsatile flow of blood after needle insertion and this persists after the vessel is released (no longer held off) and before the syringe is attached, it usually indicates that the needle is in an artery and thus an unsafe site for injection.

Nothing should be injected until one is certain the needle is in the vein. Intra-arterial injection can result in a response varying from excitation and an increased respiratory rate to violent seizuring and death. In the event of an intra-arterial injection, every effort should be made to protect the horse from further injury. No attempt should be made to hold down a horse suffering from a violent seizure; generally this can only result in injury to those attending the animal. Once the injection reaction has subsided, veterinary assistance should be sought and the horse evaluated for any injuries that might result in permanent abnormalities.

ORAL MEDICATION
Administration of medication by mouth can be accomplished fairly easily if the horse is adequately restrained and the procedure is performed in a nonthreatening manner. Balling guns traditionally employed to deliver medications into the back of the mouth and force swallowing are not commonly used in horses. If recommended for the administration of a medication, their correct use should be carefully reviewed with the attending veterinarian. It is relatively easy to harm the horse's mouth with a balling gun if wielded improperly.

Medications in paste form can be inserted into the horse's mouth relatively easily, usually at the corner (**commissure**) of the lips. Medications can be made into paste form by mixing them with a small amount of corn syrup. The more liquid the preparation, the more likely it will run back out of the mouth. Administration of a more liquid medication (as delivered through a syringe) can be accomplished by gently inserting the tip of the syringe at the corner of the lips, and angling it back into the mouth. It is important to accomplish insertion and administration in the same motion, or the horse will start playing with the syringe and attempt to chew it. An alternate technique is to place the nondominant hand on the side of the horse's face, with the fingers on the bridge of the nose and the thumb in the corner of the mouth. This will prompt the horse to open its mouth. The medication can then be squirted between the cheek and tongue.

Most horses will spontaneously chew after the oral administration of a medication; sometimes it is advisable to hold the horse's chin in an elevated position until swallowing is completed. As with injections, care should be taken to stand in a relatively safe position when giving an oral dose of medication. Usually the best position is close to the horse and slightly in front of the shoulder.

EYE MEDICATION

Eye (**ophthalmic**) medications can be challenging to administer to horses because frequent application, often at 2- or 4-hour intervals, may be required. Also, the powerful musculature of the horse's eyelids and controlling the horse's head make this task difficult. Moreover, if the eye condition is painful, the horse will soon come to resent treatment, making the application of medication even more of a challenge. Often two people are required to administer the medication safely and effectively; in some cases it may be necessary to apply a twitch to the nose to maintain adequate control of the horse's head while parting the eyelids.

The techniques for applying ointments and solutions to the surface of the eye are very similar. The thumb and index finger are used to force the lids open. When using solutions, the lower lid should be pulled down to provide a large trough into which the liquid can be dripped. Ointments will adhere to the surface of the eye; thus the lids need merely to be separated and the ointment applied directly to the surface of the eyeball, taking care not to touch the surface of the eye with the container.

Bandaging

A variety of bandage types have been designed to treat wounds, reduce swelling, and provide support for the limb. Bandages are usually formed in layers, with each layer having a different function. Selection of material for the initial layer will depend on the nature of the surface to be covered.

The primary layer of the bandage is in direct contact with the body. The material selected for this layer should be nonadherent if it is desirable not to disturb the surface layer of the wound, adherent if removal of tissue at each bandage change is desirable. It should be absorbent if it is desirable that fluid oozing from the wound surface be removed, impermeable if it is necessary for an applied medication to remain in direct contact with the skin surface and not soak into the upper layers of the bandage. The upper layers of the bandage serve to anchor the primary layer to the body and to provide support and protection to the area.

Commercially available cotton or paper-gauze sponges (often called "3×3's" or "4×4's", depending on their size, i.e., 3 inches square or 4 inches square) are the most commonly used materials for the primary bandage layer. Whether the sponges are placed on the wound surface wet or dry will be determined by the character of the wound discharge. In a wound with a very thick discharge, wetting the sponges before application will thin the discharge and remove debris when the dried gauze is removed. Wounds with a thinner discharge are better managed with dry gauze sponges. The primary layer for clean wounds or surgical incisions should be composed of a nonadherent material, e.g., a teflon-coated surface or petroleum-jelly–impregnated gauze. Commonly available products include Telfa pads, Melolite, Release, and Adaptic.

When trying to reduce swelling (**edema**) from a limb, the primary bandage layer should be composed of an impermeable material such as Saran Wrap, which is placed over the limb after the application of an emollient mixture. Most of the commonly used mixtures (referred to as "sweats") include furacin and Epsom salts; other combinations incorporate dimethyl sulfoxide (DMSO), menthol products, camphor, and glycerin. Before mixing any of these substances a veterinarian should be contacted, because some of these ingredients have **carcinogenic** (cancer-causing) properties and must be handled very carefully. Sweats should not be left in contact with the skin for prolonged periods, as many of them will eventually blister the skin.

The secondary layer of a bandage provides some pressure support and absorptive capabilities. This layer of the bandage protects a limb, for example, from undue pressure on the flexor tendons, which can result in "bandage bows" if inappropriate pressure is applied to the limb. The thickness of the layer will be based on the requirements of the bandage. Bandages designed to absorb wound discharge, place a large amount of pressure on a limb, or support a splint should be thick to allow a distribution of pressure and a large absorptive area. When a great deal of support is supplied a Robert-Jones bandage can be fashioned by alternating layers of roll cotton with brown gauze. Roll cotton, sheet cotton, and baby diapers are the most frequently used materials for the secondary layer. As a rule, 1–1½ inches of loose pressed cotton correctly applied will provide enough protection against bandage bows.

The third layer is the bandage cover, and is the layer that secures any external splints to the limb. In bandages designed to produce very little pressure or support, a layer of brown gauze held in place by white adhesive tape will suffice. Because of its relative lack of elasticity, white tape should never completely encircle the limb unless it is applied in a "barber-pole" configuration. The use of elastic tapes such as Vet Wrap or Elastikon will increase the pressure produced by the bandage and the effective duration of the bandage as well. In bandages requiring a waterproof seal, a layer of duct tape can be used.

A basic lower-limb bandage is applied as follows. The primary layer (if covering a wound or healing surgical site) is secured to the limb with a layer of soft roll gauze, applied in overlapping fashion and being careful to avoid wrinkles in the gauze. The secondary layer is rolled over the limb from outside to inside as the bandage moves from the front to the back of the leg, and secured and tightened with a roll of brown gauze. Care should be taken that the pressure is distributed evenly over the limb when tightening the brown gauze. The bandage is completed with one of the adhesive tapes described above, based on the requirements in each particular case. If a second bandage is stacked atop this lower-limb bandage it can be used to cover structures on the upper limb. If this "stack wrap" is to be left on the limb for any length of time the pressure points will need to be protected. This can be done by cutting the tape and brown gauze as they pass over the accessory **carpal bone** (on the forelimb) or the point of the **hock** (on the hindlimb).

Bandages should be reset daily to maintain even pressure on the limb. Bandages will settle or compress with time and generally start to slip (especially stack bandages) after about 48 hours. In some circumstances the veterinarian may recommend leaving the limb bandaged for several days before changing the wrap. Usually this is necessary in order to maintain pressure over a specific region. After removal of a bandage and attention to any wound care, the limb should be massaged to facilitate circulation. If possible, washing and drying the limb will keep the skin healthy and serve to massage the tissue.

Cast Care

Occasionally wounds, surgical incisions, or fractures are better protected by a cast rather than a bandage. Commonly used casts in horses include **heel casts** (enclose the foot), **short limb casts** (the top of the cast finishes just below the knee or hock), and long limb or **full-length casts** (these finish as high up on the leg as possible toward the elbow or stifle). Management of casts at home requires diligent attention to the cast in order to prevent the development of cast sores. Pressure sores resulting from inappropriately applied casts or casts that are wearing unevenly can cause very serious problems. Pressure sores most commonly form over bony prominences, e.g., the sesamoids, accessory carpal bone, styloid process of the radius, and point of the hock. Another problem area for cast sores are the bulbs of the heels; pressure or rub sores at this location can cause considerable pain.

Regardless of the region confined in a cast, keeping the horse confined to a stall will decrease the likelihood of complications and increase the effectiveness of the cast. Casts should be evaluated several times a day to detect changes that may be occurring. It is important to remember that many of the initial changes will be subtle in nature and their recognition will be masked by the thickness of the cast material. A developing pressure sore can be detected as a localized area of increased heat on the cast surface. Surgical sites also may be associated with increased warmth of the cast surface. Other important signs that a cast may be causing a problem include changes in the use of the limb, developing lameness, swelling of the limb above the cast, decreased tolerance of the cast (e.g., chewing at the cast or pawing with the cast limb), flies collecting on the cast, and discharge from the cast. Localized discoloration of the cast surface not associated with external contamination usually means the development of a discharge beneath the cast. If flies also are consistently attracted to this spot, one can be reasonably sure that there is a problem beneath that area of the cast.

If a fiberglass cast has been placed over a draining wound to speed healing, it can be hosed off or soaked in Epsom salts to increase the interval between cast changes. In general, however, casts should be kept dry and the bottom surface evaluated for wear. Any concerns or changes in the horse's use of the limb should be immediately brought to the attention of the veterinarian.

Care of the Horse with Colic

Home management of a horse with colic is a task requiring careful observation and a cautious use of medication. Although some experienced horse owners may feel comfortable providing initial therapy, it is generally better to have a horse evaluated by a veterinarian. The following guidelines should be useful for the initial care of a colicky horse.

Careful assessment requires a stethoscope and thermometer. A thorough initial physical examination should include a rectal temperature, pulse, gut sounds (inconsistent rumbling in all areas of the abdomen is normal), and mucous membrane color. (For information on normal values, see CHAPTER 37, "SURGERY AND POSTOPERATIVE CARE.") Horses with an exceptionally high heart rate (more than 70 beats per minute), nonexistent gut sounds, extreme pain (often recumbent with violent, uncontrollable pain), full body sweat, extreme bloat, and dark-red to purple mucous membranes require immediate veterinary care. Horses exhibiting only mild signs of pain, such as pawing, repeated looking at the flank, or occasional lying down without any of the other signs of severe colic just described, can be treated cautiously with *analgesic* (pain-killing) medication. The two safest medications to keep on hand in a first-aid kit would be phenylbutazone and dipyrone. Other medications such as Banamine, Ketoprofen, Xylazine, and Detomidine should be used with extreme caution, owing to their ability to mask signs of pain until the horse is in severe trouble.

Horses with signs of abdominal pain should be held off feed until the signs of pain have resolved and normal manure has been passed. If the horse can be distracted from its pain by walking, this should be done in order to decrease the need for analgesics. When signs of pain are mild the horse is better left alone but should be observed frequently. If the signs of pain are violent in nature, consideration should be given to the safety of the horse and its handlers until a veterinarian can be called to administer appropriate care.

Although most colics are relatively simple gastrointestinal disturbances requiring either no treatment or simply a mild analgesic, some can only be managed surgically. Time lost with home remedies, home treatment, or reluctance to call a veterinarian may result in such deterioriation of a horse's condition that even with surgical treatment the horse may die. Early veterinary care can make all the difference in the outcome of a serious colic.

Care Following Colic Surgery

Convalescent care for horses following colic surgery largely depends on the underlying cause of the colic. The primary goals of home care are a gradual return to full feed, protection and care of the incision, and monitoring for the development of complications.

Return to full feed must be gradual because of the colic- and surgery-induced alterations in gut motility. The most common change is delayed passage of food through the digestive tract; because of this, a rapid return to full feed or a major change in diet will likely cause further problems. Feed should first be offered in small amounts at frequent intervals. If no further problems arise, the amount of feed can be gradually increased and the frequency of feeding decreased until the normal feeding pattern is reestablished. Normally, by the time a horse is discharged from the surgical clinic it will be receiving at least half its normal daily ration divided among three or four feedings.

Incision care is particularly important because of the position of the incision and the nature of the patient. Because the incision is at the lowest point of the abdomen it is more susceptible to swelling and also to contamination, especially if the horse is still uncomfortable and repeatedly getting up and down. The incision should be checked daily for signs of infection. Some swelling along the incision line is normally observed; however it should be cool and not painful to the touch. A firm, painful swelling with or without drainage could indicate either an infection or a reaction to the suture material. If sites of drainage have already opened and the horse is otherwise healthy, the draining sites can be cleaned and gently flushed, on at least a daily basis, with either dilute Betadine or a dilute Nolvasan solution. If the horse begins to exhibit signs of illness (depression, partial or complete inappetence, elevated heart rate, fever) associated with incisional drainage, the veterinarian should be called immediately.

Horses should be restricted to a stall, with daily hand walking, for the first 30 days after colic surgery. Opportunities for exercise can then be increased by keeping the horse in a small paddock or pen for 30 days, then in a pasture for 30 days before riding again. These precautions are designed to increase physical stress on the incision site slowly during healing, and to decrease the likelihood of hernia formation. Hernias usually occur within the first 90 days after surgery. If progressive swelling or a hernia is noted it should be examined by a veterinarian before the horse is exercised. Not all incisional hernias need to be repaired. If repair is recommended, it is better to wait five or six months for the scar tissue at the edges of the hernia to strengthen, so that when the hernia is repaired the tissue will be strong enough to hold the suture material. An additional three months of rest will be required after hernia repair before the horse can be ridden again.

Daily physical examinations after colic surgery include observation of sites that may have particular problems. Because most horses require intravenous fluids and antibiotics after surgery, catheters are normally placed into the jugular vein to avoid repeated needle puncture of the vein. In some cases, owing to the toxicity of the colic and other factors, a firm clot (**thrombosis**) may develop in the vein. For this reason the vein should be checked daily. Pain, swelling, and heat at the catheter insertion site could indicate infection and should be brought to the veterinarian's attention. Application of hot packs to bring the infection to the surface is usually the initial approach to therapy. If the horse becomes depressed or loses interest in eating the veterinarian should be called.

Laminitis (founder) may occur after colic surgery, either because of the toxins produced in the affected bowel during the colic episode, or because of the stresses associated with the colic and surgery. The pulse in the digital vessels of the feet should be evaluated daily. Increased digital pulses, abnormal warmth at the **coronary band** (band or ring of tissue along the upper edge of the hoof wall), pain on palpation of the coronary band, reluctance to walk freely, and evidence of pain when one front foot is picked up, forcing the full weight on the opposite foot, are early signs that a horse is probably foundering. Recognition of any of these changes warrants immediate veterinary attention.

Treatment of colic-associated laminitis often includes administration of phenylbutazone to reduce the amount of inflammation and to provide relief from pain. Medications such as acepromazine and isoxuprine can help increase blood flow to the foot. Additional medications may be recommended by the veterinarian, depending on the circumstance. Protection of the foot by physical means—e.g., keeping the horse on sand or loose dirt, use of foot bandages and frog pads—is aimed at distributing the pressure of the animal's weight over the entire sole, in order to reduce the likelihood of rotation of the coffin bone. Severe laminitis can be a devastating complication; early veterinary care is critical if permanent lameness is to be prevented. (*See* CHAPTER 22, "THE MUSCULOSKELETAL SYSTEM AND VARIOUS DISORDERS.")

Care After Orthopedic Injuries

Nursing care of horses that have suffered orthopedic injuries is designed to rest and protect the affected region during healing, provide passive motion to reduce stiffness and improve joint movement, slowly increase activity in the limb to stimulate strong healing, and return the horse to a degree of fitness that hopefully will prevent reinjury. Effective rehabilitation of an injured horse thus requires an active dialog between owner and veterinarian.

After acute injuries it is important to reduce swelling in the limb by the use of pressure bandages (to reduce the potential space in the tissues for fluid buildup to occur) and by the application of ice or cold water (to produce constriction of the small blood vessels responsible for fluid formation). The technique used for icing is not as important as its temperature and duration. A bucket or boot filled with an ice-water slurry should be applied to the limb for 10–15 minutes a day for the first three days after injury.

After the first three or four days the swelling is generally at its peak, so efforts should then be directed to techniques that will increase blood flow and so remove swelling. This can be accomplished by the use of warm-water hydrotherapy, sweat bandages, and pressure wraps. Restricted exercise is usually indicated in order to protect the limb from further injury. This often involves various degrees of stall confinement, wrapping, splinting, or casting, depending on the nature of the injury.

Scarring is a part of nature's way of strengthening injured tissue. Scar tissue may be very effective at stabilizing a weakened joint; however, it often leaves the joint stiff and less functional. Various techniques have been employed to decrease the stiffness associated with confinement after orthopedic injury or surgery. Passive motion has been shown to protect the range of motion in a joint, aid in the healing of cartilage defects, speed the removal of blood and bacteria from the joint, and reduce pain. Currently the only method of providing passive motion is repeated daily flexion and extension of the affected joint. Precise guidelines for passive-motion therapy in horses have not been developed; however, many orthopedic surgeons recommend at least twice-daily sessions of flexion and extension for periods of 15–20 minutes. The joint should be flexed to the point where any further flexion would cause pain.

Other methods of reducing scarring include the use of therapeutic ultrasound (to stimulate tissue remodeling) and DMSO (to limit scar-tissue formation). With time, scar tissue will remodel. During this remodeling phase, some controlled stresses should be applied at the injured site to increase the strength of the healing tissue. Various techniques have been developed to load the healing limb, including swimming, pony work, and gradual controlled exercise. Swimming is an effective method of strengthening muscle tone, increasing the range of motion in the joints, and loading an injured area without putting undue weight on the affected limb.

Veterinary instructions often involve a return to hand walking after prolonged stall confinement. This can be quite a challenge in horses with lots of energy. Oral acepromazine granules, which can be obtained from the veterinarian, may be useful during the first few days out of the stall to decrease some of this hyperactivity.

Wound Care

Wounds that cannot be closed with sutures and that do not involve vital structures (joints, tendon, nerves, or a body cavity) may be candidates for home care. If there is any suspicion that a wound involves any of these vital structures, the assistance of a veterinarian should be sought.

Decisions often have to be made before a veterinarian arrives at the site of an emergency. For example, a horse may be bleeding profusely from a wound, and action must be taken immediately. Direct pressure is the best means of reducing blood loss. If the wound is down on a leg, a pressure bandage should be applied to shut off the leaking vessels. If one of the large vessels of the upper limb or the neck is involved, firm pressure with the fingertips to stanch the bleeding can be applied until another method is available.

Basic wound care involves maintaining a clean environment and protecting the injured area until **granulation tissue** ("**proud flesh**") forms to cover and protect the wound. Before this occurs, antiseptics that are relatively non-toxic to tissue should be used in the primary layer of the bandage. Washing the wound and the mechanical action of pulling the dried gauze from the surface of the wound both act to remove dead tissue, bacteria, and foreign debris. The secondary layer of the bandage should be fashioned to provide a sufficiently large absorptive area to remove all the discharge from the wound, since this material can serve as a medium for the growth of bacteria. In areas such as the armpit or where a large pocket causes an accumulation of discharge, Scarlet oil, Preparation H, or hydrotherapy can be used to speed the formation of granulation tissue.

During the weeks and months to follow, it usually becomes necessary to decrease the formation of excessive or "exuberant" granulation tissue, especially on wounds below the carpus and tarsus. Granulation tissue can be considered exuberant if it rises above the level of the surrounding skin. Exuberant granulation tissue is undesirable because it acts to inhibit the contraction and formation of the **epithelium** (outer skin layer) that will form part of the skin that eventually covers the wound. Limiting motion at the site of the wound is a highly effective means of reducing the formation of granulation tissue. This along with the pressure provided by the bandage will help to speed the healing of the wound.

Frequent removal of granulation tissue can be performed with a sharp scalpel blade without the aid of local anesthesia, because the tissue contains no nerve endings. Cutting should begin at the *bottom* of the wound; otherwise the profuse bleeding will obstruct one's view of the remainder of the wound area. Dressings containing zinc sulfate and lead acetate (white lotion), copper sulfate (blue lotion), or corticosteroids (Panalog, Furacin with Azium) may be applied to help suppress granulation tissue. Caustic home remedies containing creosote, oil, or kerosene should be avoided because of their irritating nature.

If it is unlikely that the wound can heal completely, or if the granulation tissue becomes **fibrous** (tough, scarred), or if the thin tissue that forms over the wound is likely to be subjected to repeated trauma, then **skin grafting** (transfer of fresh skin to the site) should be considered as an alternative, in order to speed cover of the wound and provide a strong outer layer. Grafting techniques are available for equine patients and are quite varied in their expense, complexity, and cosmetic outcome.

CHAPTER 39

First Aid and Orthopedic Emergencies

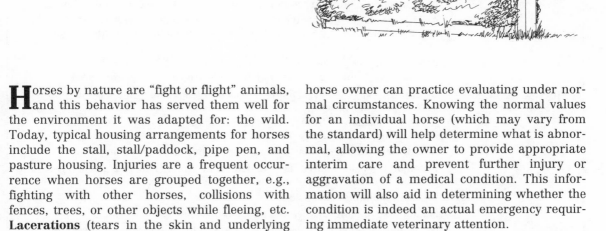

by Robin H. Kelly and Jack R. Snyder

Horses by nature are "fight or flight" animals, and this behavior has served them well for the environment it was adapted for: the wild. Today, typical housing arrangements for horses include the stall, stall/paddock, pipe pen, and pasture housing. Injuries are a frequent occurrence when horses are grouped together, e.g., fighting with other horses, collisions with fences, trees, or other objects while fleeing, etc. **Lacerations** (tears in the skin and underlying muscle), punctures, and fractures comprise the vast majority of injuries. Prompt recognition of an injury and appropriate interim treatment prior to arrival of the veterinarian can be critical for a successful outcome.

Upon discovery of an injury, it is important to determine the extent of the damage as quickly as possible. This can be done by examining the horse's entire body for swelling, lacerations, punctures, fractures, or other abnormalities. A simple and quick physical examination can provide additional information that the veterinarian will find useful to assess the degree of injury. Table 1 summarizes some of the physical parameters (and suggested normal ranges) that the

horse owner can practice evaluating under normal circumstances. Knowing the normal values for an individual horse (which may vary from the standard) will help determine what is abnormal, allowing the owner to provide appropriate interim care and prevent further injury or aggravation of a medical condition. This information will also aid in determining whether the condition is indeed an actual emergency requiring immediate veterinary attention.

Although it is in the best interest of young horses for their early years to be uninhibited and free in the pasture, the veterinarian and farrier often wince when they are called to treat such uneducated "wild hares." Some degree of ground handling and basic training is advisable so that young horses' first experiences with the farrier and veterinarian will not be completely unpleasant for all. One should not expect these professionals to bear the wear and tear of early training of a youngster!

Once it has been determined that an injury or other abnormality exists, the owner should enlist the aid of family or neighbors to care for the horse while the veterinarian is contacted.

Table 1
Normal Physical Parameters of the Horse

TEMPERATURE:
99.5–100.5°F (adults), 100.5–101.5°F (foals).
Use a large-animal thermometer, or a human rectal thermometer, held in the rectum for 2 minutes.

The temperature will normally elevate after exercise.

HEART RATE:
24–36 beats per minute (adults), 40–60 beats per minute (foals)
Obtain an inexpensive stethoscope and practice evaluating the heart sounds on the wall of the chest, just behind the elbow.

RESPIRATORY RATE:
12–24 breaths per minute (adults), 32–54 breaths per minute (foals), (may be altered with excitation, stress, or exercise).

The presence of a slight **serous** (clear) nasal discharge is normal.

Note if there is **purulent** (containing pus, whitish-yellow in color) material draining from one or both nostrils.

MUCOUS MEMBRANES:
Normally pink and moist, with a capillary refill time of 1–2 seconds. To evaluate capillary refill, squeeze the gum tissue with a finger and note the number of seconds required for the gum color to return. If you are not certain whether the gums of the horse are abnormal, compare with those of another horse.

Always check the mucous membranes in normal light or with a flashlight. Do *not* use fluorescent lighting, which can make the gums appear abnormally pale.

Abnormal gums are pale-white, blue, brick-red, or purple in color.

Capillary refill times greater than 3 seconds are considered abnormal.

PHYSICAL EXAM:
Examine closely for physical differences in the left side of the body as compared to the right side.

Check for discharges from the eyes, nostrils, mouth, rectum, vulva, sheath, wounds, abscesses, or any other evidence of trauma.

Note whether the horse has passed manure or has diarrhea on its tail.

Listen on both sides of the flank to determine whether there is normal gastrointestinal activity (a stethoscope or your ear will do).

Is there abdominal distension?

Is the horse making a concerted effort to breathe?

ATTITUDE:
Determine whether the horse is alert and bright, or dull and depressed, or whether its behavior is in some way altered from what you know as normal.

Can the horse walk and move normally? Evaluate it at the walk and trot.

Is the horse bearing its weight evenly on all four limbs?

Has the horse eaten or drunk, and is there evidence of fresh manure?

Note if the fencing/stall shows evidence of a struggle.

Be sure to check any other resident horses for similar or related injuries or problems.

Instituting appropriate therapy as rapidly as possible often dictates the success of the veterinary care obtained from the veterinarian. If the horse has a traumatic injury or has experienced significant blood loss from a laceration, puncture, or nosebleed, the horse should be kept as quiet as possible. If the horse is exhibiting signs of **colic** (abdominal pain) and is obviously in pain, it should be walked in a safe area. (*See* CHAPTER 40, "PROCEDURES FOR MEDICAL EMERGENCIES.")

If the horse appears to be in marked pain and potentially dangerous to handlers, it should be confined in a stall with sturdy walls.

With a severe limb laceration with extensive bleeding, quickly clean the injured area with an antiseptic (**betadine scrub**), attempt to wrap the limb with a thick pressure bandage firmly applied, and leave the bandage in place even if it gets soaked through. If the wound is on the body or head, apply a pressure bandage with a towel or washcloth and manually hold it in place until the veterinarian arrives. As a general rule of thumb, do not apply any ointments or wound powders to wounds that will be evaluated and potentially **sutured** (stitched together) by the veterinarian.

Suggested bandage materials that horse owners should have on hand at all times include the following:

Quilted cotton leg wraps
Pillow leg wraps
Disposable sheet cottons
Disposable 6-inch Brown gauze
Track bandages (these resemble Ace bandages)
4 × 4 gauze pads
Duct tape

Injuries to the Head, Neck, Trunk, and Body

SUPERFICIAL ABRASIONS
A superficial abrasion is any skin scrape in which the hair and superficial skin surface have been removed but there is no gap or separation of skin edges. Superficial abrasions do *not* require suture repair.

Treatment
Clean the injury with betadine scrub or a mild antibacterial soap. Dry and apply **furacin** ointment, furacin (nitro furazone ointment) spray powder, or aloe vera cream/vitamin E 1–2 times daily until healed. If the wound is on the face or top line of the body, try to keep the horse out of direct sunlight. If the abrasion is on the head or around the eyes, apply a *fly mask* (net cover for the head) for protection and to reduce irritation from sunlight, dust, wind, and flies. If swelling

develops, hot compresses or cold packs (these can be alternated) applied for 15 minutes twice a day may help. If it is certain that the wound does not involve a fracture, phenylbutazone ("**bute**") may be given as a nonsteroidal anti-inflammatory drug (**NSAID**).

Warning: More serious injuries may be present even though simple abrasions are the only obvious sign. It is always best to avoid treating minor swelling with drugs that provide pain relief, as they may mask signs of hairline (incomplete or nondisplaced complete) fractures, which may be life-threatening if they become complete fractures.

Local therapy with ice, cold water hosing, heat compresses, or pressure bandages and controlled, light exercise will achieve the same results, perhaps more slowly. Signs that might suggest a more severe bone injury would include:

- Slight lameness, which may become more obvious over 5–7 days
- Swelling or pain to the touch which persists despite local therapy
- Decrease in the normal level of activity
- Decrease in degree of weight-bearing on an affected limb

If uncertain of the course of healing, the veterinarian should be contacted.

SUPERFICIAL LACERATIONS
These are wounds with a separation of skin edges gaping 5 mm (.2 inches) or more. Lacerations involving mucocutaneous junctions (eyes, mouth, or nose) of any length, or those in other regions longer than 2 cm (.8 inches) or gaping 5 mm (.2 inches) or more should be sutured. Lacerations of smaller dimensions can be sutured as well but might not be cosmetically superior to what natural healing would accomplish. Smaller lacerations should receive the care described for abrasions (above). Lacerations involving the head are especially important to repair for cosmetic concerns. In addition, if the injury involves the eyelid it may impair function of the lid and distribution of the tear film. Even a small gap in the continuity of the lower eyelid

and interruption of its contact with the eyeball can lead to chronic tear-formation and inflammation, and potentially to ulcers of the **cornea** (the transparent outer coat of the eye).

Wound Care

Prior to arrival of the veterinarian, it is important to clean the wound (except those involving the eyes) with a mild antiseptic (**betadine soap**) and to remove any foreign debris or dirt. Warm compresses or alternation with ice-packing will help to minimize swelling. Move the patient out of direct sunlight, dust, or wind, and cover the wound with a damp towel to keep it moist and protected.

Do not apply vaseline or any sprays or caustic powders if the wound is to be sutured. Ideally, attempt to have your horse examined by a veterinarian within 6 hours. Wounds heal more quickly and with fewer complications the sooner they are sutured. With more serious lacerations (e.g., flaps hanging from the wound, or extensive muscle, bone, or joint exposure), immediate veterinary attention is necessary.

HEMATOMAS

These blood-filled cavities appear as round to oval swellings that resemble water balloons under the skin. They may appear small initially but over several days can grow considerably in size. In some cases they may be mistaken for an abscess. To differentiate between the two, an abscess will appear as a firm, painful swelling, while a hematoma is soft, fluctuant, and not painful. Hematomas usually are caused by a traumatic blow from a fixed object or a kick from another horse, resulting in bleeding from broken vessels or muscle. They are most often found on the body or neck. Once drained, hematomas normally require 2–3 weeks to heal completely, usually with minimal scar formation.

Treatment

It is best to confine the horse immediately to minimize further bleeding and extension of the hematoma into a larger area. The larger the hematoma, the greater the soft-tissue separation from the skin. Hematomas may continue to bleed depending on the size of the vessels and physical condition of the horse, and therefore it is best not to lance them until one is certain that the bleeding has stopped. Most veterinarians prefer to lance a hematoma once its size has stabilized—usually in 4 or 5 days. Once lanced, the hematoma is often packed and left open to drain. Antibiotics may be given if it is considered necessary by the veterinarian.

ABSCESSES

Abscesses appear as small swellings anywhere on the body that gradually increase in size. Most often they are firm and painful to the touch. There are many possible causes, and most abscesses are best treated by a veterinarian. Initial therapy usually consists of warm/hot compresses and application of a **poultice** (soft, often medicated paste spread on a cloth and draped over a wound) to encourage the abscess to "come to a head." Common poultice ingredients include numotizine, ichthymol, and epsom salts. If the abscess contains potentially contagious organisms, as in strangles and "pigeon fever" (*see* CHAPTER 25, "THE RESPIRATORY SYSTEM AND VARIOUS DISORDERS," and CHAPTER 31, "BACTERIAL DISEASES"), it is best that the veterinarian remove a small amount of material from the abscess for culture and identification. Care should be taken to isolate the animal from others in case it is contagious. Once the abscess has been lanced it should be cleaned and packed and allowed to drain (preventing premature closure of the wound). Antibiotics may be administered depending on the nature of the infectious process and the potential for contagion.

DEEP LACERATIONS

Serious wounds such as these have large gaps between the skin edges, particularly those involving large flaps of skin separated from the underlying tissue or defects in the deeper muscle layers. Deep lacerations are an emergency and require immediate attention. Upon contacting the veterinarian, clearly communicate the extent and location of the injury, approximate dimensions of the wound, degree of separation of the wound edges, and amount of blood loss. If the veterinarian is not available within the hour, it is important to obtain a referral to another practitioner who can provide immediate care. Timely assistance is especially important with lacerations involving a flap or significant separation of the skin from its underlying blood supply. The longer flaps are left unattended, the poorer the prognosis for salvage of the skin, and the more likely the post-operative complications (skin grafting, extensive bandaging, and so forth).

Wound Care

As with superficial lacerations, warm compresses and careful antiseptic cleaning are important. Attempt to replace the flap and tissues back into their normal anatomic orientation, in order to restore the blood supply and keep the tissues moist and warm. If necessary, keep the patient as quiet as possible; often, providing food is all that is needed. Have at least one person hold the horse while the compresses are applied. Use a bucket of clean, warm water and a clean towel or washcloth. It may be necessary to apply compresses until the veterinarian arrives, and for this reason a sufficient number of people should be brought in to assist in the procedure. If the flaps have been stripped from their underlying blood supply and tissue attachments, they become dry and cold; surgical repair is certain to fail.

Do not apply any ointments or spray powders to wounds that will be treated by the veterinarian as they may compromise wound healing and will require added efforts to remove. Although deeper lacerations of these regions of the body are not easy to bandage, it would be advantageous to apply pressure compresses by hand as this may ease swelling as well. It may be necessary for the veterinarian to apply a *stent bandage* to wounds that require protection from exposure or protection from self-inflicted trauma such as scratching, rubbing, or chewing. This is merely a patch or patches of gauze that are fixed in position by umbilical tape, which is laced through large open sutures placed on the skin at appropriate intervals (like a shoelace). Fly masks and 8-inch stockinettes can be used as wound protectors for head wounds and are surprisingly well tolerated.

Wound Care after Laceration Repair by the Veterinarian

Keeping wounds clean and free of an accumulation of discharge and debris is important. If there was contamination of the wound with dirt, wood, or metal, a drain may have been implanted that will require attention at least twice a day. Some veterinarians prefer warm compresses and advocate daily expression of the wound edges, checking for accumulation of tissue fluids or pus; others prefer that the wound be kept clean but undisturbed. Antibiotics are often administered because most wounds are considered contaminated to some extent. Most veterinarians dispense oral trimethoprim-sulfa preparations, which are relatively palatable to horses when mixed with alfalfa meal or a bran mash/grain/applesauce mix. More discriminating patients may require oral dosing, with the tablets dissolved in a small amount of water mixed with Karo syrup and administered through a syringe.

Injuries to the Limbs

SUPERFICIAL LACERATIONS

Treatment is similar to that for superficial lacerations of other areas of the body, with some exceptions:

Lacerations, even of a minor nature, may result in extensive localized swelling, particularly in horses that are stall-confined. As a result injured horses may exhibit varying degrees of lameness or sensitivity to **palpation** (feeling with the hands or fingers). It is advisable to bandage or apply leg wraps to injured horses that are stall-confined and in particular those that have previously exhibited a tendency toward swelling after injury.

For lacerations that have been sutured, it is always advisable to apply a clean leg wrap to prevent swelling and protect the wound from manure contamination. Wounds that have been sutured often become itchy, particularly if the wound accumulates fluid under the skin edge or debris caked on the skin surface. Protecting the wound from chewing, rubbing, or manure contamination is especially important in younger horses. Once the sutures have been removed, the wound will often heal uneventfully. It will, however, require daily bandage changes to prevent **dehiscence** (breakdown of the healing site) and irritation from chewing or rubbing. Sterile surgical wounds require a full 6 weeks to heal; contaminated lacerations are likely to take at least as long. Wound protection will probably be necessary for at least 3–4 weeks, and in cases where the wound edges are not closed (owing to flap failure or excessive swelling), the development of **granulation tissue** (newly formed, velvety tissue, rich in blood vessels, known as "proud flesh") is most likely an end-result. Formation of granulation tissue can significantly prolong postoperative care and expense and lead to residual scarring.

Some seemingly small lacerations of the limbs may require a lengthy time to heal, owing to a delay in early attention or treatment, contamination, exposure to the elements, or extensive swelling. If left unattended and exposed, these wounds may develop an infiltration of granulation tissue that will impede the ability to repair the wound surgically and cosmetically.

Injuries resulting from kicks or from a traumatic blow may be more serious than they seem at first. If a horse has a small laceration on a limb below the knee and hock (where there is minimal soft-tissue protection) and exhibits a severe to non–weight-bearing lameness with or without swelling, it should be stall-confined and veterinary attention sought immediately. Severe kick injuries can result in hairline or nondisplaced-complete fractures that can have disastrous results if undetected. Some horses with severe injuries may not exhibit any obvious clinical signs. *It is wise to avoid the use of phenylbutazone or other anti-inflammatory medications in wounds that may involve a more serious injury.* Treatment for swelling may include leg wraps, Naquasone boluses (dispensed by the veterinarian to assist in reducing swelling), and local anti-inflammatory therapy (cold/warm compresses). Such treatment will provide therapeutic management without masking pain. Horses with hairline fractures or nondisplaced fractures may aggravate their condition if they are medicated and thus become more active than their injuries can tolerate.

DEEP LACERATIONS

Deep lacerations of the limbs require immediate veterinary attention. Determining the extent of injury as soon as possible is essential, owing to the presence of numerous tendon, ligament, tendon sheath, and joint spaces. Wounds extending into tendon sheaths or joints usually result in severe lameness and moderate temperature elevations 38.9–40°C (102–104°F). They will often require rapid referral to a surgical center for **lavage** (flushing) to remove infected cellular debris. Postoperative care may require additional flushes and extensive intravenous antibiotic therapy for at least 7–10 days, followed by a course of oral antibiotics for approximately 3 weeks. Unfortunately, these wounds can be very difficult to treat even in the best of circumstances. It is thus important to indicate the severity of the injury when contacting the veterinarian, by providing accurate assessments of the horse's body temperature, degree of lameness, presence of swelling, extent and location of the injury, and duration of clinical signs.

Deep lacerations that do not involve joints, tendons, or ligaments but simply result in skin separation should be repaired as discussed above and maintained with postoperative wraps until healed.

Deep lacerations involving the front of the leg below the knee or hock will require laceration repair, postoperative leg wraps, and stall confinement. If the extensor tendons have been lacerated, suture repair is usually not attempted; instead, splinting to immobilize the region is preferred. Splinting often utilizes wide PVC (polyvinyl chloride) irrigation pipe placed over the front of the bandage and secured with elastikon or duct tape. Effective immobilization of the extensor tendons is achieved by fixing the joint above and below (fetlock and knee) in a heavy bandage with splinting from the pastern to mid-radius. Splinting will also allow wounds to fill in more rapidly when soft tissue is lost around the tendon and motion inhibits healing.

Some of the materials that it may be useful to stock, in the event of laceration injuries, include the following:

Granulation tissue stimulators:
   Furacin ointment
   Scarletoil
   Moist saline bandages

Granulation tissue inhibitors:
   Betadine solution
   White lotion
   Baking soda powder
   Panalog ointment
   Hydrocortisone ointment

Bandage material (disposable):
   Sheet cottons 30 × 36-inch
   Brown gauze, 6-inch
   Vet wrap, 4-inch
   4 × 4 gauze pads
   Duct tape
   Elastikon
   Large PVC pipe for splints

Bandage material (nondisposable):
   Quilted cotton leg wraps
   Track bandages, 6-inch
   Easy Boot

Wounds in which a large amount of soft tissue has been lost will need to fill in with granulation tissue and must be kept clean and moist during the regenerative process. Protection with a bandage requiring daily or every-other-day bandage changes is necessary to keep the exposed tissues from drying out. An alternative to daily bandage changes is the application of a cast, to serve several purposes: protection, maintenance of a moist environment, and rigid immobilization. Casts can be left on for varying periods of time, depending on the extent of the injury, tolerance of the patient, cast comfort, and clinician preference.

DEEP LACERATIONS INVOLVING THE HINDLIMB FLEXOR TENDONS
When tendons are lacerated, immediate attention is required. The wound should be cleaned, a bandage applied, and the horse confined in a stall. Determine whether the injured leg is lower than the opposite leg at the level of the fetlock, and whether the toe is tipping up. The veterinarian will flush the wound, evaluate the degree of tendon injury, and remove the dead tissue. Lacerations over the tendons are usually not sutured, owing to the extent of contamination which can result in breakdown of the suture repair.

If the superficial digital flexor tendon (SDFT) is partially lacerated, a wedge shoe can be applied to elevate the heel and decrease strain on the tendon. A flattened roll of elastikon may be used as a temporary heel elevator if the fetlock is significantly dropped or if the toe of the foot is tipping up.

Severe lacerations of the SDFT and deep digital flexor tendon (DDFT) usually result in some elevation of the toe and drop of the fetlock. Affected horses are severely injured and are unlikely to recover their athletic potential. If the intent is to salvage the horse for breeding purposes, application of a hand-made board splint will place the fetlock/pastern/hoof in flexion and place the weight-bearing load on the point of the toe and bony column rather than the tendons. Affected horses should be splinted immediately and referred to a surgical center for evaluation. Severe lacerations involving extensive damage to tendons and possibly ligaments may be better stabilized prior to referral by application of a temporary cast for transport.

SPLINTS FOR FRACTURES
With many fractures, damage continues to occur after the original injury owing to lack of stabilization of the broken bone(s). The most important action an owner can take is immediate immobilization of the fracture site and protection of the injury from contamination. Attempt to keep the horse quiet and do not move it from the location it is in until the limb is adequately stabilized. *Never sedate the horse,* as this will often compromise coordination and reduce pain sensation—which may result in greater physical activity and potentially greater damage. Pain relief may be provided with nonsteroidal anti-inflammatory drugs, but if the veterinarian is already on the way, it is better to wait.

If the intent is to refer the patient to a surgical center for repair, it is always best to have the fracture evaluated by the local veterinarian and stabilized for transport. Often the best method of accomplishing this is to apply a temporary cast. If there is an open wound associated with the fracture injury, it is imperative that the wound be quickly cleaned and bandaged to protect the injury from further contamination.

Fractures that do not have a wound or opening can quickly become open and contaminated if the patient flails about. Thus stabilization should be attempted as soon as possible. Generally, splints should be at least 4–6 inches wide (the wider the better). Use thick PVC pipe which is split in thirds (so the surface placed next to the bandage will lie flat). Avoid using broomsticks or sharp materials composed of metal. As a general principle, one wants to stabilize the joint above and below the location of the fracture.

Fractures of the Skull

FRACTURES INVOLVING THE TEETH
Generally these require X-ray evaluation and surgical stabilization using wires and occasionally pins. Surgical repair is normally done under general anesthesia, but can occasionally be done with the horse standing. The teeth can be placed back into position and secured with surgical wire. Fractures of the lower jaw may require additional immobilization with pins. Fractures involving the teeth have an excellent prognosis and merely require postoperative antibiotics, nonsteroidal anti-inflammatory drugs, and mouth flushes.

FRACTURES OF THE SKULL PROPER
Simple fractures appearing as a crush injury over the front of the face can have an excellent cosmetic result, provided the wound is evaluated and repaired quickly. The fracture fragments are elevated and secured in position using a combination of wires, screws, and small plates. Postoperative care usually involves antibiotics and flushes if the wound is left open, wound care if it is closed. Head wraps with an 8-inch stockinette will protect the wound from contamination by dust and debris.

Fractures of the Neck

The neck should be suspected as the location of injury if a horse presents with hindlimb paraly-

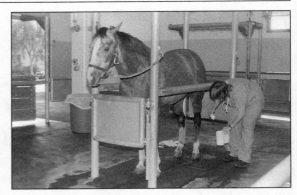

Photo by Mordecai Siegal.

sis or moderate to severe incoordination of sudden onset. Fractures of the neck are usually the result of a fall or trauma from a head-on collision with a fixed object. Often the forelimbs have reduced sensation and the horse may be unable to rise. Affected horses have a very poor prognosis for recovery.

Fractures of the Forelimb

COFFIN BONE FRACTURES
The hoof forms a natural cast but one will need to apply corrective shoeing to stabilize the hoof wall. Options for shoeing include an egg bar shoe with a full rim metal pad, or a regular shoe with a metal pad (14-ga. sheet metal) welded to the shoe and stabilized with at least three clips drawn up on the toe and quarters. Until an accurate diagnosis by X ray can be made, it is recommended to stall-confine the horse, keep it as quiet as possible, and avoid the use of phenylbutazone. Coffin bone fractures must be differentiated from hoof abscesses, which may present with identical signs.

PASTERN FRACTURES
Keep the horse as quiet as possible and do not move it until the injury has been splinted by the veterinarian. Apply a firm, heavy bandage with wide PVC pipe placed over it on the front surface, from the knee to the ground. If the horse is to be transported to a referral center and there is any concern that the horse may not be calm, a cast may be the best method of temporary stabi-

lization. If a cast is applied, it will need to enclose the hoof and extend up to the knee.

Fetlock Dislocation/Fracture of the Distal Cannon Bone

Similar to treatment for pastern fractures (*see* above).

CANNON BONE FRACTURES

It is especially important to protect the fracture from further damage and contamination. A bandage and splint can be applied as far above the knee as possible. Two splints should be applied at 90-degree angles to one another on the front and outside of the leg. Be sure to extend the splints to the ground surface, as contact with the ground will aid stabilization. Bandage material should be at least 3 inches thick, and can be composed of several layers of pillow wraps or quilted cotton with track bandages. Apply all materials as firmly as possible and stagger the wraps so that the first set extends from the **coronary band** (ring of vascular tissue along the upper edge of the hoof wall) to the knee and the second set extends from the knee towards the elbow. The bandages should overlap so that the lower wrap is under the upper wrap and will effectively hold the upper one in position. Apply the PVC splints with elastikon tape as tightly as possible to the front surface and outside surface of the wrap.

KNEE FRACTURES

Same splinting technique as for the cannon bone.

FRACTURES OF THE RADIUS

A thick bandage should be applied along with a splint as for the cannon bone, except that the outside splint should be much longer and extend up along the outside of the elbow and shoulder. These splints will need extensive taping to stabilize them.

FRACTURES OF THE ELBOW AND HUMERUS (SHOULDER)

Wrap a heavy bandage just below the elbow and place the splint along the back of the leg up to the elbow (but not right over the fracture). This splint will place the knee in a fixed position and will help prevent the elbow from dropping.

Fractures of the Hindlimb

The principles are the same as for the forelimb, except that with cannon bone fractures of the hindlimb, it is better to place the splint along the back of the limb.

CHAPTER 40

Procedures
for Medical
Emergencies

**by Robin H. Kelly and
Jack R. Snyder**

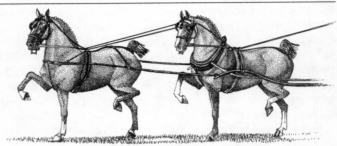

Choke

Choke is an obstruction or blockage of the **esophagus** (the hollow tube running from the throat to the stomach). It is the most common disorder of the esophagus in horses. Choke typically occurs in greedy eaters and in older horses or ponies. Affected horses often have dental problems, such as sharp enamel points or moderate to severe gum disease. The classical clinical signs of choke include a green, frothy discharge from both nostrils, coughing, gagging, distress, and evidence of abdominal pain.

WHAT TO DO
Remove feed immediately and place the horse in a stall without bedding, feed, or water. If practical, tie the horse's head up to a normal position and keep the stable area quiet. Contact the veterinarian immediately. It is wise to have the horse evaluated early, although the veterinarian may recommend giving the horse a little time to see if the obstruction will pass on its own. This is preferable to the potential damage a stomach tube and **lavage** (flushing) may produce if the

obstruction has been present for a time.

In many cases the obstruction will pass within several hours. The horse will become noticeably more comfortable and the nasal discharge will subside. Despite apparent resolution of the problem, the horse should be examined to determine if there is any damage to the surface layer of the esophagus. A potential complication of choke is **aspiration pneumonia**, in which feed material is inhaled into the lungs and produces an infection. Listening to the horse's lung sounds through the chest wall, using a stethoscope, will help in determining whether aspiration pneumonia is present. Aspiration pneumonia normally requires antibiotic administration as part of its treatment.

If the obstruction does not pass, the veterinarian will examine the esophagus through an **endoscope** (long flexible viewing tube connected to a video apparatus). At the same time the teeth should be evaluated for periodontal disease, poor dentition, and enamel points. If the obstruction is still present, the veterinarian will pass a stomach tube and gently flush the obstruction with warm water. This will often dislodge the obstruction and allow it to pass into the stomach.

Horses with choke are at risk for future obstructions, and the veterinarian will advise on appropriate dietary adjustments and post-treatment care. After the initiating cause has been resolved, the diet should consist of water-softened pellets until the irritation to the surface of the esophagus has subsided. **Sucralfate** (sulfinated compound used to coat the damaged tissue) is often administered to treat surface damage, with gradual adjustment back to a normal diet if treatment is successful (i.e., if reobstruction does not occur). If the obstruction recurs, further diagnostics may need to be pursued to determine the underlying cause of the problem.

Colic

Colic in its broadest sense refers to abdominal pain, which can be caused by a number of conditions, including bloating and obstruction (*see* CHAPTER 26, "THE DIGESTIVE SYSTEM AND VARIOUS DISORDERS"). Typical clinical signs of colic include:

- Decrease in appetite
- Depression or other change in normal attitude
- Demonstration of pain (pawing the ground, lying down, rolling, changes in facial expression, body posture)
- Decrease in manure output
- Change in manure consistency, presence of mucus

On physical examination the temperature is typically normal. The heart rate is usually elevated:

- Mild colic: 36–48 beats per minute (bpm)
- Moderate colic: 48–60 bpm
- Severe colic: 60+ bpm (80–120 bpm, life-threatening)

With serious colic the mucous membranes (gums, etc.) will be white, blue, brick-red, or purple. (Capillary refill time greater than 4 seconds is a sign of severely compromised circulation. (*See* CHAPTER 39, "FIRST AID AND ORTHOPEDIC EMERGENCIES" under "MUCOUS MEMBRANES," page 388, for the technique to rate capillary refill time.) The motility of the intestines is usually reduced, although it may be increased with **enteritis** (inflammation of the small intestine). Bloating of the abdomen may signify an obstruction or twist in the bowel.

The degree of pain may be difficult to assess, because some horses are stoic and have a high threshold for pain while others wince at the slightest cramp. Overall it is better to have a horse that is sensitive to pain, as it will more quickly alert the owner of a potential problem.

WHAT TO DO

Call a veterinarian *immediately*. Do not attempt to diagnose the underlying problem or its severity without the assistance of an experienced professional. Avoid administering medications unless absolutely necessary, since many drugs may mask enough of the clinical signs to obscure important information. Keep the horse walking to avoid rolling and also to provide some pain relief. Allow only experienced handlers near the horse; human injuries can result from the unpredictability of animals in pain.

On arrival the veterinarian will perform a physical examination prior to administering any medications. A stomach tube will be passed to determine whether intestinal contents are flowing from the small intestine back into the stomach—a sign of intestinal obstruction. A rectal examination will be performed to palpate portions of the bowel and assess their position, the presence of distension, malpositioning of abdominal organs (e.g., spleen), and to determine the nature of the manure (or its absence). The results of these examinations will provide the veterinarian with a general picture of the underlying problem and a recommendation for treatment or referral will then be made.

If there is no intestinal obstruction or malpositioning of organs and the clinical signs are mild, the veterinarian may recommend conservative management, based on the following possible diagnoses:

- An impaction (sand, feed)
- Mild spasmodic colic
- Presence of sand in the manure
- Suspicion of intestinal parasites
- Mild deydration/constipation

Initial treatment will probably include:

- Pain medication in low doses
- Administration of mineral oil through a stomach tube
- Light exercise (hand walking)
- Decrease in feed (if an impaction is suspected)
- Intravenous fluids (if a more severe impaction is suspected)

A specific period of time will be allotted to allow the above therapy to resolve the clinical signs. Low doses of medications normally are given to avoid masking a more serious problem that may not yet be clinically apparent.

If more serious abnormalities exist, the pain medication administered will provide relief for a relatively short period of time. Typically, the horse will again become uncomfortable or the prior signs will resume. The horse should continue to be monitored by evaluating the heart rate, respiratory rate, mucous membrane color and refill time, presence of abdominal bloating (if increasing), appetite, manure output or lack thereof, and degree of pain. The horse should be checked on a 2–4 hour basis over the next 24 hours; the veterinarian should be called if further abnormalities develop.

Many colics initially appear simple and resolve with minimal therapy. Subsequent resumption of clinical signs may indicate that a minor problem is becoming more severe, or that an obstruction exists and now will require surgery to correct. Signs of increasing severity cannot be ignored and will become life-threatening if they are not treated or if the horse is not referred to a surgical facility.

If the pain appears to increase, contact the veterinarian immediately and consider referral to a surgical facility as quickly as possible. If the horse is passing fluid back from the intestine into the stomach, it is wise to transport the horse with a stomach tube taped in place so that the stomach can continue to be decompressed. Intravenous fluids can be administered if the veterinarian is concerned about the horse's hydration status. Ideally the patient should be stabilized prior to transport but referred as quickly as possible to ensure the best surgical outcome. If necessary fluids can be administered in the trailer and pain medications provided before departure. Plan to stop every half hour to change the intravenous fluid bags in order to avoid bleeding from the indwelling catheter. If the transport time is short (1–2 hours), giving fluids in transit is probably not necessary unless severe dehydration is present.

Diarrhea

Diarrhea can be caused by bacterial or viral infections or by metabolic imbalances. Typical clinical signs include:

- Elevated temperature (38.3–40.5°C, 101–105°F)
- Brick-red or "muddy" mucous membranes with a prolonged capillary refill time (2–4 seconds)
- Increased gut motility (may be intermittently decreased in some horses)
- Increased output of watery, smelly manure
- Depression
- Often a decreased appetite

Some horses with diarrhea become severely dehydrated and will require large volumes of intravenous fluids to make up for the fluid lost in the feces. **Propulsive diarrhea** (squirting watery diarrhea from the rectum) may become a life-threatening emergency if not evaluated and treated quickly. Often these horses become **septic** (develop a widespread infection owing to absorption of gastrointestinal bacteria across a damaged gut wall) and will require extensive care with intravenous fluids, antibiotics, anti-inflammatory medications, and activated charcoal (to coat the intestine and decrease the absorption of toxins from the bowel). Many affected horses are at risk for developing secondary complications, such as colic, *laminitis* (see below), and **endotoxemia** (presence of bacterial toxins in the blood). Management depends on the cause and severity of clinical signs. Milder signs of diarrhea may be due to parasitic infestations, stress, bacterial infections, dietary changes, foreign material irritating the bowel, dehydration, mild colic episodes, and antibiotic therapy.

TREATMENT
Intravenous fluids should be given if dehydration is present, antibiotics if infection is a concern, and anti-inflammatory medications if inflammation or endotoxemia is suspected. Oat hay should be fed to provide roughage and reduce the moisture in the manure. Kaopectate or Pepto-Bismol can be used to coat the intestinal tract and reduce the absorption of toxins. Severe cases ideally should be referred to an intensive-care facility. These cases can be very difficult to manage and, as with colics, may become expensive to treat as well.

Myositis ("Tying-Up," Exertional Myopathy)

Muscle diseases caused by exertion are seen most frequently in performance horses. They are usually the result of exercise following a period of inactivity during which the horse was maintained on a full ration high in carbohydrate (i.e., grain). A similar condition is seen in unfit horses that have received inadequate conditioning for the exercise attempted. (See "EXERTIONAL MYOPATHIES" in CHAPTER 22, "THE MUSCULOSKELETAL SYSTEM AND VARIOUS DISORDERS," page 208.)

The typical clinical sign of **myositis** (muscle inflammation) is a stiffening of the gait while the horse is being worked. Most often this occurs as the horse is being warmed up or cooled out, and more commonly in extremes of either cold or hot weather. Some horses will cramp in the hind end and not be able to walk forward. Others merely appear stiff but may break out in a full sweat. Some exhibit mild to moderate signs of colic and may try to lie down or roll while fully tacked.

TREATMENT
It is best not to move the horse from its position. Remove all tack and blanket the horse even if

the ambient temperature is mild. Contact the veterinarian immediately. The veterinarian will attempt to determine the extent of muscle damage and whether the horse is dehydrated. Most often affected horses are agitated and uncomfortable. *As long as significant dehydration is not a factor,* nonsteroidal anti-inflammatory drugs and symptomatic care are indicated. If dehydration exists, nonsteroidal anti-inflammatory drugs can cause kidney damage. In general it is always recommended that a horse be adequately hydrated prior to administering any medications.

When attempting to recondition the horse after an adequate period of convalescence, be sure to warm up and cool out the horse very slowly. If it appears to stiffen and cramp, stop at once and follow the same procedures as before. On repeated episodes, more severe complications may occur—so condition carefully and slowly.

Laminitis (Founder)

Laminitis in simplest terms is an inflammatory process affecting the **laminae**, the structures that serve to attach the coffin bone to the hoof wall. Many factors can produce this disease, and treatment and prognosis vary depending on the underlying cause and the extent of damage to the affected tissue. (See "DISORDERS OF THE FOOT" in CHAPTER 22, "THE MUSCULOSKELETAL SYSTEM AND VARIOUS DISORDERS," page 214.) Typically, bony changes affecting the coffin bone are initiated by a specific disease process, with loosening and rotation of the bone within the hoof usually evident within 48 hours. The wide range in prognosis reflects the varied degree of rotation, drop of the foot within the hoof capsule, secondary complications, and pain threshold of the horse.

Among the more common factors causing laminitis are:

- Grass or grain overload
- Ingestion of cold water after exercise
- Overingestion of inappropriate feeds (e.g., pig feed)
- Excessive trauma to the feet ("road founder")
- Systemic infections

- Hormonal abnormalities
- Metabolic or gastrointestinal diseases

Clinical signs include:

- A stiff-legged gait with the fore feet stretched out in front and the hind feet tucked under the abdomen
- Strong, pounding pulse palpated along the back of the pasterns
- Moderate to severe sensitivity of the soles of the feet with hoof testers
- Palpable heat in the hoof wall (severe cases)
- Unwillingness to move at all

Horses in the acute stage of laminitis must be evaluated by a veterinarian. If the inciting cause can be determined, treatment will clearly be aimed at resolving it. Dehydration may also be a factor and can complicate treatment, since primary care often consists of pain relief with nonsteroidal anti-inflammatory drugs. Once the patient is better hydrated, phenylbutazone or flunixin meglumine (Banamine) (anti-inflammatory drugs) may be administered to make the horse more comfortable and combat endotoxemia (bacterial toxins in the blood). Minimizing exercise is the current aim of management, along with provision of deep bedding (combination of shavings and straw) for extra padding and comfort. Foot wraps for protection of the sole may be beneficial for horses in whom trauma and severe bruising may be a factor, but care must be taken to avoid excessive sole pressure which may aggravate the condition. If a systemic infection is driving the laminitis, antibiotics and nonsteroidal anti-inflammatory drugs are indicated. Intravenous dimethylsulfoxide may be recommended as an aid in controlling inflammation.

The aims of long-term care are to prevent aggravation of the condition and to provide corrective shoeing. Early corrective shoeing is aimed at providing heel support, sole protection, and short toes. Corrective shoes should not be applied in the acute stages of laminitis because further damage can be inflicted by the process of shoeing. Shoes can be applied once the horse has been stabilized. Egg bar shoes with pads, reverse shoes with or without pads, sneakers and regular shoes with wedge pads, are among the various shoe types currently in use. (See "CARE OF THE FEET" in CHAPTER 3, "EQUINE HUSBANDRY," page 50.)

Each case of laminitis is different, with its own unique factors and management that may or may not apply to any other case. The prognosis varies depending on the cause, age of the horse, and complications. *Once a horse develops any degree of laminitis, its feet will never be the same.* Although they may recover fully and enjoy many years of usefulness, affected horses will exhibit abnormal hoof-wall growth and whiteline changes. Chronic mild lameness may persist despite corrective shoeing; typically such horses demonstrate tenderness prior to shoeing (as their toes get longer) and just after shoeing (since the sole was trimmed thinner).

Injuries to the Eyes

Eye injuries are fairly common in horses and as can be imagined they require immediate attention. Clinical signs are not always obvious because horses tend to normally droop their eyelids and many owners may not realize that an ocular problem exists. When feeding a horse or just on a daily basis, it is a good idea to check its eyes for abnormalities. Note whether both eyes are open to the same extent and whether the lids appear "sleepy." The **cornea** (transparent outer coat of the eye) of each eye should appear clear, and the **pupil** (black, central opening through which light penetrates into the inner reaches of the eye) and **iris** (circular, pigmented structure surrounding the pupil) should both be visible. (*See* CHAPTER 19, "THE EYE AND VARIOUS DISORDERS.")

Ocular abnormalities are often subtle and may not be noticed until the underlying disease process is considerably advanced. The sooner an abnormality is noticed and diagnosed, the better the outlook for repair. Severe ulcers of the cornea, for example, can progress to the point where an infection is so severe that it perforates the eyeball, resulting in blindness and necessitating in many cases removal of the eye (**enucleation**). Often an injury may be minor but the degree of pain experienced by the horse may result in further trauma and damage. Horses often will scratch or rub a body part that is painful, and so self-inflicted trauma can become a significant factor.

CONJUNCTIVITIS

This is usually a minor inflammatory reaction affecting the mucous membrane lining socket of the eyeball and the inner surface of the eyelids. These areas can become inflamed and reddened secondary to trauma, infection, or presence of a foreign body (dust, dirt, plant material, debris). Contact the veterinarian to evaluate the eye, even if you are able to remove the foreign body. A thorough eye exam should always be performed to be certain that a corneal ulcer or other abnormality has not developed.

Never apply any eye ointment (or any other kind of ointment) to an eye without the advice and direction of a veterinarian. Treating an eye inappropriately with ointment containing a steroidal anti-inflammatory agent (e.g., hydrocortisone) may encourage a simple, subclinical ulcer to progress and possibly even perforate, resulting in loss of the eye.

If a foreign body is clearly evident, it may be possible to remove it gently with a soft cotton Q-tip, taking great care to avoid scratching the cornea. If the foreign body resists removal, allow a veterinarian to do it. Foxtails, splinters, and dirt are the most common objects usually found and they can incite a very strong inflammatory response when lodged in the eye. It takes very little time for an affected eye to become swollen and inflamed. What owners usually see is an eye that has swollen shut or has a bulging conjunctiva. A horse with such an eye will require significant sedation and pain relief. Staining the surface of the cornea to determine if an ulcer is present will be an important aspect of the veterinary examination. Once the foreign body has been removed and the eye itself has been evaluated, the lid and conjunctiva should be treated with appropriate ointments and local therapy (hot/cold compresses 2–3 times daily), systemic anti-inflammatory medication, and protection with a fly mask or head gear.

CORNEAL ULCERS

Although they often occur secondary to ocular injury, ulcers may also represent the primary problem and always require immediate attention. Superficial ulcers may not be obvious to an untrained observer and must be stained with a fluorescent dye for their full extent to be made visible. Treatment consists primarily of antibiotics applied to the eye, and anti-inflammatory drugs (if necessary) to prevent rubbing and scratching. For more severe ulcers, a bacterial and/or fungal culture of the cornea is recommended. Severe ulcers may be accompanied by other abnormalities (e.g., uveitis) that may require treatment as well. The ulcer may heal but if uveitis is left unchecked, the inflammatory complications may compromise vision. If the pupil of the affected eye is significantly constricted in comparison to the pupil of the normal eye, uveitis is becoming a factor. The pupil should be dilated to reduce the inflammatory reaction and for pain relief. This will necessitate keeping the horse indoors, protected from sunlight, until the pupil recovers its normal dimensions.

When an eye is adequately dilated, the pupil will be round and roughly the size of a quarter. Once the pupil is dilated, expect the eye to require approximately 2–3 weeks to return to normal size. While the pupil is dilated the patient must be kept in the shade and protection provided with a fly mask or goggles. Turnout at dusk or dawn may be done as long as the ulcer is uncomplicated. More severe or deeper ulcers will require diligent care and may be more effectively treated at a referral center. Such ulcers are best managed by a veterinary ophthalmologist—a veterinarian trained specifically in treating problems of the animal eye.

Superficial corneal ulcers have an excellent prognosis so long as they are treated quickly. Once ulcers have become more serious, treatment and prognosis become more protracted and complicated. It is thus important to be vigilant in observing horses' eyes on one's daily rounds, in order to pick up any abnormality and have it evaluated in a timely fashion.

Note: Horses wearing fly masks—particularly in pasture—must be checked on a regular basis as they may develop ulcers despite the protection. Unless masks are removed daily, ulcers may go unobserved and progress to a severe stage before the damage is discovered. As a rule, take masks off at night to avoid this potential complication.

UVEITIS

Uveitis (inflammation of the cellular layer of the eye that contains the iris) occurs usually secondary to a local injury (severe corneal ulcer or trauma) or a systemic illness. Signs commonly include a reddened, inflamed eye, squinting, and a painful, cloudy or white cornea. Usually the signs reflect the duration of the disease as well as its frequency of occurrence. More chronic abnormalities may reflect the cyclical nature of some cases of uveitis, e.g., "moon blindness." In many cases uveitis has been present but undetected for varied periods of time and more chronic changes may be present. Chronic changes include a droopy eyelid with moderate to severe tearing or rubbing, constricted pupil, and an opaque sheen to the cornea. These conditions dictate immediate veterinary attention. Resist the urge to apply any medication until the veterinarian has established the nature of the problem. It is best to bring the patient into the shade, especially if light-sensitive (**photophobic**), and apply a fly mask to reduce light irritation.

The veterinarian may recommend warm/cold compresses and nonsteroidal anti-inflammatory drugs to ease the swelling. Atropine to dilate the pupil and antibiotics may also be given. Once the underlying ulcer or infection has been treated and controlled, steroids may be given to aid in reducing the inflammation within the eye. (*See* CHAPTER 19, "THE EYE AND VARIOUS DISORDERS.")

Adverse Vaccine Reactions

Vaccines are given to produce an immune response in order to stimulate the production of protective antibody and immune lymphocytes (*see* CHAPTER 29, "THE IMMUNE SYSTEM AND VARIOUS DISORDERS," and APPENDIX B, "VACCINATIONS AND INFECTIOUS DISEASE CONTROL"). A common misconception is that horses receiving vaccinations should not experience any side-effects. If that were the case, it could be argued that the resulting immune response is potentially ineffectual! What needs to be determined, in cases where a reaction to a vaccine is suspected, is whether the reaction is due to the vaccine or is secondary to an infection. A normal vaccine reaction consists of mild swelling and local sensitivity at the site of the injection. The sensitivity may persist for several days and in some uncommon cases may require hot/cold compresses to resolve. Abnormal reactions to a vaccine include:

- Extensive swelling (may get larger than a cantaloupe, and continue to expand)
- Fever of 40°C (104°F) or greater
- Signficant abnormalities of gait
- Severe body soreness

Horses experiencing severe vaccine reactions may have them again after future injections. Such reactions thus should be anticipated and can be treated prophylactically by giving **phenylbutazone** (an anti-inflammatory drug) before and after vaccination. Occasionally, horses may develop life-threatening reactions in which abscesses and localized cell death result. Certainly these reactions are rare, but if significant reactions have occurred in the past, it is wise to vaccinate a horse in a body region that drains well. It may also be argued that only those vaccines that are absolutely necessary be administered to horses in which the disease being vaccinated against poses less of a threat than a vaccine reaction.

CHAPTER 41

Poisonous Plants

by Murray E. Fowler

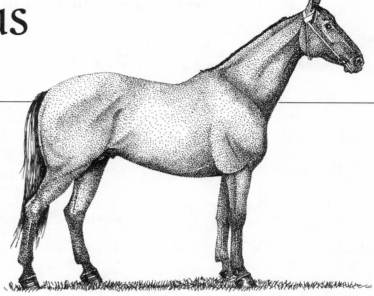

Plant poisoning is an uncommon occurrence in horses. Nevertheless, toxic plants such as yellow star thistle and oleander are so widely distributed that owners should always be on the alert for them and take appropriate precautions to protect their horses. Although horses may be exposed to poisonous plants in various ways, poisoning usually occurs only when basic management principles have been neglected.

Why Horses Eat Poisonous Plants

As a general rule, poisonous plants are not palatable; horses eat them only when available forage is insufficient. When a pasture has been overgrazed and poisonous plants are present, horses may resort to eating them even if their taste is unpleasant. Hungry horses introduced into a new corral or pasture may eat whatever foliage they first encounter. Horses may avoid eating green shrubby plants in or near their corrals, but if cuttings from those same plants are allowed to wilt and are tossed where horses can get at them, danger looms.

An especially hazardous practice is the feed-ing of grass clippings. On first glance it may seem perfectly natural to feed green grass to an animal; grass clippings, however, may contain leaves of toxic garden ornamentals, such as ole-ander. Moreover, piled grass clippings quickly begin to ferment and may cause a serious gaseous colic if ingested. This is almost a breed hazard in ponies, which often develop acute *laminitis* ("founder") from such an episode (*see* CHAPTER 22, "THE MUSCULOSKELETAL SYSTEM AND VARIOUS DISORDERS").

Owners must be particularly cautious of feed-ing pelleted or cubed products to their horses. Poor-quality, weedy hay may be converted into such products by unscrupulous producers; unfortunately the buyer can no longer assess quality when the feed is in such a form. (*See* CHAPTER 7, "FEEDING HORSES.") Neither can the horse detect weeds or poisonous plants in pel-lets or cubes. Similar considerations may also hold for baled hay. The integrity of the hay pro-ducer and dealer is the only assurance the buyer has that manufactured feeds are of top quality.

Owners may be excessively critical of plants in or near corrals and pastures but neglect to be

Table 1
Plants That May Cause Poisoning While on a Trek or Packing Trip

Common Name	Scientific Name	Signs of Poisoning	Sites to Avoid	Plant Characteristics
Rhododendron	*Rhododendron* spp.	Severe colic, diarrhea	Don't picket horses near shrubs	Wild species have large leaves and flowers
Azalea	*Rhododendron* spp.	Same as for rhododendrons	Same as for rhododendrons	Same as for rhododendrons
Death camas	*Zigadenus* spp.	Colic, frothing at the mouth, convulsions	Meadows and open slopes in the late spring and early summer	Large, grass-like leaves; Flowers multiple, white, lily-like
Labrador tea	*Ledum glandulosum*	Same as for rhododendrons	Edges of meadows at high mountain elevations	Short shrub with white flowers
Black laurel, mountain laurel	*Leucothoe davisii*	Same as for rhododendrons	Same as for rhododendrons	Short shrub with white, bell-shaped flowers

concerned about potentially dangerous ornamentals around the house or farmyard. It is not unusual for horses to escape from corrals and begin nibbling on nearby shrubs. Just a small amount of one such shrub, the yew (*Taxus* **spp**. [multiple species]), can kill a horse.

A prime use of pleasure horses is for a wilderness experience. Riding and pack horses, burros, and mules will become hungry during a prolonged trek and may eat any forage available at rest stops or campsites. Table 1 lists some shrubs and plants that should be identified lest a pleasure trip become a tragedy.

It should also be mentioned that horses unfortunately may acquire a taste for an otherwise unpalatable plant. Initially a horse may be forced through hunger to eat a toxic plant such as yellow star thistle. Later it may inexplicably seek out the plant despite the presence of abundant lush pasture.

Where to Look for Poisonous Plants

One must be continually on the alert to spot unfamiliar plants in the horse's environment. Encroaching vegetation at the margins of a well-

managed pasture may evade the watchful eyes of the owner. Similarly, toxic plants may appear in first-cutting alfalfa hay or oat hay; in waste areas along gullies, washes, abandoned roads, and field; around water tanks, ponds, sluggish streams, and standing water; along fence rows and conservation strips; in woodlots, especially at the margins; and in the barrow pits and verges of roads and railroad tracks. Poisonous plants may be seasonal in occurrence, and foreign plant seeds may be carried in by irrigation systems. Pastures should be walked and examined periodically for unfamiliar foliage.

Recognition and Identification of Poisonous Plants

Tables 2 through 5 list poisonous plants of different categories. It is not necessary to be a botanist to identify plants, but it does require an interest and some effort. Owners should become knowledgeable about the common plants found in their area, either through reading or instruction. If a particular identification is doubtful, a specimen of the suspect plant can be taken to the Cooperative Agricultural Extension office in the local county

Table 2
Some Common Plants Poisonous for Horses

Common Name	Scientific Name	Signs of Poisoning	Trouble Spots	Plant Characteristics
Oleander	*Nerium oleander*	Diarrhea, colic, irregular heartbeat	Roadsides, farmyards, plant cuttings	Ornamental shrub with long, linear leaves
Yellow star thistle	*Centaurea solstitialis*	Inability to chew, starvation	Grows extensively in waste places and poorly managed pastures	Yellow flowering head with star-burst thorns
Russian knapweed	*Centaurea repens*	Same as for Yellow Star	Same as for Yellow Star	Purple-to-lavender flowers, minimal thorns
Common groundsel	*Senecio vulgaris*	Head-pushing, incoordination, jaundice	As a weed in first-cutting alfalfa hay	White puff-ball flowering heads
Fiddleneck, fireweed	*Amsinckia intermedia*	Same as for groundsel	Weed in first-cutting alfalfa hay and oat hay	Yellow flowers on one side of an uncurling stalk, giving the impression of a violin neck
Castor bean	*Ricinus communis*	Severe diarrhea, colic, shock	Ornamental, but grows wild in waste places. Seeds are the dangerous part	Round, prickly seed pods. Leaves large and shaped like a hand
Bracken fern	*Pteridium aquilinum*	Incoordination, weakness	Mountain pastures Regrowth on burnt ranges	Robust fern with three divisions of the frond
Locoweed	*Astragalus* spp. *Oxytropis* spp.	Incoordination, falling, aimless wandering	Localized sites in foothills	Compound leaflets, pealike flowers. Seeds in a pod
Jimsonweed, thorn apple	*Datura stramonium*	Incoordination, rapid pulse, convulsions	Fields, pastures, waste places	Large white, tubular flowers. Wavy leaves. Fruit in spiny pods
Yew	*Taxus* spp.	Acute collapse and rapid death	Ornamental, evergreen shrub. Grown as a hedge	Needles dark green above, light green below. Seed in a red, fleshy cup
Tree tobacco	*Nicotiana glauca*	Excitement, tremors, shaking, paralysis	Waste places, abandoned lots	Large, light green leaves. Long tubular, yellow flowers

Table 2 (cont.)
Some Common Plants Poisonous for Horses

Common Name	Scientific Name	Signs of Poisoning	Trouble Spots	Plant Characteristics
St. John's-wort	*Hypericum perforatum*	Photosensitization	Perennial herb in pastures, roadsides, dry soil	Yellow flowers with many stamens. Leaves opposite, dotted
Rattlebox	*Crotalaria* spp.	Incoordination, walking in circles, jaundice	Roadsides, fields	Annual or perennial legume with yellow flowers
Sudan grass, sorghum	*Sorghum vulgare*	Incoordination of the hind end, incontinence, bladder infection	Planted for pasture, hay, or silage	Tall, robust grass

Table 3
Some Ornamental Plants, Shrubs, and Trees Potentially Poisonous for Horses

Common Name	Scientific Name	Clinical Signs	Plant Characteristics
Black locust	*Robinia pseudoacacia*	Colic, depression, convulsions	Shrub to a large tree. Leaves compound and flower pea-like. Fruit a long pod
Oleander	*Nerium oleander*	Colic, diarrhea, sweating, irregular heartbeat	Leaves long and linear. Flowers in spring, summer, fall
Foxglove	*Digitalis* spp.	Same	Large, bell-shaped, multi-colored flowers. Grows in moist, cool gardens and in the wild
Yew	*Taxus* spp.	Sudden collapse and death	Needles dark green above, light green below. Seed in red, fleshy cup
Red maple	*Acer rubrum*	Loss of appetite, depression, anemia, jaundice	Wilted maple leaves are the source of poison
Black walnut	*Juglans nigra*	Laminitis (founder)	Shavings and sawdust bedding are the source of poison
Lantana	*Lantana camara*	Jaundice, liver failure	Yellow-to-lavender flowers

Table 4
Some Plants That Are Mechanically Injurious to Horses

Common Name	Scientific Name	Type of Injury
Foxtail, wild barley	*Hordeum* spp.	Sharp awns get into eyes, ears, nostrils, mouth, around teeth, alongside tongue
Yellow bristle grass	*Setaria lutescens* *Setaria glauca*	Sharp, brittle awns penetrate and break off in the mucous membranes of the mouth, producing ulcers
Cocklebur	*Xanthium strumarium*	Becomes entangled in mane and tail
Beggar's ticks	*Bidens frondosa*	Becomes entangled in hair
Tarweed	*Hemizonia* spp.	Tarry resin sticks to the hair of the legs and face, accumulating filth

seat. The office may also have extension bulletins available that describe specific poisonous plants. If no one in the office is able to identify a particular specimen, it can be taken or sent to an herbarium for a positive identification.

Recognition of Poisoning

There is no generic syndrome of poisoning. The chemicals found in poisonous plants may affect one or all organ systems of the body. Although diarrhea, weakness, incoordination, and convulsions are commonly observed in cases of poisoning, such signs may be caused by infectious or parasitic diseases as well. Diagnosis of poisoning frequently is made after eliminating the more common or other likely disorders. Because there are essentially no specific treatments for plant poisonings in horses, the veterinarian can only treat the general signs and provide good nursing care.

In the case of plant poisoning, prevention is truly much more important than therapy, which all too often may be futile. Close and frequent surveillance of the environment is a major component of prevention. Provision of adequate

Table 5
Some Plant Poisonings Affecting Cattle, Sheep, or Goats, But Rarely Horses

Larkspur (*Delphinium* spp.)

Spoiled yellow sweet clover hay (*Melilotus officinalis*)

Nitrate poisoning

Cyanide poisoning

Chokecherry (*Prunus* spp.)

Milkweed (*Asclepias* spp.)

Water hemlock (*Cicuta douglasii*)

Poison hemlock (*Conium maculatum*)

Black nightshade (*Solanum nigrum*)

Oaks, scrub oak (*Quercus* spp.)

palatable forage is also essential. Select a reliable feed dealer, but constantly check on the quality of forages that are provided. Pastures should be surveyed often for unfamiliar and potentially toxic plants.

PART VIII

Appendices

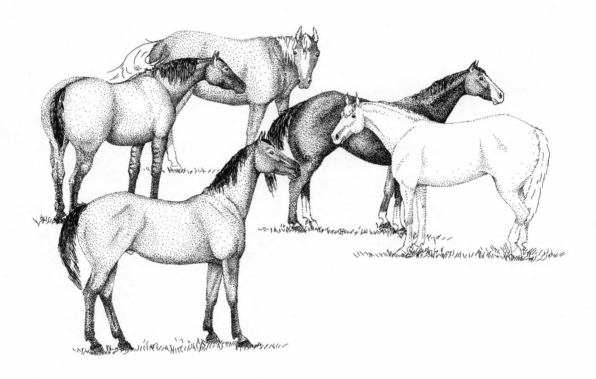

To God I speak Spanish,
to women Italian,
to men French,
and to my horse German.

CHARLES V, 1500–1558, ATTRIBUTED

Zoonotic Diseases: From Horses to People

by Bruno B. Chomel

The horse has always been close to Man. Its domestication led to the conquest of the world by the ancient tribes of Huns and of the New World by the conquistadors. Despite the massive regression of equine populations in the developed countries, the use of horses for leisure activities is still very popular. Unfortunately, horses can carry **zoonoses**, i.e., infectious diseases that can be transmitted to people. In many instances horses serve as a reservoir or amplifier of the infection. Although diseases such as glanders, a devastating bacterial infection that plagued armies for centuries, have almost been eradicated from the earth, several major infectious or parasitic diseases can still be transmitted by horses.

The frequency of occurrence of zoonoses transmitted from horses to human beings is rather difficult to estimate and depends on several factors, including:

- Number of infected animals
- Geographic distribution of the infectious agent
- Mode of transmission of the agent
- Existing measures of prevention

A brief review of horse-associated human diseases will be useful to provide objective information for horse owners and for general equine care and management.

Viral Zoonoses

Among the large variety of viral diseases affecting horses, rabies is one of the major diseases that is particularly dangerous for human beings. In the Americas, horses are also affected by several arboviral infections, such as the equine encephalitides, and can serve as a reservoir for arboviral (viruses transmitted by mosquitoes and ticks) infection of mosquitoes. (*See* CHAPTER 30, "VIRAL DISEASES.")

RABIES

Although the frequency of occurrence of *rabies* in horses is low (less than 1% of all diagnosed rabid animals), approximately 45–50 cases are reported annually in the United States. In southern Ontario, Canada, over 700 cases were reported between 1970 and 1990. The most important wildlife reservoirs of the rabies virus are foxes and skunks in the northeastern United States and southern Canada, and raccoons in the southeastern and Atlantic regions. In the central United States and California skunks are the primary rabies reservoir. Bat rabies, widespread throughout North America, can also be transmitted accidentally to horses.

A spectrum of clinical signs, ranging from paralysis to abnormal behavior, has been reported in rabid horses. Exposure of horses to a suspected rabid animal is rarely witnessed. Because of the vagueness of its early clinical signs, rabies often is suspected only late in its clinical evolution. Thus the number of persons exposed to a rabid horse is often high; postexposure rabies treatment of several dozen individuals is quite common. Fortunately, no human death from exposure to a rabid horse has occurred in North America.

In horses, the **incubation period** (time between exposure and the onset of clinical signs) for rabies averages between 2 and 4 weeks (range: 2 weeks to 3 months). Clinical signs of disease at the time of initial examination usually include weakness of the hindquarters, lameness, and **colic** (abdominal pain). After an excitation period, paralytic signs occur that cause difficulty in swallowing, followed by incoordination of the extremities. In all cases there is a change in behavior. Because neurologic signs always progress with rabies, other possible diagnoses should be considered if the signs have not worsened in 5 days. Horses affected with rabies usually die within a week of the onset of clinical signs.

Rabies vaccination is recommended for horses living in areas where wildlife rabies is a problem. Because many horses are kept as pets or are in close contact with human beings, vaccination may serve to establish an "immune barrier" between people and wildlife populations. Two **inactivated** ("killed") rabies vaccines are currently licensed for use in horses in the United States. Horses must be at least 3 months of age or older at the time of their first inoculation, and should receive a booster dose annually. (*See* APPENDIX B, "VACCINATIONS.")

THE EQUINE ENCEPHALITIDES

Arboviral diseases have worldwide impact, especially in tropical and subtropical countries. The viruses causing equine **encephalomyelitis** (inflammation of the brain and spinal cord) have been isolated only in the western hemisphere. The first record of *eastern equine encephalomyelitis* (**EEE**) in the United States was made in 1831 by a physician who described an episode of neurologic disease in horses in Massachusetts. *Western equine encephalomyelitis* (**WEE**) was first recognized in the western United States in 1847, while *Venezuelan equine encephalomyelitis* (**VEE**) was first described in northern South America in the 1920s. Clinical signs of the equine encephalitides range from inapparent infections to a mild or severe, and frequently fatal, neurologic disorder. For the first few days a nonspecific fever is observed, which is soon followed by profound depression and stupor, or in some cases hyperexcitability. (*See* CHAPTER 30, "VIRAL DISEASES.")

Human beings can become infected with EEE virus, WEE virus, and some subtypes of VEE virus. The clinical syndrome in people can vary from a mild influenzalike illness to severe brain disease. Deaths have been reported primarily in children and the elderly. Direct transmission from horses to human beings usually does not occur; rather, the disease agent is carried by mosquitoes feeding on both horses and people. Human cases are frequently reported during outbreaks of the equine disease.

Horses are the most important amplifiers and indicators of outbreaks of VEE virus activity. Important wildlife reservoirs include birds (for EEE and WEE viruses), rodents (for WEE and VEE viruses), and several species of mosquitoes (for all three viruses). Recent EEE outbreaks in Florida, Georgia, and South Carolina have resulted in both equine and human cases, owing to heavy spring rains that led to exceptionally large mosquito populations. In 1994 health departments in 20 states reported 100 presumptive or confirmed human cases of arbovirus disease to the Centers for Disease Control and Prevention (CDC), including 2 WEE cases and 1 EEE case. A major outbreak of VEE occurred in

South America in 1995, with an estimated 13,000 human cases in Venezuela and 45,000 human cases in Colombia. Hundreds of horses died. Cases in humans and horses were also reported in El Salvador and Panama in the fall of 1995.

Effective preventive measures are based on:

- Destruction of adult mosquitoes
- Destruction of mosquito breeding sites
- Avoidance of outdoor activity at night (particularly at dusk and dawn) in affected areas
- Application of mosquito repellents
- Wearing of long-sleeved shirts and long pants

Safe and effective EEE and WEE virus vaccines for horses are commercially available and should be administered regularly to horses living in affected areas. (*See* APPENDIX B, "VACCINATIONS AND INFECTIOUS DISEASE CONTROL.")

VESICULAR STOMATITIS

Vesicular stomatitis (**VS**), a viral disease of cattle and horses, is limited to the Western Hemisphere. It is found primarily in the forested plains of tropical and subtropical areas of the Americas. In horses the disease is characterized by a short incubation period (2–4 days), followed by a brief period of fever and the appearance of **papules** (minute, firm, well-demarcated elevations of the skin) and **vesicles** (blisters) in the mouth. Affected animals usually recover within a week. In people the incubation period is only 1–2 days. Influenzalike symptoms (fever, headaches, muscle aches) lasting for a few days are characteristic. Most human cases have been diagnosed in laboratory personnel but infections can also occur naturally in the field. People in contact with affected animals should wear protective clothing and gloves. (*See* CHAPTER 30, "VIRAL DISEASES.")

INFLUENZA

Equine *influenza* is caused by two different subtypes of type A influenza virus, referred to as *H7N7* and *H3N8*. Although transmission of equine influenza from horses to people has *not* been observed under natural conditions, experimental infection of human volunteers with H3N8 virus has resulted in an influenzalike illness, with virus recoverable for the first 6 days after infection. Conversely, horses exposed to the Hong Kong strain of human influenza virus (known as *H3N2*) developed a mild **febrile** (characterized by fever) illness, with virus readily recoverable for up to 5 days after infection. Antibody surveys in the United States and Great Britain have shown that human populations in the past have been exposed to equine H3N8 or a similar virus. To date, however, the zoonotic aspects of equine influenza remain controversial. (*See* CHAPTER 30, "VIRAL DISEASES," and APPENDIX B, "VACCINATIONS AND INFECTIOUS DISEASE CONTROL.")

EQUINE MORBILLIVIRUS DISEASE

A new zoonotic disease occurred in 1994 in Australia involving a paramyxovirus similar to the measles and canine distemper viruses. Equine cases were reported in Thoroughbred horses on two premises in the Brisbane area of Queensland. Between September 7 and 23, 1994, 14 horses (13 on one premise and 1 on another) were humanely destroyed after becoming seriously ill. Clinical signs included fever, incoordination, rapid and labored respiration, sweating, congested mucous membranes, severe depression, and a bloody discharge from the mouth and nostrils. Severe lung **edema** (swelling) was a consistent finding on necropsy examination.

Ominously, the trainer in charge of some of the diseased horses became ill and subsequently died of a similar respiratory condition. The trainer had been in direct contact with the horses. At the time the animals were clinically ill, the trainer had apparently force-fed the horses, introducing his hand and arm, on which there were abrasions, into the horses' mouths. A stable hand also became ill, but has since fully recovered.

Other viral conditions (African horse sickness, equine influenza, equine herpesvirus) were ruled out, as was hantavirus (suspected because of the clinical signs in the trainer, and because one of the affected farms had a significant rat infestation, with droppings and urine present in the horse feed). The affected trainer was reported often to have tasted the horses' feed during mixing. The trainer's clinical signs were also suggestive of legionnaire's disease, but this too was ruled out.

The new virus, called *equine morbillivirus* (**EMV**), was isolated at the Australian Animal Health Laboratory. Antibodies specific for the virus were detected in the deceased trainer, the recovered stable hand, and a private veterinary practitioner in attendance during the early stages of the disease outbreak, but who remained clinically unaffected. It was possible to reproduce the disease experimentally in horses through inoculation of tissues from affected horses as well as through virus grown in cell culture.

Studies suggest that EMV does not spread easily among horses and is not considered highly infectious for humans. However, persons handling ill horses need to exercise basic hygienic precautions. During the outbreak five premises were placed under quarantine. All sick horses that were not destroyed have since recovered.

A new human case of EMV infection was reported in the fall of 1995, when a 35-year-old farmer near Mackay in northern Queensland died. About a year before his death the farmer had developed **meningoencephalitis** (inflammation of the brain and its outer layers). He had assisted at necropsies of two horses that, at the time, had been diagnosed with other illnesses. Laboratory tests on tissues from one of the horses confirmed that it was infected with EMV.

Bacterial Zoonoses

SALMONELLOSIS
In horses, *salmonellosis* is an infectious disease that can result in diarrhea, **septicemia** (presence of bacteria in the blood, accompanied by related clinical signs), and death. Some horses, however, may shed *Salmonella* bacteria without developing any clinical signs. Surveys in Great Britain and the United States indicate that *Salmonella typhimurium* is the most common type isolated from horses. The frequent finding of this bacterium in riding horses and ponies

may be related to their being kept in fields contaminated by seagull droppings, which contain a wide variety of *Salmonella* types. Stress and other debilitating factors are frequently associated with outbreaks of salmonellosis in horses. Several infections acquired in veterinary hospitals have been reported, some of them associated with human contaminations.

Salmonellosis is a zoonotic disease causing a risk of infection to human beings who handle horses and to other animals housed where equine salmonellosis is a problem. Direct transmission of *Salmonella* from sick horses to people has been reported in the United States and France. Symptoms of salmonellosis in people include fever, vomiting, diarrhea, and dehydration. Identification of the *Salmonella* type from fecal samples of both horses and people is needed to determine the origin of an outbreak. Antibiotic sensitivity testing must also be performed because many *Salmonella* strains (especially *S. typhimurium*) are resistant to several different antibiotics. All contaminated facilities must be thoroughly cleansed, preferably with hot pressurized water, to remove all traces of feces and animal tissue, and then disinfected with any of several approved products (which can be obtained from, or recommended by, the consulting veterinarian).

OTHER BACTERIAL ZOONOSES
Several other bacterial zoonoses, some of them producing very severe illness in human beings, occur in horses but are either very rare and geographically restricted (such as glanders, brucellosis, and anthrax), or are relatively more difficult to transmit to people (leptospirosis, melioidosis). (*See* CHAPTER 31, "BACTERIAL DISEASES.")

Glanders
Once a worldwide disease of equids, glanders is caused by *Pseudomonas mallei*. This disease is now very rare and restricted to certain parts of the Middle East (Turkey, Iraq) and Asia (India, Mongolia). Glanders occurs chiefly in a chronic form in horses, but is almost always an acute disease in donkeys and mules. In people, as well as in animals, *Pseudomonas mallei* tends to localize in the lungs and mucous membranes of

the nasal passages, larynx, and trachea. **Pulmonary nodules** (enlargements or lumps within the lungs) and ulcerations of the **mucous membranes** (lubricating membranes lining the internal surfaces of body cavities) of the upper respiratory tract are characteristic of the disease. **Pneumonia** (inflammation of the lungs, characterized by the filling of air spaces with fluid) and related problems are common. In the skin form of glanders, nodules, ulcers exuding an oily fluid, and swollen lymph nodes and lymphatic vessels are the major clinical signs. People can contract the infection by direct contact with infected horses.

Brucellosis

Brucellosis is a rare disease seen in horses sharing pasture or housing with cattle or pigs infected with *Brucella* bacteria. It usually manifests itself in the form of a **fistulous bursitis** (inflammation of *bursae* [fluid-filled sacs found at certain places in the tissues where friction is a problem] accompanied by draining tracts). Human beings can contract the infection from horses having open, infected lesions.

Anthrax

Anthrax is caused by a spore-forming bacterium, *Bacillus anthracis*. Horses grazing in areas where anthrax has been a problem can become infected. An epidemic of human (716 cases, 88 deaths) and animal anthrax raged in the African country of Chad from September to December, 1988, infecting more than 50% of the donkey and horse population. In people the most common clinical form of anthrax is **cutaneous** (involving the skin) anthrax. After an incubation period of 2–5 days, a small papule develops and evolves into a blister. In a few days the clear blister fluid becomes dark. When the blister is ruptured, a sharp-walled, depressed ulcer crater with a centrally developing, black **eschar** (sloughing of tissue) is seen. Horses are afflicted with an acute form of anthrax, characterized by **enteritis** (inflammation of the small intestine), colic, high fever, depression, and death within 2–4 days. Infection through insect bites may occur, and was a suggested explanation for the intensity of the outbreak among donkeys in Chad. A hot, painful, **subcutaneous** (beneath the skin) swelling appears at the site of the bite and spreads to the throat, abdomen, and groin. Vaccination of horses in affected areas is considered an appropriate preventive measure. Penicillin therapy, if provided early enough, can be effective in curing the disease in both horses and people.

Leptospirosis

Human cases of **leptospirosis** are relatively rare in the United States (less than 100 cases per year in the last 10 years). Leptospirosis is primarily a water-borne illness, with rodents acting as major reservoirs of infection with the causative *leptospires* (spiral-shaped bacteria belonging to the *spirochete* group). Human beings are accidental hosts who become infected through occupational or recreational exposure. Horses can be infected with several different leptospires but most infections are inapparent. **Periodic ophthalmia,** an ocular disorder, is one of the major complications of leptospirosis in horses (*see* CHAPTER 19, "THE EYE AND VARIOUS DISORDERS"). Direct human contamination from infected horses has not been definitively proven to occur.

Melioidosis

Melioidosis is caused by *Pseudomonas pseudomallei*, a **saprophitic** (living on dead and decaying matter) bacterium found in certain soils and waters, especially in southeast Asia and Africa. Various animal species, including sheep, goats, horses, swine, and monkeys, are susceptible to infection. Clinical cases in horses (as well as in a few human beings) were reported in the late 1970s and early 1980s in France. The clinical spectrum of melioidosis in horses and people is very wide, ranging from inapparent infection to a rapidly fatal septicemia. Direct transmission from horses to people has not been reported; however, infected horses may contribute to contamination of the environment with the causative bacterium. Antibiotics can provide an effective treatment.

Tuberculosis

Tuberculosis is a very rare disease in horses, but can potentially be transmitted to people when it does occur. Horses may become infected with *Mycobacterium bovis* (the primary agent of bovine tuberculosis) in countries where cattle infection is high.

Pasteurellosis and Other Bite-Transmitted Zoonoses

Horse bites are often severe and infection of the bite site with bacteria such as *Pasteurella multocida* can occur. *Actinobacillus lignieresii* and an *Actinobacillus equuli*-like bacterium were isolated from an infected horse bite in a 22-year-old stable foreman, while *Actinobacillus suis* was recovered from a bite injury in a 35-year-old man who had been attacked by a horse. Interestingly, suspected *Lyme disease* transmission to a 24-year-old man who was bitten while tending sick horses—horses with high levels of antibody to the causative agent of Lyme disease, *Borrelia burgdorferi*—has been reported in Belgium. (*See* CHAPTER 31, "BACTERIAL DISEASES.")

Fungal Zoonoses

RINGWORM

Ringworm, also known as **dermatophytosis**, is a common, transmissible, superficial fungus infection of animals (including horses) and human beings. It affects primarily the hair, skin, and nails. The fungi most commonly causing ringworm in horses are *Trichophyton equinum*, *Trichophyton mentagrophytes*, and *Microsporum equinum* (the latter being infrequently found in the Americas). *Microsporum canis* (the common ringworm fungus of dogs) and *Microsporum gypseum* (a ringworm fungus found in the soil) are also often isolated from horses. Ringworm lesions are circular and hairless, with the affected skin being thickened and covered with scales. Treatment is based on administration of an appropriate antifungal medication (**griseofulvin**). Thorough scrubbing of boxes and grooming equipment and disposal of bedding and blankets of affected horses are effective control measures. (*See* CHAPTER 17, "THE SKIN AND VARIOUS DISORDERS.")

Parasitic Zoonoses

TRICHINOSIS

Trichinosis is a serious, occasionally fatal food-borne disease of human beings, but usually does not produce recognizable clinical signs in other species. It is caused by *Trichinella spiralis*, a parasitic worm whose larval forms are found in muscle tissue. When the (raw or undercooked) muscle is eaten, the larvae are liberated and mature in the small intestine, where the adults reproduce and produce offspring. In the mid–1970s and 1980s, large outbreaks of trichinosis occurred in Italy and France that were associated with the consumption of raw or undercooked horsemeat imported from the United States and eastern Europe. Clinical symptoms in affected human beings are variable, but can include muscle pain, skin eruptions, fever, difficult respiration, and ocular swelling.

HYDATID DISEASE (ECHINOCOCCOSIS)

Hydatid disease (also called *echinococcosis*) of human beings is only rarely diagnosed in the United States, but is of importance because of its potentially fatal outcome. The disease is characterized by the development of large, **cystic** (fluid-filled) structures called *hydatid cysts* in various tissues of the body. The cysts contain maturing stages of the causative tapeworm, *Echinococcus granulosus*. Dogs carry the adult tapeworm within the intestinal tract, from which eggs are shed in the feces.

Echinococcus granulosus is present in the western United States, Alaska, and Mexico. In Great Britain two strains of *Echinococcus granulosus* occur, an equine strain whose life cycle involves horses and dogs, and an **ovine** (sheep) strain that circulates between sheep and dogs. Doubts exist about the equine strain's infectivity for human beings. Because consumption of horsemeat is not traditional in Great Britain, the risk of human contamination is very limited.

Vaccinations and Infectious Disease Control

by W. David Wilson and Jeffrey E. Barlough

Control programs for infectious diseases are essential for maximizing the health, productivity, and performance of horses. Disease in an individual animal or an outbreak of disease in a group can result when horses are exposed to a dose of an infectious disease agent sufficient to overwhelm the immunity acquired by previous exposure or vaccination. Control programs should be aimed at reducing the quantity of infectious disease agent in the horses' environment, minimizing factors such as stress that erode disease resistance, and maximizing factors such as vaccination that enhance disease resistance. Programs relying solely on vaccination for protection against infectious disease often fail or are only marginally successful, because a tenuous degree of resistance can be overpowered by a massive exposure to the disease agent. Proper feed and dental care, hygiene, housing, pasture management, parasite and fly control, training and exercise routines, transportation practices, and other components of management all interact to one degree or another in promoting effective infectious disease control.

General Considerations

The frequency of infectious disease problems in horses tends to rise as the numbers and concentration of horses on a farm increase. Problems can result as well from movement of horses on and off the farm and from external environmental and management conditions. Conditions on breeding farms, at race tracks, and in show-horse and performance-horse barns are virtually perfect for the introduction and transmission of infectious disease agents, particularly those affecting the respiratory tract.

On breeding farms the addition of horses from outside sources, the intermingling of horses of different ages, and the high number of young susceptible horses and pregnant mares pose particular problems and can serve to illustrate some important principles of infectious disease control. For instance, the chances of acquiring an infection can be minimized by segregating horses according to their age and function. Weanlings, yearlings, horses in training, and visiting mares should be kept entirely apart from a farm's resident mares and their foals.

Visiting horses should be tested negative for *equine infectious anemia* (**EIA**) (*see* CHAPTER 30, "VIRAL DISEASES.") and should receive all appropriate immunizations and be dewormed before being received onto the premises. While on the farm they should be housed in barns and paddocks distinct from those occupied by the resident horses.

All new arrivals should be received initially into an isolation barn physically separated from the remainder of the farm. Separate equipment, and preferably separate personnel, should be reserved for this facility. During an initial 30-day quarantine period, new horses should be monitored closely for signs of infectious disease. Monitoring should always include daily recording of the rectal temperature. Any preventive health care measures that were not performed before arrival should be completed during quarantine.

Pregnant mares being sent to a distant breeding farm should be transported 6 to 8 weeks before they are due to foal. This will provide sufficient time for them to become exposed to the infectious disease agents present on the breeding farm and to mount proper immune responses against them. By the time the foals are delivered the mares will have concentrated antibodies to the disease agents in the **colostrum** (first milk) and thus be able to pass this temporary protection (**maternal immunity**) on to their offspring (*see* below and CHAPTER 29, "THE IMMUNE SYSTEM AND VARIOUS DISORDERS"). Recently foaled mares being transported short distances for breeding purposes can be shipped during *estrus* (heat), without the attendant foal, and returned home on the same day in order to reduce the risk of the foal's acquiring an infection.

Any horse exhibiting signs of a potentially contagious illness should be placed in isolation until at least 10 days beyond complete disappearance of those signs, in order to reduce the risk of disease spread to other susceptible horses on the farm. If separate personnel are unavailable to care for a horse in isolation, the horse should be attended to only after all the other horses on the farm have been cared for. A stall that has housed a sick horse should be thoroughly cleansed, disinfected, allowed to dry, and kept vacant for as long as possible before use by another horse.

Vaccination represents an important component of an overall infectious disease control program for horses. The risk of infection with any specific disease agent varies from farm to farm, so control programs must be tailored to each individual operation. A veterinarian can assist the horse owner in developing a comprehensive immunization program appropriate for his or her particular circumstances. From the outset the owner's expectations of success should be realistic, keeping in mind the efficacy of the vaccines currently available as well as the level of management the owner is willing to devote to the endeavor.

Vaccination involves the injection of infectious disease agents that have been either weakened (**attenuated**) or completely *inactivated*, such that they are incapable of inducing disease yet retain their characteristic surface structures to which the immune system of the horse can respond. The response to vaccination usually involves the production of **antibodies** and immune cells called **lymphocytes** and often mimics very closely the immune response that develops during recovery from natural infection. (*See* CHAPTER 29, "THE IMMUNE SYSTEM AND VARIOUS DISORDERS.") For most **inactivated** ("killed") vaccines, two or more initial doses of vaccine are required to provide a sufficient level of immunity. Over time this immunity gradually wanes, however, necessitating "booster" doses of vaccine at periodic intervals. The time interval between boosters depends on the particuar disease agent in question and the type of vaccine used. Tetanus toxoid, for example, is a highly effective vaccine and induces an immunity that persists for at least a year. By contrast, current vaccines against equine influenza virus induce a much less durable immunity lasting only a few months. This discrepancy is partly explained by the fact that even natural infection with influenza virus or other disease agents affecting the respiratory tract in general does not induce a long-lasting immune response. Moreover, because the most common method by which vaccines are administered (by the **intramuscular** (**IM**) route, i.e., into the muscle) is an unnatural route of infection for most disease agents, vaccination is unlikely to provide a more durable immunity than that resulting from natural infection.

Completion of the primary immunization series and injection of booster doses should be timed to precede potential exposure. Whenever possible, all horses in a herd should be vaccinated according to the same schedule. This will maximize the level of immunity delivered to the herd and establish transmission "blocks," i.e., immunized animals that are much less likely to pass the infectious disease agent on to other horses, effectively blocking its transmission within the herd. This has the added benefit of aiding protection of horses responding poorly to vaccination, since the overall amount and spread of the disease agent in the herd will be reduced (owing to individual variation in immune responses, all animals in any given population are not protected to an equal degree or for an equal length of time following vaccination).

Manufacturers' recommendations regarding the storage and handling of vaccines should be followed closely unless otherwise advised. Good record-keeping is also a must. Handwritten individual records are usually appropriate for smaller operations, while calendar-based computerized systems are highly recommended for improving efficiency and accuracy in larger herds. Copies of immunization and health-maintenance records should accompany all horses leaving a farm for sales, breeding, or training.

Some horses develop localized muscle swelling and soreness and/or transient clinical signs (fever, lethargy, inappetence) after being vaccinated. Thus as a general rule it is not advisable to vaccinate horses within 7 to 10 days of an event.

Horses can also receive protection against infectious disease through the administration of pre-formed antibodies, either by injection of **antiserum** (serum containing high levels of antibody specific for a particular disease agent of interest) obtained from an immunized horse, or by absorption through the digestive tract of antibodies present in colostrum (as occurs in newborn foals). Administration of antiserum can provide immediate protection in emergency situations; however, the antibodies in antiserum have a defined lifetime in the circulation and will slowly disappear, leaving the animal once again susceptible to infection. Some horses may mount an immune response against the antiserum itself and develop an illness known as **serum sickness.** Repeated administration of an antiserum such as tetanus antitoxin (*see* below) should thus be avoided.

The antibodies present in colostrum are essential for the protection of newborn foals against infectious disease. This natural means of defense can be enhanced in immunization programs by giving booster doses of vaccine to mares during the final 6 weeks of pregnancy to increase the levels of colostral antibody. The duration of protection provided by antibodies in colostrum varies from 6 weeks to about 6 months, depending on the disease agent involved and the quantity of antibody absorbed by the foal. Unfortunately, this antibody cannot discriminate between the actual disease agent and a modified version of the agent as present in a vaccine. Thus, maternal immunity can interfere with vaccination of foals by "soaking up" a particular vaccine component and making it unavailable to the foal's own immune system. One way to get around this problem is to delay initial immunizations until colostral antibodies have fallen below this inhibitory level. This approach is commonly taken when the risk of infection is low, as with rabies or with influenza in isolated herds. When the risk of infection is high, as with influenza on large breeding farms, immunizations are started earlier and given at intervals throughout the period during which maternal immunity is waning (in such instances it is thus necessary to administer more than two doses of vaccine in the primary series). By giving such an extended series of initial vaccinations the inhibitory effects of maternal immunity are minimized, while at the same time the period during which the foals are most susceptible to natural infection is made as brief as possible.

The Vaccines

TETANUS

Tetanus is an acute, often fatal disease caused by a **neurotoxin** (toxin targeting the nervous system) produced by the spore-forming bacterium *Clostridium tetani*. This organism is a normal resident of the soil and may also be found in small numbers in the intestinal tract and feces of people, horses, and other animals. *Spores* (highly resistant, thick-walled "resting stage" formed by certain bacteria to ensure their survival during periods of unfavorable environmental conditions) can persist in the environment for many years, resulting in repeated exposure of horses and people on farms. Spore contamination of dead or dying tissue in a penetrating wound is the most common means by which tetanus is induced. The spores **germinate** (grow into mature bacterial forms) soon after entering the wound. Germination is followed by production of the neurotoxin, called **tetanospasmin**, which affects neuromuscular responses in different areas of the body. The toxin blocks nerve impulses that normally inhibit muscle contractions. As a result the large muscle groups are trapped in a state of constant contraction characterized by prolonged, painful spasms. (*See* CHAPTER 31, "BACTERIAL DISEASES.")

All horses should be vaccinated against tetanus using **tetanus toxoid** (an attenuated form of the toxin). Available tetanus toxoid products are relatively inexpensive, safe, and induce a solid, durable immunity. Primary immunization involves the administration of two IM doses given 1 month apart, followed by a yearly booster. The annual booster for pregnant mares should be given 4 to 6 weeks before foaling in order to protect the mares should they sustain trauma during foaling and to provide protection for the foal in the colostrum. The two-dose primary vaccination series for foals should begin at 3 to 4 months of age. Vaccinated horses that have sustained a wound or have had surgery more than 4 months after their last tetanus inoculation should be boosted.

Antiserum containing antibodies against tetanus toxin, a product known as **tetanus antitoxin,** is available to provide immediate protection. Tetanus antitoxin is normally reserved for use in unvaccinated horses that have sustained an injury and in newborn foals born to unvaccinated mares.

EQUINE ENCEPHALOMYELITIS (SLEEPING SICKNESS)

In the United States equine encephalomyelitis is caused by either eastern equine encephalomyelitis virus (EEE virus) or western equine encephalomyelitis virus (WEE virus). Venezuelan equine encephalomyelitis (VEE) caused by VEE virus, which occurs in South and Central America, has not been diagnosed in the United States for more than 20 years. All three encephalomyelitis viruses are transmitted from wild birds and rodents (which serve as reservoirs) to horses by mosquitoes and occasionally by other bloodsucking insects. The viruses replicate in internal organs and spread through the blood circulation to infect blood vessels of the nervous system, leading to severe neurologic dysfunction. The mortality rate is high, ranging from approximately 50 percent for WEE to 70–90 percent for EEE and VEE. (*See* CHAPTER 24, "THE NERVOUS SYSTEM AND VARIOUS DISORDERS," and CHAPTER 30, "VIRAL DISEASES.")

Vaccines containing the EEE and WEE viruses provide effective control and are highly recommended for use in all horses residing in areas of the country where the viruses occur. Primary immunization consists of two IM doses of inactivated, combination EEE/WEE vaccine given 3 to 4 weeks apart. Annual booster vaccinations are recommended in the spring, just prior to the peak insect season. (Veterinarians in southern states where mosquitoes remain active year-round often prefer to immunize horses twice a year in order to ensure uniform protection).

Booster vaccination of pregnant mares 4 to 6 weeks before foaling will provide colostral protection for foals for 6 to 7 months. In areas of the country where mosquitoes die off during winter, primary immunization of foals delivered late in the breeding season can be postponed until the next spring. Otherwise, foal vaccinations should begin at 3 to 4 months of age. Foals vaccinated before this should be boosted at 6 months and 1 year to ensure adequate protection.

Although vaccines are available to protect horses against VEE virus, immunization against this agent is not routinely practiced in most areas of the country. The recent outbreak of VEE in southern Mexico, however, has prompted a recommendation that horses living in the southern border country of California, Arizona, New Mexico, and Texas be immunized against VEE virus.

EQUINE INFLUENZA

Equine influenza is one of the most common infectious respiratory diseases of horses. It is a highly contagious viral illness, spreading with lightninglike speed once it has entered a group of horses. Typical signs include fever, lethargy, depression, inappetence, a frequent dry, harsh cough, and a watery nasal discharge that may become cloudy after a few days if secondary bacterial infection develops.

Control of equine influenza is complicated by the fact that immunity following natural infection persists for little more than a year at most. Moreover, influenza viruses are subject to a process of **antigenic drift,** wherein the surface structures of the viruses (which the immune system uses for recognition) are constantly changing in an effort to evade host immune defenses. This reduces the degree and duration of protection conferred by previous infection or vaccination, allowing horses to become susceptible again within a relatively brief span of time. (*See* CHAPTER 30, "VIRAL DISEASES.")

Current influenza virus vaccines, all of which are inactivated and given by the IM route, do not induce an immunity equal to that resulting from natural infection. In addition, federal regulations governing vaccine testing make it an expensive and time-consuming task for vaccine manufacturers to update their vaccines regularly so that they will include the most relevant field strains of virus. Consequently the virus strains found in many influenza vaccines may not be representative of the strains currently in circulation. This can result in a less-than-optimal level of protection and necessitates frequent booster immunizations at intervals as short as 2 to 4 months. (Vaccinating less frequently than this will not prevent infection but can mitigate the severity of clinical signs.)

Vaccination against equine influenza virus is highly recommended for horses having signifi-

cant exposure to horses from outside facilities. The primary series of immunizations involves two IM doses of vaccine 3 to 4 weeks apart. Booster vaccinations should be given thereafter at intervals of 2 to 12 months, depending on the age of the horse, the risk of acquiring influenza virus infection, and the length of time during which the risk of exposure is high. For optimal protection, booster immunizations of young competitive horses should be given at intervals of 3 months, while a broader interval of 4 to 6 months is probably adequate for mature horses over 5 years of age that have been on a regular influenza vaccination program for several years.

Horses not having contact with outside horses except for brief, relatively defined periods may be vaccinated to maximize immunity at the time of likely exposure. For example, horses traveling to shows or other events only during the summer months should receive a booster dose 2 to 4 weeks before transport, with a follow-up booster 3 months later if conditions involving possible exposure are prolonged.

On breeding farms all mature horses should be revaccinated at intervals of 4 to 6 months, with boosters given to pregnant broodmares 4 to 6 weeks before foaling. Foals born to previously exposed but unvaccinated mares will normally be protected by maternal immunity for several months. This immunity may however block a foal's own immune response to influenza virus vaccine given before 6 months of age (*see* above). Thus programs for primary influenza immunization of foals will depend on the vaccination status of the mares and on the risk of exposure.

In foals born to vaccinated mares and kept isolated from contact with outside horses, the primary series of immunizations can be delayed until 6 months of age. Otherwise, primary vaccination should be initiated at 3 to 4 months of age, with boosters given at intervals of 4 to 6 weeks until the foal is 7 months old. Foals born to unvaccinated mares can be vaccinated as early as 1 month of age if the risk of exposure is high; under normal circumstances, however, it is prudent to adhere strictly to manufacturers' directions and begin the primary immunization series at 3 to 6 months of age.

EQUINE HERPESVIRUS (RHINOPNEUMONITIS)

Rhinopneumonitis is now known to represent two separate diseases caused by two different viruses, equine herpesvirus type 1 (EHV–1) and equine herpesvirus type 4 (EHV–4), both of which infect the respiratory tract. Clinical signs range from mild fever and a transient nasal discharge to a more severe influenza-like illness characterized by high fever, inappetence, lethargy, malaise, nasal discharge, and cough. Secondary bacterial infections often occur and can lead to bacterial pneumonia. One of the two viruses, EHV–1, also causes abortion in pregnant mares, birth of weak nonviable foals, and a paralytic neurologic disorder.

As with herpesviruses in other species, equine herpesviruses can remain dormant or **latent** in chronic carrier horses. Chronic carriers do not exhibit clinical signs but excrete virus under stressful circumstances, e.g., weaning, overcrowding, transportation, or concurrent illness. This seriously compromises efforts at control and explains why outbreaks of EHV–1 or EHV–4 can occur in "closed" herds in which no new horses have been introduced. (*See* CHAPTER 24, "THE NERVOUS SYSTEM AND VARIOUS DISORDERS," and CHAPTER 30, "VIRAL DISEASES.")

There are two major indications for vaccination of horses against equine herpesviruses:

- Prevention of EHV–1 abortion in pregnant mares
- Prevention of respiratory disease (**rhinopneumonitis**) in foals, weanlings, yearlings, and young performance and show horses at risk of exposure (owing to high levels of stress and contact with outside horses)

Although the current vaccines do not provide absolute protection, they do apparently modify the incidence and severity of illness and limit the occurrence of abortion outbreaks ("abortion storms"). It is strongly recommended that all pregnant mares be vaccinated during the fifth, seventh, and ninth months of pregnancy using an approved, inactivated EHV–1 vaccine (some veterinarians recommend an additional dose during the third month). Vaccination of mares using an inactivated EHV–1/EHV–4 vaccine at the time of breeding and again a month before foaling is also commonly practiced and recommended. Stallions and barren mares should be boosted before the start of the breeding season and again 6 months later, if not bred or pregnant.

The primary immunization series for foals involves administration of two or three doses of inactivated EHV–1/EHV–4 vaccine, or attenuated EHV–1 vaccine, 4 to 6 weeks apart, beginning at 3 to 5 months of age. Although manufacturers' recommendations specify booster vaccinations at 6- to 12-month intervals, immunity following vaccination appears to be short-lived; as a precaution it is recommended that foals, young horses, and performance or show horses at high risk of exposure be boosted at 3-month intervals instead (as for equine influenza).

The advantages of intensive vaccination programs against EHV–1 and EHV–4 in foals and young horses should always be weighed against the disadvantages. Some veterinarians and horse owners prefer to manage periodic herpesviral respiratory disease rather than subject their young horses to such frequent booster immunizations. Others have found that the incidence of pneumonia in foals and upper respiratory tract infections in yearlings and young horses in training is reduced by intensive vaccination against EHV–1, EHV–4, and equine influenza virus. Combination vaccines containing both influenza virus and the two herpesviruses are convenient for boosting high-risk horses. Frequent booster vaccination of nonpregnant mature horses (except those on breeding farms) with herpesvirus vaccines is generally not indicated.

STRANGLES

Strangles is a highly contagious bacterial disease caused by *Streptococcus equi* and is most often a problem on breeding farms, affecting mainly young horses (weanlings and yearlings). Also known as **distemper**, it is spread by direct contact with affected horses or healthy carriers, or by indirect contact with contaminated materials (water troughs, feed bunks, stalls, pastures, trailers, tack, grooming equipment, etc.). The causative bacterium infects the surface lining of the upper respiratory tract, inducing a severe inflammatory response characterized clinically by a sore throat, pain on eating, and a copious nasal discharge. The organism then spreads to the lymph nodes of the head, jaw, and throat, causing enlargement of the nodes (**lymphadenopathy**) and the formation of **abscesses** (walled-off lesions filled with pus) that drain a creamy white pus onto the skin surface. The enlarged lymph nodes may cause compression of the throat area, resulting in swallowing problems or respiratory difficulties (hence the name "strangles"). (*See* Chapter 31, "Bacterial Diseases.")

Several inactivated vaccines are currently available, but none is completely effective in preventing strangles (although they do reduce the overall incidence and severity of illness in a herd). All strangles vaccines have a tendency to cause reactions at the inoculation site, particularly if given in the neck muscles. As a result vaccination against strangles is not routinely recommended except on certain premises, particularly breeding farms where the disease is a persistent problem, or in individual horses that are being transported to a high-risk facility.

For primary immunization manufacturers' recommendations specify two or three doses be given at intervals of 2 to 4 weeks, followed by an annual booster. In this author's opinion, protection against strangles can be improved by using a three-dose primary series with boosters at 6-month intervals. On breeding farms, efforts should concentrate on preventing infection in foals and weanlings by vaccinating broodmares during the final 4 to 6 weeks of pregnancy, and by initiating the primary series in foals at 3 to 4 months of age, with an additional dose at 6 months or at weaning. Routine strangles vaccination of pleasure or performance horses at low risk of exposure to *Streptococcus equi* is not recommended, except if the risk of exposure is high.

RABIES

Rabies is a disease primarily of bats and carnivores, the latter including the domestic dog and cat. Rabid animals excrete large quantities of rabies virus in their saliva, accounting for the primary means by which the virus is transmitted, i.e., by the bite of an infected animal. For both animals and people, rabies is an inevitably fatal illness once clinical signs have appeared.

Rabies is only infrequently encountered in horses. When it does occur, it is usually the result of a bite from an infected wildlife host. Wildlife species serving as natural reservoirs for infection vary in different regions of North America, and include skunks, raccoons, foxes, badgers, and bats. The bites are most often delivered to the muzzle, face, and lower legs. Following infection the virus migrates up the nerves to the brain, where it causes a rapidly progressive, invariably fatal **encephalitis** (inflammation of the brain). (*See* Chapter 24, "The Nervous System and Various Disorders," Chapter 30, "Viral Diseases," and Appendix A, "Zoonotic Diseases: From Horses to People.")

Horses maintained in rural (particularly wooded) areas where rabies is known to occur in the local wildlife are at risk and should be vaccinated. Several rabies vaccines, all containing inactivated virus for IM injection, are approved for use in horses and appear to be safe and effective. Manufacturers' recommendations specify primary vaccination of horses aged 3 months or older with a single dose of vaccine, followed by a second dose at 1 year of age with annual boosters thereafter. However, this author prefers to begin the primary series by administration of two doses 1 month apart.

Rabies vaccination of pregnant mares is not currently recommended, pending further safety studies of vaccination during pregnancy. Mares should therefore receive their immunizations prior to breeding.

POTOMAC HORSE FEVER

Potomac horse fever, also known as **equine monocytic ehrlichiosis**, is caused by the rickettsial bacterium *Ehrlichia risticii*, which is probably transmitted by ticks. Although it remains most prevalent in the eastern states, particularly near the larger waterways, Potomac horse fever is known to occur in other areas of the United States as well as in Canada and Europe. The incidence of the disease is seasonal, cases occurring between late spring and early autumn in temperate areas with the majority in July, August, and September.

There may be sporadic individual cases or outbreaks involving several horses. Clinical signs include fever, inappetence, depression, reduced or absent intestinal sounds, mild to profuse diarrhea, colic, and dehydration. Twenty to 36 percent of affected horses die or are destroyed because of serious complications. (*See* CHAPTER 31, "BACTERIAL DISEASES.")

Once cases of Potomac horse fever have been verified on a farm or in a particular geographic region, it is likely that cases will continue to occur in subsequent years. Vaccination with one of several available inactivated vaccines is strongly recommended for horses residing in or traveling to such areas. A two-dose primary series administered 3 to 4 weeks apart will produce peak protection 3 to 4 weeks after the second dose. Booster immunizations at 6- to 12-month intervals are usually recommended by vaccine manufacturers; however, a vaccination interval of 6 months or less is recommended in highly affected areas because the protection following vaccination is incomplete and short-lived. (At best 80 percent of vaccinated horses will be protected from most clinical signs, although disease severity and mortality tend to be greatly reduced in those that do become ill).

Vaccination should be timed to precede peak exposure during the summer months (in the midwestern and eastern states) or in autumn, winter, and spring (California coastal foothill areas). Available vaccines have been approved for use in stallions and pregnant mares and can be given one month before foaling. In geographic areas of high incidence foal immunizations should begin at 3 to 4 months of age. Additional doses should be given at monthly intervals up to 5 months of age to ensure that a primary response is achieved, i.e., to avoid blocking of the response by maternal immunity.

BOTULISM

Botulism is a rare disease caused by neurotoxins produced by the spore-forming soil bacterium *Clostridium botulinum*. These neurotoxins are the most potent biological toxins known and act by blocking the transmission of nerve impulses,

resulting in weakness progressing to paralysis, inability to swallow, and often death. Three forms of botulism are seen in horses: *toxicoinfectious botulism* ("**shaker foal syndrome**"), **forage poisoning**, and **wound botulism.** Shaker foal syndrome occurs following ingestion of *Clostridium botulinum* spores and their transformation into mature, toxin-producing bacterial forms in the intestinal tract of **susceptible foals** (foals without sufficient immunity), while forage poisoning results from the ingestion of preformed toxin produced in decaying plant material or animal carcasses. Wound botulism is caused by germination of spores and toxin production in contaminated wounds. (*See* CHAPTER 31, "BACTERIAL DISEASES.")

Of the eight distinct toxins produced by subtypes of *Clostridium botulinum*, types B and C are associated with the majority of botulism outbreaks in horses. A vaccine against *Clostridium botulinum* type B has been approved for immunizing horses in the United States. It is used chiefly to prevent shaker foal syndrome, which is a significant problem in foals between 2 weeks and 8 months of age in Kentucky and the mid-Atlantic region (almost all cases of shaker foal syndrome are caused by type B toxin). For primary immunization in problem areas, pregnant mares should be vaccinated during pregnancy using a series of three doses, each given a month apart, with the final dose 2 to 4 weeks before foaling. The goal is to ensure optimal protection of the foal through maternal immunity. In subsequent pregnancies, mares can be booster-vaccinated with a single dose 1 month before foaling.

Currently there are no vaccines available approved for use in horses to prevent botulism due to *Clostridium botulinum* type C or other toxin types.

EQUINE VIRAL ARTERITIS

Equine viral arteritis (EVA) is characterized by early fetal death or abortion in pregnant mares, and influenza-like signs and swellings of the eyelids, face, limbs, trunk, and genital areas in other horses. Many horses, particularly Standardbreds, may become infected without exhibiting clinical signs. The most important means of spread in breeding stock involves sexual transmission to

Table 1
Suggested Immunization Schedule for Horses[1]

DISEASE	FOALS AND WEANLINGS	YEARLINGS[2]	PERFORMANCE HORSES[2]	PLEASURE HORSES[2]	BROOD MARES	COMMENTS
Tetanus	1st dose: 3–4 months 2nd dose: 4–5 months	Annual	Annual	Annual	Annual, 4–6 weeks before foaling	Conveniently administered in combination with EEE, WEE, influenza, or PHF
Encephalomyelitis (EEE, WEE)	1st dose: 3–4 months 2nd dose: 4–5 months	Annual, in spring	Annual, in spring	Annual, in spring	Annual, 4–6 weeks before foaling	Conveniently administered in combination with tetanus, influenza, or PHF
Influenza	1st dose: 3–6 months 2nd dose: 4–7 months 3rd dose: 5–8 months (see TEXT) Repeat at 3-month intervals	Every 3 months	Every 3 months	Biannual, with added boosters prior to likely exposure	At least biannual, with one booster timed 4–6 weeks before foaling	A series of at least 3 doses is recommended for primary immunization of foals (see text). Use combination vaccines for pre-foaling and spring boosters
Rhinopneumonitis[3] (EHV–1 and EHV–4)	1st dose: 2–3 months 2nd dose: 3–4 months 3rd dose: 4–5 months (see TEXT) Repeat at 3-month intervals	Every 3 months	Every 3 months	Optional; biannual if elected	5th, 7th, 9th months of pregnancy (inactivated EHV–1 vaccine)	If primary series is started before 3 months of age, a 3-dose primary series is necessary. Vaccination of mares pre-breeding and 4–6 weeks pre-foaling with EHV–1 and EHV–4 is also recommended

[1] Recommendations for the major vaccine types used in horses. All horses should be vaccinated against tetanus and encephalomyelitis. Use of other vaccines depends on the individual risk of infection.

[2] Assuming the primary series was completed during foalhood; otherwise, follow label directions for primary immunization.

[3] Stallions and barren mares should follow the same program as brood mares, with biannual rhinopneumonitis booster vaccination substituted for the rhinopneumonitis program recommended for pregnant mares. Products containing EHV–4 may be indicated in foals, weanlings, yearlings, performance horses, and pleasure horses because a large proportion of EHV respiratory infections are caused by EHV–4.

Table 1 (cont.)
Suggested Immunization Schedule for Horses[1]

DISEASE	FOALS AND WEANLINGS	YEARLINGS	PERFOR-MANCE HORSES[2]	PLEASURE HORSES[2]	BROOD MARES	COMMENTS
Rabies	1st dose: 3–4 months 2nd dose: 4–5 months	Annual	Annual	Annual	Annual, before breeding	Rabies vaccination recommended in areas where wildlife rabies is a problem
Strangles	1st dose: 8–12 weeks 2nd dose: 11–15 weeks 3rd dose: 14–18 weeks (depending on product used) 4th dose: weaning (6–8 months)	Biannual	Optional; biannual if risk is high	Optional; biannual if risk is high	Biannual, with one dose timed 4–6 weeks before foaling	Use in conditions or circumstances where risk of exposure is high
Potomac horse fever (PHF)	1st dose: 3–4 months 2nd dose: 4–5 months (*see* TEXT)	Biannual	Biannual	Biannual	Biannual, with one dose timed 4–6 weeks before foaling	PHF vaccination recommended only in known risk areas. Foals from vaccinated mares should be vaccinated at monthly intervals up to 6 months of age to ensure protection

[1] Recommendations for the major vaccine types used in horses. All horses should be vaccinated against tetanus and encephalomyelitis. Use of other vaccines depends on the individual risk of infection.

[2] Assuming the primary series was completed during foalhood; otherwise, follow label directions for primary immunization.

[3] Stallions and barren mares should follow the same program as brood mares, with biannual rhinopneumonitis booster vaccination substituted for the rhinopneumonitis program recommended for pregnant mares. Products containing EHV–4 may be indicated in foals, weanlings, yearlings, performance horses, and pleasure horses because a large proportion of EHV respiratory infections are caused by EHV–4.

mares in the semen of healthy carrier stallions. (*See* CHAPTER 30, "VIRAL DISEASES.")

During outbreaks of EVA in the 1980s, an attenuated EVA vaccine was used to protect mares being bred to carrier stallions and to prevent infection of uninfected stallions. Many countries will not import horses having a positive blood test for antibodies to EVA virus. Because the antibody response resulting from vaccination is indistinguishable from that produced by natural infection, EVA vaccination will complicate blood-testing of horses for export. Vaccination of mares and uninfected stallions before the breeding season is performed only under special circumstances and should be coordinated through the appropriate state and United States Department of Agriculture veterinary officials.

ANTHRAX

Anthrax is a rapidly fatal illness caused by multiplication and spread of the bacterium *Bacillus anthracis* following ingestion of soil-borne spores of the organism. The disease is encountered only in certain geographic regions of the world where soil conditions are favorable for the bacterium's survival. (*See* CHAPTER 31, "BACTERIAL DISEASES.") Because anthrax occurs only rarely in horses and the approved vaccines may be associated with undesirable side-effects, vaccination is practiced only in rare circumstances when horses are pastured in a known contaminated area. A primary series of two doses given 2 to 3 weeks apart followed by annual boosters appears to provide adequate protection.

APPENDIX C
Diagnostic Tests

by Joseph G. Zinkl

Often the veterinarian may recommend that laboratory tests be performed on one or more biological samples obtained from an equine patient. Areas of diagnostic testing that the veterinarian may be interested in include: clinical pathology (including hematology, serum chemistry, urinalysis, and cytology), pathology, microbiology (including bacteriology, parasitology, and virology), immunology, radiology, pharmacology and drug testing, toxicology, and feed nutrient testing. The veterinarian may perform some diagnostic tests in his or her own hospital, but may need to submit some samples to diagnostic laboratories having the more sophisticated equipment required for certain assays. In most respects these diagnostic laboratories utilize the same equipment as laboratories processing human samples submitted by physicians. Although laboratories that handle primarily human samples have the equipment, techology, and personnel to perform such tests, laboratories that deal exclusively with veterinary samples offer several advantages:

- Veterinary diagnostic laboratories are usually under the direction of a veterinary clinical pathologist with advanced training in animal diagnostics.
- The technologists working in these laboratories usually have special expertise in animal diagnostics.
- Besides providing accurate information and efficient service, veterinary diagnostic laboratories provide expert consultation service.

There are many reasons for performing laboratory tests. Veterinarians most often use such tests to make or confirm a clinical diagnosis. The results of laboratory tests may also alter the veterinarian's approach to the treatment of an ill horse by suggesting a new, different, or additional diagnosis. Laboratory tests can be used to gauge the success of therapy and to detect complications arising from therapy. Laboratory tests can aid the veterinarian in assessing the health of an apparently normal horse during routine physical examination or pre-sale soundness examination. Sometimes, laboratory tests are required by regulatory agencies so that horses may be transported from one location to another, particularly for interstate shipment. Laboratory tests may be required by equine registry groups for verifying the parentage of foals. Results of laboratory tests can also be used to determine if an equine athlete has any abnormality that may detrimentally affect performance. In some cases, tests for certain drugs that may alter performance are required by agencies in charge of equine athletic events. Finally, it may be necessary in certain situations to test for natural or man-made poisons.

Hematology

Hematology is the study of blood and the blood-forming organs. The most common hematologic test is the **hemogram**, also known as a **complete blood count** or **CBC**. A CBC is performed on blood that is withdrawn from a vein and placed in a vial containing a substance (an **anticoagulant**) that prevents the blood from clotting. In horses, the jugular vein located on the lower side of the neck is usually the vein from which blood samples are obtained. A CBC provides information on red blood cells (**erythrocytes**), white blood cells (**leukocytes**), and blood **platelets** (cells important for blood clotting), as well as certain components of *plasma*, the fluid portion of the blood.

Red Blood Cell Parameters
The red blood cells (**RBCs**) are small disk-shaped cells containing the red pigment **hemoglobin**, which is responsible for transporting oxygen from the lungs to the tissues. The total number of RBCs, their hemoglobin content, and the percentage of total blood volume (**packed cell volume** or **PCV**; also called the **hematocrit**) they occupy are included in the CBC report. In general, RBC counts, hemoglobin concentrations, and PCVs are higher in light-breed horses used for sport and transportation (so-called "hot-blooded" horses) than in heavy-breed working horses ("cold-blooded" horses, draft horses) used for traction.

The RBC parameters are most useful for the detection and diagnosis of **anemia** (low RBC count, reduced PCV, or reduced hemoglobin levels). Many diseases can cause anemia. Severe anemia can be life-threatening, but mild anemia may not be recognized in horses kept as pets (the performance of anemic working or athletic horses will be affected significantly, however). Injuries in which large amounts of blood are lost also result in anemia. Horses may suffer internal blood loss into the intestines or body cavities. Horses poisoned by certain **rodenticides** (rodent poisons) that prevent the blood from clotting may bleed sufficiently to develop anemia. Some parasites also can cause anemia. Equine infectious anemia virus, a retrovirus that produces a lifelong infection in horses, causes an anemia that can recur at periodic intervals for years. Many chronic illnesses such as strangles and internal abscesses cause relatively minor anemias that probably contribute to the malaise affected horses often exhibit.

The RBC parameters are also used to evaluate the fitness of performance horses. Elevated RBC counts, hemoglobin concentrations, and PCVs are often found in horses well trained for short-duration events such as track racing. Conversely, lower levels may be found in fit horses used for long-term activities such as endurance racing or trail riding.

White Blood Cell Parameters
White blood cells (**WBCs**) or leukocytes are larger than RBCs and are responsible for fighting infection. WBCs thus represent an essential component of the immune system. Five different types of WBCs are enumerated in the CBC by total cell counts and by the percentages of the different cells present (*differential WBC count*): *neutrophils, lymphocytes, monocytes, eosinophils*, and *basophils*. These cells have many functions. Neutrophils and monocytes kill and digest bacteria, fungi, other infectious agents, and foreign debris. Lymphocytes produce *antibodies* (specialized proteins that bind to foreign material and alert immune cells to its presence) and act in other ways to maintain the immune system. Eosinophils and basophils play important roles in inflammatory and allergic conditions.

An increase in the number of neutrophils in

the blood is found in inflammatory or infectious diseases. As the horse overcomes an infection, the neutrophil count decreases. Some severe conditions, particularly inflammatory diseases of the intestinal tract, may produce extremely low leukocyte counts involving especially neutrophils and lymphocytes.

Lymphocyte counts may be increased in horses that are producing large quantities of antibody. Young horses in general have higher lymphocyte counts than do older horses, perhaps because they are actively manufacturing antibodies to organisms in their environment. Lymphocyte counts are decreased in foals with severe combined immune deficiency (**SCID** or **CID**), an inherited disease of Arabians and some other breeds. *Leukemia* occasionally occurs in horses, and can be diagnosed by finding the cancerous leukocytes in the blood. Leukemia involving lymphocytes is the most frequently diagnosed form of equine leukemia. (*See* Chapter 34, "Cancer.")

OTHER PARAMETERS

The CBC also contains a platelet count and fibrinogen concentration. Platelets are the smallest cells in the blood. They respond very rapidly to injuries that cause bleeding, by adhering to ruptured blood vessel walls and helping form a seal or **clot**. This is done with the aid of several other noncellular blood constituents, one of which is **fibrinogen**, a clotting factor that is converted into its active form (**fibrin**) by an enzyme called **thrombin**. Decreases in either the platelet count or fibrinogen concentration indicate that a horse may not be capable of preventing hemorrhage should it be traumatized. Other substances important for clotting may be tested for in order to detect inherited clotting conditions such as hemophilia or to diagnose poisoning by some rodenticide poisons that cause bleeding.

The *plasma protein* concentration is also reported on the CBC. This parameter is helpful for evaluating a horse's hydration, immune, and nutritional status.

Serum Chemistry

Serum chemistry tests are often performed on horses. For these tests the liquid portion of the blood, either **serum** (plasma minus fibrinogen) or plasma, is separated from the blood cells, and the concentrations of various substances and activities of certain enzymes in the fluid are determined. Often the veterinarian will have the laboratory run a panel of serum chemistry tests in which several results are determined on a single sample. Such a screening procedure is used to evaluate the function and integrity of many different organs and tissues, such as the liver, kidneys, muscles, lungs, and some of the **endocrine** (hormone-producing) organs.

Sometimes, individual tests or small panels of tests are run in order to evaluate specific tissues or organs, or to obtain information on the severity of a particular disease condition. The severity of muscle damage as well as how rapidly a horse is recovering from an injury can be evaluated by measuring levels of the serum enzymes *aspartate transferase (AST)* and *creatine kinase (CK)*. Kidney damage may be indicated when a horse's *blood urea nitrogen (BUN)*, *creatinine*, and *calcium* concentrations are increased. Liver disease is suggested when there is an increase in *bilirubin* (a yellow bile pigment, representing a breakdown product of recycled hemoglobin from RBCs) and increased activity of the enzymes *alkaline phosphatase (ALP)*, *gamma glutamyl transferase (GGT)*, and AST. Reproductive hormone analyses are used to determine the stage of the estrous cycle in broodmares, to evaluate reproductive failure in mares and stallions, and to determine if a mare is pregnant. These latter tests are most useful when they are used in conjunction with other reproductive examination procedures.

Urinalysis

Laboratory evaluation of urine is known as **urinalysis**. Urinalysis provides information on the urinary tract (kidneys, ureters, bladder, and urethra), and may also be useful for assessing conditions affecting other body systems. Urine from horses with properly functioning kidneys usually has a cloudy appearance, owing to the presence of calcium carbonate crystals (which form because horses normally excrete calcium and bicarbonate through the kidneys). The ability of the kidneys to regulate water balance is determined by measuring the urine **specific gravity,** an estimate of how concentrated or dilute a urine sample is. Because the kidneys must function properly to produce highly concentrated urine when fluid intake is low (for water conservation) and, conversely, must also allow for the elimination of surplus fluid by making the urine very dilute, measurement of urine specific gravity can provide an evaluation of kidney function.

Infection and inflammation of the urinary bladder can be evaluated by examining a small amount of urine *sediment* through a microscope. The sediment is obtained by **centrifuging** (spinning at high speed) a urine sample in a tube and collecting the material that is pelleted out at the bottom of the tube. In cases of **cystitis** (inflammation of the urinary bladder), white blood cells and bacteria may be identified in the sediment. When evidence of infection of the urinary tract is discovered, the urine is usually cultured (*see* "Microbiology" below) in order to isolate and identify the causative bacterium so that appropriate antibiotic therapy can be administered.

Equine athletes suffering significant muscle damage may have darkly-colored urine. A test to determine if the urine contains **myoglobin**, the respiratory pigment of muscles, can be used to confirm that muscle damage has occurred.

Cytology

The microscopic evaluation of fluid or tissue smears, known as *cytology*, can be useful for determining the cause of many lesions or diseases. Frequently the material submitted for examination has been **aspirated** from the tissue or body cavity in question by drawing it through a fine-gauge needle into a syringe (**fine-needle aspirate** or **aspiration smear**). This procedure offers fairly rapid results and is often the preferred routine screening test for preliminary or definitive identification of inflammatory, infected, or cancerous lesions.

Analysis of abdominal fluid obtained from horses with colic can be useful for determining the cause and severity of the colic, and often helps the veterinarian and owner come to a decision regarding medical or surgical treatment. Samples from the respiratory tract, including tracheal and bronchial washes and fluid obtained from the chest cavity, can aid in determining the cause of a pneumonia and whether a horse has developed **pleuritis** (inflammation of the **pleura**, the thin transparent membrane covering the lungs and lining the inside of the chest cavity). Infection of the uterus, a frequent cause of reproductive failure in mares, can be evaluated by microscopic examination of fluid taken from the uterus. Samples from the joints are used to determine if lesions in the joints are the cause of lameness. Bacterial culture of the fluid is often performed in order to identify the underlying cause and initiate specific therapy.

Microscopic evaluation of fluids and tissues is useful for the diagnosis of cancer. Horses may develop a number of different cancers, including melanoma, malignant lymphoma, squamous cell carcinoma, and several types of leukemia (*see* Chapter 34, "Cancer"). Malignant lymphoma may arise in lymph nodes or in the chest and/or abdominal cavities. Melanoma can occur in the skin and is particularly prevalent in gray horses. It may **metastasize** (spread) to the lymph nodes and body cavities. Squamous cell carcinomas can arise in the skin, penis, or stomach. Samples from bone marrow are examined to diagnose some leukemias. Smears of samples taken from these different tissues thus are useful for diagnosing these and other cancers. Generally, a veterinary clinical pathologist with special training in cytology is asked to evaluate these types of smears.

Parasitology

A fecal examination is frequently performed to determine if a horse is carrying intestinal parasites, and occasionally to identify parasites such as lungworms that may be present in other body tissues. Horses can become infected with a variety of different parasites. The most important intestinal parasites of horses are the nematode worms known as *strongyles*. During their migration through the tissues, strongyles can produce lesions in the walls of abdominal arteries—lesions that can lead to intestinal injury and severe colic. Veterinarians often examine feces for parasites in order to help owners develop effective antiparasite programs, which usually include the timely administration of **anthelmintics** (deworming medications) and implementation of grazing practices that minimize exposure to the infective forms of the various parasites. (*See* Chapter 33, "Internal Parasites.")

Microbiology

Bacterial infections are often diagnosed by a combination of methods involving the microscopic examination of fluids or tissues, and culture of microorganisms on agar plates or in various microbiological broths. Usually, a small amount of the material to be cultured is smeared onto a glass microscope slide and stained with **Gram stain**, a routine stain used for the laboratory identification of bacteria. A Gram stain is performed to determine the shape, size, and staining characteristics of the organisms(s) under study. The veterinarian may initiate antibiotic therapy based on this early, tentative identification, but may modify this therapy once an absolute identification of the bacterium and its antibiotic sensitivity can be made (*see* below).

Laboratory culture of bacteria entails mixing or inoculating a specimen onto a solid (**agar**) or liquid (**broth**) medium, which contains special ingredients either to enhance or inhibit the growth of certain types of organisms. The growth characteristics of the organisms found after 24–48 hours of incubation allow for a more exact identification. Bacterial colonies grown on solid media are identified on the basis of their size, shape, color, and other characteristics. Cultures are often incubated both **aerobically** (in the presence of oxygen) and **anaerobically** (in the absence of oxygen) to determine if the organism requires oxygen for growth. Special media can be used to determine other metabolic characteristics of the organisms as well.

In addition to culture for the purpose of identification, *antibiotic sensitivity testing* can be performed to determine the effect of different antibiotics on the growth of the bacterium involved. If it is found that the organism is resis-

tant to the antibiotic initially chosen for therapy, a more appropriate selection can then be made based on the results of the sensitivity testing.

Virology

Viruses can be identified in several ways. Because most viruses are too small to be seen through a light microscope it is necessary to use an electron microscope to view them. Considerable time and effort are required to process tissues or other material for electron microscopy. Occasionally it is necessary to visualize a virus in the electron microscope in order to identify and classify it. Far more commonly, viruses are identified by **isolating** (growing) them in *cell cultures* in the laboratory. Cell cultures are composed of sheets of cells of various types, that are grown in plastic or glass containers. Some viruses can be isolated in several different cell culture types, while others are more fastidious and require very specific cells and conditions for growth. Identification is often made on the basis of the physical appearance of the virus by electron microscopy, characteristics of its growth in cell culture, and inhibition of growth by specific antibodies.

Virus isolation is an expensive and time-consuming procedure, and far too impractical for routine use in private veterinary hospitals. Many commercial, governmental, and university veterinary diagnostic facilities, however, are equipped to handle samples for virus isolation.

Immunology

The techniques of immunology are employed in many of the diagnostic disciplines. The serum of newborn foals is often tested to determine if a sufficient amount of antibody has been transferred from the mare through the **colostrum** ("first milk"). Relatively rapid tests are available for this, but actual quantitation of the antibody requires more elaborate methods. Quantitation of antibody is also used to diagnose severe combined immune deficiency syndrome (SCID, CID) of Arabian and other foals. Sometimes antibody quantitation is used to determine if a horse has a chronic infectious disorder, such as the fungal disease *coccidiomycosis* ("valley fever"), or a rare cancer of plasma cells called *multiple myeloma*. (*See* CHAPTER 29, "THE IMMUNE SYSTEM AND VARIOUS DISORDERS.")

Immunologic methods are often used to determine if a horse has been exposed to a specific infectious disease agent or to an **allergen** (substance inducing allergic reaction). The *Coggins test*, for example, is used to detect antibodies to equine infectious anemia (EIA) virus (*see* CHAPTER 30, "VIRAL DISEASES"). A positive Coggins test in an adult horse indicates that the horse has been exposed to EIA virus and is probably a carrier. Other tests are available for detecting antibodies to a host of other disease agents as well.

Sometimes the veterinarian may draw two blood samples at an interval of 2–4 weeks in order to determine if amount of antibody to a particular disease agent has increased during the interval. The finding of such a rising **titer** (antibody level) to a particular agent suggests that the horse has responded immunologically to it, implying that a recent infection with that agent has occurred.

Genetic Testing

Immunologic methods can be used for blood typing and serum protein identification. Some horse registries require that the blood type and serum protein profile of a newborn foal be compared to those of the alleged parents in order to verify parentage. While the results of these tests do not provide absolute proof of specific parentage, they rule out so many possibilities that the chances of a mistaken identification are rare. Blood typing is also used to select the most appropriate blood donor to use for a transfusion.

Neonatal isoerythrolysis (NI; hemolytic disease of the newborn) is a condition similar to the *Rh syndrome* of human babies. It develops when a mare with antibodies to a surface component of her foal's RBCs transfers those antibodies in her colostrum to the foal. The result is destruction of the foal's RBCs. The RBC surface component is inherited from the stallion. Usually the mare develops antibodies to it when blood from a previous fetus accidentally reaches her tissues or blood. Blood typing of the mare and stallion and tests to detect antibodies to stallion or foal RBC surface components can aid in predicting whether a foal will develop NI. If the tests suggest that NI is a possibility, the owner and veterinarian can be prepared to prevent the newborn from nursing (and thus ingesting the antibodies) by muzzling the foal for about 48 hours. The foal can be given frozen, stored colostrum from a mare free of the damaging antibodies. The veterinarian may also be able to give the foal transfusions of compatible blood or initiate total blood exchange using blood of the appropriate type. Knowledge of the blood type of mares and stallions can be used to select matings that will decrease the risk of NI. (*See* CHAPTER 14, "CONGENITAL AND INHERITED DISORDERS," and CHAPTER 29, "THE IMMUNE SYSTEM AND VARIOUS DISORDERS.")

Technology involving *deoxyribonucleic acid (DNA)*, the genetic material of living organisms, is now being used for parentage identification and for diagnosing certain inherited diseases. Detection of genes that code for inherited disorders is now in use in human beings. Recently, the first test to detect the gene for *hyperkalemic periodic paralysis (HYPP)* in Quarter Horses has been developed (*see* CHAPTER 14, "CONGENITAL AND INHERITED DISORDERS"). This and other laboratory tests detecting genes causing inherited disorders will undoubtedly become more widely available in the coming years.

Radiology, Ultrasonography, and Endoscopy

Radiographs or X rays are taken by exposing special photographic films to X rays that pass from an X-ray machine through an animal's body and strike the film emulsion. Many veterinarians practicing equine medicine have portable radiographic equipment for farm calls, and large-animal veterinary hospitals have stationary equipment for taking radiographs. Generally, portable machines are limited to radiographing limbs and joints because they do not have the power of stationary equipment. Radiographs produce a rather detailed black-and-white image of bones and soft tissue. Fractures of bones, pneumonia, increased fluid in tissues, inflammation of joints and tissue, tumors, and displaced organs can be detected by an examination of radiographs.

Recently, **ultrasonography** (*diagnostic ultrasound*) has become an important diagnostic tool for veterinarians. Ultrasonography detects objects by recording sounds that are passed into the body and then "echoed" back by organs and tissues. Diagnostic ultrasound is particularly useful for diagnosing pregnancy, tumors, and foreign bodies in the intestinal tract, and for evaluating heart function.

Endoscopy is used to visualize internal body parts directly, through the use of specialized lighting and magnification devices housed within rigid or flexible tubes (**endoscopes**). Endoscopes can be inserted and guided into such areas as the nasal cavity, trachea, or accessible regions of the gastrointestinal tract such as the stomach. Endoscopy is particularly useful for locating lesions and obtaining samples for culture, cytology, or biopsy.

Toxicology

A great number of tests can be used to identify poisons. For some poisons the tests are relatively simple and can be performed in a small laboratory; other tests, however, require sophisticated and expensive equipment.

Heavy metals such as lead are poisonous to horses, and their detection in blood, urine, or tissues is used, along with the history and clinical features, to diagnose lead poisoning. Pesticides, particularly *organophosphate* and *carbamate* insecticides, are also toxic. Confirmation of the diagnosis usually requires documentation of decreased *acetylcholinesterase* activity in serum, blood, or brain tissue. Because there are many organophosphate and carbamate insecticides, determining the specific insecticide responsible for an incident requires identification of the chemical in stomach contents, tissues, or feed.

Horses may be poisoned by rodenticides that act on the blood-clotting mechanism. Horses may accidentally ingest rodenticides because the poisons are often formulated in a grain bait. Diagnosis of anticoagulant poisoning can be made by documenting prolonged blood-clotting times. Elaborate methods are required to identify the specific rodenticide involved.

Horses may ingest poisonous plants found in pastures or feed. Often veterinarians or other specialists are able to identify the plants in pastures or portions of the plants in hay. However, when the plants are incorporated into pellets or cubes, laboratory tests may be needed to detect the toxic substance(s). Poisonous plants can produce a constellation of clinical signs and affect many body tissues. For example, oleander causes heart problems, *pyrrolizidine alkaloids* such as those found in tansy ragwort, fiddleneck, and some other plants cause liver degeneration, and yellow star thistle causes softening and liquefaction of specific areas of the brain. (*See* CHAPTER 41, "POISONOUS PLANTS.")

Pharmacology and Drug Testing

Horses competing in athletic events are frequently tested for drugs that may alter their performance. Urine or blood must be collected by certified personnel and placed in special containers. A regular "chain of possession" must be maintained from the time of collection until the samples are analyzed at the laboratory. Often samples are divided at the laboratory, one portion being stored for analysis at a later date, if necessary, to settle disputes or to confirm results. Laboratories that perform these types of tests are under the jurisdiction of regulatory agencies and are mandated to implement quality-assurance programs. Occasionally, "spiked" samples are submitted in a blind fashion in order to run an independent check on results. In addition, divided samples may be run independently and the separate analyses compared for accuracy.

Nutrition Testing

Nutrient analyses are occasionally run on feed samples. Most frequently the mineral content is assessed to determine if there is a need to supplement a horse with certain **trace minerals** (minerals that are required in the diet in very minute amounts) (*see* CHAPTER 6, "EQUINE

NUTRITIONAL REQUIREMENTS"). A few tests are run on blood samples to detect deficiencies of certain nutrients, e.g., decreased *glutathione peroxidase* activity in RBCs suggests a deficiency of selenium. Vitamin B_1 (**thiamine**) deficiency can be detected by another test run on RBCs. Many laboratories perform these and other nutrition tests. Some tests are run by feed companies, while others are performed by agricultural agencies of the government, such as the United States Department of Agriculture (USDA), or by private testing laboratories.

Transporting Horses

by Barbara L. Smith

In this highly mobile age, transport is nearly a way of life for horses that breed, show, or compete in athletic events. Fortunately most horses adapt well to transport. For some, however, being moved from one place to another can be a very stressful event. Factors in the transport environment that can contribute to stress include confinement, the motion of the trailer, withholding of food and/or water, separation from the herd, and exposure to unfamiliar horses. Horses stressed by transport are more susceptible to a variety of diseases, particularly pneumonia, colic, diarrhea, and **laminitis** (founder)—not to mention acute injuries caused by frantic behavior within the trailer. Not only are these problems costly in terms of medical care and lost revenue, but they also reduce the quality of life for an afflicted horse. Thus it is important for horses' own welfare that the stresses of transport be minimized.

What Constitutes Stress?

An animal is stressed when it is required to make abnormal or extreme adjustments in phys-iology or behavior in order to cope with adverse aspects of its environment or method of management. Stress has no discrete or common cause, nor is there a precise way to measure it. Relatively little is actually known about managing horses during transport in order to reduce stress. Most of the available information is anecdotal, with little or no scientific evidence to validate the opinions expressed. There are no regulations in the United States governing the interior intrastate transport of horses by road; thus owners are left with little but their own common sense when managing the transport of their horses.

How Do Horses Adapt to Transport?

As with any other change in environment, horses must be given time to become accustomed to a new mode of transport. There are many makes and models of transport vehicles for horses, ranging from one-horse trailers to 12-horse commercial vans. A horse that has been transported only in large commercial vehicles will likely have a very different experience if transported in a smaller two-horse trailer. Becoming accustomed to the new mode of transport may involve several sessions of loading and unloading with the unfamiliar trailer until the procedures can be performed quietly and without a struggle. Once this has been accomplished the horse can be transported for increasing lengths of time, beginning with very short trips and incrementally lengthening them as the horse adapts. The length of time required for a horse to adjust to a transport environment is highly variable, depending on the horse's age, behavior, health status, and previous transport experiences. The ideal time to adapt a horse to transport is before weaning.

TRANQUILIZERS

Tranquilizing a horse prior to loading or transport is generally not recommended, particularly for lengthy distances, because some horses become more excited when exposed to a stressful situation while tranquilized. Transport is an athletic effort for horses that requires continuous foot movements to maintain balance, and using tranquilizers may result in incoordination. Tranquilizers may also interfere with a horse's ability to regulate its body temperature, so their use should be particularly avoided during extremes in environmental temperatures. The exception to this rule would be a horse experiencing severe pain (i.e., colic) that requires sedation to minimize suffering during transport to a veterinary facility. Tranquilizers administered in low doses can be used to relieve the anxiety or apprehension associated with loading or traveling for short distances, however.

DRIVING

A careless driver can make even the quietest horse a nervous or even frantic traveler. Rapid accelerations, decelerations, and turns should be avoided, as the horse often does not have time to adjust its stance to balance itself. Taking a ride in the trailer will allow a driver to appreciate good driving habits, and also demonstrate how dramatically movements and the roughness of the road are amplified in the back of the trailer. Placing a glass of water on the dashboard of the towing vehicle is one good way for the driver to monitor the smoothness of accelerations, decelerations, and turns.

TEMPERATURE INSIDE VERSUS OUTSIDE THE TRAILER

On hot days (temperatures greater than 32°C or 90°F) it is important not to keep horses in a trailer for long periods after loading when the trailer is not moving. Temperatures within a loaded trailer usually average 5–8°C (10–15°F) higher than the outside ambient temperature. If prolonged stops are unavoidable during transport, the trailer should be parked in a shady location and/or the horses unloaded.

How Do Horses Respond to Transport?

FACE FORWARD OR BACKWARD?

Because rapid deceleration (braking) often cannot be avoided, it has been proposed that horses may prefer traveling with the head facing away from the direction of travel, i.e., toward the back of the trailer. The rationale for this theory is that horses traveling face forward must carry the head and neck in uncomfortable and, therefore, stressful positions in order to balance themselves, particularly during rapid decelerations. Moreover, they must balance their hindquarters in an unnatural position by standing with their hind limbs splayed out. Were horses facing the rear of the trailer instead of the front, presumably they could balance themselves more comfortably.

Research conducted at the University of California, Davis, has shown that although many (but not all) horses selected rear-facing transport when given the choice, some persistently preferred to face forward. Nevertheless, heart rates (an indicator of excitement, associated with stress) when horses were transported face forward were not statistically different from heart rates during rear-facing transport. These studies concluded that horses were not measurably less stressed when forced to travel in the direction they preferred to face (i.e., backward) than when forced to travel facing forward.

It is possible that a horse that does not travel comfortably and quietly when facing forward may travel more quietly when allowed to face rearward. Conventional two-horse trailers are not designed for rear-facing travel, because the axles do not properly balance the redistributed weight. Stock trailers are often suitable for horses preferring rear-facing transport, and usually are large enough for horses to turn around comfortably when loose inside. Rear-facing two-horse trailers are also available for use.

HEALTH STATUS

A horse in good physical condition will be much less likely to succumb to transport-associated illness than a horse with an obvious or even **subclinical** (not exhibiting clinical signs) illness. Studies have demonstrated that horses recently exposed to a respiratory virus prior to transport are more likely to develop pneumonia after transport. Prior to lengthy travel, horses should be examined by a veterinarian to assess their health status. (Such an examination is *required* prior to issuing a health certificate for interstate transport.) Horses with obvious or even subtle illness should not be transported until recovery is complete, with the obvious exception of horses requiring transport to a veterinary facility for emergency care.

Management During Transport

FEEDING AND WATERING

There are no data available concerning feeding and watering practices during transport. Most owners provide their horses with hay to eat while being transported, particularly when traveling long distances. Because it is difficult to provide water continuously, it may be necessary to stop periodically to offer water. Horses often will not drink water from unfamiliar sources, so if at all possible the water should be taken along. The frequency of stops depends on the horse's age, health status, and environmental conditions. Horses may require more frequent watering stops on hotter days. Some horses normally do not eat or drink at all while traveling, and they will need to be monitored closely during and after the trip for any signs of illness.

FREQUENCY OF REST STOPS

There is no available information about frequency or duration of rest stops during long-distance travel. The interval between rest stops and the duration of stops are often left to the driver's discretion. Many people feel it is important to unload horses periodically to allow them to stretch their limbs. There is probably no harm in this, but whether or not it is necessary for the health of the horses is unknown. Stopping trailer movement periodically will however give horses a rest from the constant weight-shifting they must perform in order to maintain balance during transport.

Transporting Horses Under Special Circumstances

TRANSPORTING MARES WITH FOALS

Many foals will follow their dam into the trailer with little or no struggle. The mare should be tied inside the trailer, with the center partition of the trailer removed so that the foal may nurse, move around, or lie down comfortably.

TRANSPORTING STALLIONS

Stallions should be transported alone whenever possible. If this is not feasible, the stallion should be loaded first and unloaded last. If it is necessary to transport a stallion with mares, rubbing Vicks Vaporub® on the stallion's nostrils will prevent it from smelling the mares. There should be a solid partition between the stallion and the other horses.

TRANSPORTING HORSES WITH FRACTURED LIMBS

A major objective in transporting a horse with a fractured limb is to avoid causing further damage to the leg. This is accomplished by minimizing the need for the horse to use the fractured limb. Prior to loading, the fractured limb should be properly **splinted** (have a bracing apparatus placed over the fractured area to prevent movement of the broken pieces). To minimize the distance the horse must walk on the injured limb, the transport vehicle should be brought to the horse.

Horses with forelimb fractures should be transported facing the rear of the trailer, so that the weight of the body is supported by the two sound rear limbs during rapid decelerations. Standard forward-facing two-horse trailers cannot be utilized for rear-facing travel, so if a rear-facing trailer or van is not available, a stock trailer should be equipped with a rigid partition before loading the injured horse. Horses with hindlimb fractures should be loaded facing forward for the same reason.

During transport the injured horse should be strictly confined with chest and rump bars, with partitions to squeeze the horse into as small a space as possible. This allows the patient to lean on the partitions for added support to maintain balance, resulting in less dependence on the injured limb. Transporting the horse without partitions may cause it to inflict trauma on the already injured leg as the animal tries to balance itself. If possible the horse's head should be tied very loosely, so the horse may use its head to help balance itself (confining the head may result in increased body sway). Foals with limb fractures should be transported with the dam and with an attendant, if possible.

TRANSPORTING PREGNANT MARES

Stress has been suggested as a cause of early pregnancy loss in mares, owing to fluctuations in blood hormone levels. However, it has been shown that the incidence of early embryonic death in pregnant mares (up to 38 days of pregnancy) is not different between transported mares and nontransported mares. No data are available on pregnancy loss due to transport in later-term mares.

Suggestions for Safe Transport of Horses

Listed below are several factors to keep in mind when transporting horses by road:

- Before loading, closely inspect the trailer for tire wear and damage and rotted or loose floorboards. Trailer lights, safety chains, and brakes should also be inspected. Wheel bearings should be checked at least once a year, especially if the trailer is in heavy use.
- Always bring one extra halter and lead rope for each horse transported. Leather halters are easily broken if a horse pulls back forcibly, so the spare halter should be made of nylon.
- Emergency equipment may come in useful; it should include bandaging material, a flashlight, extra feed and water, extra buckets, wire cutters, knife, twitch, and jumper cables.
- A citizen's-band radio or cellular telephone is handy and somewhat comforting to have in the towing vehicle when traveling, for use in an emergency, particularly if the driver is traveling without an assistant.
- Be sure the ground around the truck and trailer is safe for loading and unloading.
- When loading an inexperienced horse, lead the horse into the trailer from the opposite side of the partition, i.e., when loading a horse into the left side, lead it on the right side, and vice versa. If possible, train the horse to enter the trailer without need of a person leading it inside. If someone must lead the horse into the trailer, be sure that the escape door is open in case a quick exit is necessary.
- When hauling a single horse, place it on the left side of the trailer.
- Secure the rump bar or chain before tying the horse inside. When unloading, untie the horse before opening the back of the trailer.
- Tie the horse with a quick-release knot. The rope should be loose enough to allow the horse to use its head for balance, but not loose enough for it to become tangled.
- During rest stops, remove manure from the trailer. This will help minimize the horse's exposure to bacteria, particulates, and manure gases within the trailer. Bedding the trailer with shavings or straw should be avoided because this may increase the amount of dust a horse breathes in during transport.
- Be sure the trailer is well ventilated. Good ventilation may help minimize the threat of respiratory disease in transported horses.
- Avoid sudden starts, stops, and turns while driving.

Glossary

Compiled by Jeffrey E. Barlough

abiotrophy. Progressive loss of function of a tissue or organ.

abnormal host. A host infected with a parasite normally found in another host species.

abscess. A walled-off lesion filled with pus.

acariasis. General term for a mite infestation.

accommodation. Ability of the lens to change its shape in order to focus vision effectively on objects at different distances from the eye.

acetabulum. The "cup" or "socket" portion of the hip joint.

acetylcholine (ACh). Messenger molecule released from axon terminals by a nerve impulse; responsible for transmission of the nerve impulse across the *synaptic cleft* to the muscle fiber supplied by the nerve.

acetylcholinesterase. Enzyme capable of breaking down acetylcholine.

acidosis. Systemic condition characterized by abnormally acid blood.

actin. A vital protein component of muscle, one of the proteins responsible for muscle contraction.

actinic keratoses. Single or multiple, firm, elevated, plaque- or papulelike skin lesions that result from excessive exposure to sunlight; considered to be precancerous lesions.

actinomycosis. Pus-producing diseases caused by bacteria of the genus *Actinomyces*.

active immunization. Vaccination.

acute. Of short duration and relatively severe; having a rapid onset.

Addison's disease. Hypoadrenocorticism; insufficient secretory activity by the adrenal cortex.

adenocarcinoma. Any malignant tumor originating in glandular tissue.

adenoma. Any benign tumor originating in glandular tissue.

adenosine triphosphate (ATP). The major form of energy used by cells in the body.

adhesion. A fusion or sticking together of surfaces.

adipsia. The absence of thirst; avoidance of drinking.

adjuvant. Substance that nonspecifically stimulates immune responses; used in inactivated vaccines to prolong the immune response to vaccine components.

adjuvant chemotherapy. Use of anticancer drugs following surgical or radiation treatments in an effort to destroy residual (microscopic) tumor cells that may have been left behind.

adrenal cortex. The outer layer of the adrenal glands.

adrenal glands. Glands located adjacent to the kidneys, involved in the secretion of several important hormones including cortisol, corticosterone, aldosterone, and epinephrine (adrenaline).

adrenaline (epinephrine). A hormone secreted by the adrenal glands; it acts to increase blood sugar levels and blood pressure and to accelerate the heart rate.

adrenocorticotropic hormone (ACTH). A hormone produced by the pituitary gland in the brain; it exerts a controlling function over the cortex (external portion) of the adrenal glands.

adsorb. To bind to a surface.

adulticide. Medication to kill adult worms.

aerobic. Requiring the presence of oxygen to grow.

aerosol exposure. Exposure to an infectious agent by means of contaminated moisture droplets drifting in the air.

aerosol therapy. Treatment in which drug therapy (antibiotic or other compound) is delivered by misting or spraying the drug into the airways, usually by means of a funnel or cone placed over the nose; useful in treating pneumonia and certain other respiratory ailments. Also called *nebulization*.

African horse sickness. Acute, severe to mild, insect-transmitted disease characterized by fever and signs of cardiac or pulmonary insufficiency; caused by an orbivirus in the Reoviridae family of RNA viruses.

alanine aminotransferase (ALT, SGPT). A liver-cell enzyme; increased levels in the bloodstream are indicative of liver-cell injury.

albumin. A major protein component of the blood plasma, important in maintaining osmotic pressure within the blood vasculature and as a transport protein for many substances.

aldosterone. A hormone secreted by the adrenal cortex; important in the regulation of sodium and potassium levels and, in turn, in retaining water within the body.

algae (singular: alga). Single-celled organisms that include seaweed, many fresh-water plants, and certain opportunistic pathogens such as *Prototheca*.

allele. An alternative form of a given gene. For each gene there are two alleles, one on each chromosome of a chromosome pair. One allele is inherited from the mother, the other from the father.

allergen. Any substance that can induce an allergic reaction.

allergenic. Inducing allergy.

allergic bronchitis. Allergic inflammation of the bronchi.

allergic contact dermatitis. An uncommon skin disease caused by a hypersensitivity reaction, as occurs in hikers and backpackers following contact with poison ivy or poison oak.

allergy. A hypersensitive state of the immune response, wherein exposure to a particular substance (an allergen) results in a noxious and sometimes physically harmful immunologic response.

allograft. Tissue graft obtained from an individual of the same species as the recipient.

alopecia. Absence or loss of hair.

alveoli (singular: alveolus). Small air sacs comprising the innermost structure of the lungs. It is through the delicate walls of the alveoli that gas exchange occurs between the blood (flowing through the pulmonary capillaries) and the inhaled or exhaled air.

ambulatory. Involving locomotion; able to walk.

amino acids. Nitrogen-containing molecules that form the structural backbone of proteins. All amino acids contain both an amino group (NH_2) and a carboxyl group (COOH).

ammonia. A waste product of protein metabolism; normally excreted through the kidneys.

amnion. The placental membrane immediately surrounding the foal.

amylase. Enzyme produced by the salivary glands and pancreas that breaks down carbohydrates.

amyloid. An insoluble protein substance that causes disease (amyloidosis) when deposited in large quantities in tissues.

amyloidosis. Disease process characterized by deposition of amyloid in various tissues of the body, including the kidneys.

anabolism. The body's conversion of simple substances to more complex compounds.

anaerobic. Able to grow in the absence of oxygen.

anagen. The phase of hair follicle activity during which hair is actively being produced.

analgesics. Pain-killing medications.

anal sphincter. The circular band or ring of muscle that controls the release of feces from the anus.

anamnestic response. Immunologic memory; the ability of the immune system to "remember" a foreign substance to which it has been exposed, and to produce an even more effective response to it upon subsequent reexposure.

anaphylactic reaction (anaphylaxis). A rapidly developing, exaggerated (and sometimes life-threatening) allergic reaction.

anatomy. The study of body structure.

androgen. Male sex hormone; e.g., testosterone.

anemia. Low red blood cell count, reduced hemoglobin levels, or reduced volume of packed red cells.

anestrus. The sexually inactive period between two estrus cycles.

angioedema. Recurrent wheals or welts in the skin, caused by dilation and/or increased permeability of capillaries.

angiography. The radiographic visualization of blood vessels, accomplished by the intravenous injection of a contrast medium that allows the shape and course of the vessels to be delineated on X-ray examination.

angiosarcoma. Tumor of blood or lymphatic vessels.

ankyloblepharon. Failure of one or both eyelids of the newborn to open at the appropriate time.

ankylosis. The immobility and consolidation of a joint, secondary to trauma, infection, or surgery.

annular ligaments. Ligaments that function to maintain tendon alignment where the tendons cross a joint.

anorectic. Having no appetite.

anorexia. Loss of appetite; inappetence.

antemortem. Before death.

anterior chamber. The fluid-filled space at the front of the eye, situated between the cornea and the iris.

anterior uvea. The iris and ciliary body of the eye.

anterior uveitis. Inflammation of the iris and ciliary body of the eye.

anthelmintic. Any deworming medication.

anthrax. A rapidly fatal illness caused by multiplication and spread of the bacterium *Bacillus anthracis* following ingestion of the bacterial spores.

antibiotic. A chemical substance produced by microorganisms that is capable of inhibiting or killing other microorganisms; many antibiotics are used medically for the treatment of serious bacterial infections. Examples of antibiotics include penicillin, tetracycline, and gentamicin.

antibiotic sensitivity testing. Laboratory test procedure for identifying the sensitivity or resistance of a bacterial isolate to several antibiotics.

antibodies (immunoglobulins). Specialized proteins produced by cells of the immune system in response to the presence of foreign material (bacteria, viruses, toxins, etc.); antibodies are capable of binding to the foreign material and thus alerting other immune cells to its presence.

anticoagulant. Chemical that prevents blood from clotting.

antidiuretic hormone (ADH). Pituitary gland hormone that controls water resorption by the kidneys, urine production and concentration, and water balance; also called *vasopressin*.

antiemetics. Medications for controlling vomiting.

antifungal. A chemical substance produced by microorganisms or by other means, useful in the treatment of fungal infections.

antigen. A substance capable of inducing a specific immune response in the body, by binding to a specific antibody; can be a property of bacteria, viruses, other foreign proteins, or even host tissue cells.

antigenic. Having the properties of an antigen.

antimicrobial. Killing or suppressing the growth of microorganisms; also, any antibiotic or antifungal medication.

antinuclear antibody (ANA) test. Test that detects autoantibodies against the DNA of cell nuclei; used as an aid in the diagnosis of systemic lupus erythematosus (SLE, lupus).

antioxidants. Substances such as vitamin E and selenium that protect cells against damage caused by by-products of normal metabolic processes.

antiserum. Serum that contains high levels of antibodies specific for a particular antigen of interest.

antispasmodics. Medications to prevent spasms of the gastrointestinal tract.

antitussives. Cough suppressants.

anuria. Complete cessation of urine production.

aorta. The great vessel arising from the left ventricle of the heart, that feeds blood through the arterial system into the body.

aortic stenosis. Constriction (abnormal narrowing) of the connection between the left ventricle and the aorta.

aortic valve. The semilunar valve on the left side of the heart; also called the *aortic semilunar outflow valve*.

aplasia. Imperfect development or absence of a tissue or organ.

apnea. Cessation of breathing.

apocrine cyst. Cyst caused by obstruction of a sweat gland.

apocrine sweat glands. Sweat glands that empty their contents into an associated hair follicle.

appendicular skeleton. That portion of the skeleton composed of the bones forming the limbs and pelvis.

aqueous humor. The fluid occupying the anterior and posterior chambers of the eye.

Arabian fading syndrome. Juvenile Arabian leukoderma.

arachidonic acid. An essential fatty acid found in animal fats; a precursor in the biosynthesis of compounds such as the prostaglandins.

arborize. To branch.

area centralis. Specialized area of the retina, near the optic disc, that possesses an abundance of cone photoreceptors and is largely responsible for the most precise and accurate vision.

argasid ticks. Soft-bodied ticks; distinguished from *ixodid* (hard-bodied) ticks.

arrhythmia. Any abnormal irregularity of the heartbeat caused by an electrical disorder in the heart.

arteries. Thick, muscular vessels that drive oxygenated blood from the heart toward the tissues.

arterioles. Small arteries.

arteritis. Inflammation of an artery.

arthritis. Joint inflammation.

arthropathy. Any joint disease.

arthropod. An invertebrate organism with a hard outer skeleton (exoskeleton) and a segmented body; examples include insects, spiders, and crustaceans.

arthroscopic surgery. Surgery using a tubular instrument (*arthroscope*) for examining and carrying out surgical procedures within a joint, without the need for an extensive incision.

arthrospores. Infective units of the filamentous mold form of the fungal pathogen *Coccidioides immitis*, the cause of coccidioidomycosis ("valley fever").

articular cartilage. Cartilage found within joint structures.

articulate. To connect at a movable joint.

ascariasis. Any ascarid infestation.

ascarid. A type of roundworm.

ascites. The accumulation of fluid within the abdominal cavity.

ascorbic acid. Vitamin C.

aspartate aminotransferase (AST, SGOT). A liver-cell enzyme that is also found in muscle cells and red blood cells.

aspermogenesis. Failure to produce sperm.

asphyxia. Suffocation.

aspirate. The removal of fluid from a tissue or cavity by means of a syringe and needle.

aspiration pneumonia. Pneumonia caused by accidental inhalation of food or other material into the lungs.

aspiration smear. Diagnostic procedure in which fluid, containing cells, is withdrawn from a tissue or body cavity and then smeared onto a glass microscope slide for examination.

asymptomatic. Not exhibiting clinical signs.

ataxia. Incoordination.

atherosclerosis. Vascular disease associated with high blood pressure and high cholesterol and fats in people; exceptionally rare in animals.

atopic dermatitis. Heritable hypersensitivity to pollens or other environmental allergens, which results clinically in immunologic and inflammatory reactions in the skin.

atopy. An inherited predisposition toward the development of allergy.

atresia. Congenital absence or occlusion of an orifice or tubular organ.

atrial fibrillation. Arrhythmia characterized by irregular, disorganized, chaotic changes in the electrical activity of the upper chambers of the heart, resulting in abnormal contractions.

atrial septal defect. Rare congenital defect characterized by the presence of a hole in the wall or *septum* separating the left and right atria of the heart.

atrioventricular (AV) node. The heart region electrically connecting the atria and ventricles; it slows the conduction of the depolarization wave so that a short period of time is interposed between atrial and ventricular contractions.

atrioventricular (AV) valves. The heart valves that separate each atrium from its corresponding ventricle. The AV valve on the right side of the heart is known as the *tricuspid* valve, and the corresponding valve on the left side is called the *mitral* valve.

atrium (plural: atria). One of the two upper chambers of the heart.

atrophy. Shrinking or wasting of a tissue or organ.

atropine. An alkaloid drug that relaxes smooth muscle, increases the heart rate, and in the eye causes dilation of the pupil.

auditory ossicles. Tiny bones in the middle ear that are responsible for transmitting the vibrations of the eardrum to the inner ear.

aural flat warts (aural plaques). Skin warts found on the ears of horses greater than a year of age; caused by a papillomavirus.

auscult, auscultate. To listen to the inner sounds of the chest or abdomen with the aid of a stethoscope.

autoanalyzers. Automated equipment for performing serum chemistry panels.

autoantibody. An antibody directed against "self," i.e., against the body.

autoimmune response. An inappropriate immune response, directed against the body's own tissues.

autonomic nervous system. That part of the nervous system involved in the regulation of the heartbeat, glandular secretions, and smooth muscle contraction and relaxation, and generally not subject to conscious control.

autonomously. Uncontrollably.

autosomal. Referring to any of the chromosomes excluding the sex chromosomes.

aversion conditioning. Learned avoidance of unpleasant situations, such as an encounter with an electric fence.

avidin. A constituent protein of egg whites that can impair absorption of the vitamin *biotin*.

avulsion. A pulling or tearing away.

axial skeleton. That portion of the skeleton composed of the skull, vertebrae, ribs, and *sternum* (breastbone).

axillary nodular necrosis. Uncommon, sporadic skin disease characterized by the development of nodules in the *axillary* region ("armpit").

axon. The fingerlike extension of a nerve cell, along which the nerve impulse travels.

axon terminals. Branchings of a nerve axon within muscle, forming neuromuscular junctions with the myofibers supplied by the nerve.

azotemia. An elevation of blood urea nitrogen (BUN) and creatinine levels in the bloodstream.

azoturia. Presence of excessive quantities of nitrogen waste products in the urine, caused by the excessive breakdown of muscle tissue.

B lymphocytes (B cells). Lymphocytes that upon proper stimulation by an antigen transform into plasma cells, which produce antibody to the antigen.

babesiosis. Any of several diseases caused by protozoa of the genus *Babesia*.

Bacillus Calmette-Guerin (BCG). A live, avirulent bacterial cell preparation of the bovine tuberculosis organism, *Mycobacterium bovis*; useful for immunizing people against tuberculosis and for nonspecifically stimulating the immune system.

bacteremia. Presence of bacteria in the bloodstream.

bacteria (singular: bacterium). Minute, single-celled organisms ubiquitous in the environment; they contain a cell wall and a nucleus lacking a delimiting membrane, and divide by *binary fission* (the parental cell dividing into two approximately equal daughter cells).

bacterial endocarditis. Inflammation of the lining of the heart, caused by bacterial infection of one or more heart valves.

bacterin. Any killed bacterial vaccine.

bacteriology. The study of bacteria.

balanitis. Inflammation of the penis.

balanoposthitis. Inflammation of the penis and prepuce.

barium. Metallic element commonly used as a contrast medium in radiology, particularly useful for examining disorders of the gastrointestinal tract. The barium is first swallowed by the patient and X-ray films are then taken. The general structure and movements of the gastrointestinal tract become visible owing to the inability of the X-ray beam to penetrate the contrast medium.

basal cell layer. The bottom cell layer of the *epidermis* (the outermost layer of the skin).

basal cell tumor. Benign tumor of basal cells, present in the basal cell layer of the *epidermis* (the outermost layer of the skin).

basidiobolomycosis. A form of phycomycosis caused by *Basidiobolus*; occurs only rarely in the United States.

basophil. A specialized white blood cell containing histamine and serotonin.

basophilic. Staining dark blue.

"bastard" strangles. In strangles, formation of abscesses in areas other than the head and neck.

bean. Common term for *urethral diverticular concretion*.

Bence-Jones proteins. Immunoglobulins or immunoglobulin fragments detected in blood and sometimes urine in patients with multiple myeloma.

benign. Not malignant; a tumor that is not cancerous (i.e., will not spread).

beta blockers. Drugs that block beta-adrenergic nerve impulses; important in treating *tachycardias* (abnormally rapid heart rates).

beta cells. Cells within the islets of Langerhans in the endocrine pancreas; they are the source of the hormone *insulin*.

bicipital bursitis. Inflammation of the *bicipital bursa*, located underneath the biceps tendon.

big head. Colloquial term for nutritional secondary hyperparathyroidism.

bilateral. Occurring on both sides.

bilaterally symmetrical. Occurring simultaneously in approximately the same place on each side of the body.

bile. Fluid produced by the liver and deposited in the

small intestine through the bile ducts, for the purpose of aiding the digestion of nutrients.

bile acids. Steroid acids made from cholesterol, they are components of bile.

bile duct. Duct that discharges digestive fluids (*bile*) from the liver into the small intestine.

bilirubin. A yellow bile pigment, a breakdown product of recycled hemoglobin from red blood cells; the pigment causing jaundice.

binary fission. Method of bacterial and protozoal multiplication wherein the parental cell divides into two approximately equal daughter cells.

binocular fixation. The ability, particularly well developed in primates, to focus both eyes on a single object.

biological response modifiers. Substances such as the interferons and the interleukins that modify immune responses.

biological vector. A vector in which a developmental stage of a particular parasite necessarily occurs.

biopsy. The procedure by which a small sample of tissue is obtained for microscopic examination or culture, for the purpose of making a medical diagnosis.

blastocyst. An early stage of the developing embryo.

blepharitis. Inflammatory disease of the eyelids.

blepharospasm. Spasm of the eyelid musculature, causing squinting.

blind spot. That portion of the visual field behind the line of sight, that cannot be seen without changing eye and head position.

blind staggers. Common name for *leukoencephalomalacia*.

bloat. Distension of the stomach.

blood. The fluid and its component cells, that circulate through the blood vessels and carry oxygen and other nutrients to body cells.

blood plasma. The liquid fraction of the blood (as opposed to blood cells).

blood smear. A thin layer of blood smeared on a glass slide, stained, and viewed under a microscope; used to identify the maturity and type of blood cells present and to detect any abnormalities of those cells.

blood-typing. Laboratory procedure by which the red blood cells in a blood sample are identified as belonging to one of several blood groups.

blood urea nitrogen (BUN). A measure of the nitrogenous waste products circulating in the blood; elevated levels are usually indicative of kidney malfunction.

blood vessels. Arteries, arterioles, veins, venules, capillaries: the conduits for the transport of blood throughout the body.

bog spavin. Chronic swelling of the upper joint of the hock; most commonly caused by *osteochondritis dissecans (OCD)*.

boil. A deep-seated bacterial infection of a hair follicle, producing a painful skin nodule containing pus; also called a *furuncle*.

bone marrow. The soft inner tissue of bones, containing the blood-forming elements (precursor cells of the red and white blood cells and blood platelets) of the circulatory system.

bone plating. Method of fracture repair wherein the bone fragments are replaced in their original location and held in place with a perforated metal plate (*bone plate*), which is attached to the fragments with small screws.

bone spavin. Degenerative arthritis of the lower joints of the hocks; the most common cause of hindlimb lameness in horses.

bony orbit. The bones of the skull that house and protect the eyeball.

booster. Any dose of vaccine given subsequent to the initial dose, or subsequent to natural exposure, and designed to maintain the immune state or improve it.

borborygmus. Gurgling noises caused by the rapid movement of gas through the intestines.

Borna disease. Rare, highly fatal disease of horses and sheep in Germany and Switzerland; caused by an RNA virus that thus far has proved extremely difficult to characterize or classify.

botryomycosis. Type of wound infection caused by *Staphylococcus aureus* that occurs following trauma; common sites include the lower extremities and scrotum.

bots. The larvae of hairy, beelike flies of the genus *Gasterophilus*; they are often found in the stomach of the horse.

botulinal toxin. The neurotoxin produced in botulism.

botulism. A rare disease caused by a neurotoxin produced by the bacterium *Clostridium botulinum*; it targets the neuromuscular nerve endings, producing a flaccid paralysis.

brachygnathism. Condition wherein the lower jaw is shorter than the upper jaw, placing the lower incisor teeth farther behind the upper incisor teeth.

brachytherapy. Radiation therapy technique wherein a radioactive device is inserted into a tumor and left in place for a period of time, during which the radiation slowly kills the tumor cells.

bradycardia. Abnormally slow heart rate.

bradyzoites. Dormant, encysted forms of the parasite *Toxoplasma gondii*.

brain stem. Portion of the brain containing nerve centers that control the heart rate, respiratory rate and pattern, and level of consciousness.

bran disease. Generalized disorder caused primarily by a deficiency of calcium in the diet in the face of a phosphorus excess.

breakdown injury. Rupture of the suspensory apparatus, i.e., loss of one or more supporting structures of the fetlock.

breech presentation. Birth in which the fetus is delivered rear-end first.

broken wind. Common name for *chronic obstructive pulmonary disease*.

bronchi. The larger air passages leading from the trachea and branching within the lungs.

bronchioles. Smaller branches of air passages leading from the bronchi to the alveoli (the small air sacs within the lungs, through the walls of which gas exchange between the blood and air occurs).

bronchoconstriction. Narrowing of the larger airways.

bronchodilators. Drugs that cause expansion of vital airways in the lungs, allowing for improved respiration.

bronchopneumonia. Lung inflammation that is initiated within the bronchioles.

bronchoscopy. Endoscopic examination of the trachea and bronchi.

bucked shins. Painful condition caused by inflammation and hemorrhage over the front surface of the cannon bone; a common injury of 2- and 3-year-old race horses.

budding. Form of asexual reproduction in certain protozoa wherein a dividing cell divides into two unequal parts, the larger part being considered the parent and the smaller one the bud.

bulbourethral glands. Glands that produce the fluid portion of the semen.

bulla. A large vesicle.

bullous pemphigoid. A very rare autoimmune skin disease characterized by the production of autoantibodies and the development of vesicles and bullae beneath the epidermis.

buphthalmos. Gross enlargement of the eyeball.

bursa. Fluid-filled sac or saclike cavity, situated over pressure points in tissues where friction from repeated movement might develop.

bursitis. Inflammation of a bursa.

buttress foot. An advanced form of degenerative arthritis, caused by new bone growth in the region of the extensor process of the coffin bone.

cachexia. Seriously poor health; malnutrition and wasting.

caesarean section. Delivery of a fetus by surgically removing it from the uterus.

calcaneus. Heel bone.

calcification centers. Areas of bone deposit and change within bone tissue.

calcitonin. A calcium-regulating hormone produced by the thyroid gland.

calcium channel blockers. Drugs useful in treating *tachycardias* (abnormally rapid heart rates).

calculus (plural: calculi). Dental *tartar*, the mineralized concretions of salivary calcium and phosphorus salts and tooth-surface plaque; also, a urinary stone.

calculogenic. Stone-forming.

calorie. Unit defined as the amount of energy needed to raise the temperature of 1 gram of water 1 degree Celsius (centigrade). However, the larger *kilocalorie* is usually referred to as a "calorie" in the nonscientific community.

cancellous bone. Bone tissue having a spongy or latticelike internal structure; an example is the bone marrow.

cancer. The general term for any malignant tumor.

candidiasis. A relatively uncommon infection of skin and mucous membranes of the oral cavity, respiratory tract, and genital area of horses, caused by yeast of the genus *Candida*.

canker. Chronic overgrowth of the horn-producing tissues of the foot, occurring most commonly in horses housed under unsanitary conditions.

cannon bone. The third metacarpal bone, above the fetlock joint.

cannon keratosis. Seborrhea affecting the front surface of the rear cannon bone.

cannula. A tube inserted into a duct or body cavity, for the purpose either of infusing or removing fluid.

cantharidin. The toxin in blister beetles responsible for blister beetle poisoning in horses.

capillaries. The smallest blood vessels. They permeate the tissues, serving as microscopic extensions of arterioles and venules; through their semipermeable walls, fluids, nutrients, and waste gases are exchanged between the blood and the tissues.

capped hock. Traumatic bursitis over the point of the hock, usually caused by the horse's kicking a solid structure.

caps. Remnants of deciduous premolar teeth that are left behind when the permanent premolars erupt.

carbuncle. A deep-seated skin infection containing many pockets of pus.

carcinogen. Any cancer-causing substance, such as asbestos, nickel, alcohol, or tobacco.

carcinoma. A cancer (malignant tumor) of epithelial cells.

cardiac. Pertaining to the heart.

cardiac arrest. Cessation of the heartbeat.

cardiac catheterization. The passing of a catheter through a peripheral blood vessel and inside the heart, either for diagnostic or therapeutic purposes.

cardiac insufficiency. Heart failure.

cardiac muscle. Specialized type of muscle found only in the heart.

cardiac tamponade. Acute compression of the heart, caused by filling of the pericardial sac with fluid or blood.

cardiac ultrasound. Examination of the heart by means of ultrasonic sound waves, for the purpose of disease diagnosis; also known as *echocardiography*.

cardiogenic shock. Shock caused by a diseased heart that has become so dysfunctional that it can no longer pump sufficient blood to the body.

cardiomyopathy. Enlargement of the heart, caused either by a thickening or thinning of the heart muscle.

cardiopulmonary bypass. Open-heart surgery wherein a heart-lung machine oxygenates and pumps blood while the heart is stopped.

cardiovascular system. The heart and blood vessels of the body.

carnivores. Meat eaters.

carpal canal syndrome. Annular ligament constriction on the back side of the carpus, causing lameness.

cartilage. Specialized connective tissue especially important in bone growth and the formation of joints.

Caslick's operation. Surgical procedure to decrease the aspiration of air and contaminants into the female reproductive tract.

castration. Surgical removal of the testes; sterilization of the male.

casts. Solid, tubular deposits in the urine, usually cast off from the walls of kidney tubules.

catabolism. The body's breakdown of complex molecules, such as protein and fat, to simpler compounds.

cataract. Lens opacity in the eye, affecting vision.

catecholamines. Compounds secreted by the adrenal medulla, the most notable of which is epinephrine (adrenaline).

cathartics. Drugs to induce evacuation of the bowel.

catheter. A flexible tubular instrument for insertion into a blood vessel or body cavity.

cauda equina. The nerve roots at the termination of the spinal cord.

caudal. To the rear of; toward the tail.

cecum. The first segment of the large intestine, consisting of a large dilated pouch.

cell. The most basic functioning unit of living organisms, composed of a nucleus, cytoplasm, organelles, and other constituents. Cells are the fundamental building blocks of tissues and in their nuclei contain all the genetic information necessary for the growth and differentiation of a complete organism.

cellular differentiation. The process by which cells mature into specialized, fully functioning units.

cellular (cell-mediated) immune response. The mounting of a cytotoxic T cell/macrophage/natural killer (NK) cell immune response to an antigen.

cellulitis. Diffuse inflammation resulting from (usually bacterial) infection of deep connective tissue, sometimes forming an abscess.

cementum. Specialized type of connective tissue that covers the tooth roots.

central nervous system (CNS). The brain and spinal cord.

centrifuge. To spin in order to separate the light and heavier particulates in a fluid sample; a machine for performing this procedure.

cercaria. Tadpolelike larval form of flukes that arises from the *redia* stage.

cerebellar abiotrophy. Inherited disorder seen in some Arabian family lines, characterized by a progressive loss of neurons in the cerebellum.

cerebellar hypoplasia. Underdevelopment of the cerebellum, manifested clinically by incoordination.

cerebellum. Portion of the brain concerned with motor function, balance, and the coordination of movement.

cerebrospinal fluid (CSF). Fluid bathing the surfaces of the brain and spinal cord.

cerebrum. Portion of the brain concerned with conscious thought, perceptions, and learned skills.

ceruminous glands. Glands that produce the waxy coating of the ear canal.

cervical. Pertaining to the neck.

cervical spondylosis. Degenerative and proliferative disease of the neck vertebrae.

cervix. Oval-shaped mass in the female reproductive tract whose opening connects the uterus with the vagina.

cestocidal. Able to kill tapeworms.

cestodes. Tapeworms; internal parasites having a head unit (*scolex*) and numerous body segments (*proglottids*).

cheekteeth. General term for the premolar and molar teeth.

chemosis. Excessive swelling of the conjunctiva (membranes covering the inner surface of the eyelids).

choke. Physical obstruction of the esophagus.

choline. A B vitamin important for proper function of the nervous system and for preventing fat deposition in the liver.

chondroids. Pus in the guttural pouch that, over time, has becomed thickened into variously sized, cheesy concretions.

chondrosarcoma. A malignant tumor of cartilage.

chorioretinitis. Inflammation of the choroid and retina of the eye.

choroid. Thin, pigmented middle layer of the eye containing nerves and blood vessels; it supplies blood to the retina.

chromosomes. The very large and complex molecules of DNA that occur in the nucleus of every cell and that carry the genetic information needed to make every protein in the body.

chronic. Long-term; of lengthy duration; persisting over a long period.

chronic carrier state. Situation in which an animal or human being maintains (carries) an infectious disease agent for a prolonged period of time.

chronic interstitial nephritis. Chronic, progressive destruction of the kidneys, marked by a reduction in kidney size and scarring of kidney tissue.

chronic obstructive pulmonary disease (COPD). Term referring to a number of conditions leading to chronic or recurrent obstruction of airflow within the lung; also called *heaves* or *broken wind*.

chronic pharyngeal lymphoid hyperplasia (CPLH). An abnormal increase in size of the lymphocyte-rich tissues lining the pharynx, analogous to *tonsillitis* of children; also referred to as *chronic pharyngitis* or *follicular pharyngitis*.

cicatrization. Scar-tissue formation.

cilia (singular: cilium). Minute, hairlike cellular processes lining much of the respiratory tract; their rhythmic beating movements, in concert with an overlying layer of mucus, effect removal of debris and other foreign material from the airways.

ciliary body. The circular muscle located directly behind the iris of the eye.

cirrhosis. Liver disease characterized by replacement of functioning liver cells by scar tissue.

classical conditioning. The association between a stimulus and a response.

cleft palate. Birth defect characterized by an abnormal connection between the oral cavity and the nasal cavity; as a result, small amounts of milk often may be seen dripping from the nostrils when the foal suckles.

clitoris. Small mound of erectile tissue in the female reproductive tract; the female analog of the male penis.

club foot. In horses, a flexural deformity of the coffin joint resulting in a raised heel; not to be confused with the club foot deformity of human beings.

coagulation. Blood clotting.

cobalamin. Cobalt-containing component of vitamin B_{12}.

coccidioidomycosis. The main systemic fungal infection of importance in horses in the United States, characterized by chronic weight loss, persistent coughing, musculoskeletal and/or abdominal pain, intermittent fever, and superficial abscesses; caused by *Coccidioides immitis*.

cochlea. Curled bone in the inner ear which contains the *organ of Corti*, the actual organ of hearing.

codominant alleles. Genes wherein both members of an allelic pair are fully expressed.

coffin bone. The *distal phalanx* or toe of the forelimb, incorporated within the hoof.

Coggins test. Test for detection of antibody to equine infectious anemia (EIA) virus.

coitus. Sexual intercourse.

colic. Acute abdominal pain.

colitis. Inflammation of the large bowel (colon); contrasts with *enteritis* (inflammation of the small intestine).

collagen. Protein constituent of connective tissue.

coloboma. A defect of any tissue of the eye.

colon. The portion of the large intestine connecting the cecum (lowermost portion of the small intestine) with the rectum.

colonoscopy. Endoscopic examination of the colon.

color flow Doppler echocardiography. Technique using sound waves to examine the direction and velocity of blood flow within the heart and great vessels, allowing the cardiologist to observe directly the regions of abnormal blood flow that develop in association with most common cardiac abnormalities.

colostrum ("first milk"). Milk produced by the mare during the first day or two after the birth of her foal; it is high in protein and protective antibodies (maternal immunity).

coma. Unconsciousness from which one cannot be aroused.

comatose. Unconscious and unable to be aroused.

comminuted fracture. Fracture in which the affected bone is broken or crushed into small fragments.

commissure of the lips. The corner of the mouth.

complement system. A specialized series of blood proteins whose major role is to disrupt the surface structure of microbes and altered body cells, resulting in their destruction.

complete blood count (CBC). Blood analysis containing an enumeration of the number of red and white blood cells per unit of blood volume, the proportions of the different white blood cell types, and the amount of hemoglobin present.

compound fracture. Fracture that breaks through the skin; open fracture.

computerized axial tomography (CAT scan). Highly specialized diagnostic X-ray technique that produces cross-sectional images of the inside of the body.

concentrates. Rich sources of individual nutrients that are used to enhance the quality of the diet.

conceptus. Embryo or fetus plus the accompanying extraembryonic membranes.

concussion. A violent blow to the head, usually resulting in the loss of consciousness.

cones. Photoreceptor cells in the retina of the eye that are responsible for color vision and visual acuity.

conformation. The overall physical appearance of a horse, reflecting the arrangement of muscle, bone, and other body tissues.

congenital. Present at birth.

congenital hypotrichosis. Hairlessness.

congenital stationary night blindness. An hereditary abnormality of vision affecting Appaloosas.

congenital testicular hypoplasia. Underdevelopment of the testicles.

congestive heart failure. Syndrome caused by the inadequate pumping of blood by the heart.

conidiobolomycosis. A form of phycomycosis caused by *Conidiobolus coronatus*, characterized by a thick nasal discharge, coughing, respiratory difficulty, and halitosis (bad breath).

conjunctiva. Mucous membrane lining the eyelids and covering the white surface (*sclera*) of the eyball.

conjunctivitis. Inflammation of the conjunctiva.

connective tissue. A general term encompassing the different types of supportive tissues that hold together many body structures.

constitutional signs. Generalized clinical signs, such as inappetence, lethargy, weight loss.

contagious equine metritis. Highly contagious disease characterized by inflammation of the female genital tract and production of a thin, profuse, grayish-white discharge from the vulva; caused by a bacterium, *Taylorella equigenitallium*.

continuous heart murmur. A murmur that is present during both contraction and relaxation of heart muscle.

contracted tendons. A developmental orthopedic disease of foals, associated with rapid growth rates and high planes of nutrition.

contralateral. On the opposite side.

contusion. A bruise.

convulsions. Seizures.

Coombs' test. An immunologic procedure for the detection of autoantibody attached to red blood cells; also called an *antiglobulin test*; important in disease diagnosis as well as in cross-matching blood samples for transfusion purposes.

coprophagy. The eating of feces.

cor pulmonale. Disease of the right side of the heart caused by increased pressure within the pulmonary artery.

coracidium. Free-swimming larval form of pseudophyllidean tapeworms.

core biopsy. Biopsy obtained from an awake patient using local anesthesia and a specialized small-bore biopsy needle.

cornea. The transparent outer coat of the eye.

cornified. Converted into hardened tissue; *keratinized*.

corns. Chronic lesions found in the sole of the foot, at the angle formed by the wall and the bar of the sole.

cornstalk disease. Common name for *leukoencephalomalacia*.

coronary band. Ring of vascular tissue along the upper edge of the hoof wall from which the horn of the hoof grows.

coronitis. Inflammation of the coronary band.

corpora nigra. A row of dark protuberances normally present along the upper border of the equine iris; also called *granula iridica*.

corpus luteum (plural: corpora lutea). Ovarian follicle after discharge of the *ovum* (egg); it secretes the hormone *progesterone*.

cortex. Outer layer of an organ (kidney, adrenal gland, brain) or hair shaft; contrasted with *medulla*.

corticosteroids. Steroid hormones (cortisol, corticosterone, etc.) produced by the cortex of the adrenal gland. Corticosteroids elevate blood sugar, increase fat and protein breakdown, and exert an anti-inflammatory effect on conditions such as arthritis and dermatitis.

corticosterone. A corticosteroid hormone.

cortisol. A corticosteroid hormone.

cortisone. A corticosteroid hormone (a precursor of cortisol) found in small quantities in the adrenal cortex.

cranial. Toward the head; pertaining to the head.

cranial nerves. Nerves originating largely in the brain stem that control the facial muscles and certain specialized activities of the head (sight, smell, hearing).

creatine kinase (CK). A muscle-specific enzyme found in serum; determination of CK levels represents a useful tool for the diagnosis of muscle disorders.

creatinine. Nitrogen-containing compound generated from the breakdown of ingested proteins.

creep feed. Feed provided in a separate area where the foal can eat without interference from the mare.

cremaster muscle. Muscle that suspends the testicle.

cribbing. A stable vice in which the horse places its upper teeth on the edge of a feeder or fence, arches its neck, inhales, and often produces a grunt or belching sound.

cross-match. Procedure by which blood samples from donor and recipient are tested before blood transfusion, in order to determine compatibility.

cross-ties. Fixed lines attached to each side of the halter.

croup. Hindquarters; area between the hips and the point of the buttocks.

crown. The portion of a tooth that lies above the gum line.

cryogen. Any substance, such as liquid nitrogen, used to produce extreme cold during *cryosurgery.*

cryosurgery. A procedure by which local application of intense cold (freezing) is used to destroy unwanted tissue.

cryptorchidism. Developmental defect wherein one or both of the testicles has not descended into the scrotum.

cryptosporidiosis. Diarrheal disease of debilitated or immunodeficient foals, caused by a protozoan, *Cryptosporidium parvum.*

Culicoides hypersensitivity. Allergic skin disease caused by the bites of midges of the genus *Culicoides*; also known as *Queensland itch* and *sweet itch.*

cunean bursitis. Inflammation of the *cunean bursa* underneath the *cunean tendon*, which travels over the front and inside of the hock.

curb. Inflammation and thickening of the plantar ligament (the ligament that courses along the back of the *calcaneus* bone in the hock).

Cushing's disease. Hyperactivity of the adrenal cortex, representing the most common endocrine disorder of horses.

cusps. The sharp points of the tooth crown.

cutaneous. Pertaining to the skin.

cutaneous habronemiasis. A skin disease of horses caused by stomach worms (*Habronema* spp.); also called *summer sores.*

cutaneous horns. Projections of hardened skin.

cutaneous onchocerciasis. Skin disease caused by *Onchocerca cervicalis*, a threadworm that 'ives in the nuchal ligament of the neck.

cuticle. The outermost layer of a hair shaft; also, the thick, noncellular covering on the surface of a roundworm (*nematode*) parasite.

cyanocobalamin. Vitamin B_{12}.

cyanosis. A bluish discoloration of the skin and mucous membranes, resulting ultimately from a deficiency of oxygen in the blood.

cyst. Simple, saclike cavity that can develop in any of a number of different body tissues; it usually contains fluid or a semisolid, cheesy or doughy material.

cystadenoma. A benign tumor of cystic and glandular structures.

cystitis. Inflammation of the urinary bladder, often occurring secondary to diseases causing incomplete emptying of the bladder.

cytokines. "Messenger molecules" by which cells of the immune system signal and instruct one another; the interferons and the interleukins are examples.

cytologic examination, cytology. The microscopic examination of cells obtained by scraping, aspiration, or biopsy, for the purpose of disease diagnosis.

cytoplasm. Cell protoplasm; the fluid and particulates within a cell, exclusive of the cell nucleus.

cytotoxic. Harmful to cells.

cytotoxic T cells. T lymphocytes that are responsible for tracking down and eliminating altered or infected body cells.

deciduous teeth. "Milk teeth," the temporary teeth that are lost to make way for the permanent teeth.

definitive host. Host in or on which a parasite reaches sexual maturity or undergoes sexual reproduction.

degenerative joint disease. Term for a group of disorders resulting in progressive deterioration of the articular cartilage of a joint, accompanied by bone proliferation around the joint margins and thickening of the soft tissues of the joint; also called *degenerative arthritis.*

degranulation. Release of granules from a cell.

dehiscence. Breakdown of healing at a wound or suture site.

dehydration. Loss of body water, occurring when the intake of water is insufficient to cover water losses.

demarcated. Having sharp borders.

dematiaceous fungi. Dark, pigmented fungi represented by the genera *Drechslera, Alternaria*, and others.

dementia. Mental deterioration.

dendrites. Short threadlike extensions of a nerve cell; they act to receive nerve impulses from adjacent nerve cells.

density. The concentration of a nutrient in a feed.

dental float. Veterinary instrument for grinding down enamel points.

dentin. The tooth layer lying between the inner *pulp* (containing the tooth's blood and nerve supply) and the overlying *enamel.*

deoxygenated. Having a low oxygen content; said of venous blood.

deoxyribonucleic acid (DNA). The genetic material of living cellular organisms and of certain viruses.

depigmentation. Localized loss of normal skin color.

depolarization. A change from a negative to a positive charge, generating an electrical wave (as in the production of the heartbeat).

dermal papilla. Structure at the base of each hair follicle that, with the associated *hair matrix cells*, is responsible for the production of hair.

dermatitis. Any inflammatory skin disease.

dermatomycosis. Any fungal skin infection.

dermatophilosis. Relatively sporadic skin disease caused by an unusual threadlike bacterium, *Dermatophilus congolensis*; also known as *streptothricosis* and *rain-scald*.

dermatophytes. Fungi causing ringworm.

dermatophytosis. Ringworm.

dermatosis. Any skin disease, particularly one without an inflammatory component.

dermis. The middle and thickest major layer of the skin; composed of connective tissue fibers and a ground substance, it lies just beneath the *epidermis*, the outermost layer of the skin.

dermoid. A misplaced piece of skin found on the conjunctiva as a congenital lesion; it may also involve the cornea.

desmitis. Inflammation of a ligament.

detoxification. Reduction in toxic properties of compounds.

detrusor. Smooth muscle layer of the bladder wall; contraction of the detrusor results in voiding of urine.

dextrose. Glucose; blood sugar.

diabetes mellitus. Diabetes, a chronic disease caused by either insufficient production of insulin by the islets of Langerhans in the pancreas, or by resistance of target tissues to the effects of insulin. Diabetes results in an inability of cells to utilize glucose (blood sugar), with widespread adverse effects owing to impaired utilization of carbohydrates, fats, and proteins by the body.

diabetic ketoacidosis. Serious, life-threatening complication of untreated or poorly treated diabetes mellitus, characterized by the buildup of ketone bodies in the circulation and a fall in blood pH, i.e., increasing acidity of the blood.

diaphragm. The large muscle used for breathing which separates the abdominal and chest cavities.

diaphragmatic hernia. Rupture of the diaphragm, with movement of some of the abdominal contents into the chest cavity.

diaphysis. The central shaft of a long bone.

diarrhea. An increase in the fluid content, volume, or frequency of bowel movements.

diastole. The relaxation/filling phase of the heartbeat, following *systole*.

diastolic blood pressure. The pressure that occurs when the heart is not pumping blood into the arterial system (i.e., during the relaxation period between contractions).

diastolic heart murmur. Murmur that is present only during *diastole* (the relaxation phase of the heartbeat).

diestrus. The quiescent period between one estrus period and the next; also called *interestrus*.

differential white blood cell count. Total white blood cell (WBC) counts and percentages of different WBC types present; component part of a complete blood count (CBC).

differentiation. The development of cellular specialization as cells mature.

digestible carbohydrates. Sugars and starches.

digestible energy (DE). For a feed, the sum of the digestible carbohydrate, protein, fat, and fiber; also called *total digestible nutrients (TDN)*.

digestion. The breakdown of larger substances into smaller subunits, which can be more readily carried into the body for use in energy production and the construction of body tissues.

digital pressure. Pressure applied by the fingers.

digital pulse. The pulse as felt in the digital arteries of the feet; important for the detection of *laminitis* (founder).

digoxin. Medication that increases the strength of the heartbeat while decreasing the heart rate; used most often for the treatment of congestive heart failure.

dilated. Enlarged or widened; expanded.

dilated fixed pupil. Pupil that does not contract.

dilation. Expansion.

direct life cycle. With regard to parasites, a life cycle that can be completed without the participation of an intermediate host.

discospondylitis. Inflammation of an intervertebral disk.

dispensable amino acids. Amino acids that can be synthesized by the body so long as a source of nitrogen is present in the diet.

disseminated intravascular coagulation (DIC). A bleeding disorder characterized by the excessive utilization of blood-clotting factors, due to widespread clotting within blood vessels; the resultant hemorrhaging often represents a terminal event in a number of diseases.

distal. Farther, more distant.

distemper. Alternative name for *strangles*.

disuse atrophy. Loss of muscle mass because of muscle disuse.

diuretic. Any drug that promotes urination.

diurnal. Having a daily cycle or rhythm.

DNA. Deoxyribonucleic acid, the genetic material of living cellular organisms and of certain viruses.

dominant gene. A gene capable of expressing its trait even when carried by only one member of a chromosome pair.

Doppler echocardiography. Technique using sound waves to examine the direction and velocity of blood flow within the heart and great vessels.

dorsal. Pertaining to the back; toward the back.

duct. Tiny tube or passageway.

ductus arteriosus. Blood vessel normally present during fetal life that allows blood to bypass the lungs, which of course are nonfunctional at this time; the ductus normally closes shortly after birth.

duodenum. The first part of the small intestine, connecting the stomach with the jejunum.

dysgerminoma. Malignant but extremely rare tumor of the ovary.

dysphagia. Difficult or painful swallowing.

dysplasia. Any abnormality in the size, shape, or development of cells.

dyspnea. Difficulty breathing; labored breathing.

dystocia. Difficult birth.

dysuria. Painful or difficult urination.

eardrum. Translucent membrane between the outer and middle ear which vibrates in response to sound vibrations transmitted down the ear canal; also called *tympanic membrane*.

eccrine sweat glands. Sweat glands that empty their contents directly onto the skin surface.

echinococcosis. Hydatid disease.

echocardiography. Examination of the heart by means of ultrasonic sound waves, for the purpose of disease diagnosis; also known as *cardiac ultrasound*.

eclampsia. Calcium deficiency in a lactating mare.

ectoparasite. External parasite; examples include ticks, fleas, and mites.

ectopic. In or at an abnormal site; not in the normal position.

edema. The accumulation of abnormally large quantities of fluid in the intercellular tissue spaces (spaces between cells); *pulmonary edema* refers specifically to fluid buildup in the lungs.

edematous. Swollen with fluid.

effusion. Fluid escaping into a body cavity or tissue.

elastin. Protein found in elastic connective tissue fibers that imparts flexibility to the tissue.

elective surgery. Surgery that is medically necessary but need not be performed immediately.

electrocardiogram (ECG). Examination of the electrical activity of the heart, for the purpose of disease diagnosis. The ECG records the size and direction of the waves of depolarization that spread across the heart during muscle contraction and relaxation.

electroencephalography (EEG). Examination of the electrical activity of the brain, for the purpose of disease diagnosis.

electrolytes. Simple, inorganic salts that act as charged particles in water solutions, i.e., they are able to conduct electricity; examples include sodium, potassium, and chloride.

electromyography (EMG). Examination of the electrical activity within a muscle at rest or during voluntary or evoked muscular contractions, for the purpose of disease diagnosis.

electrophoresis. Separation of components of a mixture by their differing migration in an applied electric field.

electroretinogram (ERG). Examination of the electrical activity of the *retina* (light-sensitive layer of cells at the back of the eye), for the purpose of disease diagnosis.

electrosurgery. Surgical techniques (such as electrocautery) wherein electrical methods are used to remove tissue and/or seal broken blood vessels to alleviate hemorrhage.

ELISA. *E*nzyme-*l*inked *i*mmuno*s*orbent *a*ssay; any of the many highly sensitive color-based test methods for detecting either antibody or antigen in blood, serum, or plasma.

embolism. Sudden blockage of an artery by a blood clot.

embryonic vesicle. The fertilized egg (embryo) with its surrounding fluid and membranes.

emetics. Drugs used to induce vomiting.

enamel. The thin, calcium-rich outer surface of the teeth, overlying the harder *dentin* layer; it functions to resist wear.

enamel hypoplasia. Underdevelopment or incomplete development of the enamel layer of a tooth.

enamel points. Sharp points that develop in the enamel of the teeth, owing to the normal positioning and growth of the teeth in the mouth; the sharp points can be ground down with a special instrument called a *dental float*.

endocarditis. Inflammation of the innermost lining of the heart (*endocardium*), usually caused by bacterial infection of one or more heart valves.

endocardium. A thin serous membrane, the innermost lining of the chambers of the heart.

endocrine glands. Glands that secrete their contents directly into the blood or interstitial fluid (the fluid surrounding cells).

endocrinology. The study of hormones and hormone-producing glands.

endocrinopathy. Hormonal imbalance leading to disease.

endogenous. Originating within the body.

endometritis. Inflammation of the innermost lining of the uterus; the leading cause of infertility in broodmares.

endoparasite. Any parasite found inside the host, chiefly in the gastrointestinal tract.

endoscopy. Procedure wherein tubelike viewing apparatus (an endoscope) is inserted into an orifice or body cavity, for the purpose of examining the internal portions of that cavity or a hollow organ.

endospore. The type of spore produced during the *spherule* stage of the life cycle of the fungus *Coccidioides immitis*, the cause of coccidioidomycosis ("valley fever").

endotracheal tube. A plastic tube for breathing, commonly inserted into the trachea during general anesthesia.

energy density. The amount of energy contained in a given quantity of food.

enophthalmos. Recession of the eye deep within the orbit.

enteric. Referring to the small intestine.

enteritis. Inflammation of the small intestine; contrasts with *colitis* (inflammation of the large intestine).

enterolith. Stony concretion that develops in the large intestine.

entropion. Turning in of an eyelid.

enucleation. Surgical removal of the eyeball.

enzootic. Widespread in a population and always present, but producing disease in only relatively few animals; said of infectious disease agents.

enzyme. Any of a myriad number of different proteins produced by cells, capable of accelerating biochemical reactions occurring within the cells.

eosinophil. A white blood cell that contains granules readily stained with eosin; functions in the allergic reaction to parasitic infections.

epicardium. The outermost membrane of the surface of the heart.

epidermal appendages. Collectively the hair follicles, sweat glands, and sebaceous glands.

epidermis. The outermost layer of the skin.

epidermoid cyst. Follicular cyst.

epididymis. In the male, the duct connecting the testis to the vas deferens; used for the storage, maturation, and movement of sperm.

epilation. Plucking of hair by the roots.

epilepsy. Brain disorder resulting in seizures.

epinephrine (adrenaline). A hormone secreted by the adrenal glands; it acts to increase blood sugar levels and blood pressure and to accelerate the heart rate.

epiphysis. Either end of a long bone.

episiotomy. Surgical enlargement of the vulvar opening.

epistaxis. Bleeding from the nostril; nosebleed.

epitheliogenesis imperfecta. A rare, lethal skin defect of draft-horse foals; inherited as an autosomal recessive disorder.

epithelium. Cellular covering of the internal and external surfaces of the body.

epizootic. Attacking many animals over a short period of time, with resulting high morbidity (high percentage of animals becoming ill); said of infectious disease agents. Also, an acute disease outbreak.

equids. Members of the horse family.

equine coital exanthema. Disease characterized by painful wartlike lesions on the skin of the vulva and perineum or on the shaft of the penis; caused by equine herpesvirus type 3.

equine collagenolytic granuloma. The most common nodular skin disease of horses, possibly caused by a hypersensitivity to insect bites; also called *nodular necrobiosis.*

equine degenerative myeloencephalopathy. Chronic, progressive disease of young horses, characterized by abnormalities of gait; the cause is thought to be related to a vitamin E deficiency and is associated with lack of green forage or the feeding of heat-processed pelleted rations.

equine granulocytic ehrlichiosis. Tick-transmitted disease characterized by fever, depression, reluctance to move, depressed white blood cell and platelet counts, and lower-limb swelling; caused by a rickettsia, *Ehrlichia equi.*

equine herpesvirus myeloencephalitis. Inflammatory disorder of the brain and spinal cord, caused by the abortion-inducing strain of equine herpesvirus type 1.

equine infectious anemia (EIA). One of the most important viral diseases of horses, caused by a retrovirus; it is a chronic infection resulting in a persistent (lifelong) carrier state with periodic exacerbations of anemic illness; also called *swamp fever.*

equine influenza. Very important viral respiratory disease of horses caused by subtypes (A_1 and A_2) of equine influenza virus, an orthomyxovirus.

equine monocytic ehrlichiosis. Potomac horse fever.

equine protozoal myeloencephalitis. Inflammatory disorder of the brain and spinal cord, caused by a poorly characterized protozoan parasite tentatively designated *Sarcocystis neurona.*

equine viral arteritis (EVA). Contagious viral disease of horses causing fever, ocular and respiratory signs, fluid distension or swelling of the limbs, and abortion.

equine viral encephalomyelitis. Inflammation of the brain and spinal cord, caused by eastern equine encephalomyelitis (EEE) virus, western equine encephalomyelitis (WEE) virus, or Venezuelan equine encephalomyelitis (VEE) virus.

equine viral papillomatosis. Disease characterized by the development of papillomas (warts) on the muzzle, around the lips, or on the extremities; caused by equine papillomavirus, a member of the Papovaviridae family of DNA viruses.

erectile tissue. Tissue capable of erection, i.e., stiffening following engorgement of blood; found in the penis of the male and the clitoris of the female.

erosion. A superficial denudation of the skin involving only the epidermis.

eructation. Forceful, retrograde expulsion of air from the stomach; "burping" or "belching."

erythema. Reddening of the skin, due to congestion of the underlying capillaries.

erythema chronicum migrans. A skin reaction seen in human beings with Lyme borreliosis.

erythema multiforme, epidermal type. An uncommon but highly characteristic skin disease with a proposed immunologic basis.

erythrocyte. Red blood cell, the carrier of oxygen in the blood.

erythropoietin. A hormone produced by the kidneys that stimulates red blood cell production in the bone marrow.

esophagitis. Inflammation of the esophagus.

esophagus. The muscular tube extending from the pharynx (back of the mouth) to the stomach.

essential amino acids. Amino acids that cannot be synthesized in sufficient quantities by the body and therefore must be provided in the diet.

essential fatty acids. Fatty acids that have structural functions in cell membranes and serve as precursors for *prostaglandins.*

estrogens. General term for female sex hormones.

estrus. "Heat"; a recurrent period of varying length, during which the mare produces a watery secretion from the genital tract, becomes sexually receptive to the stallion, and ovulates.

etiology. The cause of a disease.

eumycotic mycetoma. A swollen, progressing, tumorlike lesion caused by certain species of fungi.

eustachian tube. Short canal that connects the middle ear with the back of the throat.

euthanasia. Humane killing; putting to sleep.

excise. To cut out; remove surgically.

excisional biopsy. Biopsy sample representing an entire (small) lesion, removed surgically both as diagnosis and treatment.

exertional myopathies. Muscle diseases caused by exertion; these include *azoturia, tying-up,* and *endurance-related myopathy.*

exhaustive disease syndrome. Condition seen in endurance horses, three-day event horses, and horses on long trail rides; characterized by a significant level of dehydration, owing both to massive losses of fluid and electrolytes in sweat and to decreased fluid intake.

exocrine glands. Glands that secrete their contents through ducts (tiny tubes).

exogenous. Originating outside the body.

exostosis. A benign growth protruding from the surface of a bone.

expiration. The act of breathing air out; exhalation.

extender. Fluid added to collected semen to increase or "extend" the volume.

external urethral sphincter. Sphincter located at the junction of the bladder and urethra.

extragonadal. External to the testes.

extraocular. External to the eyeball.

exudate. A high-protein fluid derived from blood and deposited in tissues or on tissue surfaces, usually as a result of inflammation.

fabella (plural: fabellae). Small sesamoid bone occasionally found in the area of the knee.

facultative parasite. A parasite whose life cycle can be completed without a parasitic phase, but which may optionally include a parasitic phase under certain circumstances.

fallopian tubes. Uterine tubes or oviducts.

familial. Running in a family line; occurring in a family line with greater frequency than by chance alone.

farcy. A form of glanders that affects the skin; characterized by nodules, ulcers, and swollen lymph nodes and lymphatic channels, most often involving the legs or abdomen.

fasciae (singular: fascia). Sheets of fibrous tissue that ensheath the muscles and define their shape.

fasciculations. Frequent small, localized muscle contractions.

fat-soluble vitamins. Vitamins A, D, E, and K.

febrile. Having a fever.

fecal flotation. Laboratory procedure for identification of parasite eggs in a fecal specimen.

feminization. Development of certain female sex characteristics in a male.

femur. Thigh bone.

feral. Wild; untamed.

fermentable. Able to be digested by intestinal microorganisms.

fetal resorption. Disintegration of the fetus while in the uterus.

fetlock joint. The joint between the long pastern bone and the cannon bone.

fever. A rise in body temperature caused by a change in the thermoregulatory set-point in the brain; usually caused by disease.

fibrin. An insoluble protein that forms the nucleus of a blood clot.

fibrinogen. Clotting factor in the blood, is converted into its active form (fibrin) by the enzyme *thrombin*.

fibroblast. Immature fibrocyte.

fibrosarcoma. A malignant tumor of connective tissue cells.

fibrosis. Formation of fibrous tissue; scarring.

fibrous tissue. Tough connective tissue.

fibrous tunic. The outer layer of the eyeball.

filamentous. Threadlike.

flagging. Rhythmic up-and-down movements of the stallion's tail during ejaculation.

flatulence. Presence of excessive air or gas within the intestinal tract.

flehmen reaction. A unique behavior wherein the horse extends its head and curls back the upper lip while drawing air into the nasal cavity; usually expressed by a stallion attempting to detect *estrus* ("heat") in a mare.

flora. The population of microorganisms (bacteria, viruses, fungi, protozoa) normally resident within an individual host, or within a certain portion of the host (e.g., the intestinal tract).

fluorescein. A fluorane dye used for, among other things, identifying ulcers on the cornea.

foal heat. A mare's first heat period after the birth of a foal.

foal heat scours. A normal physiological diarrhea occurring during the first heat cycle of a mare after foaling.

focal ventral midline dermatitis. A frequently encountered skin disease of horses kept in close proximity to cattle; probably caused by the bites of horn flies.

follicle-stimulating hormone (FSH). Hormone produced by the pituitary gland, that stimulates the development of ovarian follicles in the female and sperm production in the male.

follicular cyst. Cyst originating within a hair follicle; also called *epidermoid* cyst.

follicular pharyngitis. Alternative name for *chronic pharyngeal lymphoid hyperplasia*.

follicular sheath. Long tubelike structure through which a hair passes through the *dermis* (middle layer of the skin) and exits to the skin surface.

folliculitis. Inflammation of one or more hair follicles.

forage poisoning. Form of botulism in horses caused by ingestion of botulinal toxin produced by *Clostridium botulinum* in decaying plant material.

forage disease. Common name for *leukoencephalomalacia*.

founder. Common name for *laminitis*.

frog. Thickened, horny area located in the middle of the sole of the foot.

frozen-section biopsy. Biopsy sample frozen and cut for immediate examination and diagnosis, as during exploratory surgery.

fulminant. Sudden and intense.

fundus. General term for the back of the eye.

fungal tumor. Eumycotic mycetoma.

fungi (singular: fungus). A large group of organisms characterized by the presence of a rigid cell wall and the absence of chlorophyll, and whose primary purpose is the decomposition of organic material; examples include the yeasts and molds, mushrooms, smuts, and rusts.

Galvayne's groove. A dark line that forms on the outside of the corner incisor teeth; its length and appearance are useful in aging a horse.

gametes. Reproductive cells, each containing a single set of chromosomes; *ova* (eggs) in the female and *spermatozoa* (sperm) in the male.

gametogamy. Sexual reproduction involving the formation of male and female reproductive cells which fuse to form a *zygote*; also called *syngamy*.

gangrene. Death and decay of tissue, usually owing to the loss of blood supply and subsequent invasion by bacteria.

gas colic. Colic caused by overconsumption of lush grass feed, resulting in excessive gas production in the intestine.

gaskin. The portion of the hind limb below the stifle.

gastric. Pertaining to the stomach.

gastritis. Inflammation of the stomach.

gastroesophageal sphincter. Sphincter located between the esophagus and the stomach.

gastroscopy. Endoscopic examination of the stomach.

gastrula. An early stage of the developing embryo that follows the *blastula* stage.

gauge. A measure of the diameter of an injection needle.

gelding. Castrated male horse.

gene linkage. Phenomenon wherein genes located on the same chromosome tend to be inherited together more often than they are split apart.

genera. Plural form of *genus*.

genes. The individual units of inheritance, composed of stretches of DNA found along the *chromosomes* within the nucleus of every cell.

genome. The total genetic information of an individual cell or virus.

genotype. The genetic makeup of a given physical trait; also, the total genetic makeup of an individual organism.

genus (plural: genera). One of the major classifying categories of taxonomy, further divided into species or subgenera.

geriatrics. Branch of medical science concerned with the diseases, disabilities, and care of aged patients.

gestation. The full period of pregnancy, from fertilization of the egg by a spermatozoon until birth.

giardiasis. Chronic diarrhea caused by the protozoan *Giardia*.

gingiva. The gums of the mouth.

gingivitis. Inflammation of the gums.

gland. Collection of cells that produces secretions or excretions of a specialized character.

glanders. An ancient and once worldwide bacterial disease of equids, now rare and restricted to certain areas of the Middle East and Asia; caused by *Pseudomonas mallei*.

glans penis. The cap-shaped termination of the penile shaft.

glaucoma. Group of diseases caused by increased pressure within the eyeball, which damages the optic nerve and can result in blindness.

globe. The eyeball.

glomerular filtration rate (GFR). Rate at which the kidney glomeruli filter the blood passing through them.

glomerulonephritis. An inflammatory disease involving the capillaries (small blood vessels) of the kidney glomeruli.

glomerulus (plural: glomeruli). Any one of the many tiny clusters of blood vessels within the kidney; they filter waste products from the blood and excrete them in the form of urine, which is transported to the bladder for elimination.

glucocorticoids. Steroid hormones such as cortisol that are produced by the cortex of the adrenal gland; they elevate blood sugar levels, increase fat and protein breakdown and the secretion of stomach acid, and exert an anti-inflammatory effect on conditions such as arthritis and dermatitis.

glucose. Blood sugar, the body's most important fuel molecule.

glucosuria. Spillage of glucose into the urine, as in diabetes mellitus.

glycogen. Animal starch; a complex carbohydrate stored primarily in the liver and muscles, and broken down into its component glucose (sugar) molecules whenever they are needed by the body.

goiter. An enlarged thyroid gland.

goitrogen. Any substance that causes goiter.

gonadal hypoplasia. Underdevelopment of the gonads (*testes* or *ovaries*).

gonadotropin-releasing hormone (GnRH). Hormone released from the hypothalamus of the brain, that triggers the release of luteinizing hormone (LH) and follicle-stimulating hormone (FSH) from the pituitary gland.

gonads. *Ovaries* (in the mare) and *testes* (in the stallion); the reproductive glands that produce *ova* (eggs) in the female and *spermatozoa* (sperm) in the male, as well as the sex hormones *progesterone* and *estrogen* (ovaries), and *testosterone* (testes).

gossypol. A toxic fatty acid that can be found in cottonseed meal.

Gram stain. A routine stain used for the laboratory identification of bacteria.

granula iridica. Corpora nigra.

granular cell layer. A layer of cells within the *epidermis*, the outermost layer of the skin; it lies above the prickle cell layer and below the horny layer.

granulation tissue. Newly formed, velvety tissue, rich in blood vessels but lacking nerve endings, that develops at the site of a healing wound; "proud flesh."

granule. A tiny grain or particle.

granulocytes. White blood cells that contain stainable granules; examples include *neutrophils*, *eosinophils*, and *basophils*.

granulocytic leukemia. Cancer of granulocytes.

granuloma. Lesion indicative of a chronic inflammatory response, characterized by the accumulation of white blood cells around an offending agent for the purpose of walling off the agent from the rest of the body.

granulosa cells. The cells that surround the developing ovarian follicle.

gravel. Common term describing drainage at the coronary band of the foot; caused by infection that migrates up the hoof wall and breaks out as an abscess at the coronary band.

grease heel. General term for a variety of inflammatory skin conditions affecting the pastern region.

gross appearance. Appearance as viewed by the unaided (naked) eye; as opposed to microscopic appearance.

growth hormone (GH). Hormone produced by the pituitary gland; it controls the rate of body growth.

guttural pouch. In horses, an internal sac that represents an outgrowth of the *eustachian tube*, the short canal that connects the middle ear with the back of the throat and that acts to equalize pressure within the ear.

guttural pouch empyema. Accumulation of the pus in the guttural pouch, often a complication of *strangles*.

guttural pouch mycosis. Fungal infection of the guttural pouch, usually caused by fungi of the genus *Aspergillus*.

guttural pouch tympany. Distension of the guttural pouch.

gymkhana. Athletic event.

habituation. Learning process wherein the response to a repeated stimulus gradually declines, resulting eventually in the total absence of the response; becoming desensitized.

hair bulb. The deepest portion of the hair follicle; its cells are referred to as *hair matrix cells*.

hair follicle. The structural unit of hair production within the skin, containing two major components, the *follicular sheath* and the *hair bulb*; two major types exist, *simple* follicles and *compound* follicles.

hair matrix cells. Cells at the base of the hair follicles that together with the *dermal papilla* are responsible for the production of hair.

hair matrixoma. Benign skin tumor arising from cells at the base of hair follicles (hair matrix cells).

hair root. The lower, anchoring structure of a hair.

hair shaft. The upper, free portion of a hair; as distinguished from the hair root.

hard palate. Bone and tissue composing the roof of the mouth, separating the nasal cavity from the oral cavity.

head-nodding. A stable vice characterized by a repetitive bobbing motion of the head, usually performed alone in a stall while in a drowsy state of consciousness.

head-shaking. A normal behavior that developed as a defense mechanism against irritating and often biting insects.

heart murmur. An abnormal heart sound produced when blood flows too rapidly or too chaotically through a portion of the heart; a common sign of heart disease.

heart rate. The heart's rate of contraction (*systole*) and relaxation (*diastole*).

heaves. Common term for *chronic obstructive pulmonary disease*.

helminthosis. Any parasitic worm infestation.

helminths. Parasitic worms.

helper T cells. T lymphocytes that have a major role in assisting other lymphocytes, known as B cells, to produce antibody against an antigen.

hemagglutinins. Autoantibodies directed against the body's own red blood cells.

hemangioma. Benign tumor of newly formed blood vessels.

hemangiosarcoma. Malignant tumor of blood vessels and associated tissue.

hemarthrosis. Bleeding into a joint.

hematinics. Compounds that improve the quality of the blood; "blood builders."

hematocrit. The percentage of red blood cells in a specified volume of whole blood; measurement of the hematocrit is performed to check for anemia; also called *packed cell volume (PCV)*.

hematologic. Referring to the blood and/or blood cells.

hematopoiesis. The production of new red blood cells.

hematuria. Presence of blood in the urine.

hemeralopia. "Day blindness," a disorder of the retina characterized by blindness during the day but partial return of vision in dim light.

hemoglobin. An iron-containing pigment found in red blood cells; it serves as the carrier of oxygen to the tissues.

hemoglobinuria. Presence of hemoglobin in the urine; "red water."

hemogram. Results of blood examination including red blood cell count, packed cell volume (PCV) or *hematocrit*, and total and differential white blood cell counts.

hemolysis. Red blood cell destruction.

hemolytic. Characterized by red blood cell destruction.

hemolytic disease of the newborn. Neonatal isoerythrolysis.

hemophilia A. Recessive, X-linked bleeding disorder characterized by a deficiency of clotting factor VIII; the most common bleeding disorder of horses.

hemoptysis. Coughing up blood.

hemorrhage. Bleeding.

hemorrhagic diathesis. Disease condition in which an abnormal bleeding tendency exists, as in *disseminated intravascular coagulation (DIC)*.

hemorrhagic enteritis. Inflammation of the intestine accompanied by bleeding in the intestinal tract.

hemorrhagic shock. Shock caused by severe bleeding (usually from trauma) resulting in depletion of blood from the circulatory system, so that less oxygen is transported from the lungs to the tissues.

hemospermia. Blood in the semen.

hemothorax. Pooling of blood in the chest cavity.

heparin. An anticoagulant; it prevents blood clotting by indirectly inhibiting the formation of *fibrin* (the chief protein component of blood clots).

hepatic. Pertaining to the liver.

hepatic lipidosis. Abnormal accumulation of fat in liver cells.

hepatic necrosis. Liver-cell death.

hepatomegaly. Enlargement of the liver.

hepatopathy. Any disease of the liver, particularly one characterized by degenerative changes.

hepatosplenomegaly. Enlargement of the liver and spleen.

hereditary multiple exostosis. Inherited bone disorder characterized by the development of numerous small projections along the bones, resulting in an abnormal bony contour.

hermaphroditism. Presence of male and female sex organs in the same individual.

hernia. Protrusion of an organ or tissue through an abnormal fissure; rupture.

heterozygous. Having inherited a different allele from each parent, at a given locus on a chromosome; contrasted with *homozygous*, in which the same allele for a given trait is inherited from both parents.

high ringbone. Ringbone affecting the pastern joint.

hinny. Animal produced by crossing a jennet (female donkey) with an equine stallion.

histamine. Powerful molecule produced by mast cells and basophils, that is responsible for an army of unpleasant effects seen in allergy; it causes contraction of smooth muscle and dilation of capillaries and increases the heart rate, among other actions.

histiocyte. A tissue macrophage.

histiocytoma. Benign skin tumor composed of *histiocytes* (tissue macrophages).

histology. The microscopic examination of normal tissue.

histopathology. The microscopic examination of diseased tissue.

hobbling. Tieing the legs together.

hock joint. Position in the hind limb where the tibia joins the tarsal bones; equivalent to the human ankle and heel.

holocrine secretion. Type of secretion in a gland wherein each entire gland cell disintegrates, with the cell contents becoming the secretion.

homogeneous. Uniform.

homozygous. Having inherited the same allele for a particular trait from both parents.

hormone. Any molecule produced by an organ or tissue, usually in extremely small quantities, that has a specific regulatory effect on the activity of another organ or tissue.

Horner's syndrome. A specific set of clinical signs—constriction of the pupils, protrusion of the third eyelid, drooping of the upper eyelid, sweating of the face and neck on the affected side—resulting from partial interruption of the nerve supply to the eyes and head.

horny layer. A cell layer of the *epidermis*, the outermost layer of the skin; it is composed entirely of tightly adherent, dead *keratinocytes* containing abundant quantities of *keratin*.

host. The living organism in or on which a parasite resides.

human chorionic gonadotropin (hCG). Hormone produced by the placenta that can stimulate ovulation.

humoral immune response. The mounting of an antibody response to an antigen by the immune system.

hydatid disease. Disease of humans caused by the tapeworms *Echinococcus granulosus* and *Echinococcus multilocularis*; characterized by the production in the tissues of large, fluid-filled structures (*hydatid cysts*), in which the parasite undergoes a further process of maturation.

hydrocephalus. Cerebrospinal fluid accumulation within the brain.

hydrometra. Accumulation of watery fluid within the uterus.

hydrophilic. Having the property of attracting or absorbing water molecules.

hydrotherapy. Use of water externally as a therapeutic measure.

hygroma. Fluid-filled sac or cyst, most often caused by trauma.

hymen. Membranous tissue partially or completely covering the external opening of the vagina in virgin mares.

hyper-. A prefix meaning *above* or *beyond*; excessive.

hyperammonemia. Abnormally elevated ammonia levels in the blood.

hyperandrogenism. Excessive production of male sex hormones.

hypercalcemia. Abnormally elevated levels of calcium in the blood.

hyperchloremia. Abnormally elevated levels of chloride in the blood.

hyperelastosis cutis. Skin disease of Quarter Horses, characterized by a lack of subcutaneous attachment of the skin to the underlying tissues.

hyperemia. Reddening caused by increased blood flow.

hyperestrogenism. Excessive production of the female sex hormone *estrogen*.

hyperglycemia. Abnormally elevated levels of glucose (blood sugar) in the blood.

hyperhidrosis. Excessive sweating.

hyperkalemia. Abnormally elevated levels of potassium in the blood.

hyperkalemic periodic paralysis (HYPP). Genetic disease of Quarter Horses and derived breeds (Paints, Appaloosas), characterized by sporadic episodes of generalized muscle tremors and stiffness accompanied by elevated serum levels of potassium.

hyperkeratosis. Abnormal overgrowth of the horny layer of the epidermis.

hyperlipidemia. Abnormally elevated levels of fat in the blood.

hypernatremia. Abnormally elevated levels of sodium in the blood.

hyperparathyroidism. Hyperactivity of one or more parathyroid glands.

hyperphosphatemia. Abnormally elevated levels of phosphorus in the bloodstream.

hyperpigmentation. Localized, abnormal darkening of the normal skin color.

hyperplasia. Overgrowth due to an abnormal increase in the number of cells in a given tissue; contrasted with *hypertrophy*.

hyperprogestinism. Excessive production of the hormone *progesterone*.

hypersensitivity vasculitis. An abnormal immunologic reaction targeted at blood-vessel walls.

hypertension. Abnormally elevated blood pressure.

hyperthermia. Abnormally elevated body temperature; also, a method of heating tumors to lethal temperatures in an attempt to kill tumor cells.

hyperthyroidism. Abnormally increased activity of the thyroid gland, with elevated secretion of thyroid hormones; has not been reported to occur spontaneously in the horse.

hypertrophy. Overgrowth due to an abnormal increase in the size of cells in a given tissue; contrasted with *hyperplasia*.

hyphema. Bleeding into the anterior chamber of the eye.

hypo-. A prefix meaning *below* or *under*; deficient.

hypoadrenocorticism. Addison's disease; insufficient secretion of steroid hormones from the adrenal cortex.

hypoalbuminemia. Abnormally low levels of the protein *albumin* in the blood, often reflecting abnormally low body stores of protein.

hypoallergenic. Minimizing allergic reactions.

hypocalcemia. Abnormally low levels of calcium in the blood.

hypochloremia. Abnormally low levels of chloride in the blood.

hypodermis. Alternative name for *subcutis*.

hypoglycemia. Abnormally low levels of glucose (blood sugar) in the blood.

hypokalemia. Abnormally low levels of potassium in the blood.

hypoluteoidism. Sterility in the female caused by insufficient secretion of the hormone *progesterone*.

hyponatremia. Abnormally low levels of sodium in the blood.

hypoparathyroidism. Insufficient secretion of parathyroid hormone (PTH) from the parathyroid glands.

hypoperfusion. Reduced blood flow.

hypophosphatemia. Abnormally low levels of phosphorus in the blood.

hypoplasia. Underdevelopment or incomplete development of a given tissue.

hypoproteinemia. Abnormally low level of plasma proteins in the blood.

hypopyon. Accumulation of white blood cells (pus) in the anterior chamber of the eye.

hypostatic gene. A gene whose expression is masked by another gene.

hypothalamus. The part of the brain concerned with operation of much of the autonomic (unconscious) nervous system, the production of specific hormones that are subsequently stored in and released by the pituitary gland, and the regulation of body temperature, sleep cycles, and food and water intake.

hypothermia. Abnormally low body temperature; cooling of the body to slow metabolism.

hypothyroidism. Abnormally decreased thyroid function.

hypotrichosis. Condition characterized by a sparse hair coat.

hypovolemia. Abnormally decreased volume of circulating blood; can lead to shock.

hypoxemia. Abnormally low blood oxygen levels

hypoxia. Oxygen deprivation.

iatrogenic. Arising as a complication of medical treatment.

idiopathic. Having no known cause.

ileocecal orifice. The point at which the small intestine joins the large intestine.

ileus. Loss of normal intestinal motility.

immune complex. Antibody attached to (complexed with) an antigen.

immune-mediated, immunologically mediated. Refers to any condition in which the deleterious effects are caused wholly or in part by components of the immune system.

immunization. The administration of a vaccine in order to produce protective immunity against the infectious disease agent(s) present in the vaccine.

immunofluorescence assay (IFA). Assay technique for the detection of antigen or antibody using antibodies labeled with a fluorescent dye.

immunoglobulins (antibodies). Specialized proteins produced by plasma cells (end-stage B lymphocytes) in response to the presence of foreign material (bacteria, viruses, toxins, etc.). Antibodies are capable of binding to the foreign material and thus alerting other immune cells to its presence. Often abbreviated *Ig*, there are five major classes: IgG, IgM, IgA, IgE, and IgD. In horses a subset of IgG known as IgG(T) is involved in the immune response to parasites and tetanus toxoid.

immunotherapy. The use of medications that boost the immune response, to assist in the treatment of a disease.

impaction colic. Colic resulting in blockage of the intestine; can result from excessive consumption of grain or lush pasture, or ingestion of foreign material.

in utero. Within the uterus.

inactivated ("killed") vaccine. A vaccine in which the infectious agent has been modified in some way (most often chemically) so that it no longer can infect and replicate within the host, but nevertheless is still capable of stimulating an immune response.

inappetence. Lack of appetite; *anorexia*.

incisional biopsy. Biopsy sample representing a portion of a larger lesion.

incisional hernia. A defect in a healing incision wound that results in a bulging out of the underlying tissues.

incisors. The front teeth.

incontinence. Loss of voluntary control over urination or defecation.

incubation period. The time between exposure to an infectious disease agent and the onset of clinical signs of disease.

indirect life cycle. With regard to parasites, a life cycle that can only be completed with the participation of an intermediate host.

infarct. Localized tissue death resulting from obstruction of the blood supply to the affected site.

infective stage. The specific stage in the life cycle of a parasite that is able to initiate an infection in a definitive or intermediate host.

infertility. Diminished ability to produce offspring.

inflammation. Protective response, often localized, involving white blood cells and other components of the body, wherein a disease agent or other irritant factor is sequestered and attempts made to destroy it or neutralize its effects.

ingesta. Ingested food.

inguinal. Pertaining to the groin area.

inguinal canal, inguinal ring. An opening deep within the groin area for passage of the spermatic cord or the round ligament of the uterus.

inhalation pneumonia. Pneumonia caused by inhalation of noxious fumes, as during a house or forest fire.

innervation. The distribution of nerves to a particular tissue or body part.

insoluble fibers. Dietary fibers such as cellulose and wheat bran; they are good bulk-forming agents and are only poorly fermented (digested) by bacteria in the large intestine.

inspiration. The act of breathing air in; inhalation.

insulin. Critically important hormone produced by the beta cells of the endocrine pancreas; responsible for regulating the blood concentration of glucose, the body's most important fuel molecule.

insulin-dependent diabetes mellitus. Diabetes mellitus characterized by an inability to utilize blood glucose because of inadequate amounts of circulating insulin.

insulinlike growth factors. Alternative name for *somatomedins*.

integument. The skin.

interestrus. Diestrus; the quiescent period between one heat period and the next.

interferons. A specialized group of protein molecules capable of inhibiting virus replication and the growth of tumor cells, and of modulating the activities of certain components of the immune system.

intermediate host. A host that (usually) is essential to the life cycle of a parasite and in which the parasite undergoes development to juvenile but not mature stages.

intersexuality. Having characteristics of both sexes intermingling in the same individual.

interstitial fluid. The fluid surrounding cells.

intervertebral disks. Cartilaginous, cushioning structures positioned between the vertebrae of the spinal column.

intoxication. Poisoning.

intracranial. Within the skull.

intramuscular (IM). A route of injection (into the muscle).

intraocular pressure. The pressure within the eye.

intromission. Insertion of the penis of the male into the vagina of the female during intercourse.

intubation. Insertion of a breathing tube into the trachea during anesthesia.

intussusception. Prolapse ("telescoping") of one section of bowel into an adjoining section.

involution. Period of repair in which there is a return to normal size and composition, as of the uterus following birth and expulsion of the placenta.

ionize. To separate into ions (charged atoms).

ionizing radiation. Radiation capable of ionizing matter; examples include X rays and radioactive isotopes of elements such as radon, cesium, and strontium.

iridocyclitis. Inflammation of the iris and ciliary body of the eye.

iris (plural: irides). The circular, pigmented structure located behind the cornea; by expanding or contracting its central opening, or *pupil*, it regulates the amount of light penetrating the inner reaches of the eye.

irritant contact dermatitis. Uncommon inflammatory skin disease caused by direct contact with an irritating concentration of an offending substance.

ischemic injury. Injury caused by loss of blood supply to a tissue.

islets of Langerhans. The endocrine cells of the pancreas; the *beta cells* within the islets of Langerhans are the source of the critically important hormone *insulin*.

ixodid ticks. Hard-bodied ticks; distinguished from *argasid* (soft-bodied) ticks.

jack. A male donkey.

jaundice. Yellow discoloration of the skin and mucous membranes, caused by the deposition of bile pigment; most commonly a result of liver and/or bile-duct disease.

jejunum. The middle (and longest) portion of the small intestine, situated between the duodenum and the ileum.

jennet. A female donkey.

joint capsule. Thin, saclike structure that envelopes a joint and contains within it all the elements of the joint, such as the articular cartilage, synovial membrane, synovial fluid, etc.

juvenile Arabian leukoderma. A depigmenting syndrome seen in young Arabian horses; also called *Arabian fading syndrome* and *pinky syndrome*.

karyotype. A magnified photographic array of the *chromosomes* derived from an individual cell.

keratectomy. Surgical removal of a portion of the cornea.

keratin. An insoluble, sulfur-rich protein that represents the principal component of skin, hair, and nails (hooves).

keratinization. The process whereby keratinocytes in the epidermis mature to form the outer, horny layer of the skin.

keratinocytes. Skin cells that produce *keratin*; they are the major cell type of the *epidermis*, the outermost layer of the skin.

keratitis. Inflammation of the cornea.

keratolytic. Capable of causing softening and peeling of the outer (horny) layer of the skin.

keratoma. Slowly growing tumor of the underlying structures of the hoof wall.

ketone bodies, ketones. Organic compounds produced by fatty acid and carbohydrate metabolism in the liver; elevated (toxic) levels are often produced in individuals with diabetes mellitus.

ketonuria. Spillage of ketone bodies (ketones) into the urine in *diabetic ketoacidosis*.

kicking chains. Restraint device placed on the hind leg above the fetlock to discourage kicking.

kidney. Either of the two bean-shaped organs in the lower abdominal cavity that are responsible for filtering toxic waste products from the blood, producing the important hormone *erythroipoietin*, and maintaining the body's water and electrolyte balance.

kilocalorie (kcal). Unit defined as the amount of energy required to raise the temperature of 1 kilogram of water 1 degree Celsius (centigrade); the "large" calorie; commonly called simply *Calorie*.

kilogram. One thousand grams (2.2 pounds).

labia. The external lips or folds of the vulva of the female.

labile. Chemically unstable; easily destroyed.

lacerations. Tears in the skin and underlying muscle.

lacrimal gland. Tear gland.

lactated Ringer's solution. A sterile salt solution for (usually intravenous, but sometimes subcutaneous) administration containing sodium lactate, sodium chloride, potassium chloride, and calcium chloride; given to restore fluid and electrolyte balance.

lactation. The production of milk by the mare.

lactose. Milk sugar.

lagophthalmos. An inability to close the eyelids completely.

laminitis. Inflammation of the *laminae* of the foot, which serve to attach the coffin bone to the hoof wall; also known as *founder*.

Langerhans cells. Cells found in the *epidermis*, the outermost layer of the skin, that are important in generating immune responses in the skin.

laparoscopy. Visual inspection of the interior of the abdominal cavity with a specialized instrument (a *laparoscope*), inserted through the body wall.

larvae (singular: larva). Immature forms or stages in the life cycle of certain small animals, such as insects or parasites.

laryngeal hemiplegia. Paralysis affecting one side of the larynx, caused by damage to either of the two recurrent laryngeal nerves; also called *roaring*.

laryngitis. Inflammation of the larynx.

laryngoscopy. Visual examination of the larynx.

larynx. Muscular, cartilage-containing structure comprising the upper part of the respiratory tract between the pharynx and trachea, and containing the vocal chords; the "voice-box."

latent infection. Dormant stage of certain infections during which the infectious agent is known to be present but is not actively replicating and cannot be detected by usual means.

lateral. Closer to the side than to the midline of the body.

lavage. Irrigation or flushing out.

laxity. Looseness.

lecithin. Fatty acid-rich constituent of the outer surface of cell membranes; also called *phosphatidylcholine*.

leiomyoma. Benign tumor of smooth muscle cells.

leiomyosarcoma. Malignant tumor of smooth muscle cells.

lens. Transparent refractive structure that finely focuses images onto the retina for clear and sharp vision.

leptospires. Spiral-shaped bacteria belonging to the *spirochete* group.

leptospirosis. Bacterial disease caused by *leptospires* (spiral-shaped bacteria).

lesion. Any disease-induced abnormality of tissue structure or tissue function.

lethargy. An abnormal state of drowsiness or dullness.

leukocoria. A whitening of the pupil of the eye.

leukocytes. White blood cells.

leukocytosis. Increase in the number of circulating white blood cells.

leukoderma. Whitening of the skin, often in localized patches.

leukoencephalomalacia. Degenerative brain disorder, apparently caused by a toxin produced by the mold *Fusarium moniliforme*; also called *cornstalk disease*, *moldy corn poisoning*, *forage disease*, and *blind staggers*.

leukopenia. Reduction in the number of circulating white blood cells.

leukotrichia. Abnormal whitening of the hair, often in localized patches.

leukotrienes. Compounds that act as modulators of allergic and inflammatory reactions.

Leydig cells. Specialized cells in the testes that produce the male sex hormone *testosterone*.

libido. Sexual drive.

ligament. Strengthening band of fibrous tissue, for supporting and stabilizing a joint structure.

ligate. To bind or tie off.

limbus. The line of demarcation between the cornea and sclera of the eye.

linoleic acid. An essential fatty acid acquired from vegetable sources; important in the biosynthesis of cell membranes.

lipase. An enzyme that breaks down fat.

lipid(s). Fat(s).

lipid film. A layering of fat.

lipidosis. Abnormal accumulation of fat within cells.

lipoma. Benign tumor of fat cells.

liposarcoma. Malignant tumor of fat cells.

lobulated. Divided into small lobes or *lobules*.

lockjaw. Synonym for *trismus*, a clinical sign of tetanus.

locus (plural: loci). The site on a chromosome where a specific gene is located.

lordosis. Downward curvature of the lumbar spine; "swayback."

low ringbone. Ringbone affecting the coffin joint.

lumbosacral. Pertaining to the lower back region

lumen. The interior of a blood vessel or tubular organ, such as the intestine.

luteal phase. In the reproductive cycle, the period during which the ovarian follicle converts to a *corpus luteum* and secretes the hormone *progesterone*.

luteinization. Conversion of the ovarian follicle to a *corpus luteum*.

luteinizing hormone (LH). Hormone produced by the pituitary gland; together with follicle-stimulating hormone (FSH) it assists in causing ovulation and inducing production of the hormone *estrogen*.

luxation. Dislocation of a joint; also, total displacement of the lens of the eye from its normal position.

Lyme borreliosis, Lyme disease. An infectious arthritis of people and dogs caused by a spirochete bacterium, *Borrelia burgdorferi*; whether this organism is the cause of any significant disorder in horses remains controversial at this time.

lymph. Generally clear fluid drained from tissues, that circulates within the lymphatic vessels and contains fats, proteins, and specialized cells (lymphocytes).

lymphadenitis. Inflammation of one or more lymph nodes.

lymphadenopathy. Enlargement of one or more lymph nodes, as from inflammation, infection, or cancer.

lymph node. Any of the body's many nodular accumulations of lymphoid cells; they are interconnected by means of lymphatic vessels.

lymph-node aspirate. Sample of fluid and cells from deep within a lymph node, obtained using a needle and syringe.

lymphocyte. A type of white blood cell capable of responding to the presence of foreign material in the body; lymphocytes play a central role in directing and coordinating immune responses.

lymphocytic thyroiditis. Immune-mediated inflammation of the thyroid gland.

lymphocytosis. Abnormal increase in the number of circulating lymphocytes.

lymphoma, lymphosarcoma. Malignant tumor of lymphocytes.

maceration. Softening or dissolution of skin cell layers, resulting from overexposure to moisture or topical medications.

macrophage. A specialized white blood cell of central importance to the body; it ingests cellular debris and foreign material, destroys ingested microorganisms, processes ingested antigens as an initial step in the induction of a specific immune response, and synthesizes a number of important enzymes, coagulation factors, and messenger molecules; also referred to as a *mononuclear phagocyte*.

macule. A discolored area of skin that is not elevated above the skin surface.

malabsorption. Faulty absorption of nutrients by the intestine.

malassimilation. Defective transport of one or more nutrients from the intestinal contents across the intestinal wall.

maldigestion. Faulty digestion.

malignant. Capable of spreading and invading other tissues; said of tumors.

mammary gland. Breast.

mandible. The lower jaw.

mane-chewing. A stable vice exhibited primarily by yearlings and two-year-olds.

mania. Frantic behavior.

mast cell. A specialized, granule-containing cell found in the skin and lining of the inner body surfaces; it plays a central role in the development of allergy.

mastication. The action of chewing.

mastitis. Inflammation of one or more mammary glands.

mastocytosis. Abnormal infiltration of mast cells into a body tissue.

maternal immunity. A form of temporary immunity that is passed from the mare to the foal *in utero* (in the uterus) and/or after birth in the colostrum and milk; primarily antibody, maternal immunity serves to protect the foal until its own immune defenses become fully operative.

maxilla. The upper jaw.

mechanical vector. A vector that merely serves physically to transport a parasite from one host to another.

meconium. The contents of the foal's first bowel movement.

medial. Closer to the midline of the body.

medial canthus. The inner corner of the eye.

medulla. The innermost part of an organ (kidney, adrenal gland, brain) or hair shaft; contrasted with *cortex*.

megacalorie (mcal). One thousand kilocalories; a useful term for quantifying the energy in a ration.

megakaryocyte. A giant cell found in the bone marrow; it is the precursor of the blood platelets.

meiosis. Process involved in the formation of *gametes* (reproductive cells), wherein cell division produces new cells (*spermatozoa* and *ova*) containing only one set of chromosomes.

melanin. Dark pigment of skin and hair.

melanoblasts. Immature melanin-forming cells that originate early in fetal life.

melanocyte-stimulating hormone (MSH). Hormone produced by the pituitary gland that mediates the deposition of *melanin* (dark pigment of skin and hair) in the body.

melanocytes. Cells of the *epidermis*, the outermost layer of the skin, that produce the skin pigment *melanin*.

melanoma. A (usually) malignant tumor of pigmented skin cells.

melanotrichia. Abnormal darkening of the hair color.

melena. Dark, pitchy stool caused by bleeding into the digestive tract.

melioidosis. A glanderslike disease caused by *Pseudomonas pseudomallei*, characterized by the development of nodules in internal organs; not known to occur in the United States.

meninges. The three protective membranes surrounding the brain and spinal cord; specifically, the *dura mater*, *pia mater*, and *arachnoid*.

meningitis. Inflammation of the *meninges*.

meront. Alternative term for *schizont*.

merozoites. The daughter cells resulting from either

schizogony or *endodyogeny* (asexual forms of reproduction in certain protozoa).

mesenteric. Pertaining to the *mesentery*, the membrane that lines the abdominal organs and attaches them to the body wall.

mesovarium. Fold of tissue that holds the ovaries in place.

metabolic energy (ME). The caloric content of a diet; can be roughly estimated from the *proximate analysis*.

metabolic water. Water the body obtains from solid food and the breakdown of ingested fat, carbohydrate, and protein.

metabolism. All the life-sustaining biochemical processes in the body; the conversion of nutrients into energy.

metabolites. By-products of metabolism.

metabolizable energy (ME). The difference between the gross energy of a food and the energy that is lost in urine and feces.

metacercaria. Infective larval form of flukes that arises from the *cercaria* stage.

metaphysis. The region immediately beneath the growth plate (*epiphysis*) of a bone.

metastasis. Spread of tumor cells from the primary tumor site to distant body sites; a characteristic of malignant tumors.

metestrus. In the estrus cycle, the period of subsidence of follicular activity that follows estrus ("heat").

metritis. Inflammation of the uterus.

microbe. Any minute living organism, particularly one capable of causing disease; viruses, because they are not living organisms, technically are not considered "microbes," but are more correctly referred to by a term such as "infectious agent."

microvasculature. The smallest blood vessels (capillaries).

miller's disease. Colloquial term for nutritional secondary hyperparathyroidism.

mineralocorticoids. Corticosteroids whose primary function is regulation of water and electrolyte balance; they act by retaining sodium and excreting potassium within the kidney tubules.

minimal inhibitory concentration (MIC). Laboratory test procedure for determining the sensitivity or resistance of a bacterial isolate to several antibiotics.

miotic. Any ophthalmic medication that causes the pupil to contract.

miracidium. Free-living larval form in the life cycle of flukes.

miticide. Any medication that kills mites.

mitochondria (singular: mitochondrion). Specialized structures within body cells that are responsible for producing energy.

mitosis. Process wherein a body cell divides into two exact copies of itself, each new cell receiving two complete sets of chromosomes.

mitotic. Actively undergoing cell division.

mitral regurgitation. Partial backflow of blood through a dysfunctioning mitral valve.

mitral valve. The atrioventricular valve on the left side of the heart.

modified-live virus. Attenuated (weakened) virus that no longer produces clinical disease in the host but retains the ability to induce a protective immune response, and can be used as a vaccine; technically a misnomer, since viruses are not living organisms.

molars. The large grinding teeth.

moldy corn poisoning. Common name for *leukoencephalomalacia*.

monensin. Feed additive for cattle and poultry; toxic for horses.

monocular fixation. Focusing of one eye on an object.

monocyte. Nondescript white blood cell found in the circulation, which converts into an active *macrophage* upon entry into tissue.

moon blindness. Periodic ophthalmia.

morphogenesis. The progressive development of form and shape of an organism, or of an individual organ or tissue within the organism.

morphology. The shape and structure of an organ or of an entire organism.

motile. Capable of movement.

motility. Ability to move.

motoneuron. A nerve cell that supplies myofibers in skeletal muscle.

motor unit. The basic functional and anatomical organization of nerves and muscle fibers within skeletal muscle.

mucociliary escalator. A coordinated and forceful wave-like movement of the *cilia* lining the air passageways from the trachea to the bronchioles; essential for the normal removal of mucus and inhaled particulate matter and bacteria.

mucocutaneous junctions. Areas where mucous membranes and skin adjoin, such as the lip margins.

mucoid. Resembling mucus.

mucometra. Presence of mucus in the uterus.

mucosal-associated lymphoid tissue (MALT). Lymphoid tissue associated with the linings of the digestive, respiratory, and urogenital tracts.

mucous membranes. Lubricating membranes lining the internal surfaces of body cavities, such as the mouth, digestive tract, respiratory tract, and urinary tract.

mucus. Slimy substance secreted by certain membranes (mucous membranes); contains a variety of secretions, salts, and cells.

multilocular. Having many compartments.

multiple myeloma. An uncommon malignant tumor of plasma cells arising from the bone marrow.

murmur. An abnormal heart sound produced when blood flows too rapidly or too chaotically through a portion of the heart; a common sign of heart disease.

mutation. A permanent genetic change, sometimes resulting in altered structure or function.

mycetoma. General term for a swollen, progressing, tumorlike skin lesion caused either by fungi or certain bacteria.

mycology. The study of fungi.

mycoplasmas. Microscopic organisms closely related to bacteria that are ubiquitous inhabitants of the respiratory and genital tracts.

mydriatic. Any ophthalmic medication that dilates the pupil.

myelin. Fatty substance forming the outer tunic (*myelin sheath*) around many nerve axons; facilitates the conduction of nerve impulses along the axons.

myelogenous. Originating within the bone marrow.

myelopathy. General term for any degenerative disorder affecting the spinal cord.

myiasis. Infestation of body tissue by fly maggots.

myocarditis. Inflammatory heart-muscle disease.

myocardium. The muscular layer of the heart; heart muscle.

myoclonus. Involuntary rapid, jerky twitching or contraction of muscles.

myofibers. Muscle fibers.

myofibrils. Slender threadlike structures, bundles of which make up each muscle fiber.

myofilaments. Smaller threadlike elements making up the myofibrils of muscles.

myoglobin. The oxygen-transporting pigment of muscle tissue.

myoglobinuria. Presence of myoglobin in the urine.

myonecrosis. Muscle-cell death.

myopathy. General term for any muscle disorder.

myosin. A vital protein component of muscle, one of the proteins responsible for muscle contraction.

myositis. Muscle inflammation.

nanogram. One billionth of a gram.

nares (singular: naris). The two halves of the nasal passages; also, the external and internal openings of the nasal passages.

nasal septum. Vertical dividing wall that separates the two nasal passages or *nares*.

nasal turbinates. Delicate, scroll-like, rolled bony structures within the nasal cavity that filter, warm, and humidify inhaled air; also referred to simply as *turbinates*.

nasopharynx. The rear portion of the pharynx, above the soft palate.

natural killer (NK) cells. Specialized lymphocytes that are important in detecting and eliminating tumor cells and virus-infected cells.

navicular disease. Lameness caused by damage to the navicular bone; one of the most common causes of intermittent forelimb lameness in the horse.

necrolysis. Separation or peeling of tissue caused by cell death.

necropsy. Examination of an animal after death; postmortem; autopsy on an animal.

necrosis. Cell death.

necrotic. Composed of dead cells.

necrotizing. Causing cell death.

negative reinforcement. In training, the use of an unpleasant stimulus, such as a whip or bit, if a task is not performed.

Negri bodies. Intracellular inclusion bodies sometimes found in brain cells of animals or humans with rabies.

nematode. General term for a roundworm.

neonatal. Newborn.

neonatal isoerythrolysis. Acute hemolytic anemia of the newborn caused by ingestion of antibodies in the mare's colostrum and milk that are directed against the neonate's red blood cells; also called *hemolytic disease of the newborn*.

neonatal maladjustment syndrome. Disease or group of diseases of foals characterized by progressive neurologic dysfunction.

neoplasia. Uncontrolled, progressive proliferation of cells under conditions that normally should be restrictive of cell growth; formation of a tumor.

neoplasm. Tumor.

neovascularization. Growth of new blood vessels into an abnormal site, such as a tumor.

nephritis. Kidney inflammation.

nephrolith. Kidney stone.

nephrons. The microscopic, functional units of the kidney.

nephrosclerosis. Scarring of kidney tissue; a principal cause of the normal, progressive deterioration of kidney function that accompanies aging.

nephrotic syndrome. Abnormal fluid retention as edema or ascites, resulting from glomerular disease of the kidneys.

nervous tunic. Retina; innermost layer of the eye.

neurectomy. Surgical cutting of a nerve to relieve pain.

neuritis. Inflammation of a nerve.

neurofibroma. Benign tumor of the nervous system arising from Schwann cells.

neuroma. Tumor arising from a nerve.

neuromuscular junctions. The intimate connections between muscle cells and adjacent nerve cells, representing a specialized extension of the *sarcolemma*.

neuromyopathy. General term for any disorder affecting both neurons and muscle fibers.

neuron. An individual nerve cell.

neuropathy. Any disorder of the peripheral nervous system.

neurotoxin. Any toxin targeting the nervous system.

neutropenia. An abnormal decrease in the number of circulating neutrophils.

neutrophil. A type of white blood cell capable of engulfing and destroying bacteria and other disease agents, immune complexes, and cell debris.

neutrophilia. An abnormal increase in the number of circulating neutrophils.

nit. Louse egg.

nocardiosis. Bacterial infection caused by members of the genus *Nocardia*; in horses *Nocardia* is most often a cause of local wound infections.

nodular. Characterized by nodules.

nodular necrobiosis. Equine collagenolytic granuloma.

nodule. A large papule; small lump.

nosocomial infection. An infection acquired in the hospital environment.

nuchal ligament. A large, strong band of connective tissue that provides support for the neck.

nucleic acids. General term for deoxyribonucleic acid (DNA) and ribonucleic acid (RNA), DNA serving as the genetic material of all living organisms and some viruses.

nucleotide. An individual unit of DNA.

nulliparous. Having never given birth.

nutritional secondary hyperparathyroidism. Disease caused by an imbalance in the quantities of calcium and phosphorus in the diet, resulting in a net withdrawal of calcium from the bones; also called "big head" or "millers' disease."

nystagmus. Rapid, involuntary, rhythmic eye movements, often indicative of central nevous system dysfunction.

obligatory parasite. A parasite whose life cycle cannot be completed without a parasitic phase at some stage.

occlude. To close off or obstruct.

occlusion. The fit or "bite" of the upper and lower teeth together when in contact following closure of the mouth.

ocular. Pertaining to the eyes.

olecranon. The point of the elbow.

olecranon bursitis. Bursitis caused by repeated trauma to the point of the elbow; also called *shoe boil*.

olfactory. Pertaining to smell.

olfactory nerves. Nerves found in the nasal turbinates in which the sense of smell originates.

oliguria. Reduction in the amount of urine excreted.

omphalophlebitis. Infection (usually bacterial) of the veins of the umbilical cord in the newborn; "navel ill."

oncogenesis. The process of tumor development.

oncologist. Cancer specialist.

oocyte. Developing egg cell (ovum) in the ovary.

oocyst. An encapsulated *ovum* (egg) of a sporozoan parasite such as *Toxoplasma gondii*, usually excreted in the feces.

opacification. Loss of transparency.

opacity. An opaque area or spot, as in the lens or cornea of the eye.

open reduction. Any procedure to repair a fracture wherein the broken bone is exposed surgically.

operant conditioning. "Trial and error" learning, usually involving a reward.

ophthalmoscope. Instrument for viewing the interior of the eye.

opportunistic pathogen. Any organism that is able to induce disease only if the host's immune or other defenses are compromised.

optic disk. That portion of the optic nerve visible at the surface of the retina; also called *optic nerve head*.

optic nerve. Literally an extension of the brain, which reaches to the back of the eye (*retina*) and transmits signals derived from light energy that are translated into a visual image by the brain.

optic neuritis. Inflammation of the optic nerve.

orchitis. Inflammatory disease of the testicle.

organ of Corti. The spiral-shaped organ of hearing within the inner ear, containing specialized sensory receptors.

oropharynx. The back of the throat; tonsillar area, between the soft palate and epiglottis.

osselets. Puffiness around the fetlock joint.

osseous. Bony.

ossicles. Very small bones.

ossification. The formation of bone.

ossifying myopathy. Condition most commonly affecting the hindlimbs of the horse, in which scarring and/or bone formation occurs within injured muscles.

osteitis. Inflammation of a bone.

osteoblast. A bone-forming cell.

osteochondritis dissecans (OCD). Cartilage disorder characterized by the presence of large flaps of cartilage or loose cartilaginous bodies within a joint.

osteochondrosis. A disorder of growing cartilage that may affect either the growth plate or the articular cartilage.

osteocyte. Cell type in bone that, in response to certain hormones, is responsible for maintaining normal calcium and phosphorus levels in the bloodstream.

osteomyelitis. Infection of a bone accompanied by pus formation; usually caused by bacteria.

osteopenia. Loss of bone calcium.

osteoporosis. Thinning and weakening of bone.

osteosarcoma. A malignant tumor of bone.

osteotomy. Surgical cutting of bone.

otitis externa. Inflammation of the outer ear.

otitis interna. Inflammation of the inner ear; also called *labyrinthitis*.

otitis media. Inflammation of the middle ear; also called *tympanitis*.

ovarian follicle. An *ovum* (egg) and its surrounding cells.

ovariectomy. Surgical removal of one or both ovaries.

ovaries. Paired organs of the female responsible for the production of *ova* (eggs).

ovariohysterectomy. Surgical removal of the uterus and ovaries.

overo. Recessive equine coat-color pattern, consisting of a colored base coat with white patches and colored legs. The white markings are more irregular than the colored patches of the tobiano. White does not cross the back and the head is mostly white.

oviducts. Uterine or fallopian tubes.

ovotestes. Abnormal gonads containing both testicular and ovarian tissue.

ovulation. Release of an egg from an ovary.

ovum (plural: ova). Egg.

oxidation. The cellular "burning" of glucose, amino acids, and fatty acids to produce energy in the form of *adenosine triphosphate (ATP)*, the major form of energy used by cells.

oxygenated. Filled with oxygen; said of arterial blood.

oxytocin. A hormone formed in the hypothalamic region of the brain and stored in the pituitary gland; it stimulates contraction of the uterus and milk ejection from the mammary glands.

pacemaker. Nerve tissue that controls the heart's rate of contraction and relaxation; also known as the *sinoatrial node*. An *artificial pacemaker* is an electrical device implanted surgically to treat abnormally slow heart rhythms (*bradycardias*).

packed cell volume (PCV). A measurement of the volume of red blood cells in relation to the volume of blood fluid, expressed as a percentage; also called the *hematocrit*.

palliation. Alleviation of clinical signs in the absence of specific treatment of the underlying disorder.

palmar digital neurectomy. Permanent nerve block performed to relieve navicular disease.

palpable. Detectable by touch or feeling.

palpate. To examine by feeling with the hands and fingers.

palpebral. Pertaining to an eyelid.

palsy. Paralysis.

pancytopenia. Condition wherein red blood cell, white blood cell, and platelet cell numbers are all decreased in the circulation.

papilledema. Swelling of the optic nerve.

papilloma. Wart.

papule. A minute, firm, well-demarcated elevation of the skin.

paralysis. Total absence of voluntary movement in a muscle or set of muscles.

paranasal sinuses. Nasal chambers that act to filter, warm, and humidify incoming air.

parasite. Any organism that is dependent in some manner for its continued existence on another organism (its host), most often to the detriment of the host.

parasitemia. Presence of a parasite in the blood circulation.

parasitology. The study of parasites.

paratenic host. An "optional" host in a parasite's life cycle in which juvenile stages may persist but do not develop.

parathyroid glands. Twin, small pairs of endocrine glands located adjacent to the thyroid gland; they secrete parathyroid hormone (PTH), which is essential for the regulation of calcium and phosphorus balance in the body.

parathyroid hormone (PTH). Hormone secreted by the parathyroid glands that regulates the metabolism of calcium and phosphorus in the body.

parenteral. By injection (i.e., not by the oral route); injectable.

paresis. Diminished ability to move a muscle or a body part voluntarily.

parietal pleura. Thin transparent membrane that forms the inner lining of the chest cavity.

paroxysm. A sudden bout.

parrot mouth. Dental malformation consisting of an overshot jaw; actually caused by a shortening of the lower jaw.

parturition. The act of giving birth.

pastern folliculitis. The most commonly encountered pus-forming skin infection in the horse, caused by *Staphylococcus aureus*.

pastern joint. The joint between the short pastern bone and the long pastern bone.

patch. A large macule.

patella. Knee cap, a small triangular *sesamoid bone* located in front of the knee.

patellar luxation. Congenital displacement of the kneecap (*patella*); rare in horses.

patent. Unobstructed, open.

patent ductus arteriosus (PDA). Abnormal persistence after birth of an embryonic blood vessel connecting the pulmonary artery to the aorta; only rarely seen in horses.

patent infection. With regard to parasites, an infection in a definitive host that results in the appearance of products of the parasite's reproduction (eggs, larvae, etc.).

patent urachus. Abnormal persistence of the urachus after birth.

pathogen. Any microbial agent capable of causing disease.

pathogenesis. The cellular, biochemical, and pathological mechanism(s) underlying the development of a disease.

pathogenic. Able to cause disease.

pathogenicity. The relative ability of an organism to cause disease.

pedal osteitis. Increased vascularization and demineralization affecting the coffin bone, usually secondary to inflammation resulting from repeated, excessive concussion on the sole.

pedicle. A small stalk or stem.

pedunculated. Situated on a stalk.

pelvic flexure. Area of the large intestine where the intestine narrows and folds back on itself.

pelvic symphysis. The joint formed by the union of the two halves of the pubic bone of the pelvis.

pelvis. Hip.

pemphigus foliaceus. Autoimmune skin disease characterized by autoantibody production and the subsequent development of vesicles and pustules in the superficial layers of the skin.

penicillins. A large group of antibiotics derived primarily from fungi of the genus *Penicillium*; of pivotal importance in the treatment of diseases caused by certain bacteria such as the streptococci, clostridia, and spirochetes, penicillins interfere with the vital synthesis of bacterial cell walls.

peptide. A short chain of amino acids; peptides form the building blocks of proteins.

peptide hormones. Hormones manufactured by the body from amino acids, sometimes with the addition of carbohydrates (sugars).

peracute. Of extremely rapid onset.

percutaneous needle biopsy. Technique by which a sample of organ tissue is obtained for examination by maneuvering a biopsy needle through the skin and into the organ of interest.

perianal. In the region of the anus.

pericardial effusion. Abnormal accumulation of fluid in the pericardial sac.

pericarditis. Inflammation or infection of the pericardium.

pericardium. The thin, membranous sac that surrounds the heart, stabilizing its position and protecting it from disease affecting nearby structures.

perinatal period. The period shortly before and after birth.

perineum. Region between the thighs encompassing the anus and genitalia.

periocular. Pertaining to the area around the eye.

periodic ophthalmia. Recurrent inflammation of the eye associated with an abnormal immunologic reaction to leptospires (spiral-shaped bacteria) or threadworms; also known as *recurrent uveitis* or *moon blindness*.

periodontal ligament. Structure composed of tiny fibers that serves to attach the tooth root to the bone of the jaw.

periorbit. Eye socket.

periosteal stripping. The most common surgery for correction of angular limb deformities in foals.

periosteum. The highly sensitive connective tissue sheathing the bones; it contains a rich blood supply and provides for the nutrition, growth, repair, and protection of the underlying bone.

peripheral nervous system (PNS). The cranial, spinal, and peripheral nerves and their connections to muscle or to sensory receptors.

peristalsis. Muscular movements of the intestinal tract that function to propel contents longitudinally through the tract.

permeability. Leakiness; ability to be penetrated.

pH. A measure of the hydrogen ion concentration of a solution, reflective of acidity (pH below 7) or alkalinity (pH above 7), with a pH value of 7 representing neutrality.

phaeohyphomycosis. An uncommon chronic infection of the subcutaneous tissues caused by dark, pigmented fungi (*dematiaceous* fungi).

phagocyte. Any cell type (such as a neutrophil or macrophage) able to engulf and digest minute particulate matter.

phalanx (plural: phalanges). General term for any bone forming part of a finger or toe.

pharyngeal. Pertaining to the pharynx.

pharyngitis. Inflammation of the pharynx; "sore throat."

pharynx. Area extending from the rear of the mouth and nasal passages to the larynx and esophagus.

phenotype. The visible, physical expression of a genetic trait, e.g., blue eyes or red hair.

pheromones. Chemical secretions that elicit a specific behavioral response (often attraction) in another individual of the same species.

phlebitis. Inflammation of a vein.

phlebotomy. Therapeutic blood-letting.

phlegm. Viscous secretion produced by the respiratory tract.

phospholipids. Fats containing phosphorus.

photoaggravated vasculitis. Specific disease unique to horses, characterized by an inflammation of blood vessels (vasculitis) that appears to be "triggered" and subsequently aggravated by exposure to sunlight.

photon. The energy unit of visible light, having characteristics both of a wave as well as a discrete particle.

photoperiod. The length of time per day that an animal is exposed to natural or artificial light.

photophobia. Visual hypersensitivity to light.

photoreceptors. Specialized light receptors (*rods* and *cones*) present in the retina of the eye.

photosensitization. Clinical syndrome resulting from excessive exposure to ultraviolet radiation (sunlight).

phycomycosis. General term describing several tropical and subtropical diseases caused by different organisms, including *Basidiobolus haptosporus* (causing basidiobolomycosis), *Conidiobolus coronatus* (causing conidiobolomycosis), and *Pythium insidiosum* (causing pythiosis).

physiology. The study of body function and metabolism.

physis (plural: physes). A growth plate of a bone; an area where new bone growth originates.

physitis. Generalized bone disease of young growing horses, characterized by enlargement of the growth plates of certain long bones and of the vertebrae of the neck.

phytates. Form of *inositol* (a sugarlike compound) found in plants; excessive amounts in the diet can interfere with the absorption of zinc from the digestive tract.

picogram. One trillionth of a gram.

piebald. Black and white (horse coloration).

pinky syndrome. Juvenile Arabian leukoderma.

pinna. The external portion or flap of the ear.

pituitary gland. Endocrine gland located at the base of

the brain, and connected to it by a narrow stalk; it stores and/or secretes many hormones of pivotal importance to body function, including growth hormone (GH), thyroid-stimulating hormone (TSH), follicle-stimulating hormone (FSH), luteinizing hormone (LH), oxytocin, prolactin, antidiuretic hormone (ADH, vasopressin), and adrenocorticotropic hormone (ACTH).

placenta. The organized tissue in the uterus joining the fetus to the mother.

placentitis. Inflammation of the placenta.

plantar ligament. Ligament that courses along the back of the *calcaneus* bone in the hock.

plaque. The mixture of oral bacteria, bacterial sugars, salivary proteins, and food and cellular debris, that accumulates on the teeth; also, a flat area in the skin.

plasma. The fluid portion of the blood (excluding the blood cells).

plasma cells. End-stage B lymphocytes (B cells), whose function is to produce antibodies.

platelets. Cell fragments released from megakaryocytes, that play an important role in blood clotting.

pleura. Thin, transparent membrane covering the lungs and lining the chest cavity.

pleural cavity. The potential space between the visceral pleura and parietal pleura.

pleural effusion. Excessive fluid accumulation in the pleural cavity.

pleuritis. Inflammation of the pleura.

pleuropneumonia. Bacterial infection secondary to pneumonia or lung abscesses.

pneumonia. An inflammatory condition of the lungs; characterized by the filling of air spaces with fluid, resulting in impaired gas exchange.

pneumothorax. Accumulation of air within the pleural cavity, inside the chest but outside the lungs, impeding the ability of the lungs to expand normally; collapsed lung.

pneumouterus. Accumulation of air inside the uterus; a consequence of pneumovagina.

pneumovagina. Aspiration of air and debris into the vagina; also known as *wind-sucking.*

poll. The back of the head.

pollakiuria. Increased frequency of urination.

polyclonal gammopathy. Increase in serum gamma globulins (blood proteins that include most of the antibody classes) that tends to be spread over a wide range of protein types.

polycythemia. An excessive number of red blood cells.

polydipsia. Excessive thirst.

polyestrous. Having more than a single estrous cycle per year.

polygenic traits. Traits that are the result of the action of more than a single gene.

polymorphism. Genetic variation.

polymorphonuclear leukocyte. Any white blood cell having a lobular nucleus, such as a neutrophil.

polyneuritis. Inflammation occurring simultaneously in more than one nerve.

polyp. A small fleshy mass projecting from the surface of a mucous membrane.

polypeptide. Any peptide containing two or more amino acids; often referred to simply as a peptide.

polyphagia. Excessive eating.

polysynovitis. Inflammation of the lining membrane of a joint.

polyuria. Excessive urination.

positive reinforcement. In training, giving a reward such as food for suitable behavior.

posterior chamber. That portion of the eye between the iris and the lens.

posterior paresis. Partial paralysis of either or both hind limbs.

posthitis. Inflammation of the prepuce.

postpartum. Occurring after birth.

postprandial. Occurring after a meal.

Potomac horse fever. A gastrointestinal disease of horses, characterized by high fever, colitis (inflammation of the large intestine), diarrhea, and dehydration; caused by a rickettsia, *Ehrlichia risticii.* The disease is also known as *equine monocytic ehrlichiosis.*

poultice. Soft, often medicated paste spread on a cloth and draped over a wound.

predilection. Preference.

premunition. Maintenance of immunity to a parasite by the persistent presence of small numbers of the parasite, usually in the gastrointestinal tract; premunition immunity wanes if the parasite is completely eliminated from the body.

prepatent period. The time elapsing between the initiation of a parasite's infection of a definitive host and the appearance of the products of parasite reproduction, e.g., eggs, larvae, etc.

prepubertal. Pertaining to the period before sexual maturity.

prepuce. Fold of skin enclosing the penis; also called the *sheath.*

prickle cell layer. A layer of cells within the *epidermis,* the outermost layer of the skin; also known as the *squamous cell layer,* it lies above the basal cell layer and below the granular cell layer.

primary hyperparathyroidism. Hyperparathyroidism resulting from excessive, relatively uncontrolled secretion of parathyroid hormone (PTH) by one or more abnormal parathyroid glands.

primary hypoparathyroidism. Hypoparathyroidism resulting from an absolute or relative deficiency of secretion of parathyroid hormone (PTH).

primary lymphoid organs. Organs in which the production and maturation of lymphocytes takes place; in horses they include the bone marrow, the mucosal-associated lymphoid tissue (MALT), and the thymus.

proestrus. In the estrus cycle, the period just before estrus.

progestogen. Any compound with progesteronelike activity.

progesterone. Hormone secreted by the corpus luteum, adrenal cortex, and placenta, whose primary function is to prepare the uterus for pregnancy; also called *progestin.*

proglottid. One of the chain of segments comprising the *strobila* or body of a tapeworm parasite.

prognathism. Condition characterized by an elongated lower jaw.

prognosis. The outlook for recovery from a disease.

prolactin. Hormone secreted by the pituitary gland that simulates and sustains lactation; also called *lactogenic hormone*.

prolapse. A bulging through or protrusion of a tissue or organ.

proliferative optic neuropathy. An incidental finding in old horses, consisting of excessive tissue growth in the area of the optic disk (at the back of the eye).

prophylaxis. Disease prevention.

proptosis. Bulging or protrusion of the eyeball from the eye socket; also called *exophthalmos*.

propulsive diarrhea. Squirting, watery diarrhea from the rectum.

prostaglandins. A group of fatty acid-derived compounds that are important as regulators of a number of physiological processes involving allergic reactions, contraction of smooth muscle, dilation of blood vessels, blood clotting, and others.

prostate gland. Gland in male mammals that surrounds the urethra where it joins the bladder and is important in the production of seminal fluid.

prostatitis. Inflammation of the prostate gland.

protein-losing enteropathy. Syndrome occurring in adult horses, characterized by weight loss in the face of a ravenous appetite; the cause is unknown but the result is a "leaky" intestine that does not absorb nutrients properly.

proteins. Molecules, composed of *amino acids*, that make up many of the structural components of the body and that are needed to maintain all normal body functions.

proteinuria. Excessive loss of protein in the urine.

proteolytic. Capable of breaking down protein.

protozoa. Simple organisms that are usually composed of a single cell; most are free-living but some are capable of producing disease in animals or humans.

proximate analysis. A measure of the nutrient content of a diet, including the maximum moisture, maximum fiber, minimum crude protein, and minimum crude fat content.

pruritus. Itchiness.

pseudohyperparathyroidism. Disorder characterized by elevated levels of blood calcium resulting from production of a parathyroid hormonelike substance by a tumor.

ptyalism. Excessive drooling; hypersalivation.

pulmonary. Pertaining to the lungs.

pulmonary edema. Noninflammatory buildup of fluid in the tissues and air spaces within the lungs.

pulmonary embolism. A detached clot from elsewhere in the body occluding a blood vessel within the lungs.

pulmonic stenosis. Congenital heart defect characterized by a narrowing (*stenosis*) of the connection between the right ventricle and the pulmonary artery.

pulmonic valve. The semilunar valve on the right side of the heart; also called the *pulmonic semilunar outflow valve*.

pulp. The blood vessels, nerves, lymphatic channels, and cells that line the pulp chamber or root canal of each tooth.

Punnett square. Checkerboard diagram for delineating possible outcomes of mating two individuals of defined genotype.

pupil. The central opening of the iris, through which light penetrates into the inner reaches of the eye.

purpura hemorrhagica. Immunologically mediated condition characterized by swelling of the limbs and widespread skin hemorrhages, varying in severity from a mild transient reaction to a severe fatal condition; associated with a number of different inciting factors, occasionally streptococcal infections.

purulent. Pus-forming.

pus. Fluid produced by an inflammatory process, containing many white blood cells.

pustule. A skin vesicle containing pus.

putrefactive. Pertaining to the normal decomposition of organic matter by microorganisms.

pyelonephritis. Any infection of the kidney involving as well the renal pelvis.

pyloric sphincter. Sphincter located between the stomach and duodenum.

pylorus. The terminal portion of the stomach, connecting it with the duodenum (first part of the small intestine).

pyoderma. General term for any skin disease in which pus is formed.

pyometra. Accumulation of pus within the uterus, resulting usually from a severe bacterial infection.

pyometritis. Purulent inflammation of the uterus.

pyothorax. Accumulation of pus within the chest; also called *thoracic empyema*.

pyrrolizidine alkaloids. Plant toxins that produce a very specific type of liver damage; the most common cause of chronic liver failure in horses in the western United States. Plants containing these toxins include groundsel, tansy ragwort, fiddleneck, rattlebox, Viper's bugloss, common heliotrope, and hound's tongue.

pythiosis. A form of phycomycosis caused by *Pythium insidosum*, characterized by itchy swellings, skin ulcerations, lymph node enlargement, and draining tracts.

quadriparesis. Partial paralysis in all four limbs.

quadruped. An animal such as the horse that walks on all four limbs.

Queensland itch. Commonly encountered skin disease of horses, caused by an allergic reaction to the bites of midges belonging to the genus *Culicoides*; also called *sweet itch*.

quidd. To drop partially chewed feed material from the mouth.

quittor. Chronic inflammatory process of the collateral cartilage of the coffin bone.

rabies. Inevitably fatal viral disease, primarily of bats and carnivores, characterized by neurologic dysfunction; caused by a rhabdovirus.

radiograph. An X ray film.

radiography. The use of X rays or gamma rays to view the internal structures of the body.

radioisotopes. Radioactive elements.

radiotherapy. Radiation therapy.

rain-scald. Common term for dermatophilosis.

recessive gene. A gene that can be expressed *only* when both members of a chromosome pair contain the same allele for a given characteristic (i.e., the same allele must be inherited from both the dam and the sire).

recombination. Genetic exchange among chromosomes, producing new combinations of genes.

rectal-vaginal fistula. A tear from the top of the vestibule (entrance to the vagina) to the floor of the rectum.

rectum. Lowermost portion of the large intestine, immediately adjacent to the anus.

recumbency. Inability to stand.

recumbent. Lying down.

recurrent uveitis. Periodic ophthalmia.

redia. Larval stage of flukes arising from the *sporocyst* stage.

reduction. The setting of a bone fracture.

reflex. In general, muscle movement orchestrated by the nervous system in response to a stimulus and without conscious (voluntary) control; an example is the knee-jerk reflex.

reflux. Backward flow.

refractive. Light-bending.

refractometer. Small hand-held device that can be used for determining how concentrated or dilute a urine sample is (a measurement referred to as urine *specific gravity*).

regurgitation. Involuntary return of undigested food to the mouth after swallowing; differs from vomiting in that it is a passive process (i.e., unaccompanied by the reflex, propulsive movements characteristic of vomiting).

renal. Pertaining to the kidneys.

renal pelvis. "Collecting funnel" deep within each kidney into which the kidney tubules drain filtrate.

reservoir host. An animal from which infection may be passed to domesticated stock or to human beings.

resorption. Biochemical dissolution or loss of tissue.

respiration. Breathing.

retching. Abdominal contractions in preparation for vomiting.

reticulated leukotrichia. A form of leukotrichia seen primarily in Quarter Horses.

retina. The light-sensitive layer of cells at the back of the eye.

retinitis. Inflammation of the retina.

retrograde. Backward.

rhabdomyoma. A benign tumor of striated muscle cells.

rhabdomyosarcoma. A malignant tumor of striated muscle cells.

rhinitis. Inflammation of the nasal passages.

rhinopneumonitis. Respiratory condition of horses caused by equine herpesvirus.

rhinoscopy. Visual examination of the nasal passages, using an endoscope, otoscope, or other instrument.

rhinosporidiosis. An uncommon disease caused by an as yet poorly characterized fungus, *Rhinosporidium seeberi*; it is a chronic localized infection characterized by the formation of polyps (fleshy masses protruding from the surface of a mucous membrane) in the nasal passages.

rhythmic segmentation. Rhythmic muscular movements of the intestinal tract that serve to delay the passage of intestinal contents until digestion and absorption have been completed.

ribonucleic acid (RNA). A nucleic acid occurring in all cells and involved in cell division, gene expression, and protein synthesis; also serves as the genetic material for some viruses.

rickettsiae (singular: rickettsia). Specialized bacteria that multiply only within host cells and that are usually transmitted to animals or human beings by lice, ticks, fleas, or mites; examples include *Ehrlichia risticii*, the cause of Potomac horse fever (equine monocytic ehrlichiosis), and *Ehrlichia equi*, the cause of equine granulocytic ehrlichiosis.

ringbone. Disorder characterized by new bone growth adjacent to either the pastern or coffin joints; caused by tearing of the collateral ligaments stabilizing the joint. *High ringbone* describes bone growth around the pastern joint, while *low ringbone* describes bone growth around the coffin joint.

ringworm. A common skin infection caused by ringworm fungi (*dermatophytes*), which invade the outer, superficial layers of the skin, hair, and nails; also called *dermatophytosis*.

RNA. See *ribonucleic acid*.

roaring. Common name for *laryngeal hemiplegia*.

rods. Photoreceptor cells in the retina of the eye that are responsible for night vision and detection of motion.

root. The portion of a tooth that lies below the gumline.

root canal. The chamber within each tooth that contains nerves, blood vessels, and lymphatic channels; also known as the *pulp chamber*.

sacroiliac joint. Joint where the pelvis connects with the spine.

sacrum. Bone formed by the fusion of the sacral vertebrae, at the lower end of the spinal column.

saline. A physiologically balanced salt solution; physiological sodium chloride solution.

salmonellosis. A primarily diarrheal disease caused by members of the bacterial genus *Salmonella*.

San Joaquin Valley fever. Coccidioidomycosis ("valley fever").

sand colic. Colic resulting when horses are fed on the ground in areas where the soil is sandy, or when they develop the vice of eating soil.

sarcoid. A skin tumor unique to horses, mules, and donkeys; lesions usually appear as small growths on a stalk or as large, broad-based masses.

sarcolemma. The outer membrane surrounding every skeletal muscle fiber.

sarcoma. General term for malignant tumors of connective-tissue cells (those cells within an organ or structure that bind it together and support it).

satiety. Appeasement of the appetite; a feeling of sufficiency or satisfaction with regard to food intake.

scapula. Shoulder-blade.

schizogony. A form of asexual reproduction seen in certain protozoa, in which the nucleus of the organism divides several times before the remainder of the cell divides; also called *multiple fission*.

schizont. A developmental stage of certain protozoa, specifically, a dividing cell undergoing *schizogony*; also called a *meront*.

Schwann cells. Large cells that are wrapped around certain nerve axons to form a *myelin sheath*, which serves to facilitate the conduction of nerve impulses along the axon.

sclera. The white outer covering of the eyeball, continuous with the cornea.

sclerotic. Hardened.

scolex. The "head" of a tapeworm parasite, armed with hooks or suckers and used for attachment and locomotion.

scotoma. A localized, disease-caused "blind spot" in the retina.

scours. Diarrhea.

scrotum. Dependent pouch of skin containing the testicles.

scutum. The hard "shield" present on the back of a hard tick.

sebaceous glands. Minute skin glands, many of which are attached to hair follicles; they secrete *sebum*, an oily secretion that lubricates and protects the skin.

seborrhea. General term used to describe clinical signs of excessive scaling, crusting, and greasiness of the skin.

sebum. The oily secretion of the sebaceous glands, containing fats, bacteria, and dead skin cells; it lubricates and protects the skin surface.

secondary lymphoid organs. Organs in which antigens are trapped and destroyed by immune-system cells; they include the lymph nodes, spleen, and portions of the bone marrow and the mucosal-associated lymphoid tissue (MALT).

seizures. Relatively brief episodes of neurologic derangement caused by abnormal bursts of electrical activity within the brain; also called *convulsions* or *fits*.

selective IgM deficiency. Immunologic disorder characterized by subnormal levels of circulating IgM; seen primarily in the Arabian and Quarter Horse breeds.

self-limiting. Said of disease, with reference to any illness that will run its (usually benign) course without the need for treatment.

semen. Thick milky fluid from the male containing the male reproductive cells or *spermatozoa* (sperm).

semicircular canals. Structures in the inner ear that are concerned with the sensation of balance.

semilunar valves. The heart valves that separate each ventricle from the great artery with which it is connected (either *aorta* or *pulmonary artery*). The semilunar valve on the right side of the heart is known as the *pulmonic* valve, and the corresponding valve on the left side is called the *aortic* valve.

seminal vesicles. Pouches attached to the urinary bladder.

seminiferous tubules. Small channels within the testes wherein the *spermatozoa* (sperm) develop.

seminoma. The most common type of testicular tumor in the horse.

septic arthritis. Inflammation of the joints caused by an infectious agent, usually bacterial.

septicemia. The presence of bacteria in the blood circulation, accompanied by related clinical signs of disease.

septic shock. Shock caused by invasion of the body by bacteria that produce substances injurious to cells such that the cells can no longer utilize oxygen.

septum (plural: septa). A dividing wall, such as that dividing the right and left sides of the heart or the right and left nasal cavities.

sequestrum (plural: sequestra). A fragment of dead bone that has broken off from the underlying normal bone tissue.

serology. The use of specialized diagnostic tests for the detection of antigens and antibodies in serum.

serotype. Variant of an infectious agent based on immunological testing.

serovar. Variant or subspecies of leptospire.

Sertoli cells. Cells within the testicular tubules that are important for nuture and development of *spermatozoa* (sperm).

serum. Blood plasma minus the clotting factor *fibrinogen*; the clear liquid that remains after the blood clots, containing many important blood proteins including antibodies (immunoglobulins).

serum alkaline phosphatase (SAP). An enzyme present in the blood that is produced in many body tissues and is of greatest diagnostic significance in diseases of the bone and liver.

serum hepatitis. An acute form of liver failure in adult horses associated in most cases with the injection of some biological product of equine origin, usually tetanus antitoxin; also called *Theiler's disease*.

sesamoid bone. Any small, nodular bone (such as the kneecap) that is located within the tendon of a muscle or the capsule of a joint.

sesamoiditis. Inflammation of the proximal sesamoid bones, sometimes involving the suspensory ligament and distal sesamoidian ligaments as well.

severe combined immune deficiency (SCID, CID). Lethal, inherited disease of Arabian foals, characterized by an absence of T- and B-lymphocytes. Approximately 2% of Arabian foals are born with this condition.

sex-linked diseases. Genetic diseases of males caused by defective genes located on the X chromosome; also called *X-linked diseases*.

sexual dimorphism. Size differences between the sexes, as seen with certain parasites.

shaker foal syndrome. Form of botulism in 2- to 8-week-old foals that occurs following ingestion of *Clostridium botulinum* spores and their transformation into mature, toxin-producing bacterial forms in the intestinal tract.

shaping. In training, the gradual refining or improvement of a task or movement.

sheared heels. Breakdown of the tissue between the bulbs of the heel, caused by the hoof wall's being out of balance.

sheath. Fold of skin enclosing the penis; prepuce.

shock. Failure of the blood vascular system to provide adequate circulation to the vital organs; circulatory collapse.

shoe boil. Common term for *olecranon bursitis*.

sialolith. Small stony concretion that forms within a duct draining a salivary gland, potentially resulting in blockage of the duct.

sidebones. Term describing *ossification* (bone formation) of the collateral cartilages of the foot; usually occurs in the forefeet of horses with poor conformation.

sign. A characteristic of a disease; "signs" are seen by observation, while "symptoms" are characteristics reported by the patient; thus, animals exhibit signs of disease, while human beings report symptoms.

sinoatrial (SA) node. A collection of specialized cardiac muscle fibers found at the junction of the right atrium and the vena cava; the heart's natural pacemaker, generating the electrical discharges that stimulate the beating and pumping of the heart.

sinus empyema. Formation of pus in the paranasal sinuses; the underlying cause in many cases is dental disease.

sinusitis. Inflammation of a sinus.

skeletal muscle. The type of muscle making up most of the muscles of movement attached to the skeleton; also known as *striated muscle*.

skewbald. White and any color other than black (horse coloration).

sleeping sickness. Common term for the depression and somnolence characteristic of equine viral encephalomyelitis.

smegma. Thick, oily or cheesy secretion that collects beneath the sheath of the penis.

smooth mouth. "Smoothing" of the tooth surfaces seen in very old horses.

smooth muscle. The type of muscle found in the walls of blood vessels and the major internal organs.

soft palate. At the rear of the mouth, the soft, fleshy posterior partition separating the nasal and oral cavities.

soft-tissue orbit. The nonbony structures (muscles, nerves, blood vessels) that lie within the bony orbit.

soluble fibers. Dietary fibers as found in fruits, oat bran, and *psyllium* (the chief component of commercial stool softeners such as "Metamucil"); they attract water and form a gel, are highly *fermentable* (able to be digested by bacteria) in the large intestine, and have been shown in people to slow emptying of the stomach and to inhibit the absorption of cholesterol.

somatomedins. Small proteins produced mainly in the liver that exert an anabolic effect on the body, resulting in proliferation of bone, cartilage, and soft tissues, and enlargement of body organs; also known as *insulinlike growth factors*.

sow mouth. Dental malformation consisting of an underextended upper jaw.

spasmodic colic. Colic characterized by increased numbers of bowel movements and episodes of pain following sudden changes in environmental temperature, diet, or activity level.

species. One of the major classifying categories of taxonomy, representing divisions of a *genus*, and sometimes further classified into subspecies.

specific gravity. A measurement of the concentration of urine in a urine sample; determined by using a small hand-held device called a *refractomer*.

spermatic cord. Combined structure extending from the groin area to the testes, through which run the *vas deferens* and a number of vessels and nerves.

spermatogenesis. The process whereby sperm cells within the testes of the stallion undergo cell divisions and cellular changes that result in the produce of mature *spermatozoa* (sperm).

spermatozoa (singular: spermatozoon). The mature reproductive cells of the male; produced by the testes, their role is to fertilize the female egg (*ovum*).

spherule. The parasitic, noninfectious stage of the fungus *Coccidioides immitis*, formed during the organism's growth phase in host tissue.

sphincter. Circular band or ring of muscle that serves to open or close a tube or orifice; analogous to a valve.

spinal nerves. Nerves arising from the spinal cord that form nerves of the peripheral nervous system.

spirochetes. Filamentous, spiral-shaped bacteria, such as the leptospires and *Borrelia*.

spleen. Large abdominal organ that removes senescent (aged) red blood cells and foreign material from the bloodstream; an important component of the immune system.

splenectomy. Surgical removal of the spleen.

splint bones. The second and fourth metacarpal bones of the forefoot, attached to the cannon bone by interosseous ligaments.

splinting. Tightening of the muscles in an area in order to avoid pain associated with muscle movement.

splints. Inflammation of the interosseous ligament that attaches the splint bones to the cannon bone.

spore. Highly resistant, thick-walled "resting stage" formed by certain bacteria, to ensure their survival during periods of unfavorable environmental conditions; it germinates quickly once favorable conditions have been restored to produce a new generation of bacteria. Also, a general term referring to the reproductive cells of certain microorganisms, particularly fungi and protozoa.

sporocyst. Larval stage of flukes that arises from the free-swimming *miracidium* stage.

sporotrichosis. An uncommon chronic, pus-forming infection caused by the dimorphic fungus *Sporothrix schenckii*.

sporozoites. In certain protozoa, the daughter cells resulting from division of a fertilized cell (*zygote*).

sprain. Joint injury involving damage to one or more ligaments, but without actual ligament rupture.

squamous cell carcinoma. A malignant skin tumor of cells within the squamous cell layer of the epidermis.

squamous cell layer. A layer of cells within the *epidermis*, the outermost layer of the skin; also known as the *prickle cell layer*, it lies above the basal cell layer and below the granular cell layer.

stall-walking. A stable vice characterized by constant circling, the horse's feet describing a roughly circular path through the bedding material on the floor of the stall.

standing heat. Behavioral estrus; the full behavioral signs of estrus.

stenosis. A constriction or narrowing of a vessel or duct.

step mouth. Abnormality of older horses characterized by a wavelike or stair-step configuration of the premolars and molars from front to back; also called *wave mouth*.

stereopsis. Depth perception.

sternal. Resting on the breastbone or *sternum*.

sternum. Breastbone.

steroid hormones. Hormones manufactured by the body from cholesterol and protein.

stertor. Noisy breathing.

stifle joint. Joint where the femur joins the tibia; equivalent to the human knee joint.

stomatitis. Inflammation of the lining of the mouth.

strangles. Extremely important, highly contagious bacterial disease of young horses caused by *Streptococcus equi*; characterized by inflammation of the pharyngeal mucous membranes, with swelling, inflammation, and abscess formation in the associated lymph nodes; also called *distemper*.

strangulation. Constriction resulting in impairment of the blood supply.

streptothricosis. Dermatophilosis.

striated muscle. Skeletal muscle.

stricture. Narrowing of the diameter of a hollow tube, usually the result of contraction caused by local tissue damage.

stridor. Loud, strained, high-pitched noise on inhalation.

stringhalt. Condition in which the horse involuntarily hyperflexes the hock as it walks; the cause is unknown.

strobila. The body of a tapeworm parasite, comparised of a chain of segments called *proglottids*.

strongyles. Nematode parasites of horses; come in two varieties, large and small strongyles. Of these, the large strongyles include some of the most important parasites of the horse.

subcutaneous (SC). Beneath the skin; a route of injection.

subcutaneous edema. Accumulation of fluid beneath the skin.

subcutis. The skin layer lying beneath the *dermis*, and composed of fat cells and strands of collagenous connective tissue; also called *hypodermis*.

subfertility. A state of being less than normally fertile, but not infertile.

subgingival. Below the gumline.

subinvolution. Partial involution (return to normal size) of an organ, as of the uterus following delivery of the fetus.

subluxation. Partial dislocation of a joint; also, a slight alteration in the position of the lens of the eye.

submandibular. Beneath the lower jaw.

sucrose. Table sugar.

sulfur granules. Yellowish clumps of bacteria mixed with dead and dying cells, commonly observed in the pus draining from lesions of actinomycosis.

summer sores. Common term for *cutaneous habronemiasis*.

suppurative. Producing pus (said of bacterial infections).

surfactant. A soaplike substance produced by specialized cells lining the alveoli of the lungs; responsible for decreasing the pressure (surface tension) within the alveoli and preventing them from collapsing during normal respiratory movements.

suture. A surgical stitch.

swamp fever. Equine infectious anemia.

sweeny. Atrophy of the supraspinatus and infraspinatus muscles, located over the *scapula* (shoulder-blade); usually caused by damage to the nerve supply to these muscles.

sweet itch. Queensland itch.

symptomatic therapy. Therapy aimed at alleviating the signs or symptoms of a disease rather than treating its underlying cause.

synaptic cleft. The space between an axon terminal and the myofiber it supplies, and across which the nerve impulse is transmitted by means of "messenger molecules" such as *acetylcholine*.

syngamy. Alternative term for *gametogamy*.

synovial fluid. Joint fluid, the material that lubricates the joint surfaces.

synovial membrane. The lining membrane of a joint.

synovitis. Inflammation of the lining membrane of a joint.

systemic. Throughout the body; pertaining to the body as a whole.

systemic lupus erythematosus (SLE). A rare, chronic, multisystemic autoimmune disorder, characterized by the production of autoantibodies to DNA and normal cellular constituents.

systole. The contraction/ejection phase of the heartbeat.

systolic blood pressure. The pressure that occurs when the heart contracts and pushes blood into the arterial system.

systolic heart murmur. Murmur that is present only during systole.

T lymphocytes (T cells). Specialized lymphocytes that mature within the thymus; two important types are cytotoxic T cells and helper T cells.

tachycardia. Abnormally fast heart rate.

tachypnea. Abnormally rapid breathing.

tachyzoites. Actively dividing form of the parasite *Toxoplasma gondii* found in the tissues of an infected animal.

tail-chewing. A stable vice exhibited primarily by yearlings and two-year-olds.

tapetum. The reflective layer in the upper half of the back of the eye.

taxonomy. The classification of organisms into different categories on the basis of their individual physical and biochemical relationships to each other.

telogen. The phase of hair follicle activity during which the follicle is resting and not producing new hair.

temporal region. Area of the head in front of the ears and lateral to the forehead.

tendinitis. Inflammation of a tendon or tendon muscle attachment; also spelled *tendonitis*.

tendon. Fibrous tissue that attaches muscle to bone.

tenosynovitis. Inflammation of the lining membrane that surrounds the tendon sheath.

tenotomy. Surgical cutting of a tendon.

teratogen. Any compound or agent that disrupts normal development *in utero*, producing defects in the developing embryo.

teratology. The study of abnormal development and congenital malformations.

teratoma. Ovarian tumor characterized by the formation of cysts as well as a bizarre combination of different embryonic tissues such as bone, cartilage, teeth, and hair.

test cross. A mating between a homozygous recessive and an animal with the phenotype of the dominant allele.

testes, testicles. Paired reproductive organs of the male wherein the *spermatozoa* (sperm) are produced.

testosterone. The principal male sex hormone, produced in the testes.

tetanospasmin. The neurotoxin produced in tetanus.

tetanus. Acute, often fatal disease caused by a neurotoxin from the bacterium *Clostridium tetani*, and characterized by violent muscle spasms and contractions, hyperreflexive responses, and "lockjaw" (*trismus*); horses are highly sensitive to the action of tetanus neurotoxin.

tetany. Seizurelike tremors caused most often by a decrease in circulating calcium levels.

tetralogy of Fallot. Congenital heart defect characterized by the presence of a ventricular septal defect (VSD) and severe pulmonic stenosis, together with an abnormally positioned aorta and thickening of the right ventricle.

tetraplegia. Paralysis of all four limbs.

thalamus. Portion of the brain that serves as a relay center for sensory information coming from the rest of the body, and for nerve impulses concerned with balance and coordination arising from the cerebellum.

Theiler's disease. Alternative name for *serum hepatitis*.

theriogenology. Study of the physiology and pathology of animal reproduction.

thermocautery. Destruction of tissue using a hot point or instrument.

thoracic. Pertaining to the chest.

thoracocentesis. Procedure in which a sterile hypodermic needle is inserted into the chest cavity in order to remove accumulated air or fluid, or to obtain a sample of fluid or lung tissue for examination.

thoracolumbar. Pertaining to the upper trunk and back.

thoroughpin. Stress on the deep digital flexor tendon, with puffiness in the web of the hock.

throatlatch. Area of the throat under which the strap of a bridle or halter passes.

thrombocytopenia. Abnormally decreased numbers of circulating blood platelets.

thromboembolism. Obstruction of a blood vessel by a clot originating at another site.

thrombophlebitis. Inflammation of a vein, accompanied by the formation of a blood clot.

thromboplastin. A protein essential for blood clotting.

thrombosis. Formation of a blood clot (*thrombus*) that results in obstruction of a blood vessel at the site of clot formation; contrasts with *embolism*, which is a blood-borne clot that lodges at a site distant from its site of formation.

thrombus. A blood clot causing obstruction of a blood vessel at the site of clot formation.

thrush. Degenerative condition of the frog of the foot, characterized by infection and blackening of the affected area; usually occurs in horses housed under unsanitary conditions.

thymus. Lymphoid organ located in the chest that produces hormones (thymopoietin, thymosin) and that regulates the maturation process of specialized lymphocytes known as T cells.

thyroid gland. Endocrine gland located on either side of the trachea that produces hormones (thyroxine, triiodothyronine) important in regulating the body's metabolic rate.

thyroid hormone. Collective name for the two major hormones produced by the thyroid gland, thyroxine (T_4) and triiodothyronine (T_3).

thyroidectomy. Removal of all or part of the thyroid gland.

thyroid-stimulating hormone (TSH). Hormone elaborated by the pituitary gland that stimulates the thyroid gland to produce the hormones thyroxine (T_4) and triiodothyronine (T_3).

thyroxine (T_4). One of two important iodine-containing hormones secreted by the thyroid gland that assist in regulating the cellular metabolic rate of the body.

titer. A quantitative measure of the concentration of an antibody or antigen in blood serum; determined in principle by making serial dilutions of serum and identifying the highest dilution at which the antibody or antigen can still be detected.

tobiano. Dominantly inherited equine coat-color pattern, expressed as a white base coat with colored patches on the body. The legs are usually white, and white normally crosses the back. The colored areas are regular, usually oval or round. The head is colored as are the flanks.

tocopherols. General term for vitamin E.

tolerance. The normal state whereby the immune system remains nonreactive or "tolerant" to the body's own cells.

torsion. A twisting.

total digestible nutrients (TDN). For a feed, the sum of the digestible carbohydrate, protein, fat, and fiber; also called *digestible energy (DE)*.

tovero. Equine coat-color pattern with characteristics of both tobiano and overo.

toxemia. Presence of toxins in the blood, accompanied by related signs of disease.

toxoplasmosis. A protozoan disease caused by *Toxoplasma gondii*.

trace minerals. Minerals that are required in the diet only in very minute amounts; for horses these usually include copper, iodine, iron, manganese, selenium, and zinc.

trachea. Cartilage-lined tubular airway that descends from the larynx into the chest and branches at its lower end into two bronchi that enter the lungs; it conducts air between the upper nasal passages and the lungs; colloquially known as the *windpipe*.

tracheitis. Inflammation of the trachea.

tracheostomy. Surgically created opening through the skin into the trachea, to allow for insertion of a tube for breathing and to clear airway obstructions.

transmammary. Through the milk or colostrum.

transplacental(ly). By way of the placenta; across the placenta.

transport host. An animal in which part of the immature phase of a parasite's life cycle is spent, but no development occurs.

transtracheal wash. Flushing of material from the trachea and bronchi for diagnostic purposes, by needle puncture and aspiration through the skin and tracheal wall.

trematodes. Flukes.

trichiasis. Condition wherein facial hair or eyelashes arising from normal sites are misdirected and contact the cornea or conjunctiva.

trichinosis. Serious, occasionally fatal food-borne disease of humans caused by a parasitic worm, *Trichinella spiralis*, whose larval forms are found in muscle tissue. When the (raw or undercooked) muscle is eaten, the larvae are liberated and mature in the small intestine, where the adults reproduce and produce offspring.

tricuspid valve. The atrioventricular valve on the right side of the heart.

triglycerides. A component of fat, consisting of fatty acids linked to glycerol.

triiodothyronine (T3). An important iodine-containing hormone secreted by the thyroid gland that assists in regulating the cellular metabolic rate of the body; much more powerful than its companion hormone thyroxine, it is considered to be the active form of thyroid hormone in tissue.

trismus. "Lockjaw," caused by spasm of the chewing muscles; seen in *tetanus*..

trochanteric bursitis. Inflammation of the bursa that lies beneath the tendon of the middle gluteal muscle as it passes over the point of the hip.

trophozoites. Motile feeding forms of the parasite *Giardia*; they multiply in the small intestine by means of *binary fission*.

truncus arteriosus. Congenital heart defect consisting of a ventricular septal defect (VSD) and a single large arterial trunk exiting both ventricles.

tuberculosis. An ancient disease of humans and animals, caused by bacteria belonging to the genus *Mycobacterium*. Most infections in horses are caused by *Mycobacterium bovis* and are characterized by fever, respiratory difficulty, inappetence, weight loss, and lymph node enlargement.

tumor. A large nodule, or obvious cancerous mass.

turgor. Skin elasticity.

Turner's syndrome. The most common chromosomal abnormality of mares, characterized by a missing X chromosome; also called *63,X gonadal dysgenesis*.

tying-up. A mild form of *azoturia*.

tympanic membrane. Eardrum.

tympany. Distension.

Tyzzer's disease. An extremely rare and highly fatal liver disease of foals caused by a spore-forming bacterium, *Bacillus piliformis*.

ulcer, ulceration. A severe sloughing of the surface of an organ or tissue, as a result of a toxic or inflammatory response at the site.

ulcerative keratitis. Inflammation of the cornea accompanied by corneal ulceration.

ulcerative lymphangitis. Uncommon condition affecting the lymphatic vessels; can be caused by either *Corynebacterium pseudotuberculosis* or *Sporothrix schenckii*, usually as the result of wound contamination. The lesions appear as nodules that develop most often on the hind legs below the hocks. The nodules eventually break down and ulcerate, releasing a thick greenish pus mixed with blood.

ultrasonography. Noninvasive diagnostic technique for visualizing the internal structures of the body by means of sound (echo) reflections; ultrasound.

ultrasound. Ultrasonography.

ultraviolet radiation. High-energy radiation existing beyond the violet region of the electromagnetic spectrum; ultraviolet rays emitted by the sun are responsible for a number of effects on the skin, including tanning, burning, and activation of vitamin D.

umbilical cord. Blood-vessel connection between the mare and the fetus.

unicellular. Single-celled.

unilateral. Occurring on only one side.

unilateral papular dermatosis. Poorly understood skin disease of Quarter Horses.

unsoundness. Any deviation in structure or function that interferes with a horse's intended use or performance.

unthrifty. Unkempt in appearance and failing to thrive.

urachus. Structure that during fetal life transports the foal's urine into the placental fluids; it normally closes off after birth.

urea. Nitrogen-containing compound generated by the breakdown of ingested proteins.

uremia. Abnormally elevated levels of urea and other nitrogenous waste products in the blood.

ureter. Membranous tube that transports urine from the kidney to the urinary bladder.

ureterolith. Urinary stone lodged in the ureter.

urethra. Membranous tube that transports urine from the urinary bladder to the exterior of the body.

urethral diverticular concretion. The accumulation of smegma into a solidified mass in the urethra, resulting in inflammation and obstruction; also called *bean*.

urethritis. Inflammation of the urethra.

urethrolith. Urinary stone lodged in the urethra.

urinalysis (UA). Panel of physicochemical tests carried out on urine, as an aid in the diagnosis of urinary-tract disorders.

urinary calculus (plural: calculi). General term for a stone lodged anywhere within the urinary tract; also known as a *urolith*.

urine. The fluid filtrate of the kidneys.

urine sediment. Urine solids obtained by centrifuging a urine sample.

urolith. General term for a urinary stone.

urolithiasis. The formation of urinary stones; uncommon in horses.

uroperitoneum. Accumulation of urine in the abdominal cavity.

urospermia. Urination during ejaculation.

urovagina. Urine "pooling" in the vagina; also called *vesicovaginal reflux*.

urticaria ("hives"). Acute, usually localized skin swelling caused by an increased permeability of capillaries, producing a net outflow of fluid into the tissue spaces; often a manifestation of an allergic process.

uterine horns. Paired branchings of the uterus leading from the body of the uterus to the uterine tubes.

uterine inversion. Protrusion of a portion of the uterus through the cervix; uterine prolapse.

uterine prolapse. Uterine inversion.

uterine torsion. Twisting of the uterus, which may occur late in pregnancy when the uterus is very enlarged.

uterine tubes. Paired *fallopian tubes* of the uterus

wherein fertilization of the eggs with sperm occurs; also called *oviducts*.

uterus. Organ in the female wherein the fertilized egg implants and develops through embryonic and fetal stages until birth; *womb*.

uvea. Cellular layer of the eye that contains blood vessels, the iris, ciliary body, and choroid.

uveitis. Inflammation of the uvea of the eye.

vacuole. Small, round to oval space or cavity within a cell.

vagina. The genital canal of the mare, extending from the cervix of the uterus outward to the vulva.

vaginitis. Inflammation of the vagina.

vaginoscopic. By means of visual inspection of the vagina, using a speculum.

valley fever. Coccidioidomycosis.

valvular degeneration. Heart disease wherein the *leaflets* or *cusps* comprising a heart valve curl back on themselves, allowing the valve to leak.

vascular. Pertaining to blood vessels.

vascular endothelium. Cells lining the inner surface of blood vessels.

vascularization. The formation of blood vessels at a tissue site.

vascularized. Supplied with blood vessels.

vascular ring defect. Abnormal retention of embryonic blood vessels in the region of the aorta.

vasculature. The blood vessels—arteries, arterioles, capillaries, venules, and veins—that traverse the body.

vasculitis. Inflammation of a blood vessel or vessels; also called *angiitis*.

vas deferens. Ducts that serve as the transport conduit for sperm from the testes to the urethra; also called *ductus deferens*.

vasectomy. Sterilization of the male by severing the testicular tubules (*vas deferens*) without removing the testes.

vasodilation. Dilation (expansion in diameter) of a blood vessel.

vasopressin. Alternative name for antidiuretic hormone (ADH).

vector. A term usually applied to insects, ticks, and mites that carry disease-causing microorganisms from an infected animal to a noninfected animal.

veins. Large, thin-walled vessels that direct dexygenated blood from the tissues back to the heart.

venipuncture. Taking a blood sample from a vein.

venous. Pertaining to veins or venules.

ventral. In a direction toward the belly surface.

ventral edema. Tissue swelling affecting the underside of the body.

ventricles. The two muscular, lower chambers of the heart, that are primarily responsible for pumping blood out of the heart; also, cavities in the brain within which is produced the *cerebrospinal fluid*.

ventricular afterload. The resistance to blood flow faced by the ventricles of the heart as they contract.

ventricular fibrillation. Rapid, repeated firing of ventricular muscle fibers without coordinated contraction of the muscle itself; can result in cardiac arrest and death.

ventricular preload. The ability of the ventricles of the heart to fill adequately during the relaxation phase (*diastole*) of the heartbeat.

ventricular septal defect (VSD). Congenital abnormality in which a hole exists in the wall (*septum*) separating the left and right ventricles of the heart; the most commonly recognized congenital heart defect of horses.

ventricular tachycardia. Abnormal condition wherein damaged or diseased heart muscle within a ventricle begins contracting on its own, which it normally does not do.

venules. Small veins.

verminous pneumonia. Pneumonia caused by parasitic worms.

vertebrae. Blocklike bones that make up the spinal column and through which the spinal cord runs.

vesicle. A circumscribed elevation of the epidermis, filled with serum; blister.

vesicovaginal reflux. The retention of incompletely voided urine in the forward portion of the vagina, next to the cervix; also called *urovagina*.

vesicular. Fluid-filled; causing blisters.

vesicular stomatitis. Disease characterized by fever and the development of vesicles (blisters) and ulcerations of the mouth, tongue, coronary band, and teats; caused by a rhabdovirus.

vestibular. Pertaining to the balance mechanism in the inner ear and brain.

vestibule. Outer portion of the vagina into which the *urethra* (the connecting tube from the urinary bladder) empties.

villi (singular: villus). Tiny hairlike projections lining the interior of the small intestine, that serve to increase greatly the surface area available for the absorption of nutrients.

viremia. Presence of virus in the bloodstream.

virilizing. Producing male characteristics.

virology. The study of viruses.

virulence. Measure of the disease-causing capacity of an infectious disease agent.

virulence factor. Any factor that enhances the ability of an infectious disease agent to infect the host and damage tissue.

viruses. Minute, nonliving infectious disease agents composed primarily of protein and nucleic acid (either RNA or DNA), and characterized by the absence of independent metabolism and an inability to replicate outside susceptible host cells.

virus isolation. Procedure of propagating a virus artificially in the laboratory; more specifically, the process of recovering a virus from a tissue or fluid sample of an infected animal or human being.

viscera (singular: viscus). Any of the large interior organs of the body.

visceral pleura. Membrane covering the surface of the organs in the chest cavity.

vitamin. General term for a number of substances required in very small quantities for the normal functioning of the body's metabolic processes.

vitiligo. Uncommon, acquired disorder of pigmentation characterized by progressive, usually well-circumscribed, areas of pigment loss in the skin.

vitreous body. Viscous fluid filling the posterior portion of the eyeball (behind the lens); also called simply *vitreous*.

vitreous chamber. The deepest chamber of the eye, behind the lens.

vomiting. The forceful ejection of contents of the stomach and upper small intestine through the mouth.

vomiting center. Portion of the brain that initiates vomiting.

vomitus. Vomited material.

vulva. The external genitalia of the female, representing the entrance to the vagina; composed of the external lips or folds (*labia*) and the *clitoris*.

walking disease. Older name for *pyrrolizidine alkaloid* intoxication.

wave mouth. Abnormality of older horses characterized by a wavelike or stair-step configuration of the premolars and molars from front to back; also called *step mouth*.

weaving. A stable vice characterized by a repetitive rocking motion made by rhythmically swinging the head and neck from side to side while transferring the weight back and forth from one foreleg to the other.

wheal. A discrete, well-circumscribed, reddened skin swelling with a flat top and steep-walled margins, produced by *edema* in the dermis; often associated with allergic reactions, i.e., *urticaria*; also called a "hive."

white muscle disease. Muscle abnormality resulting from inadequate intake of selenium or vitamin E.

windpuffs. Chronic swelling of the fetlock joint.

wind-sucking. A stable vice in which the horse flexes its neck while forcibly swallowing air; also, aspiration of air and debris into the vagina (*pneumovagina*).

withers. Ridge between the shoulder blades.

wobbler syndrome. A common cause of incoordination in young horses, particularly Thoroughbreds; results from spinal cord compression caused by a narrowing of the vertebral canal, malalignment of neck vertebrae, or excessive growth of the surrounding soft tissue; also called *wobbles*.

wolf tooth. A vestigial first premolar tooth, sometimes present.

X-linked diseases. Genetic diseases of males caused by defective genes located on the X chromosome; also called *sex-linked diseases*.

yellow star thistle poisoning. Degenerative brain disease caused by ingestion of yellow star thistle (*Centaurea solstitialis*) or Russian knapweed (*Centaurea repens*).

zona pellucida. Thick, transparent outer envelope or casing that surrounds an *ovum* (egg).

zoonosis, zoonotic disease. Any disease that can be spread between animals and human beings; examples include plague, rabies, salmonellosis, and ringworm.

zoospore. The motile, infective stage of *Dermatophilus congolensis*, the cause of a skin disorder known as *dermatophilosis*.

zygote. Fertilized *ovum* (egg).

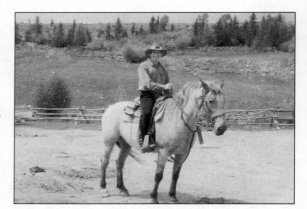

Photo by Ruth Saada.

Index